AF647706

DENTAL MICROBIOLOGY

DENTAL MICROBIOLOGY

R Panjarathinam

PhD (Bact), PhD (Medical), FZS (Cal), FNAVS
Department of Microbiology, B J Medical College
Ahmedabad, Gujarat, India

New Central Book Agency (P) Ltd

LONDON
HYDERABAD ERNAKULAM BHUBANESWAR
DELHI KOLKATA PUNE GUWAHATI

NCBA

REGD OFFICE
8/1 Chintamoni Das Lane, Kolkata 700 009, India
email: ncbapvtltd@eth.net

OVERSEAS
NCBA (UK) Ltd, 149 Park Avenue North, Northampton, NN3 2HY, UK
email: ncbauk@yahoo.com

EXPORT
NCBA Exports Pvt. Ltd, 212 Shahpur Jat, New Delhi 110 049
email: ncbaexports@ncbaindia.com

BRANCHES

208B Peacock Lane, Shahpur Jat
New Delhi 110 049
email: ncbadel@ncbapvtltd.com

Shop Nos. 3 & 4, Vinayak Towers
681/B Budhwar Peth, Appa Balwant Chowk
Pune 411 002
email: ncbapune@ncbapvtltd.com

Shop No. 15, Bharati Towers, Ground Floor
Forest Park, **Bhubaneswar** 751 001
email: ncbabub@ncbapvtltd.com

House No. 3-1-315, 1st Floor
Nimboliadda, Kachiguda, **Hyderabad** 500 027
email: ncbahydb@ncbapvtltd.com

GSS Shopping Complex, 1st Floor
Opposite College Post Office, Convent Road
Ernakulam 682 035
email: ncbaernk@ncbapvtltd.com

Radhamayee Complex (Second Floor)
Opp. S.B.I. Panbazar, Jaswanta Road
Guwahati 781 001
email: ncbaguwahati@ncbapvtltd.com

DENTAL MICROBIOLOGY • R Panjarathinam

© Copyright reserved by the Author

Publication, Distribution, and Promotion Rights reserved by the Publisher

All rights reserved. No part of the text in general, and the figures, diagrams, page layout, and cover design in particular, may be reproduced or transmitted in any form or by any means—electronic, mechanical, photocopying, recording, or by any information storage and retrieval system—without the prior written permission of the Publisher

First Published: July 2012

PUBLISHER AND TYPESETTER
New Central Book Agency (P) Ltd
8/1 Chintamoni Das Lane, Kolkata 700 009

TYPESETTER
Classic Computers, Kolkata 700 009

PRINTER
New Central Book Agency (P) Ltd
Web-Offset Division, Dhulagarh, Sankrail, Howrah

COVER DESIGNER
Soumen Paul

COVER PRINTER
Liba Graphics, Kolkata

PROOF CHECKING
Subas Maitra

PROJECT TEAM
Prabir Ghosh, Prabhat Jas, and Pradip Baidya

ISBN 978 81 7381 655 0

Price ₹ 435.00

Dedicated to
The Divine Mother
Sri Aurobindo Ashram
Pondicherry

CONTENTS

SECTION III SYSTEMATIC BACTERIOLOGY 109-213

SECTION IV VIRUSES, RICKETTSIAE AND SPIROCHAETES 217-323

SECTION VI MEDICAL MYCOLOGY 467-477

SECTION VII MEDICAL PARASITOLOGY 479-619

PREFACE

Dental care is of paramount importance for sound and healthy human life. HEALTH IS WEALTH. The paucity of books on Dental Microbiology in India has prompted the author to write a concise comprehensive book on Dental Microbiology by utilising the long-standing experience gained by teaching Medical Microbiology to medical and dental students of B. J. Medical College, Ahmedabad.

The main aim of this book is to provide a theoretical and visual aid to the identification of the causative agents (bacteria, viruses, fungi) of human diseases, serological tests, common laboratory media, instruments, laboratory animals, and to study the morphology and life cycle of medically important parasites. Revision summary of parasitology, entomology with questions and answers, glossary, technical terms are added for the special attraction of students interested in quick and ready references.

To develop a clear concept for identifying the human pathogens, microphotographs, figures and diagrammatic illustrations — both in colour and black & white — have been used to enhance the impact of this book. Emphasis has been given on features which are useful for diagnostic work — both in the laboratory and clinical practice.

It is expected that this book will be useful to dental, ophthalmic, and medical students as well as dentists, physicians, nurses and technicians.

Structural details of microscopic slides (specimens) are better revealed by fluorescence microscopy than other forms of light microscopy. The magnification of microphotographs is given as per the instrumental readings.

Both theoretical and practical studies are fully covered in lucid manner as per the University BDS Syllabus.

The study of Dental Microbiology has become more difficult to cope with, within a short time. The students need not waste their valuable time to refer to other books for further information as this book is prepared after consulting various textbooks.

The dental students can, now, acquire better up-to-date knowledge of this subject without wasting their precious time, and those students with incomplete knowledge of both theoretical and practical dental microbiology will be overwhelmed with joy after reading this unique book complete in every aspect.

R. PANJARATHINAM

ACKNOWLEDGEMENTS

I am highly grateful to Dr R C Shah, MBBS, MSc (Med), the then Director of Medical Education and Research, Gujarat state, and to Dr V V Kollali, MD (Path. Bact), DCP, Professor and Head, Department of Microbiology, BJ Medical College, Ahmedabad, for their kind permission and constant encouragement while writing this book.

I will fail in my duty if I do not acknowledge the kind initiative advise to write this book and encouragement by Dr G J Dave, BDS, MSc (Med), Professor and Head, Department of Dental Pathology, Microbiology, Gujarat Dental College, Civil Hospital campus, Ahmedabad, and Visiting Professor of Medical Microbiology, BJ Medical College, on deputation.

I wish to extend my gratitude to Shri Ramesh Aswani, microphotographer, BJ Medical College, and to Dr D N Zaveri, PhD (Med.), my ex-postgraduate student for their assistance during photography and also to my professional colleagues for their valuable cooperation.

My sincere thanks are due to my wife (Usha), my children (Rani, Bina) for their constant moral support and encouragement during the long and arduous task of preparation of the manuscript. My appreciations to New Central Book Agency (P) Ltd., Kolkata, especially to Mr. Amitabha Sen, Director, and its production staff for the excellent and elegant publication of this book.

R. PANJARATHINAM

Introduction

The prime aim of Practical Dental Microbiology is to impart a sound comprehensive practical knowledge which could help the dental students to identify accurately the causal agent of the disease in the laboratory, which may be a direct diagnostic guidance for the treatment of the patient in the ward or to diagnose indirectly the disease by serology. Besides, the students should have a clear concept of methods of collection and prompt despatch of samples to the laboratory for the microbiological investigations.

Microscope (Fig. 1.1):

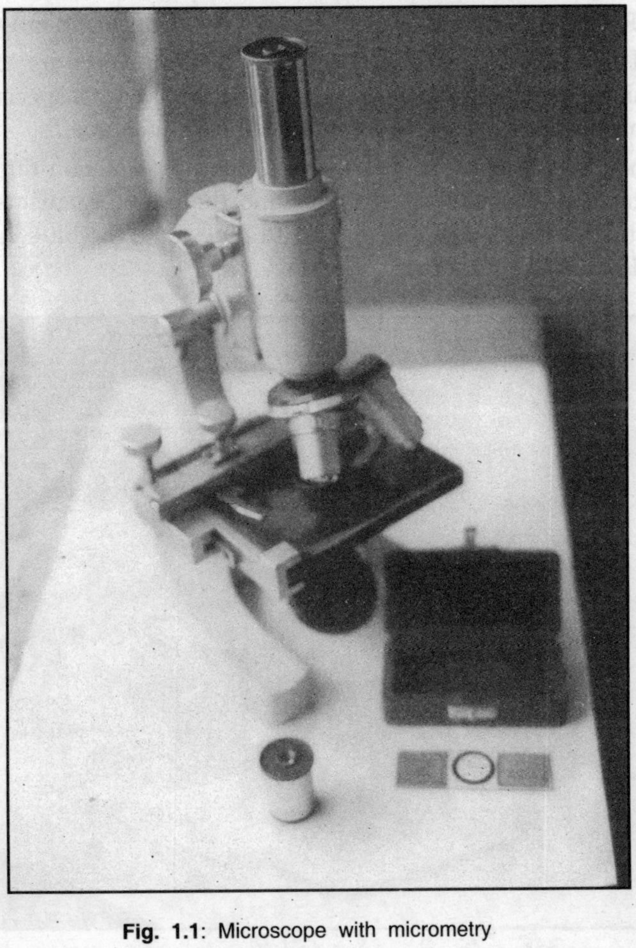

Fig. 1.1: Microscope with micrometry

The microscope is the most important routinely used instrument in the microbiology laboratory. Its magnification enables us to see the microorganisms and their structures invisible to the naked eyes. It ranges from x100, x400 to x1000. Different kinds of microscope are available.

Microscopes are of two categories : **Light** (or **Optical**) and electron—depending upon the principles on which the magnification is based. Light microscopy—in which the magnification is obtained by a system of optical lenses using light waves—includes : 1. Bright field; 2. Dark field; 3. Fluorescence; 4. Phase contrast microscope. The electron microscope uses a beam of electrons in place of light waves to produce the image. Specimens can be examined by either transmission or scanning electron microscopy. In the microbiology course, students perform most of their examinations with a bright field microscope. This is most widely used instrument for routine microscopic work. The other types of microscopy are used for special purpose or research investigation.

1. **Bright light microscopy :** In bright field microscopy, the microscopic field is brightly lighted and the microorganisms appear dark because they absorb some of the light. Ordinarily, the microorganisms do not absorb much light, but staining them with a dye greatly increases their light-absorbing ability resulting in greater contrast to colour differentiation. The ability to distinguish two adjacent points as distinct and separate is called **"Resolving power."** The resolving power of this microscope is 0.2 microns.
2. **Dark field microscopy :** In dark background, the objects are brightly illuminated. This is achieved by using the light microscope fitted with a special kind of condenser that transmits a hollow cone of light from the light source.
3. **Fluorescence microscopy :** In this method, the phenomenon fluorescence is applied with substances called fluorescent dyes and the microorganisms are stained with a fluorescent dye and then illuminated with blue light, the blue light is absorbed and the green light is emitted by the dye. (Fig. 1.2)

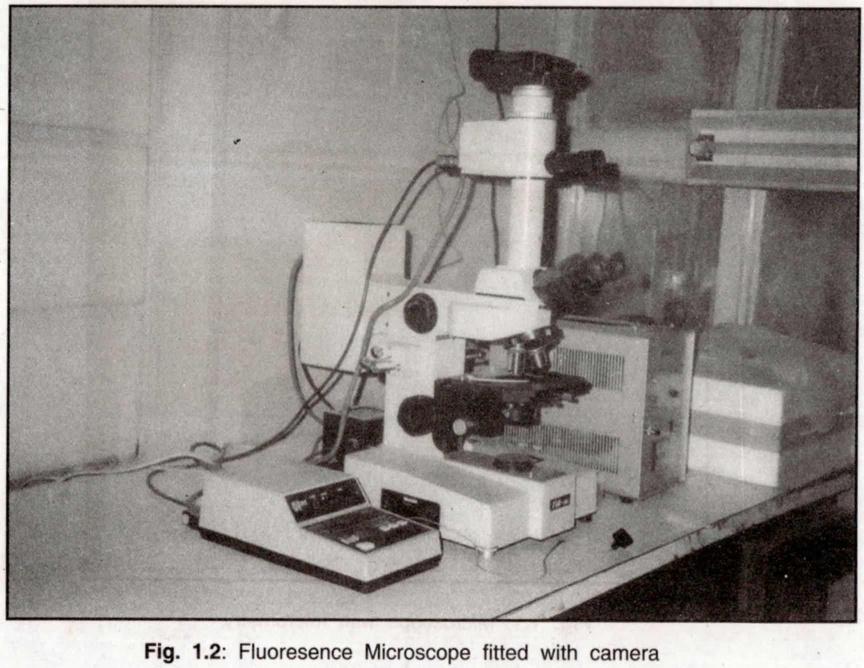

Fig. 1.2: Fluoresence Microscope fitted with camera

4. **Phase contrast microscopy:** It is useful in studying living unstained cells. It consists of a light microscope fitted with a phase contrast objective and a phase contrast condenser.

Electron microscopy : It provides tremendous useful magnification because of the much higher resolution obtainable with the extremely short wave length of the electron beam used to magnify the specimen. Electron microscope uses the electron beam and magnetic fields to produce the image, whereas the light microscope uses light waves and glass lenses.

Important regularly used parts of the light microscope can be seen in Fig. 1.1.

Use of the microscope

(i) Move the microscope so that it is directly in front of you on the laboratory table;

(ii) Use indirect sunlight or light;

(iii) Use the concave side of the mirror for artificial light;

(iv) Adjust the condenser so that it is close with the stage;

(v) Using the clips on the mechanical stage, hold the slide to be studied on the stage so that the centre of the material on the slide is directly over the lens of the condenser;

(vi) While you carefully observe the distance between the tip of the objective and the slide, lower the tip of the objective towards the slide. Do not allow the tip of any objective to touch the slide;

(vii) Focus first with low power objective whenever possible;

(viii) Look through the ocular with one eye, while keeping both eyes open;

(ix) While looking through the ocular, move the objective slowly away from the slide by turning the coarse adjustment screw **counterclockwise.**

(x) When the object is focussed with the coarse adjustment, sharpen the focus with the fine adjustment screw.

(xi) After focusing the object with low power objective, turn the high power objective into position.

(xii) To use oil immersion lens for focusing, raise the objective from the slide, place a drop of immersion oil (cedarwood oil having refractive index of glass) on the slide, swing the oil immersion objective in place and, by turning the coarse adjustment screw lower the tip of the objective into the tip of the oil;

(xiii) While looking into the ocular, focus away from the slide slowly by turning the fine adjustment screw.

(xiv) Observe very carefully all details of the specimen smear;

(xv) After completing this observation with oil immersion lens, raise the objective by screwing the coarse adjustment **counterclockwise;** wipe the excess of oil from the lens of objective or clean with dry lens paper or lens paper moistened with xylol, but **never with alcohol**—as alcohol dissolves the cementing material fixing the lens (lens paper is a very fine paper which will not scratch or damage sensitive lens).

Care of the microscope

(a) Keep the body of the microscope in a perpendicular position and two arms of the base should be pointing away from you at right angles with the edges of the table;

(b) Keep the stage clean and dry;

(c) Clean lenses with lens paper only;

(d) Use special immersion oil with the oil immersion lens and wipe away excess of oil with lens paper moistened in xylol;

(e) Carry the microscope with both hands;

(f) Place the microscope on the table gently;

(g) When you leave the microscope, clean all the lenses that you have used and swing the low objective in position over the opening of the stage.

SECTION I
GENERAL BACTERIOLOGY

1
Living Agents of Disease

In nature, both non-living and living agents do exist. The relationship of the living, agents with the environment has been named "ecology" (Gr. *aikos* — home, native land *logos* — science). The living agents are distributed everywhere in the environment as well as inside and on the surface of human body. Those living agents which produce the disease in man are called pathogenic microorganisms or "Pathogens". Though the soil is an unfavourable habitat, most of the pathogens may survive for three days to three weeks; whereas the saprophytes (non-pathogens) live for longer period in the soil.

The human body is the most suitable environment for the multiplication and production of disease by pathogenic microorganisms. Therefore, in dental microbiology, only the living agents of disease (Pathogens) are to be studied in detail as they are variable in their shape, size, structure and pathogenicity. Until the eighteenth century the classification of living organisms placed all organisms into one of two kingdoms : Plant or Animal kingdom. But in dental microbiology, we study some organisms that are predominantly plant like, others that are animal like and that are variable in size—macroscopic to electron microscopic.

	Living agents	Macroscopic	Microscopic	Electron microscopic
I.	Animal Kingdom	Helminths (worms) Arthropods (Vector)		
II.	Plant Kingdom	Nil	Fungi, spirochaete bacteria, rickettsiae, chlamydiae	All viruses

Some organisms that share characteristics common to both plants and animals are placed into a third kingdom—called Protista—to include those unicellular organisms that are typically neither plant and animals. The protists encompass bacteria, fungi and protozoa.

Viruses are not cellular organisms, therefore they are not classified as protists. Bacteria are referred to as lower protists, but others—algae, fungi and protozoa—are called higher **protists**.

Protists < Lower (bacteria)
Higher (algae, fungi and protozoa)

Electron microscopy study discovered two groups of protists : (a) one group with nucleus not bounded by nuclear membrane known as prokaryotic cells (bacteria), (b) other group with nucleus bounded with nuclear membrane called as **eukaryotic** cells (fungi, algae and protozoa).

Table 1.1. Differencees between Prokaryotic and Eukaryotic cells

Structure	Prokaryotic cells	Eukaryotic cells
A. Nucleus		
Nuclear membrane	Absent	Present
Nucleus	Absent	Present
Chromosome	One	Many
Deoxyribonucleic acid	Absent	Present
Nuclear division	By binary fission	Mitosis/Meiosis
B. Cytoplasm		
Mitochondria	Absent	Present
Golgi apparatus	Absent	Present
Endoplasmic reticulum	Absent	Present
Lysosomes	Absent	Present
Pinocytosis	Absent	Present
C. Chemical structure		
Sterol	Absent	Present
Muramic acid	Present	Absent
Diaminopimelic acid	Usually present	Absent

Micrometry : It is a method of measuring the size of microorganisms:

One thousandth (1/1000) of a metre is one millimetre (mm)

One thousandth (1/1000) of a millimetre is one micron (μ)

One thousandth (1/1000) of a micron is millimicron (mμ) or 10^{-9} metre (nanometre, nm)

One tenth (1/10) of a millimicron is Angstrom (Å) or .000,0001 mm

The unit measurement of bacteria is micron (μ).

The unit measurement of an entire virus particle is millimicron (mμ).

The unit measurement of a very small internal structure of virus (e.g. virus capsomere) is Å.

The individual virus particles (virions) vary in diameter from 300 nm to 18 nm. The largest are about half the size of the smallest bacteria and the smallest are about half the size of large protein molecules. (Vaccinia virus is 330 nm; picorna virus is 20–40 nm). Virions over 200 mμ (0.2 μ) is within the resolving power of light microscope and can be demonstrated in stained preparations. The electron microscope is the most common method of measuring the size of a virus and it can resolve a object as small as 0.3 nm (3 Å) in diameter.

The size of bacteria can be determined by micrometry.

The micrometry (Fig. 1.1) consists of a light microscope, stage micrometer and eye piece micrometer.

The stage micrometer consists of a 3 × 1 inch slide on which a millimeter scale is graduated in hundredths of millimeters. The eye piece micrometer consists of a special eye piece with a graduated scale.

The number of divisions on the eye piece scale corresponding in a definite number of divisions of the stage micrometer should first be determined when a measurement is to be made. Then the stage micrometer is removed and the object (bacteria) on the microscopic slide to be examined is focussed. The number of divisions of the eye piece scale which just cover the object is noted.

Each division of the stage micrometer is 1/100 mm or 0.01 mm.

If 100 divisions of the eye piece micrometer scale exactly covers 11 divisions of the stage micrometer, 100 eye piece divisions = 11 stage divisions = 0.11 mm.

1 eye piece division = 0.0011 mm or 1.1 μ

The stage micrometer is removed and the slide with stained bacterial smear is substituted. If the length of a bacterium covers 3 divisions of eye piece scale, i.e. 1.1 × 3 = 3.3 μ, the length of the bacterium is 3.3 μ.

Probiotics

Probiotics, derived from Greek – "for life", are live microorganisms which, when administrated in adequate amounts, confer a health benefit on the host.

There are three concepts in this definition – "Live" microorganisms and "health benefits." It has become increasingly apparent that the absence of bacteria in the intestine is unhealthy. For example, laboratory raised animals, free from germ, are often sickly with seriously under-developed immune system and vulnerable intestinal tract.

One of the best documented benefits of probiotics has been preventing eczema in babies with inherent tendency to develop allergies.

Friendly bacteria—probiotics—serve a host of biological functions important for the survival of the animal they populate. Some aid in digestion, some compete with harmful bacteria and keep them in check, some stimulate the immune system. Some control or prevent food and skin allergies in children, bacterial vaginosis and premature labour in pregnant women, inflammatory bowel disease, recurrent ear and bladder infection, *dental caries*, chronic diarrhea, and traveller's diarrhoea. They may even help to lower cholesterol in the blood and, by degrading carcinogens, thwart the development of certain cancers.

Though the health potential of probiotics has been known for about 100 years, now the interest in probiotics has exploded in the last several years in the face of surging bacterial resistance to many potential drugs.

Demonstration

Measurement of various living agents of disease by micrometry:

Fig. 1.3 **Ascaris lumbricoides** (intestinal largest roundworm) : female–20-35 cm in length by 3-6 mm in diameter.

Fig. 1.4 **Taenia saginata** (tapeworm) : 5-10 metres in length.

Fig. 1.5 **Wuchereria bancrofti** is a microscopic blood parasite which causes filariasis in man. Female – 80-100mm in length, 0.24-0.30mm in breadth.

Fig. 1.6 **Plasmodium falciparum** (malarial parasite); its trophozoite, 1.5 μ in diameter, present within the red blood corpuscles causes malaria.

Fig. 1.7 **Staphylococcus aureus,** 1 μ in diameter, arranged in cluster, causes abscess, acne, boils etc.

Fig. 1.8 **Streptococcus pyogenes,** 1 μ in diameter, arranged in chain, causes tonsillitis or septic sore throat.

Fig. 1.9 **Borrelia vincenti,** 7-18 μ long and 0.2-0.6 μ wide, causes acute ulcerative gingivitis.

Fig. 1.10 **Vibrio cholerae,** comma shaped, 1.5-3 μ × 0.5 μ, causes cholera in man.

All the above specimens observed in the practical class should be drawn in the practical notebook maintaining their relative sizes.

Answers to the following questions should be entered in the same notebook:

1. What is the magnification obtained with low power, high power, oil immersion lens and 10x ocular?
2. What is the unit measurement of bacteria, virus and internal structure of virus (capsomere)?
3. When and why oil immersion lens should be used?
4. What precautions will you take while using oil immersion lens?
5. Why alcohol should not be used to clean the objectives?
6. Why lens paper is used for wiping the objectives?
7. When you leave the microscope what objective should be in position over the opening of the stage.
8. Describe micrometry and how you will perform it.

2
Morphology of Bacteria

Bacteria can be defined briefly as minute microorganisms with a prokaryotic form of cellular organisation. They are usually unicellular, they may divide by binary fission and grow attached to one another in clusters, chains, filaments (hyphae) or a mycelium (Actinomycetales—higher bacteria). They usually measure from 0.4 to 1.5 micron, smaller than yeast, fungi and protozoa and are devoid of chlorophyll. They have rigid cell walls which cover very closely cytoplasmic membrane and are responsible for the maintenance of their characteristic shape; the shape may be: 1. spherical (Coccus); 2. rod shaped (Bacillus); 3. comma shaped (Vibrio); 4. spiral (Spirillum and Spirochaete); 5. filamentous (Actinomyces)—Fig. 2.1. Their nuclei can be seen only under electron microscope, but NOT under light microscope. A capsule which is outside the cell wall is a protective gelatinous layer, if it is too thin, it is called microcapsule. There are two filamentous appendages protruding outwards from the bacterial cell wall : (a) **flagella** which are organs of locomotion, and (b) **fimbriae** (syn, **pilli)** which are organs of adhesion. The cell wall, capsule, microcapsule, flagella and fimbriae play a special role in the process of infection. In addition to these morphological features, bacteria can be identified by the following characteristics after staining which will be performed in the next practical.

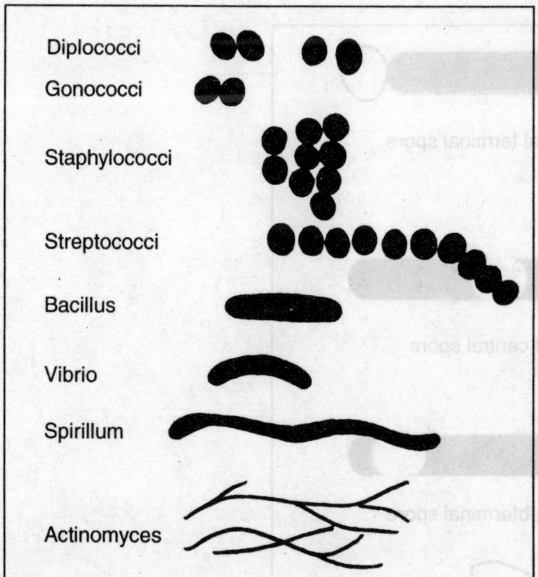

Fig. 2.1(a): Classification of bacteria

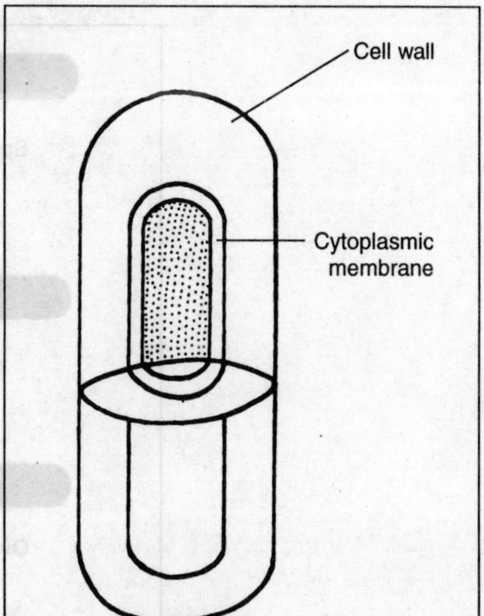

Fig. 2.1(b): Cross-section of bacteria

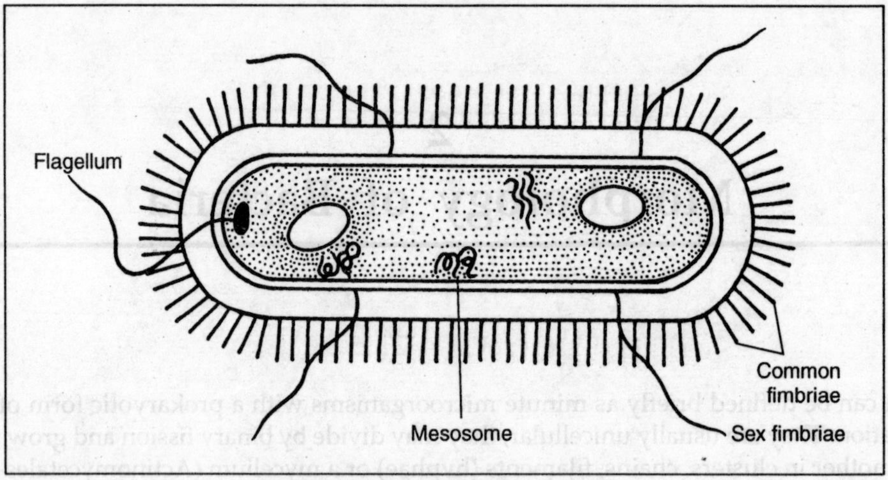

Fig. 2.1(c): Structure of bacteria

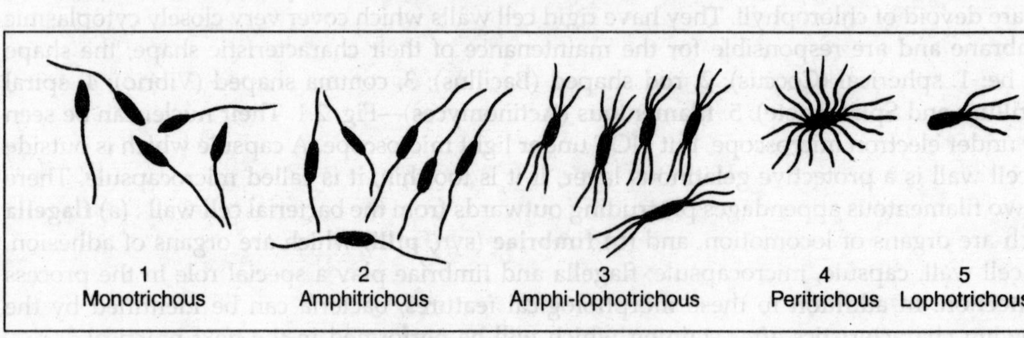

Fig. 2.1(c): Distribution of flagella

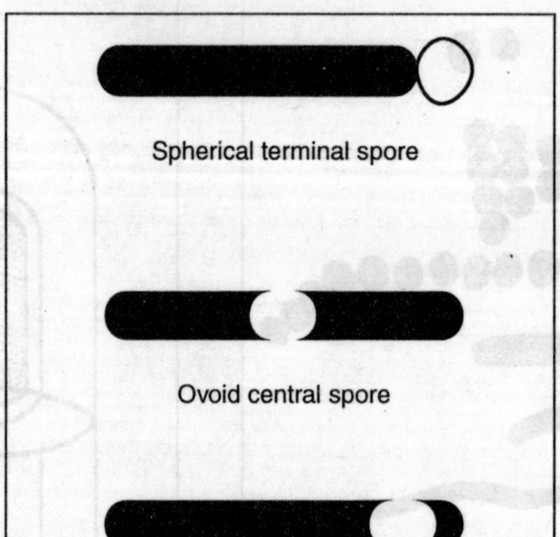

Fig. 2.1(e): Spore position (Gram's stain)

(a) SHAPE and manner of grouping of bacteria—manner of grouping or characteristic arrangement of bacteria depend upon their mode of division e.g. axis of division and tendency of the daughter cell to adhere to one another, Cocci form clusters (Staphylococci—Gr. *Staphyle,* cluster of grapes) or chains (Streptococci—Gr. *Streptos,* chain).

(b) SIZE OF BACTERIA Cocci—their size ranges from 0.4 to 2 microns in diameter, bacilli vary from 1.2 to 12 microns in length; spirilla have variable length of 114 microns. Size of bacteria can be measured by micrometry or by electron microscopy.

(c) MOTILITY of bacteria—it is due to the presence of organ of locomotion i.e. flagella—hair-like appendages. Flagella can be demonstrated by Leifson's flagellar staining. Hanging drop preparation is routinely adopted method to demonstrate the motility. Instead of using a hanging drop preparation, a film of the fluid between a microscopic slide and coverslip may be used, but in this case the edge of the coverslip should be sealed with vaseline to prevent evaporation of the fluid. Other methods are by using semi-solid agar, by agglutination with specific antisera, by dark illumination, fluorescence or electron microscopy. Spirochaetes move with the help of long filaments applied to their bodies showing rotatory cork screw-like motility. **Campylobacter jejuni, Vibrio cholerae**, and **Spirillum minus** show darting motility.

True motility of bacteria is indicated by their change in position in relation to their surroundings. It differs from Brownian movement which is a peculiar motion possessed by all fine or minute particles suspended in fluid (Table 2.1).

(d) SPORE OF BACTERIA—Bacteria can be spore (Fig. 2.1) or non-spore formers.

Practical Work

A. Hanging drop preparation

1. A glass slide with a circular concavity in its centre is used;
2. A thin ring of vaseline is outlined around the concavity by means of a matchstick dipped in vaseline (petroleum jelly);
3. With the help of a cooled sterile platinum wire loop, a loopful of fluid containing organisms was taken from bacterial suspension (or, alternatively, a small amount of culture from the surface of a solid medium is thinly emulsified in a drop of normal saline) and placed on the coverslip laid on the bench;
4. The slide is inverted over the coverslip so that it will adhere to vaseline;
5. It is quickly turned around the slide so that the coverslip is uppermost and the drop should then be "hanging" from the coverslip in the centre of concavity;
6. The slide is placed on the stage of the microscope;
7. The condenser is slightly racked down and the diaphragm is partially closed (excess of illumination renders the organisms invisible);
8. The edge of the drop of fluid is focussed with the low power objective so that it appears across the centre of the field;
9. The high power lens is turned in position and the edge of the drop is focussed; **it is advisable to use the high power dry lens, NOT the oil immersion objective** (Fig. 2.2).

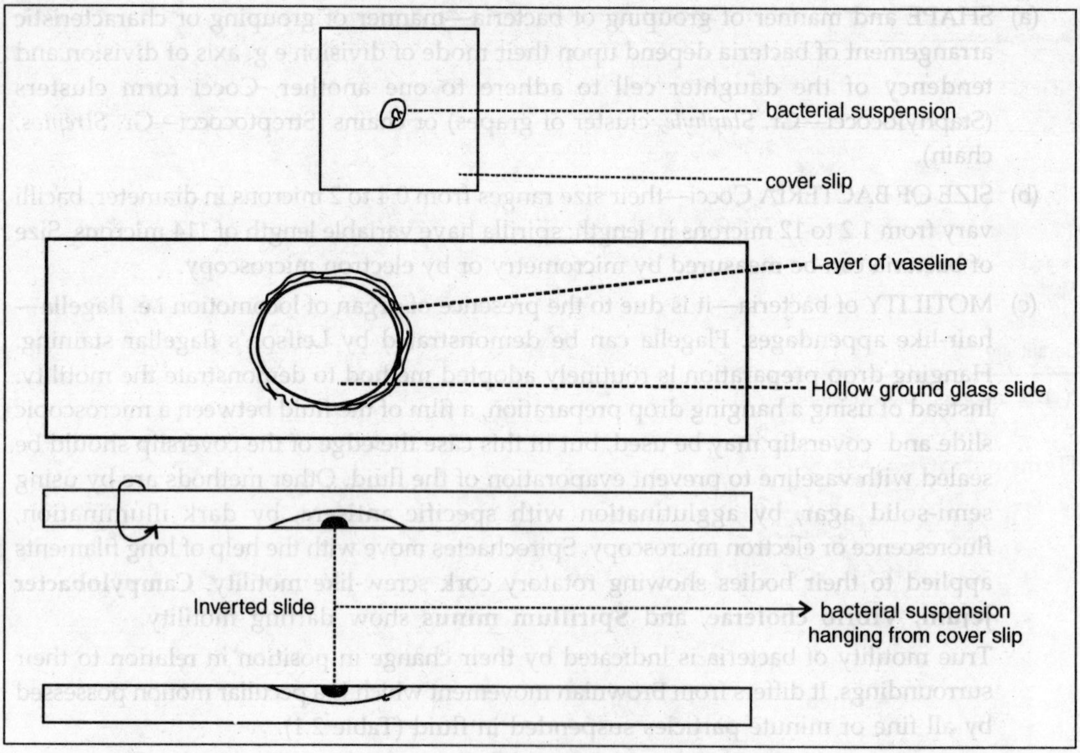

Fig. 2.2: Hanging drop preparation

Table 2.1. Motile and Non-motile bacteria

Motile	Non-motile
Escherichia coli	Shigella
Salmonella	Mycobacterium tuberculosis
Vibrio	Corynebacterium diphtheriae and diphtheroids
Pseudomonas	All cocci (staphylococci, streptococci, meningococci, gonococci, pneumococci)
Spirillum	
Treponema	
Leptospira	
Borrelia	
Clostridium tetani	Clostridium welchii
Bacillus subtilis	Bacillus anthracis

B. Simple staining method

This method shows the presence of organisms and the nature of cellular content in the exudate. The fixed smear is covered with dilute oxalated gentian violet for 2 minutes, then it is washed with running tap water for half a minute. The smear is dried between the two folds of a filter paper. Shape and arrangement of microorganisms can be studied under oil immersion objective, then the observations should be entered in the practical notebook.

Table 2.2. Characteristics of bacteria and viruses

	Bacteria	Rickettsiae	Chlamydiae	Mycoplasma	Viruses
Size	0.4-2 µm 1.2-12 µm	0.25-2 µm	200-300 nm	50-300 nm	20-500 nm
Both DNA & RNA	+	+	+	+	Either of two
Growth on artificial media	+	+	−	+	−
Intracellular replication	− *(+)	+	+	−	
Multiplication by binary fission	+	+	+	(also try ending)	−
Muramic acid in cell wall	+	+	+	+	−
Sensitivity to antibiotics	+	+	+	+	−

*(+) br abortus, Mycobacterium tuberculosis multiply intracellularly

Demonstration

- Fig. 2.2 Hanging drop preparation.
- Fig. 2.3 A smear showing cocci in chain.
- Fig. 2.4 A smear showing cocci in clusters.
- Fig. 2.5 A smear showing bacilli with no particular arrangement.
- Fig. 2.6 A smear showing bacilli in chains.
- Fig. 2.7 A smear showing comma-shaped organisms.
- Fig. 2.8 A smear showing spirochaete.

All observations should be entered in the practical notebook indicating the colour of the stain retained by the microorganisms.

Questions

1. Enumerate all the methods to demonstrate the motility of bacteria.
2. Name a non-flagellate microorganism which is motile and explain how it is motile.
3. Why should the iris diaphragm of the microscope be partially closed while demonstrating motility?
4. Name few motile bacteria.

3

Morphology of Bacteria—Staining of Bacteria

Staining is of primary importance for the recognition of bacteria, because of its ability to absorb more light and to make the bacteria quite distinct.

In addition to shape, size and motility of bacteria, other morphological characters can be studied very easily after staining. Gram stain and Ziehl Neelsen stain are routinely used methods in the microbiology laboratory. Therefore, these two techniques should be learned perfectly.

Method of smear preparation

The microscopic slides should be wiped with a clean dry cotton cloth and then freed from grease by passing it 6-12 times through blue Bunsen flame. For special purpose—such as staining of flagella—slides are cleaned with hot dichromate-sulphuric acid solution followed by flaming.

A loopful of normal saline or clean water is placed on a slide. The platinum loop (Fig. 3.1) is sterilised over the flame till red hot and a minute quantity of the culture on agar obtained

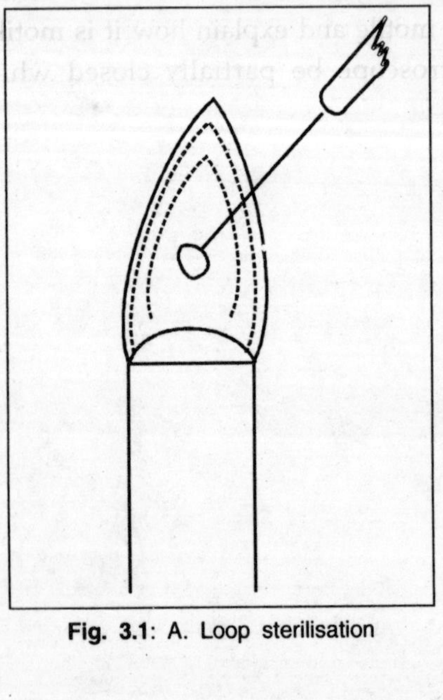

Fig. 3.1: A. Loop sterilisation

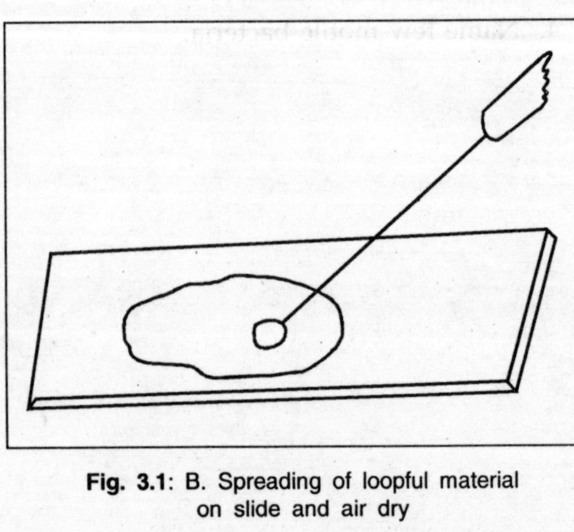

Fig. 3.1: B. Spreading of loopful material on slide and air dry

by just touching the growth is transferred to the saline drop, thoroughly emulsified, the mixture is spread evenly on the slide, dried and "fixed" by passing the dried slides three times slowly through the flame which causes coagulation of bacterial protein—rendering the bacteria to stick to the slide. The washing away of the smear is therefore prevented (Fig. 3.2).

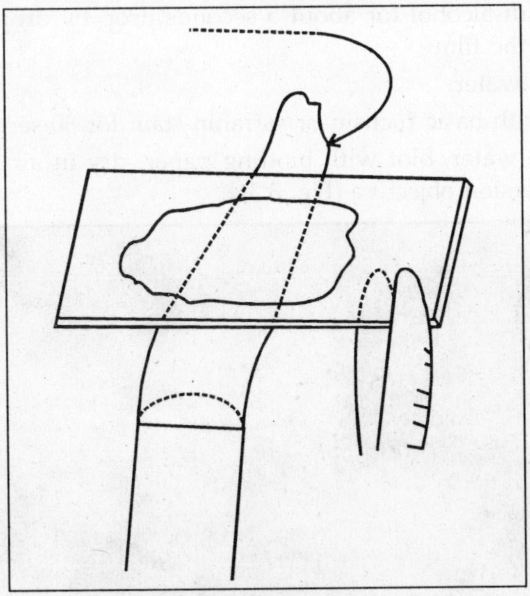

Fig. 3.2: Preparation of smear for staining

Principles of staining

1. **Gram stain** : Gram-positive organisms retain the basic dyes at higher hydrogen ion concentration (pH 2-3) than the Gram-negative bacteria. The iodine treatment enhances the cytoplasmic acid character which retains strongly the basic dye. Hence iodine acts as mordant. A dye iodine complex or "lake" is formed within the cell, which is soluble in alcohol used as decolouriser. This complex diffuses out of Gram-negative bacilli. Gram-reaction depends upon a difference in the permeability of the cell wall or the cytoplasmic membrane and the presence of a specific magnesium ribonucleate protein complex in the cell. Gram-positive staining colours the whole cell including the cell wall. If the magnesium ribonucleate is removed by autolysis or the cell wall is ruptured, the Gram-positive bacilli will become Gram-negative.
2. **Ziehl Neelsen stain** : Some bacteria like tubercle bacilli cannot be easily stained by Gram stain because of the wax-like mycolic acid (fatty acid) in their cell wall; they can be stained with a strong reagent (basic fuchsin in aqueous 5% phenol), applied with heat; but subsequently they resist decolourisation by strong acid (20% sulphuric acid) and are stained pink or red. Hence they are called "Acid fast bacilli" (AFB). Decolourised non-Acid fast organisms are counterstained with methylene blue.

Gram stain method

Before staining, the position of the smear on the slide should be confirmed by making a scratch with the help of a needle or sharp glass slide, NEVER with the fingernail which may become contaminated; the slide should be placed in such as way that the smear is on the uppermost position on the staining rack or on glass rods levelled on the laboratory sink.

1. Cover the fixed smear with crystal violet or oxalated gentian violet stain which is allowed to act for 3 minutes;
2. Pour off excess of the stain; wash away the remaining crystal violet stain with Gram's iodine and allow the Gram's iodine to act for 2 minutes;
3. Decolourise with alcohol for about 5 seconds drop by drop till the violet colour is removed from the film;
4. Wash with tap water;
5. Counterstain with basic fuchsin or safranin stain for 30 seconds;
6. Wash with tap water, blot with blotting paper, dry in air and examine the smear under oil immersion objective (Fig. 3.3).

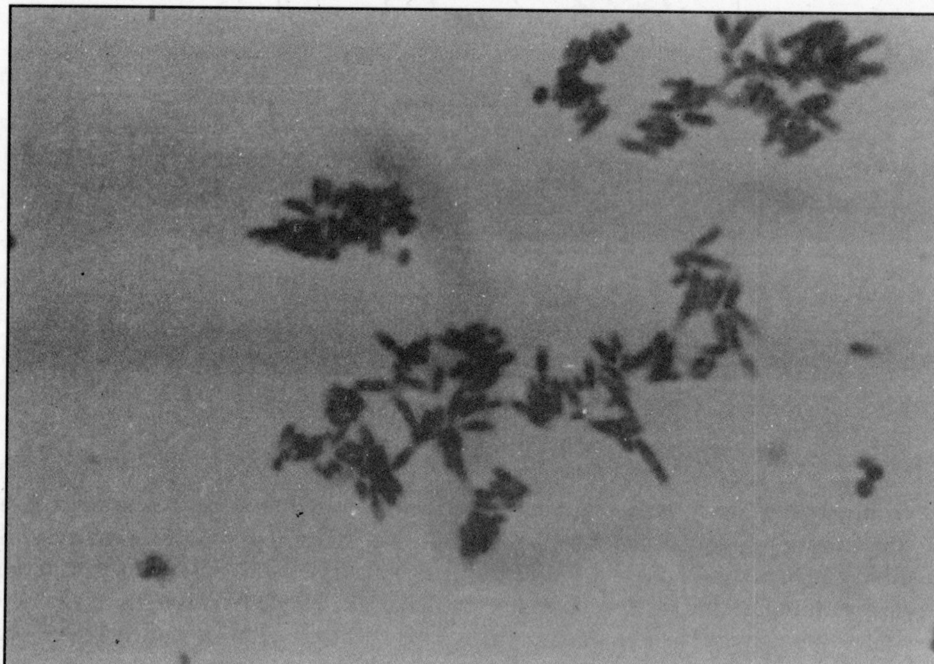

Fig. 3.3 : Gram-negative bacilli 1000X

On the basis of Gram stain, bacteria are mainly grouped into : (1) Gram-positive bacteria and Gram-negative bacteria. Gram-positive bacteria retain the gentian violet in spite of decolourisation by alcohol and stained violet, whereas Gram-negative bacteria are decolourised

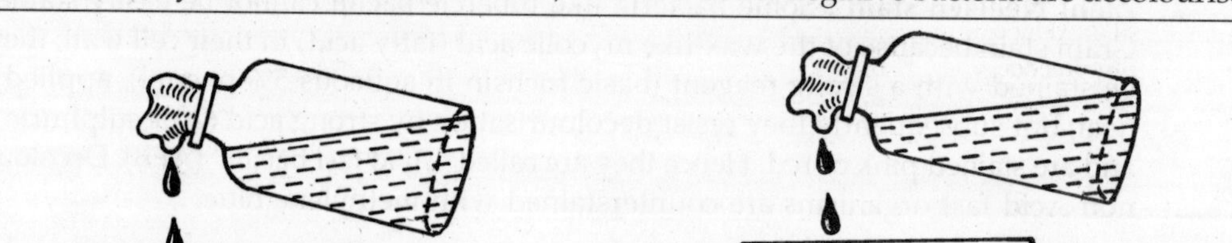

(a) Flood slide with crystal violet stain. Allow to act for 3 min.

(b) Wash off stain with Gram's Iodine. Allow to act for 2 min.

Contd.

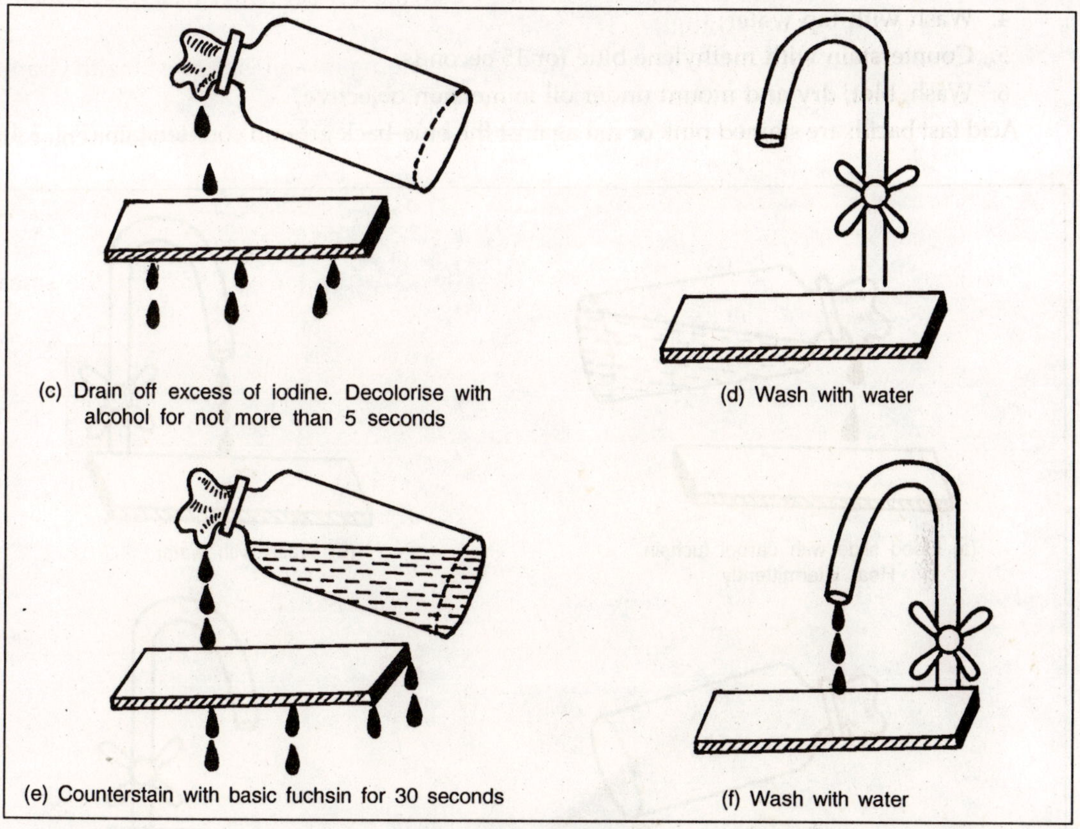

(c) Drain off excess of iodine. Decolorise with alcohol for not more than 5 seconds

(d) Wash with water

(e) Counterstain with basic fuchsin for 30 seconds

(f) Wash with water

Fig. 3.3: Gram Staining

by alcohol, loose the violet stain completely and are stained pink by the counterstain. The clinician can choose antibiotics effective against any of the groups (Table 3.1).

Table 3.1. Classification of common bacteria according to their reaction to Gram stain

Gram-positive	Gram-negative
Bacillus subtilis	Pseudomonas
Bacillus anthracis	Salmonella, Proteus
Clostridium tetani	Shigella
Clostridium welchii	Escherichia coli
Staphylococci	Vibrio cholerae
Streptococci	Brucella abortus
Pneumococci	Neisseria meningitidis
Mycobacterium tuberculosis	Neisseria gonorrhoae
Corynebacterium diphtheriae and diphtheroids	

Ziehl Neelsen method

1. Flood or fully cover the slide with carbol fuchsin and heat gently with spirit lamp from below till steam rises. Allow the stain to act for 5 minutes;
2. Wash with tap water;
3. Decolourise with 20% sulphuric acid for 1 minute till the yellowish brown or pink colour appears;

4. Wash with tap water;
5. Counterstain with methylene blue for 15 seconds;
6. Wash, blot, dry and mount under oil immersion objective.

Acid fast bacilli are stained pink or red against the blue-back ground counterstain (Fig. 3.4).

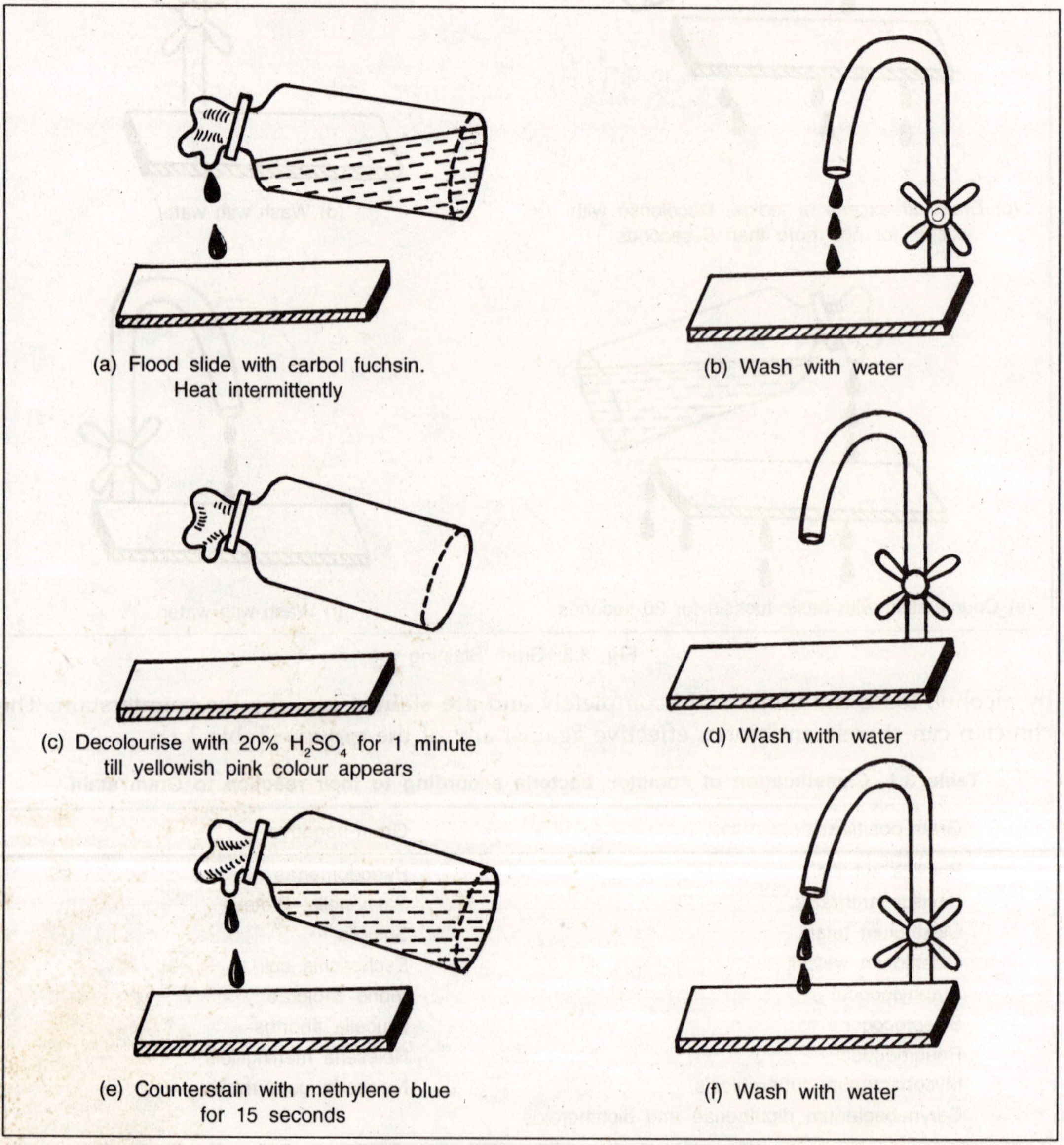

Fig. 3.4: Ziehl Neelsen method

Special staining methods : Albert or Neisser method is used to demonstrate metachromatic granules; whereas India Ink method and Leifson's method are used to observe capsules and flagella of bacteria, respectively; spores are stained by Gram's method or acid-fast stain, or malachite green stain.

Demonstration

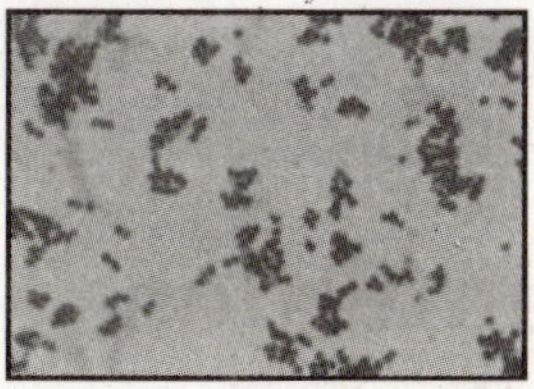

(a)

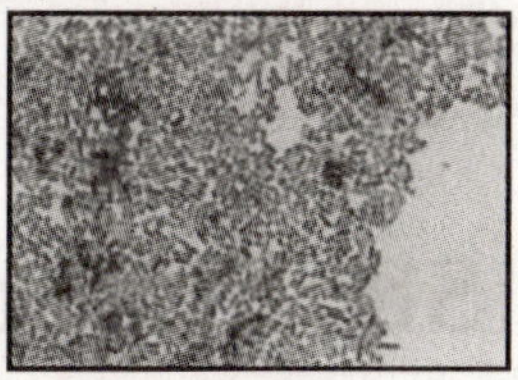

(b)

Fig. 3.5: Gram's stain smear showing (a) Gram-positive cocci (violet) and (b) Gram-negative bacilli (pink).

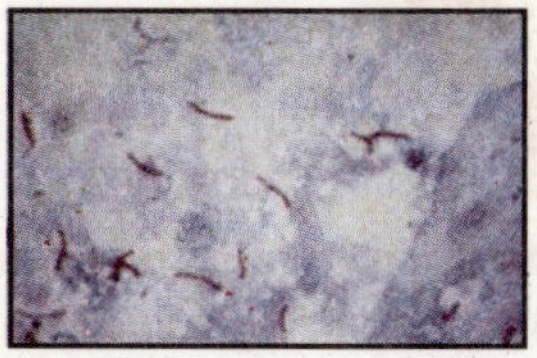

Fig. 3.6: Ziehl Neelsen stain smear showing pink or red stained acid fast bacilli and blue stained non acid-fast bacilli.

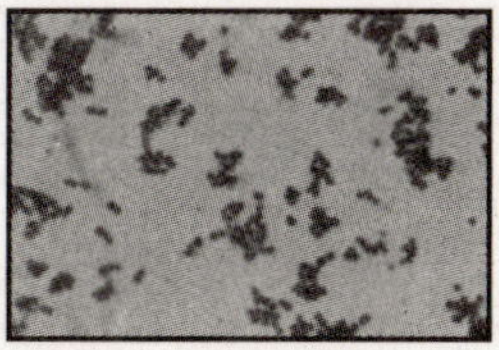

Fig. 3.7: A smear from pus (Gram stain) showing Gram-positive cocci (violet) in clusters.

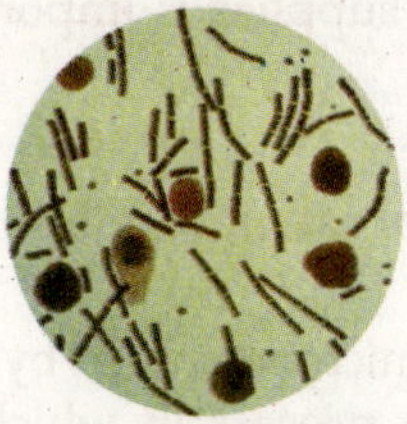

Fig. 3.8: Smear stained by Hiss's method for capsule. The capsule is stained pale bluish purple and cocci are deep violet.

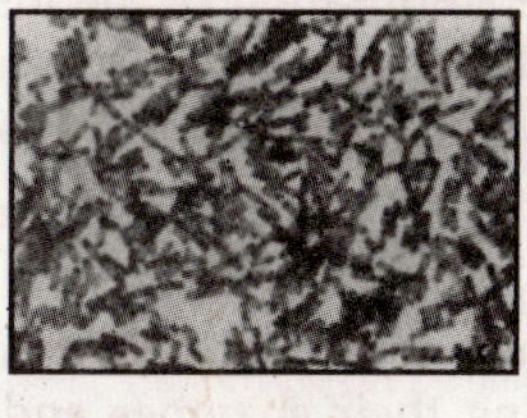

Fig. 3.9: Gram stained smear showing Gram-positive bacilli (violet) with unstained central spores.

Practical work

1. Stain the given smear by Gram's stain and study the morphology of the organisms.
2. Stain the given smear by Ziehl Neelsen method and study the morphology of organisms.
3. Your findings of the practical work and your observations during demonstration of stained permanent slides should be entered in your practical notebook.

Answers to the following questions should be entered in the practical notebook :

1. Why should the smear be fixed on the slide and how is it fixed; how will you confirm the smear is on the slide and why you should not use the fingernails to detect the position of the smear on the slide?
2. Describe the principles of Gram staining and Ziehl Neelsen method.
3. Define mordant. Name the substance acting as mordant in Gram stain and describe its function.
4. What is "lake" or dye-iodine complex?
5. When Gram-positive changes to Gram-negative?
6. Why tubercle bacilli (Mycobacterium tuberculosis) cannot be easily stained by Gram stain and why carbol-fuchsin is heated in Ziehl Neelsen method?
7. What is Acid-fast bacilli?
8. At what stage of Ziehl Neelsen method should the decolourisation with sulphuric acid be stopped?

4

Sterilisation and Disinfection
(Methods of Sterilisation)

Sterilisation is the process of freeing of an article from all living microorganisms including their spores. Sterility is an **absolute** state, while the disinfection is a relative term indicating a mere removal of pathogenic microorganisms on the article.

Sterilisation of culture media, containers and instruments is essential in microbiological work for the isolation and maintenance of pure culture. In dental, nursing practice, surgery and medicine, the sterilisation of the instruments, drugs and other supplies is important for the prevention of the spread of diseases.

Sterilisation can be effected by the following methods :

Dry heat kills the microorganisms by destructive oxidation of essential cell constituents at 160°C for 60 minutes.

Moist heat is more effective than dry heat, moist heat kills the microorganisms by coagulating and denaturing their enzymes and their structural proteins, a process in which the water participates. Heat resistant spores are killed at exposure to moist heat at 121°C for 10-30 minutes.

Chemical sterilising agents are widely used as disinfectants and antiseptics; disinfectants are potent, toxic and applied on in animate objects; antiseptics are non-toxic and used for superficial application on living tissues.

Routinely used Common Instruments for Sterilisation

Physical Methods – Dry heat

1. **Hot air oven :** The oven is heated by electricity and has a thermostat to maintain the air temperature constant (160°C for 1 hour). It is the best method to sterilise dry glass water, cotton wool plugged test tubes, Petri dishes, flasks, pipettes, swabs, powder, fat or grease). All glasswares should be dry, and wrapped in kraft paper to soak any water drop on the glassware. The oven should be loaded in such a way that the air can circulate through the load. The temperature should be raised slowly in the course of 1-2 hours to reach 160°C—which must be maintained for 1 hour. This is the **holding period.** Finally, the oven is allowed to cool gradually for 2 hours before the door is opened, otherwise the glasswares may crack due to sudden atmospheric cooling.
2. **Infrared radiation :** The infrared rays are directed on the object to be sterilised at a temperature of 180°C as a means of sterilising surgical instruments.

Moist heat

Below 100°C

1. **Constant temperature water bath**

   It is a metal box containing a heating element and a thermostat that keeps the water in the box at a constant temperature (56°C or 60°C).

   During the preparation of bacterial vaccine, the bacteria in suspension are killed in the water bath (vaccine bath) at a temperature of 60°C for 1 hour. The sterilisation of serum or body fluids containing coagulable proteins is effected at 56°C for 1 hour in water bath. The temperature above 59°C may cause inspissation (coagulation).

STERILISATION

- (A) **Physical methods**
  - HEAT
    - Dry heat
      1. Red heat
      2. Flaming
      3. Hot air Oven
      4. Infrared radiation
    - Moist heat
      - **Less than 100°C**
        1. Pasteurisation
        2. Water bath
        3. Inspissator
      - **At 100°C**
        - Arnold, Koch steam steriliser
      - **Above 100°C**
        - Autoclave
  - RADIATION
    - Non-ionising (Ultraviolet, infrared radiation)
    - ionising radiation (X-ray, gamma ray)
  - FILTRATION
    1. Berkefeld filter
    2. Chamberland filter
    3. Seitz filter
    4. Sintered glass filter
    5. Cellulose membrane filter
    6. Laminar airflow
- (B) **Chemical methods**

2. **Pasteurisation** of milk can be done by two methods :
   (a) Holder method (63°C for 30 minutes) or
   (b) Flash method (72°C for 20 seconds) in which tubercle bacilli, **Brucella abortus** and Salmonella are destroyed.
3. **Inspissator :** It consists of a water jacketed copper box. The temperature is between 75°–85°C in which the protein is completely solidified. The serum (Loeffler serum) and egg (Dorset egg or Lowenstein Jensen medium) in screw-capped (MacCartney) bottles are placed in special racks so that the tubes are in slanting position to form slopes; water vapour can enter the interior of the inspissator, the medium is kept moist, sterilised at 75°C for 45 minutes intermittently for three days and solidified.

At 100°C

Boiling water in fish kettle (100°C for 10 minutes) is sufficient to kill the non-spore forming bacilli. It does not ensure sterility and is used for rubber stoppers, instruments (scalpels, forceps, scissors), metal and glass type syringes.

Steam at 100°C is used for the sterilisation of culture media (nutrient broth and agar), but it is not as effective as autoclaving. Koch or Arnold steamer (steriliser) heated by gas or electricity is employed. It is a vertical cylinder with a conical lid having a small opening for escaping steam, i.e. steam without pressure.

Exposure at 100°C for 20-45 minutes on each of the three successive days, sometimes referred to as Fractional sterilisation (Tyndallisation), is employed to sterilise sugar media, gelatin media etc.

Above 100°C

Principle : Water boils when its vapour pressure equals the pressure of the surrounding atmosphere. This occurs at 100°C for normal atmospheric pressure (i.e. 760 mm Hg = 14.7 lb per square inch absolute pressure).

Thus, when vapour boils within a closed vessel at increased pressure, the temperature at which it boils will rise above 100°C.

This principle is employed in "Autoclave" which provides heat at temperatures above 100°C. Autoclaving is the reliable method most widely used for sterilisation of culture media and surgical supplies.

All parts of the load to be sterilised should be permeated by the steam.

1. The simple form of laboratory autoclave, the so-called "pressure cooker type" (Fig. 4.1), consists of a vertical cylinder of gun metal or stainless steel. Its size is 18 inch (45 cm) in diameter and 30 inch (75 cm). in length. The lid (or door) is fastened by screw clamps and is rendered airtight by means of asbestos washer. The cylinder contains water up to a certain level and is heated electrically below the cylinder. The bottles, tubes, culture media etc. to be sterilised are placed on a perforated tray situated above the water level. This apparatus is furnished on its lid with a discharge tap for air and steam, a pressure gauge, and a safety valve.

Direction for using the simple autoclave

Water should be sufficient in the cylinder. Insert the material to be sterilised and turn on the heater. Place the lid in position, open the discharge tap and screw down the lid. Adjust the safety valve to the required pressure. Allow the steam and air mixture to escape freely until all the air has been eliminated from the autoclave. Now close the discharge tap. The steam pressure up to 15 lb pressure per sq. inch for 121°C should be maintained for 15 minutes. This is the **holding period.** Then turn off the heater and allow the autoclave to cool until the pressure is 0 lb per sq. inch. To avoid a violent explosion, do not open the autoclave when its inside pressure is still high.

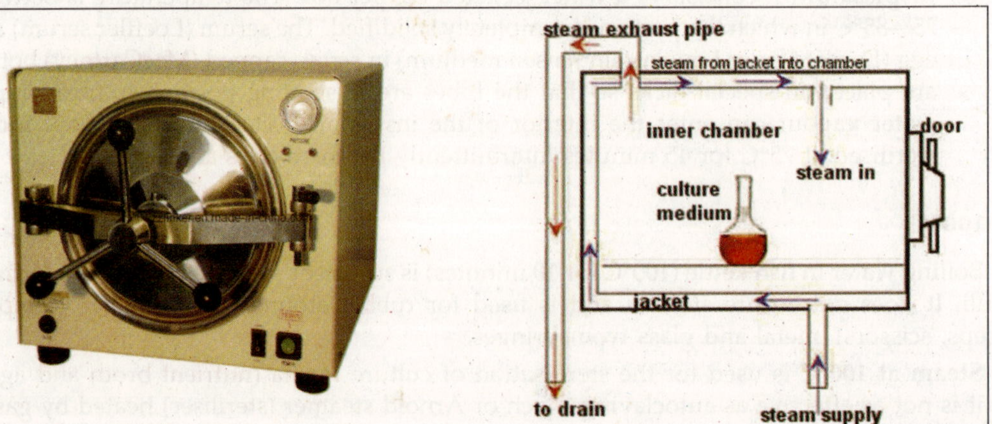

Fig. 4.1: Simple autoclave

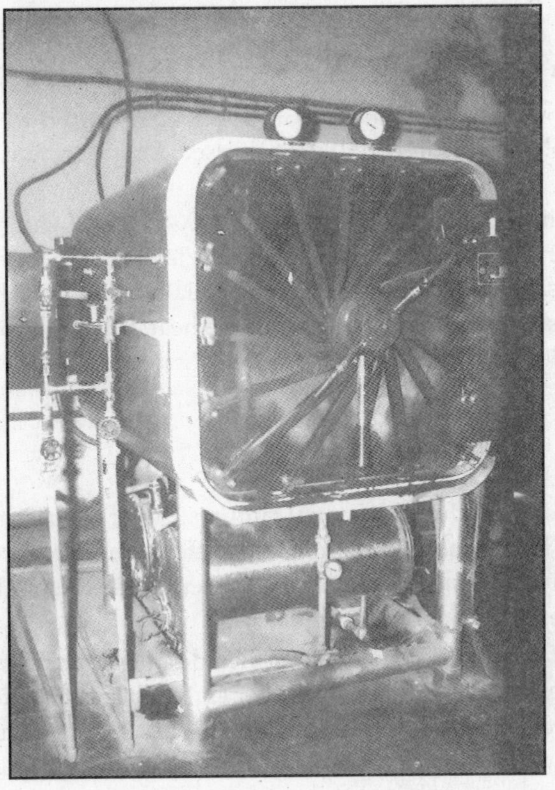

Fig. 4.2: Autoclave—Hospital Type

2. **Steam jacketed autoclave** (hospital type)

This autoclave is horizontal and is made of rustless metal. At its front is a swing door fastened by a "capstan head" which operates radially and remains locked. A pressure locked safety door is a valuable guard against a dangerous explosion through premature opening by the operator.

The hospital type autoclave (Fig. 4.2) has (a) a supply of steam from external source; (b) steam jacket; (c) a channel to discharge air and steam; (d) steam trap with thermometer to control the discharge; (e) a vacuum system to assist the drying of the load; (f) a cooling system to hasten the cooling.

To test the efficiency of autoclaving

Two methods (chemical and spore indicators) are available to detect the efficiency of autoclaving.

(1) **Chemical indicators** may be placed inside the load. Browne's steriliser control tubes contain a red solution that turns green when heated at 115°C for 25 minutes (type 1) or 15 minutes (type 2) or at 160°C for 60 minutes (type 3). **Bowie Dick tape,** applied to packs and articles in the autoclave, develops diagonal lines when exposed to the sterilising temperature for the correct time.

(2) **Spore indicators.** A preparation of dried spores of **Bacillus stearothermophilus** is placed within the load in the autoclave and after autoclaving it is tested for viability on transfer to culture media; its spores are killed at 121°C in about 12 minutes.

Radiation

Non-ionising radiation

Ultraviolet rays from suitably shielded lamps have been used to reduce the number of bacteria in the atmosphere. Infrared radiation is used for rapid mass sterilisation of glass syringes.

Ionising radiation includes high speed electrons; X-rays and gamma rays (short X-rays). In sufficient dose, these radiations are lethal to all cells including bacteria by damaging DNA. Spores are generally resistant. It is employed commercially for sterilisation of plastic syringes, rubber and catheters that are unable to withstand the heat. It is too expensive for the hospital use. This method is called **cold sterilisation.** Plastic syringes can also be sterilised by ethylene oxide gas.

Filtration

It is possible to render the fluids, bacterial cultures, sugar by passing through the special filters with pore size of less than 0.75 µm. In general, sterilising filters render liquid free from bacteria, but not from mycoplasma or virus. Thus, the serum "sterilised" by Seitz filtration must not be regarded as safe for clinical use.

Types of filter used in bacteriological work include : (a) earthenware candles (Berkefeld Chamberland); (b) asbestos disks (Seitz filter); (c) sintered glass filters; (d) in recent years, cellulose membrane filters are used to separate viruses of different sizes.

Seitz filter : It consists of a disk of an asbestos through which the fluid is filtered. The disk is inserted into the metal holder fitted to a filtering flask. Before use, the whole apparatus should be sterilised by autoclave (Fig. 4.3).

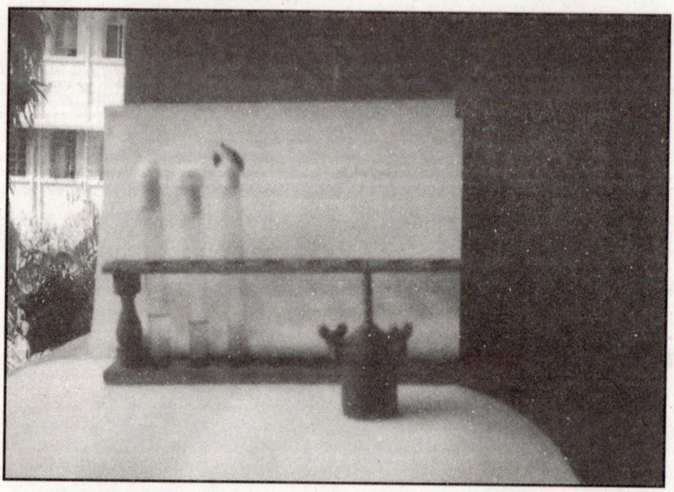

Fig. 4.3: Seitz filter in front

The development of high efficiency particulate air (HEPA) filters or fiberglass filters has made it possible to deliver clean air to an enclosure (cubicle or room). This type of air filtration together with a system of Laminar Airflow is now recommended as air disinfection and used very extensively to produce dust and bacteria-free air in vaccine sterility testing laboratory; but it is expensive.

Chemical Methods :

· Common chemical disinfectants used:

On inanimate objects		
Table, instruments	:	5% Lysol; 1-10% Formaldehyde; 2% Aqueous glutaraldehyde; 0.1% Mercury bichloride; 0.1% Quaternary ammonium compounds.
Excreta, bandages, bedpans	:	1% Sodium hypochlorite; 5% Lysol or other phenolic compounds.
Air	:	Propylene glycol or aerosol Formaldehyde vapour.
Heat labile instruments	:	Ethylene oxide gas (alkylates nucleic acid); residue gas must be removed by aeration.
On skin or wounds	:	Washing with soap and water. Soaps or detergents containing 2% hexachlorophene or 1.5% trichlorocarbanilide or chlorohexidine; 2% Tincture of iodine; 70% Ethyl alcohol 70-90% isopropyl alcohol; Povidone-iodine (water-soluble). Nitrofurazone. 0.2% Jelly or solution).
On skin or mucous membrane in candidiasis	:	Gentian violet 1 : 2,000; Nystatin cream, 100000 units/g. Candidian ointment, 0.6 mg/g. Miconazole 2% cream.
In burns	:	Silver nitrate 0.5%, Mafenide acetate cream; Silver sulfadiazine.
In dermatophytes	:	Undecyclenic acid powder, or 5-10% cream, Tolnaflate cream 1%.
In pyoderma	:	Ammoniated mercury; 2.5% ointment Bacitracin-neomycin-polymyxin ointment. Potassium permanganate, 0.01%.
In pediculosis	:	Lindane, malathion or permethrin 0.5-1%lotion.
On eyes		
Gonorrhea	:	1% Silver nitrate.
Bacterial conjunctivitis	:	Sulfacetamide ointment. Chloramphenicol ointment.

Questions

Describe in brief the following in your practical notebook:

1. The difference between sterilisation and disinfection; antiseptics and disinfectants.
2. Moist heat is preferred to dry heat; why?
3. The principles of autoclave, hot air oven, inspissator, tyndallisation.
4. The identification of all instruments with their uses and principles.
5. Hot air oven and autoclave should not be opened immediately after the holding period; give reasons.
6. Principle and use of Laminar air flow.

5

Growth Requirement of Bacteria

(Common Laboratory Media)

For rapid multiplication of bacteria in the laboratory, the following growth requirements must be provided:

(a) Food – Most pathogenic bacteria require food as source of organic carbon and nitrogen.

(b) Moisture—since bacterial cell consists of water, moisture is essential for its growth.

(c) Temperature – for each species, there is a maximum and minimum temperature at which its growth is possible. The optimum temperature for most pathogenic bacteria is 37°C.

(d) Reaction – like temperature, there is an optimum pH for each species, usually most pathogens grow well at neutral or slightly alkaline pH (7.8);

(e) Oxygen – Certain bacteria grow in presence of molecular oxygen and are called 'aerobes'; others, called "anaerobes", will grow only in absence of oxygen.

Preparation of culture media : In the laboratory, bacteria can grow on "culture media" which are mixtures of suitable food materials required for bacterial growth. After preparation, the pH of the media is adjusted by pH meter (Fig. 5.1) or comparator; the media are sterilised by autoclave and poured in Petri dish (plate), test tubes, flasks etc. They are incubated to check

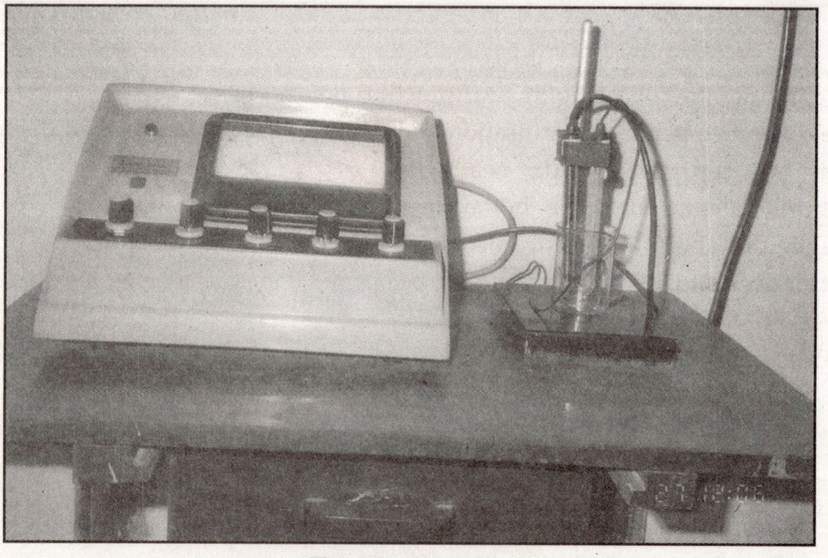

Fig. 5.1: pH meter

the sterility and, finally, they are stored in the refrigerator. For general application, the media are prepared from the base—peptone water (containing peptone, sodium chloride, water)—to which meat extract, blood, serum has been added. For solidifying the media, the agar or gelatin is added.

COMMON LABORATORY MEDIA

A. Liquid (broth)

(i) Peptone water
(ii) Nutrient broth
(iii) Glucose broth
(iv) Sugar medium
(v) Urea medium
(vi) Glycerol saline
(vii) Cary Blair
(viii) Stuart medium
(ix) Venkatraman Ramakrishnan medium

B. Solid (agar)

1. Nutrient agar
2. Blood agar
3. Chocolate agar
4. Tellurite chocolate agar
5. Loeffler serum
6. Dorset's egg medium
7. Lowenstein Jensen medium
8. MacConkey agar medium
9. Wilson and Blair medium
10. Robertson's cooked meat medium
11. Litmus milk medium
12. Triple sugar iron medium
13. Simmon's citrate medium
14. Xylose Lysine desoxycholate agar

Common Laboratory Media

1. **Peptone water :** Contains 1% peptone and 0.5% sodium chloride dissolved in water. It does not contain meat extract. The medium is colourless. Peptone water is used to study proteolytic activity of bacteria viz; formation of indole and hydrogen sulphide (H_2S). Motility of bacteria is best studied from peptone water culture; peptone water is used as a base for sugar media.

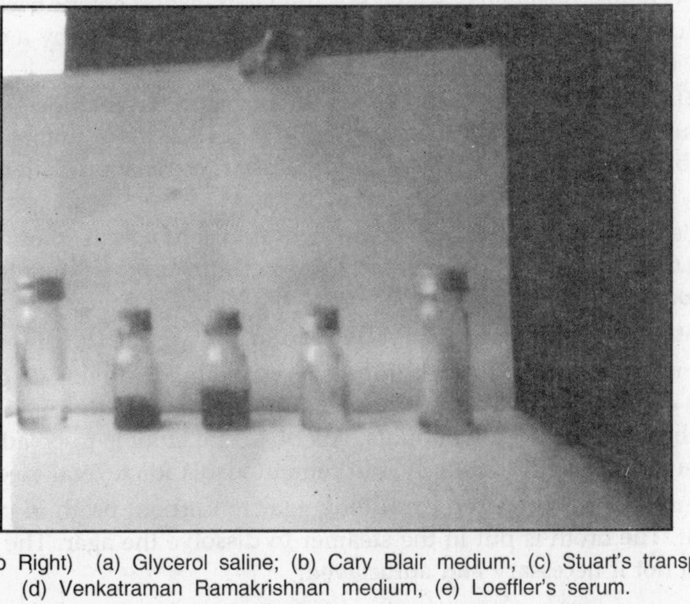

Fig. 5.2: (Left to Right) (a) Glycerol saline; (b) Cary Blair medium; (c) Stuart's transport medium (d) Venkatraman Ramakrishnan medium, (e) Loeffler's serum.

2. **Nutrient broth :** It is a pale yellow coloured liquid. The first step is to prepare the meat extract. This is done by extracting meat in cold with water. It is then heated to coagulate the dissolved proteins and filtered. The filtrate is the required meat extract. Peptone and sodium chloride are added to the above for preparation of nutrient broth. It is sterilised by autoclaving. It is a common fluid medium for non-fastidious organisms and serves as a base for preparation of solid media.
3. **Glucose broth** is a pale yellow liquid which contains basically nutrient broth to which one per cent glucose is added. It is mainly used to grow anaerobic streptococci.

   Hartley broth contains lean meat, pancreatic extract, is yellow transparent and is used for blood culture.
4. **Sugar media :** Various carbohydrates, alcohols etc. (designated as 'SUGAR') are fermented by bacteria with the formation of acid or acid and gas. Sugar media are used to study these fermentation reactions. Appropriate sugars are added to peptone water in the proportion of one per cent. A suitable indicator is also incorporated to detect the formation of acid. Usually Andrade's indicator is used which is colourless in alkaline and neutral pH and turns pink in presence of acid. To detect the production of gas, a small tube (Durham tube) is placed in an inverted position in the medium. The air is replaced by fluid during sterilisation by heat.

   Gas, if produced, is seen as a bubble at the top of the Durham tube. The sugar media are sterilised in a steam steriliser at 100°C for 20 minutes on three successive days. The common sugar media are Glucose, Sucrose, Lactose, Mannitol and Dulcitol. Note the coloured plugs to differentiate them (Glucose, blue; Sucrose, white; Mannitol, pink; lactose, red; Dulcitol, yellow or coloured beads).
5. **Urea medium :** It contains peptone, sodium chloride, glucose, buffer, 20% urea, phenol red, pH 6.8-6.9. After inoculation heavily with cultures and incubation at 37°C for 4 hrs, and then overnight at room temperature, urease at room temperature positive cultures produce purple pink colour due to a change in the colour of the indicator. Thus, urease producing organisms are identified.
6. **Glycerol Saline Transport medium :** This medium contains glycerol, sodium chloride, buffer, phenol red, water. It is used to transport enteric bacilli to the laboratory. This fluid should not be used if it becomes acid, indicated by a change in colour to yellow (Fig. 5.2(a)).
7. **Cary Blair medium :** This is a buffered solution of sodium chloride, sodium thioglycollate, disodium phosphate and calcium chloride at pH 8.4. It is a suitable transport medium for **Vibrio cholerae.** At pH 7.4, it can be used to transport Salmonella, Shigella and Campylobacter (Fig. 5.2(b)).
8. **Stuart's Transport Medium** is composed of anaerobic salt solution, methylene blue, agar 0.6% pH 7.3-7.4. This is soft agar medium used to maintain the viability of gonococci on swabs during transport to the laboratory (Fig. 5.2(c)).
9. **Venkatraman-Ramakrishnan (VR) medium.**

A simple modified form of this medium is prepared by dissolving 20 g crude sea salt and 5 g Peptone in one litre of distilled water and adjusting the pH to 8.6-8.8. It is dispensed in screw-capped bottles in 10-15 ml amounts. About 1-3 ml stool is to be added to each bottle. In this medium vibrios do not multiply, but remain viable for several weeks (Fig. 5.2(d)).

1. **Nutrient agar :** is prepared by adding agar to nutrient broth in proportion of 2 to 3 percent. The broth is put in the steamer to dissolve the agar. The agar broth fluid is filtered hot if necessary and autoclaved.

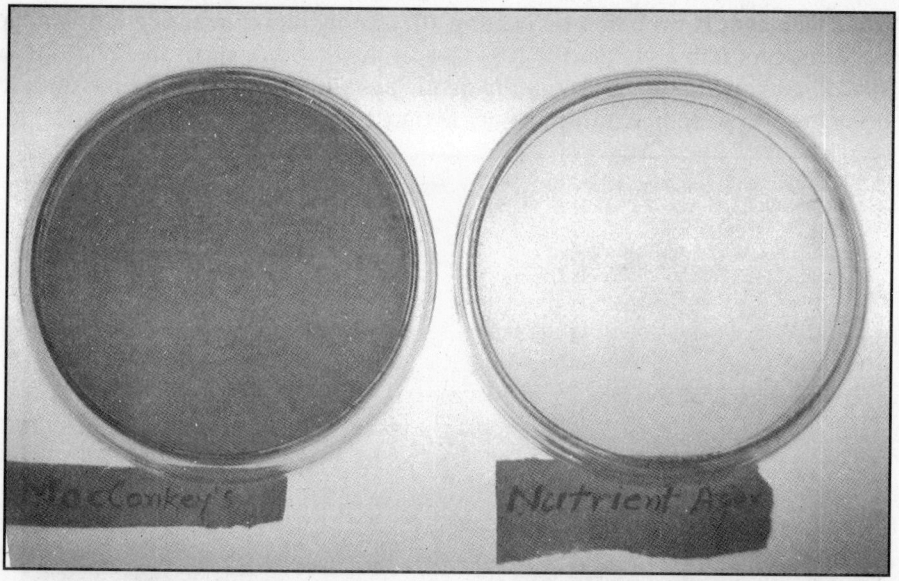

Fig. 5.3: MacConkey agar **Fig. 5.4**: Nutrient agar

It becomes solid when cooled. The medium is almost transparent. It is a common-purpose solid medium for growth of non-fastidious organisms, further, it serves as a base for the 'Enriched media' (Fig. 5.4).

2. **Blood agar :** is prepared by adding defibrinated or citrated blood to nutrient agar in the proportion of 5 to 10 per cent. Blood is collected aseptically and added to the already sterilised nutrient agar which has been melted and cooled to about 55 C. The medium is used for the cultivation of fastidious organisms which fail to grow on nutrient. Agar (Fig. 5.5).

Fig. 5.5: Blood agar

3. **Chocolate agar** is prepared by heating 10% sterile blood in sterile nutrient agar. Melt the agar, cool it in a waterbath at 75 C, add the blood & allow the medium to remain at 75 C, mixing the blood & agar by gentle agitation from time to time until the blood becomes chocolate-brown in colour, within 10 min. Then pour as slopes or plates.

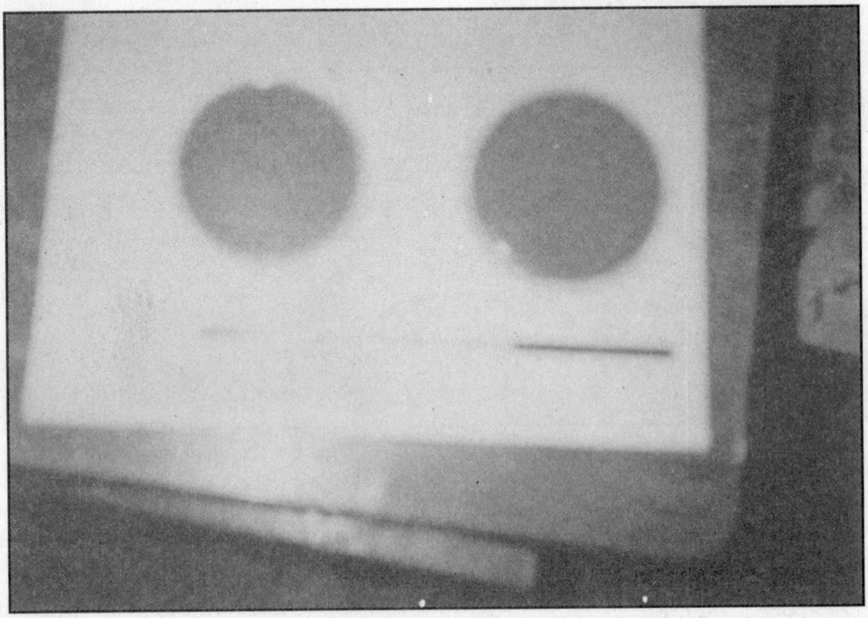

Fig. 5.7: (Left) Chocolate agar medium
Fig. 5.6: (Right) Blood agar medium

This medium is used for the cultivation of gonococci and meningococci which form greyish colonies.

4. **Tellurite Chocolate agar** : It is heated blood agar to which potassium tellurite (0.4%) has been added. It inhibits the growth of many commensal organisms likely to be present in the throat but not the diphtheria bacilli and related organisms. Moreover, these latter organisms form grey or black colonies on the medium as they reduce potassium tellurite. The medium is opaque brown in appearance.
5. **Loeffler's serum :** Consists of human or animal serum added to Glucose broth. The collection of blood and separation of serum are carried out with aseptic precautions. The medium is solidified by inspissation. The medium is opaque white in appearance. It is mostly used for cultivation of the diphtheria bacillus. It can be employed to study proteolytic activity of bacteria (liquefaction of serum) (Fig. 5.5(c)).
6. **Dorset's Egg medium** : is prepared by inspissating a mixture of whole egg fluid 3 part and saline 1 part. The medium is yellow and opaque. When glycerinated, the medium is used for cultivation of tubercle bacilli; without glycerine it is useful for the preservation of stock cultures of enteric bacilli.
7. **Lowenstein Jensen medium** : It contains a number of mineral salt, glycerine, starch, egg proteins and malachite green. The last is a bactericidal agent. This medium is used for the cultivation of tubercle bacilli.
8. **MacConkey medium :** (Bile salt lactose Neutral red agar) : It is used for the isolation of intestinal pathogens. Bile salt inhibits the growth of Gram-positive cocci. Pathogenic Gram-negative enteric bacilli (Salmonella, Shigella) do not ferment lactose and form

pale colonies. Escherichia coli (which are commensals), on the other hand, ferment lactose producing acid and, therefore, their colonies are pink. The medium is thus both an inhibitory and differentiating one. A number of media are described which work on the same principle viz, D.E.C. medium of Panja and Ghosh and Leifson's desoxycholate citrate medium etc. They differ from the basic medium described above in containing inhibitory substances other than bile salt. All appear reddish brown and transparent (Fig. 5.3).

9. **Wilson and Blair medium :** This medium is utilised for isolation of typhoid and paratyphoid organisms from heavily contaminated material like sewage. It contains sodium sulphate, Bismuth ammonium citrate and brilliant green. The last one inhibits Escherichia coli. Typhoid and paratyphoid organisms form black colonies as they reduce sulphate to sulphide in presence of glucose—precipitating insoluble bismuth sulphide (which is black). It is also a differentiating and inhibitory medium.
10. **Robertson's Cooked Meat medium :** Minced meat is boiled in alkaline water. The softened meat is then partially dried between folds of filter paper and added to nutrient broth. The medium is autoclaved for sterilisation. The medium is used for cultivation of anaerobic organisms.
11. **Litmus Milk medium :** is prepared by adding litmus solution to skimmed milk. The medium is autoclaved or boiled for sterilisation. It is used for studying proteolytic and saccharolytic activity of Clostridium welchii.
12. **Thiosulphate Citrate Bile Salt Sucrose (TCBS) medium.** This medium—containing thiosulphate, citrate, bile salt, bromothymol blue and sucrose—is available commercially and is very widely used at present. Vibrio cholerae produce large yellow convex colonies which may become green on continued incubation.
13. **Triple Sugar Iron (TSI) medium**. This medium contains glucose, lactose and sucrose, phenol red indicator (to indicate fermentation), ferrous sulphate (to demonstrate H_2S, indicated by blackening of the butt). It is orange red when uninoculated. It is used to identify the enterobacteriaceae. The glucose concentration is 1/10th of concentration of lactose and sucrose so to detect the fermentation of glucose alone. The small amount of acid produced by fermentation of glucose is oxidised rapidly in the slant which reverts to alkaline (red); in contrast, under lower O_2 tension in the butt, the acid reaction (yellow) is maintained. Free exchange of air may be permitted in the slant through the use of loose cotton plug to promote oxidation of acid produced by glucose fermentation in the slant. This reaction should be read after 24 hrs' incubation.

Interpretation of reaction

Reaction	**Carbohydrate fermented**	**Organism**
Acid slant/Acid butt	Glucose with acid and gas and lactose	Esch. coli
Alkaline slant/Acid butt	Glucose with acid, gas but not lactose and sucrose	Proteus

14. **Simmon's Citrate medium** is modified Koser's medium with agar and an indicator (bromothymol blue). It is used to test the ability of an organism to utilise citrate as the sole source of carbon and energy for growth and an ammonium salt as the sole source of nitrogen. It is also called citrate utilisation test.

Result :

Positive = Blue colour and growth of bacteria.

Negative = Original green colour and no growth.

15. **Xylose Lysine Desoxycholate (XLD) agar.** Yeast extract agar with lysine, xylose, lactose, sucrose and ferric ammonium citrate; sodium desoxycholate inhibits Gram-positive organisms, phenol red indicator. It is used to isolate and differentiate Salmonella and Shigella from other Gram-negative enteric bacilli.

Note : Wilson Blair and Lowenstein Jensen media are green. Wilson Blair, however, is usually poured in Petri dishes whereas Lowenstein Jensen medium has to be kept in screw capped bottles or tubes with parafinished plugs.

Agar agar : It is a polysaccharide prepared from a seaweed grown on the Japanese and Chinese sea coasts. It is available in dry strands or in powder forms. It has no nutrient property and is used for solidifying the media. It does not set till it is cooled to 42°C. Therefore blood, serum etc. can be added to nutrient agar at 55°C at which temperature, the medium is still fluid and there is no risk of denaturation of the serum proteins added.

Peptone is golden granuled protein powder which has the ability to support the growth of bacteria.

6
Isolation of Bacteria in Pure Culture

To determine accurately the specific causative agent of the disease, the microbiologist must isolate a single bacterium, in pure form, from other bacteria with which it is mixed, as an alchemist purifies the metal from other metals or impurities. In clinical specimens (sputum, stool, urine etc.), the mixed microorganisms are common, and may mask and confuse the diagnostic results. To avoid this confusion a pure culture is needed. The extraneous organisms may change the pH, may damage or kill the desired microorganisms. A pure culture is the one which contains only one kind of microorganism whereas a **mixed culture** contains two or more kinds of microorganism. Pure culture may be compared to a bed of roses obtained in pure culture of roses.

The methods used to isolate the bacteria in pure culture consist of separating a single living bacterial cell and allowing it to multiply in a suitable culture medium, usually in a solid medium, to form a pure colony. Bacteria multiply very rapidly, so that a single bacterial cell deposited on a solid medium gives rise to a mass which is called a colony.

1. **Streaking or Plating** (inoculation of culture media). If the material containing bacteria is streaked several times on the surface of a solid medium with a platinum loop without recharging, fewer and fewer bacterial cells will remain on the loop as successive streaks are made and, finally, it may deposit a single bacterial cell on the surface. This procedure will thus give separate colonies of the organisms present in the material (Figs. 6.1, 6.2, 6.3).

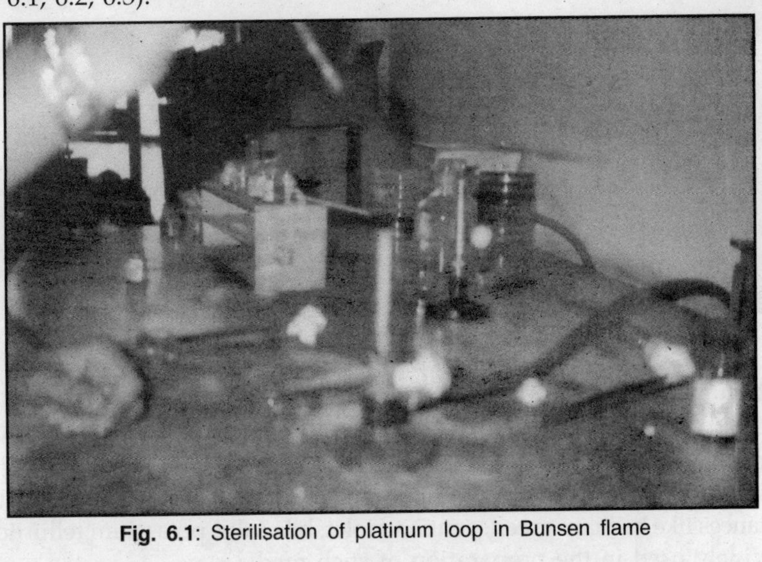

Fig. 6.1: Sterilisation of platinum loop in Bunsen flame

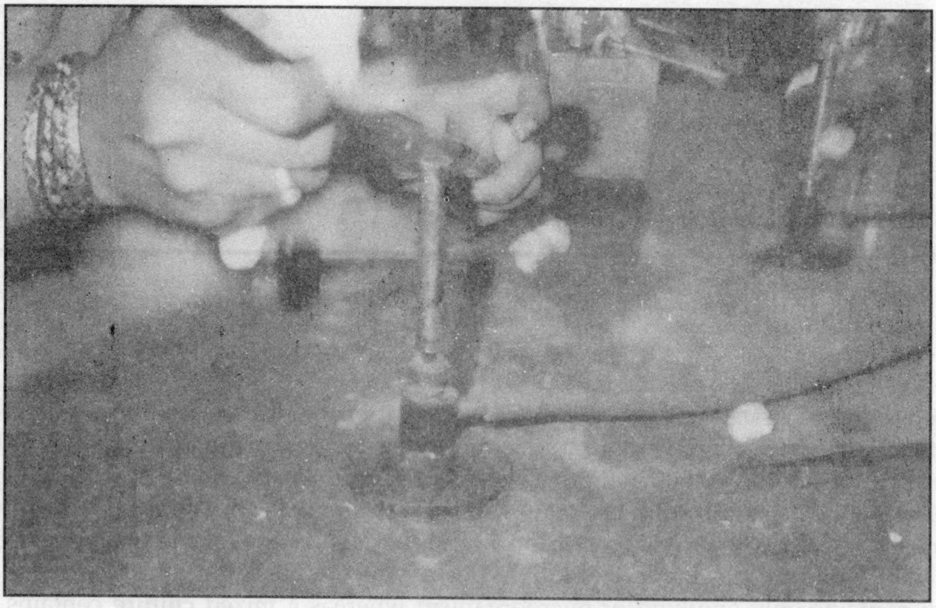

Fig. 6.2: Picking up of bacteria from culture

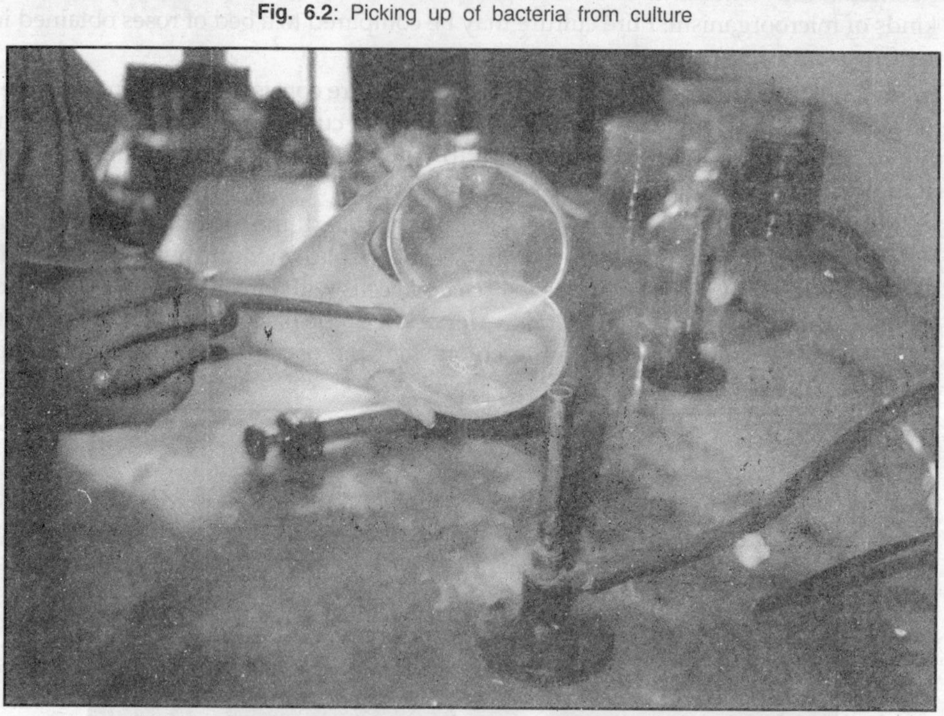

Fig. 6.3: Streaking of culture media with bacteria

2. **Dilution and Plating :** When the bacterial content of the material is expected to be high (e.g. feces), it is diluted with sterile nutrient broth or saline before plating.
3. **Use of selective medium :** Media which promote the growth of one type of organism and inhibit or retard the growth of others are known as "Selective Media". Inhibiting substances like brilliant green, gentian violet, bile salts, potassium tellurite and penicillin are widely used in the preparation of such media.

4. **Differential sterilisation by chemicals :** An example of this method is cultivation of tubercle bacilli from sputum (which contains numerous other organisms) after preliminary treatment with dilute mineral acid or alkali. In Petroff's method, the specimen of sputum is mixed with three or four times its volume of 4 per cent sodium hydroxide solution, incubated for one half to hour at 37°C and centrifuged. The deposit is neutralised, in the presence of an indicator, by dilute hydrochloric acid, and then seeded on a suitable medium. This treatment kills all other organisms except tubercle bacilli which are resistant to the action of dilute mineral acids, alkalies and other chemicals. "Antiformin" (Sodium hydroxide) can also be used instead of a dilute alkali.
5. **Differential Sterilisation by heat :** This method is employed where the organisms to be obtained in pure culture are more resistant to heat than others present in the material e.g. separation of spore bearing bacilli (which are more resistant to heat) from the non-spore bearers. The material is heated at 60°C for 30 minutes, cooled and then inoculated in a suitable medium. Only the spore bearers which have survived will grow.
6. **Inoculation of a susceptible animal :** This method is employed to isolate pathogenic microorganisms which are not easily grown on culture media or which are readily overgrown by the contaminating organisms. As example, we may quote isolation of tubercle bacilli from pus, peritoneal and pleural fluids by inoculating a guinea pig and isolation of the pneumococci from inoculating a mouse. In the later case, the contaminating organisms are rapidly killed in the animal body whereas the pathogenic organisms multiply and can be recovered in pure culture from the tissues.

7

Systematic Study of Bacteria
(Identification of Bacteria)

The identification of the bacteria isolated from a specimen may be carried out by the following studies :

1. **Morphology and Staining** serve as preliminary criteria. The Gram stained smear shows the Gram reaction, size, shape, groupings of the bacteria and intracellular position of the endospore. Special staining reaction can reveal the presence of capsule. Hanging drop wet preparation can be used to study the motility of bacteria. An unstained wet film is examined under dark ground illumination microscope to observe the exact morphology of delicate spirochaete. A smear is stained by Ziehl Neelsen method to demonstrate the acid fast staining reaction.
2. **Cultural characteristics :** The growth requirement and the appearance of colonies on media to the naked eye are further criteria to assist the identification of bacteria. A culture is a growth of bacterium on artificial nutrient medium or culture medium prepared in the laboratory. Attempts are made to grow (to cultivate or culture) the bacteria on media of different compositions (glucose, inorganic salts mixture, meat extract or meat infusion with blood) incubated under a variety of conditions (different temperatures, pH) in the presence of atmospheric oxygen (aerobically). The ability or inability to grow on medium containing a selective inhibitor (e.g. bile salt, optochin, tellurite, bacitracin, malachite green, low pH, high pH) may also be useful to identify the bacteria.

   The growth of bacteria in liquid culture medium (e.g. nutrient broth) may show :

   (1) a uniform turbidity; (2) little deposit at the bottom; (3) surface growth (pellicle formation). (Fig. 7.1a). The appearance of the discrete masses of growth or **colonies** that can be grown from isolated bacteria on the

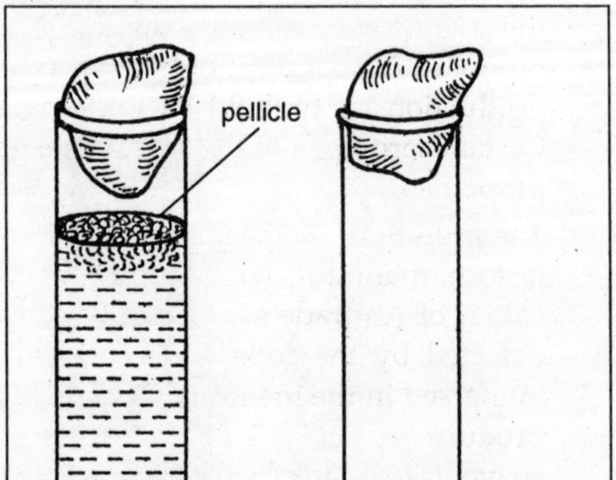

Fig. 7.1(a): Bacterial growth in liquid medium

surface of the solid medium (nutrient agar) can be used to study the size of the colonies (diameter in mm), their outline (whether circular, entire, indented or wavy or rhizoid), their elevation (low convex, high convex, flat, plateau-like, umbonate, or nodular)—Fig. 7.1b), their transparency (clear and transparent) or opaque, whether they are colourless (white or pigmented) or whether they produce any change in the medium (e.g. haemolysis in the blood agar medium).

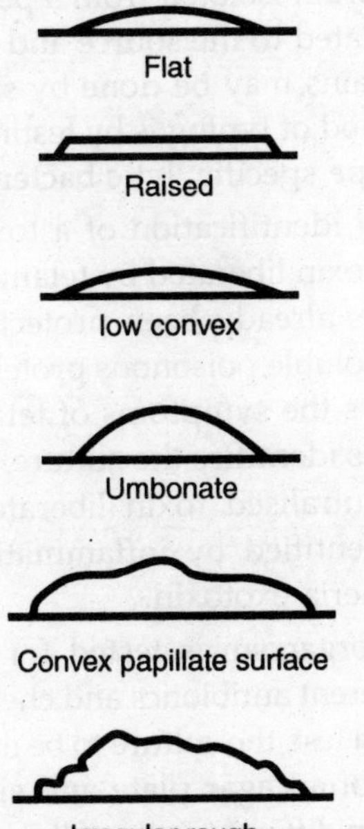

Fig. 7.1(b): Colony appearance on solid medium

3. **Biochemical reactions :** e.g. fermentation of various sugars (carbohydrates). Morphology and cultural characters may not be able to distinguish some species of bacteria; but these same species may exhibit distinct differences in their biochemical reactions e.g. typhoid and paratyphoid bacilli (glucose and mannitol are fermented without gas production by typhoid bacilli, whereas paratyphoid bacilli produce acid and gas). Certain serotypes of the salmonella group may resemble one another in fermentation properties.

   The growth of the bacteria in liquid medium will ferment particular sugars (glucose, lactose, mannitol) with the production of acid, which is detected by the changes of colour of Andrade's indicator dye incorporated in the medium; the gas production is detected by the collection of air bubble in a small inverted tube (Durham's tube) immersed in the medium. Other tests are used to find out the ability of a bacterium to produce particular end products e.g Indole, hydrogen sulphide, nitrite and certain enzymes (oxidase, catalase, urease, gelatinase, collagenase, lecithinase, lipase) in culture media.

4. **Antigenic characters :** Species or types of bacteria can be easily and distinctly identified by "specific" antibody reactions observed in serological tests performed on a glass slide. This specific antibody (antiserum) is obtained from the animal (rabbit) immunised against a particular type of microorganisms which agglutinates with the same antiserum. An unknown bacterium may thus be identified by demonstrating its reaction with one out of a number of standard known antisera. Similarly, the serum

of a person suffering from a bacterial infection may contain specific antibody. The nature of the infection may thus be diagnosed by demonstrating that the patient's serum agglutinates one out of a number of known antigens of laboratory cultures, e.g. Widal test in Typhoid fever.

5. **Typing of bacteria :** Bacteriophage sensitivity. A single bacterial pathogenic species may include different types of strains which are distinguishable in minor characters. Recognition of the type of a strain isolated from a patient may be of great importance in epidemiological studies related to the source and the spread of the infection in the community. The typing of stains may be done by special biochemical or serological tests. Another important method of typing is by testing the susceptibility of the culture to lysis by each of a set of type specific, lytic bacteriophages.
6. **Animal pathogenicity :** Final identification of a toxigenic strain of tetanus bacillus may be done by injecting the toxin liberated by tetanus bacillus into the base of the tail of two mice, one of them has already been protected by prior injection of specific antiserum to tetanus toxin (a soluble poisonous protein secreted by the tetanus bacilli). The unprotected mouse shows the symptoms of tetanus, whereas the protected one without any tetanus symptoms identifies the culture, as an organism producing toxin, as the injected antiserum neutralised toxin liberated by tetanus bacilli. Similarly, diphtheria bacillus is also identified by inflammation and necrosis of the skin of guinea pig brought by diphtheria exotoxin.
7. **Antibiotic sensitivity :** The organism is tested for its ability to grow on artificial nutrient media containing different antibiotics and chemotherapeutic agents in different concentrations. In disk diffusion test, the culture to be examined is inoculated confluently with swabs over the surface of an agar plate and six to ten paper disks containing different antibiotics are placed in different areas of the plate. Antibiotic diffuses outwards from each disk into surrounding agar. On incubation, the bacteria grow on areas of the plate except those around the antibiotic disks to which they are sensitive. The width of each growth-free "zone of inhibition" is a measure of the degree of the sensitivity of the drug.

   Information about the sensitivity patterns of strains (**antibiograms**) isolated from the patient is required as a guide to the **drug of choice for therapy** and may also be used as an epidemiological marker in tracking hospital cross-infection.

Antibiotic sensitivity Test

Subcultures of the test organisms are made in broth and incubated for 6-18 hours. Any density of inoculum may be used but in most cases the surfaces of cultures plates may be sown with broth containing approximately 100 million cells per ml. After drying the surface, the previously prepared disks of filter paper saturated with various concentrations of antibiotics are applied, the plates are incubated, and the zone of inhibition is measured. A zone of inhibition of growth around the disk may indicate that the antimicrobial agent is either bactericidal (S = bacteria are sensitive) or merely bacteriostatic (RR = bacteria are relatively resistant) or bacteria are resistant (R = resistant). If the test organism is not resistant to the antibiotic, zones of complete inhibition of the growing organism are found around the disks containing the effective antibiotic (Fig. 7.2).

Culture and sensitivity test report of diagnostic microbiological laboratory.

Culture-organism isolated. **Staphylococcus aureus.**

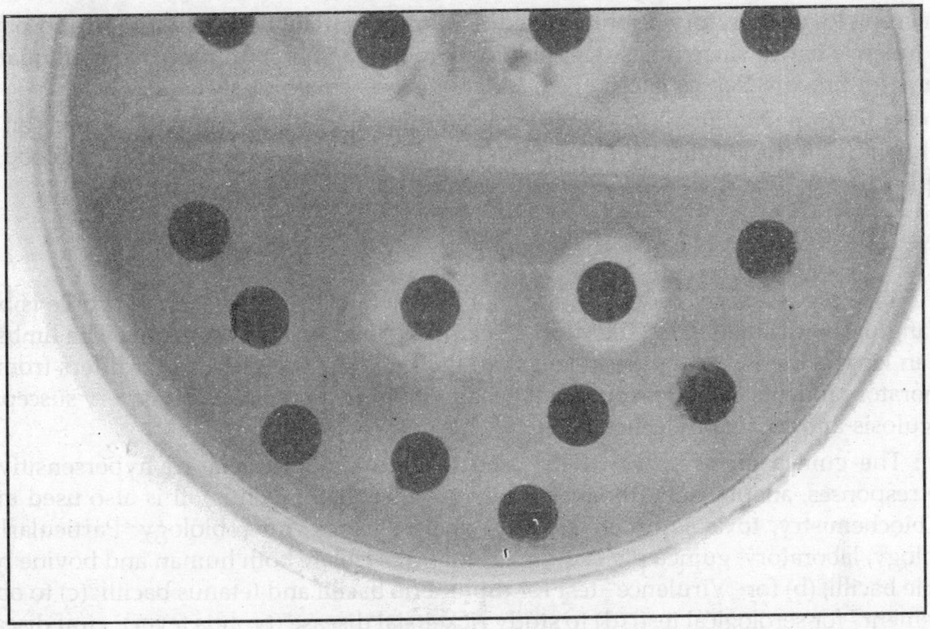

Fig. 7.2: Antibiotic sensitivity test

Sensitivity :

Penicillin	—	R
Tetracycline	—	S
Gentamycin	—	S
Streptomycin	—	RR

(R = resistant; S = sensitive; RR = relatively resistant)

Common Laboratory Animals

Animals are extensively employed in the laboratory for research purpose and for the diagnosis of the diseases.

Rabbit

The body of the rabbit is closely covered with smooth hair or fur, except at a few places (the tip of the nose, a small portion of scrotum and the inguinal spaces). The rabbit has large and erect pinnae (external ears) with readily visualised musculature. The small external opening of the mouth is bound by a clefted upper lip and an undivided lower lip. The external nostrils are ovoid in shape and are connected with the cleft in the upper lip. Prominent whiskers are present around the nose, over each eye and one or two on each cheek. The rabbit has large eyes (pink in albino rabbit) directed more laterally than those of most mammals. The hind legs are longer, muscular and powerful than forelimbs.

Use : Rabbit was used in Friedman test of pregnancy, but with the advent of more easy and refined techniques, its use for this purpose has become limited. Research areas where rabbit is experimental animal of choice include : hypertension, cardiac surgery, infectious diseases, metabolic disorders, ophthalmology. In recent times, rabbit is considered as excellent animal model for the study of gastrointestinal diseases. It is also used in serology because its large ear vein facilitates easy withdrawal of blood.

In microbiology laboratory, rabbit is used to (a) differentiate between human and bovine types of tubercle bacilli since it is susceptible only to bovine type; (b) prepare small quantity of antisera; (c) prepare Rabies vaccine; (d) isolate herpes, smallpox viruses.

Blood collection : Marginal ear vein is the preferred site of blood collection; blood can also be withdrawn from the jugular vein, the orbital sinus, for large quantity (20 ml) of blood, the cardiac puncture of anaesthetised rabbit is preferred.

Guinea Pig

The guinea pig is a short rodent, it does not have a tail. The head seen in profile is blunt and rectangular with small ears. The short thick neck emerges with the trunk. The limbs are unequal in length, the hind legs are longer than the forelegs. The guinea pig differs from the other laboratory rodents in many respects. It needs Vitamin C in the diet and is very susceptible to tuberculosis and to anaphylactic shock.

Use : The guinea pig is very widely used in immunology (delayed hypersensitivity), immune responses, anaphylactic shock and allergic encephalomyelitis). It is also used in the field of biochemistry, toxicology, physiology, pharmacology, microbiology. Particularly in microbiology, laboratory, guinea pig is quite useful (a) to isolate both human and bovine types of tubercle bacilli; (b) for "Virulence" test for diphtheria bacilli and tetanus bacilli; (c) to obtain "Complement" for serological test; (d) to study rickettsial disease (typhus fever), viral diseases.

Blood Collection : Small samples of blood (less than 0.25 ml) can be obtained by simple venesection of the marginal ear vein; large quantity by the cardiac puncture or from the metatarsal veins of anaesthetised guinea pig; repeated samples of small quantities from the orbital sinus.

Rat

The albino rat has a wide head, rough fur and long ears. The tail length is always less than the body length. It has long cylindrical body, long thin tail and very short legs. The head has a pointed snout with two silt-like nostrils, a narrow mouth with short lower jaw, and split upper lips, two small beady eyes, set so that they can look diagonally forwards and sideways, they have numerous long whiskers. It has a short neck. The trunk is slightly wider than the head.

Use : It is used mainly for research in toxicity, nutrition, cancer. In microbiology laboratory, it is used to differentiate **Yersinia pseudo-tuberculosis** from **Y. pestis** which is pathogenic only to rat. In clinical pathology, it is used for Frek (Pregnancy) test.

Blood Collection : Small blood samples can be obtained from a tail vein by snipping the tip of the tail, large quantity of blood can be collected by cardiac puncture or by orbital sinus from anaesthetised rat.

Mouse

The albino mouse is small; has a slender body with a smooth hair coat, long pointed snout, prominent round ears and long flat front teeth.

Use : It is extensively employed in the field of cancer research, toxicology, genetics, immunology, reproductive biology, diagnosis in the microbiology laboratory : (a) for the isolation of pneumococcus from sputum since the mouse is very susceptible to pneumococci; (b) for the isolation of causative organisms of relapsing fever, rat bite fever, trypanosomiasis; (c) for the isolation of viruses; (d) in clinical pathology for the Ascheim Zondek (Pregnancy) test.

(Blood samples can be collected from anaesthetised mice by cardiac puncture, tail vein puncture or tail clipping or by orbital sinus puncture).

8
Common Serological Reactions
(Serology)

Serology is the study of reaction between antigen and antibody and is grouped broadly as follows :

(1) Agglutination (in which particulate antigen is involved); and

(2) Precipitation (in which soluble antigen is involved).

1. Agglutination	2. Precipitation
(a) Widal test	(a) 1. VDRL test; 2. RPR test
(b) Weil-Felix test	(b) Kahn test
(c) Brucellosis test	(c) Wassermann test (complement fixation)
(d) Cold agglutination test	(d) Agar gel precipitation test (counter immunoelectro phoresis)
(e) Paul-Bunnel test	(e) Fluorescent antibody test
(f) Rose Waaler test or test for Rheumatoid arthritis	(f) Antinuclear factor test
(g) Latex agglutination test for Rheumatoid arthritis	(g) Antitoxin toxin neutralisation test (Skin tests)
(h) Coagglutination test	(h) Antistreptolysin-O titre
(i) Coombs' test	(i) Reverse Passive Haemagglutination (RPHA) test
(j) Blood group	(j) Enzyme Linked Immunosorbent Assay (ELISA) test
	(k) Western Blot test (ELISA and Western Blot are used respectively to screen and confirm AIDS)

Serological techniques are of considerable importance in identifying unknown antigens and detecting the presence of antibody in the serum of infected or immunised subjects.

Agglutination tests are performed by mixing a serial dilution of antiserum with a suspension of bacterial cells or particles. These methods are used to examine sera for antibodies against Salmonella and Brucella and, using standard antisera to identify the unknown organisms.

The basic principle of the techniques of agglutination tests in enteric fever (typhoid or paratyphoid) is to examine the serum quantitatively for agglutinin towards a particular organism. For this purpose, the method usually adopted is to mix varying dilutions of serum (made up in saline solution) in narrow tubes with a fixed quantity of a uniform and stable suspension of the organism or its antigen. These mixtures are kept at 37°C or 50-55°C in a water bath for a certain length of time and then examined for visible agglutination of the suspension. The agglutinated antigens tend to sediment and the reaction can also be evaluated by the amount of deposit in the tubes and clarity of the supernatant fluid. The strength can be started in terms of the highest dilutions (titres) that produce the agglutinations.

The measuring titre : The titre of an antiserum is the number of antibody units per unit volume of the original serum; thus, if the last tube, showing a reaction e.g. agglutination, contains 1 ml volume and is a dilution of 1 : 128 of the original serum, the titre of the serum is 128 units of antibody per ml of the serum.

At least 5 ml of blood should be obtained by vein puncture and the blood is immediately transferred from the syringe to a dry well stoppered sterile bottle or tube and allowed to clot; when the serum has separated, it is pipetted off.

(a) Widal test (Fig. 8.1)

In the routine laboratory diagnostic Widal reaction, the patient's serum is tested simultaneously with the antigen of each organism likely to be responsible for enteric fever in the particular region e.g. **Salmonella typhi** or **S. paratyphi** A or B or C. Additional information can be obtained by testing separately for H and O agglutinins. Thus, Widal test generally involves parallel tests with different Salmonella group or organisms and also different forms of the same organism.

In addition to the test with typhoid-paratyphoid organism, it is the practice of many laboratories to test also for Brucella melitensis agglutinins and, if considered necessary, with non-motile strains of proteus, OX19, OX2 and OXK for typhus fever, thus increasing the number of parallel tests. This is called "Triple Widal".

Master (1 : 15) dilution of the patient's serum is first prepared, thereafter a series of doubling dilutions are made in narrow tubes. Then, 0.4 ml of the bacterial antigen is added in each tube.

To observe H type (loose cotton wool) agglutination, it is usually sufficient to incubate at 37°C for 2 hours and leave for half an hour at room temperature, "Large flake" clumping or agglutination can easily be detected with naked eye. The flocculi can also sediment rapidly and the deposit is quite perceptible in the narrow tube (Dreyer's tube).

Compact agglutination of O type settles down in round bottom tubes (Felix tubes) kept in the first row of test tube rack and its readings should be made after 4 and 24 hours of incubation as these forms of reactions develop slowly. The control tube contains saline only. The clumps are small and granular, visible with the help of hand lens.

O agglutination is always positive as O antigen is common to all Salmonella. If O and H agglutinations are positive, then it is diagnosed as Typhoid—since the causative agent, **S. typhi**, contains both O and H antigens.

If AH agglutination is positive, then it is considered as paratyphoid—caused by **S. paratyphi A.**

Widal test report of diagnostic laboratory:

I. For Typhoid

		Titre	
I.	S. typhi	O - 1 : 60	
	S. typhi	H – 1 : 240	Typhoid (Positive)
	S. paratyphi A — Negative		
	S. paratyphi B — Negative		
	S. paratyphi C — Negative		

II. For Paratyphoid

I.	S. typhi	O - 1 : 60	
	S. typhi	H – Negative	
	S. paratyphi	A - 1 : 120	Paratyphoid by S. paratyphi A (positive)

S. paratyphi B — Negative
S. paratyphi C — Negative

(b) Weil-Felix Test:

It is an agglutination test which detects anti-rickettsial antibodies that cross-react with certain strains of proteus. The basis of this test is the sharing of an alkali-stable carbohydrate antigen of some rickettsial with O antigen of certain non-motile strains of proteus, P. vulgaris OX19 and OX2 and P. mirabilis OXK. False positive reaction may occur with typhoid fever, liver disease, proteus infection (UTI or other infection) etc.

Weil-Felix reaction in rickettsial diseases

Disease	Agglutination with		
	OX19	OX2	OXK
Epidemic typhus	+++	+	–
Endemic	+++	±	–
Scrub typhus	–	–	+++
Spotted typhus	++	++	–

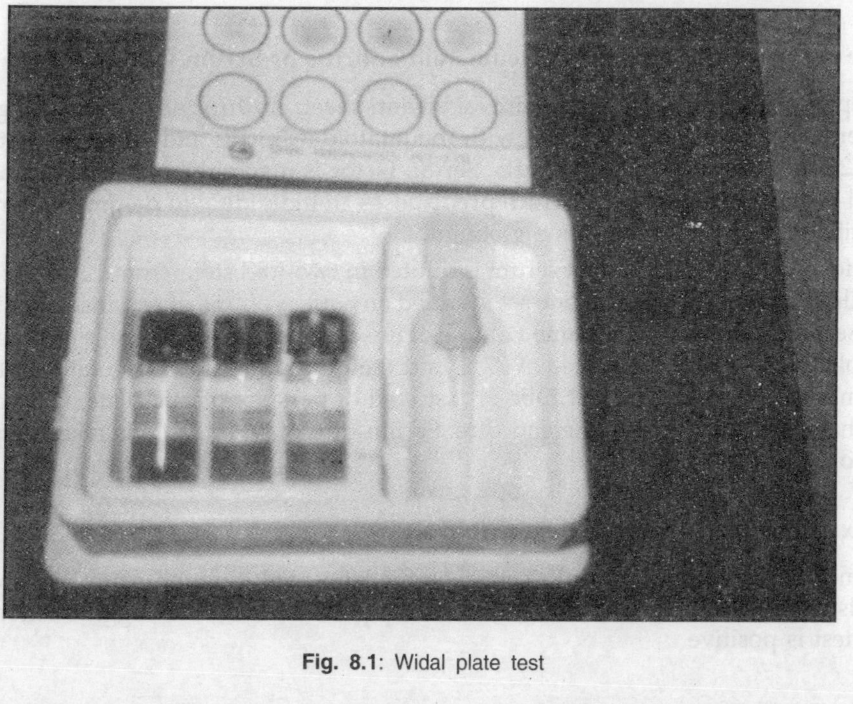

Fig. 8.1: Widal plate test

(c) Brucellosis test:

This is a tube agglutination test in which equal volumes of serial dilutions of the patient's serum and the standardised antigen (a killed suspension of a standard strain of Br. abortus) are mixed and incubated at 370°C for 24 hours or 50°C for 18 hours. A titre of 160 or more is considered significant. Most patients with acute Brucellosis develop titres of ≥ 640 by 3-4 weeks of illness.

The same agglutination technique of Widal test is also applicable to diagnose Brucellosis, Typhus fever in man. A titre of 1 : 40 or 80 International units (IU) per ml. is considered positive for Brucellosis and a titre of 200 or a peak titre of 1000-5000 is positive for Typhus fever.

(d) Cold agglutination test

In case of primary atypical pneumonia caused by **Mycoplasma hominis,** the serum may agglutinate at low temperature group O human red blood cells. To a series of doubling dilutions of patient's serum (1 : 8 to 1 : 2048) an equal volume of 0.2 per cent of suspension of washed group O human erythrocytes is added. The mixtures are kept in the refrigerator at 0°-4°C overnight. Agglutinations are observed with naked eye. A titre of 1 : 32 to 1 : 64 is considered significant.

(e) Paul-Bunnel Test

An agglutinin for sheep red blood cells is present in the serum and is of diagnostic significance during and after the attack of infectious mononucleosis.

Test : The patient's serum is heated at 55°C for 20 minutes and a series of doubling dilutions of this serum is made from 1 : 16 to 1 : 1024. The control tube contains saline only 0.5 ml of a 1 per cent suspension of saline washed sheep red blood cells is added to each tube containing diluted serum. The tube were thoroughly shaken and incubated at 37°C for four hours. Tube showing agglutination of red blood cells is the final dilution of the serum. A suggestive titre is 1 : 128; a significant titre is 1 : 256.

(f) Rose Waaler Test or Test for Rheumatoid arthritis or Serum Factor

Sheep red blood cells sensitised with rabbit anti-sheep erythrocytes serum are agglutinated by the sera of 70-80 per cent patients with rheumatoid arthiritis and positive reactions occur in some 2-5 per cent of normal subjects. Serum factor is macroglobulin which is an index of inherited metabolic disturbances which predisposes an individual to rheumatoid arthritis and is an antibody to denatured gamma globulin.

Previously inactivated patient serum is diluted in two-fold steps from 1 : 2 to 1 : 1024. Two sets of dilutions are required : to one set is added an equal volume of sensitised red blood cells and the second set receives the same volume of unsensitised red blood cells of sheep and acts as control. The tubes are incubated at 37°C and then placed in the refrigerator until the cells have completely settled. The last tube or last well of perspex plastic plate, if used, shows a definite haemagglutination as the end titre. Serum titre of 16 or more is taken as positive in rheumatoid arthritis.

(g) Latex agglutination test for rheumatoid arthritis

To one drop of diluted patient's serum on the latex agglutination plate, one drop of latex antigen is added and mixed thoroughly with the plastic stick. Latex agglutination indicates that the test is positive.

(h) Coagglutination test

Staphylococcus aureus (Cowan 1 strain) cell wall protein gets attached with Fc fragment of specific IgG molecule directed against a specific antigen and agglutinates bacteria that have that antigen. This test is of diagnostic value. This coagglutination reaction is highly specific but may not be as sensitive for detecting small quantities of antigen as latex agglutination test.

(i) Coombs' test (Anti-globulin test)

This test was devised by Coombs, Mourant and Race for detection of anti-Rh antibody. Coombs' test is of two types – direct and indirect. In direct Coombs' test, the sensitisation of RBC with incomplete antibodies takes place in vivo, as in haemolytic disease of the newborn due to Rh incompatibility, when washed RBC of infants is mixed with a drop of Coombs' serum, agglutination results. In the indirect Coombs' test, sensitisation of red cells with the antibody globulin is performed in vitro. Rh +ve RBCs are mixed with the serum to be tested for Rh-antibodies and then after washing, antiglobulin is added. If the test serum contains anti Rh-antibodies, agglutination will take place.

(j) Blood group (Fig. 8.2)

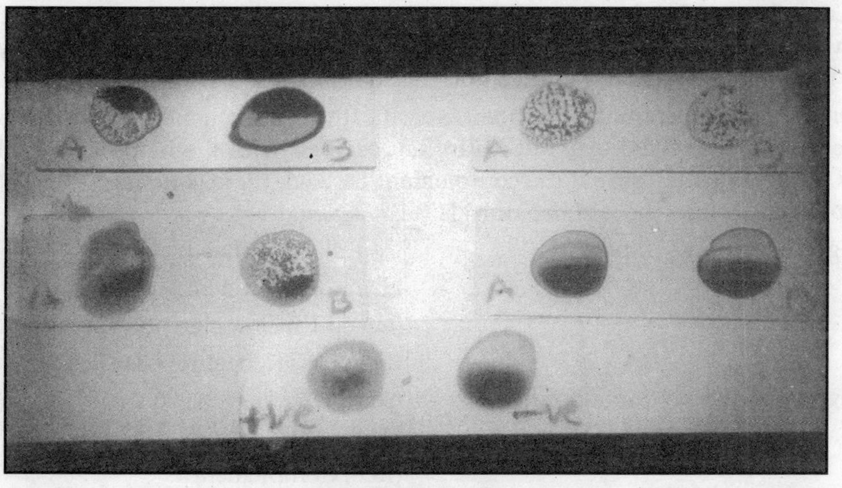

Fig. 8.2: Blood group

Precipitation

(a) 1. **Venereal Disease Research Laboratory** (VDRL) flocculation test is simple, rapid, sensitive screening test used to diagnose syphilis.

One drop (0.05 ml) of inactivated patient's serum is placed on a VDRL glass plate and one drop of diluted VDRL antigen (Cardiolipin, 0.03 per cent; Lecithin, 0.24 per cent and Cholesterol, 0.9 per cent) is added on the serum and the whole plate is rotated on VDRL rotator for 3 to 4 minutes, visible aggregation or precipitation indicates a positive reaction.

2. Rapid Plasma Reagin (RPR) card test or RPR 18 mm circle card test. Stabilised suspension of VDRL antigen and sized charcoal particles is used as RPR card antigen which reacts with patient's serum, not with CSF, to form flocculation—if positive—for syphilis. A finger prick blood is sufficient.

(b) **Kahn flocculation Test** to diagnose syphilis. The test for each serum is set up as follows :

Tube	**1**	**2**	**3**
Add diluted antigen	0.05 ml	0.025 ml	0.0125 ml
Add serum	0.15 ml	0.15 ml	0.15 ml

The tubes are shaken in a Kahn shaker machine for 3 minutes and incubated at 37°C for 20 minutes.

Then add saline	1.0 ml	0.5 ml	0.5 ml

Readings are now made after the appearance of precipitates.

The control is set up as follows :

Tube	**1**	**2**	**3**
Add diluted antigen	0.05 ml	0.025 ml	0.0125 ml
Add saline	0.15 ml	0.15 ml	0.15 ml

Shake tubes and incubate as above

Then add saline	1.0 ml	0.5 ml	0.5 ml

Reading : = large floccules at the bottom of the Kahn tube; = minute floccules just visible throughout the tube.

(c) **Complement fixation test (CFT)** is frequently employed with soluble antigen for the detection of antibody, even 0.08 µg of antibody nitrogen can be detected. It is very sensitive and specific. Both bacterial and viral infections can be diagnosed with this test.

When antigen and antibody reaction is specific, the complement is fixed. This reaction cannot be seen with the naked eye; but it can be observed with the help of haemolytic system (Sheep R.B.Cs + Haemolysin); if the complement is fixed, there is no haemolysis (Positive); if the complement is free, there is haemolysis (test is Negative).

Antigen + Antibody (Specific) + Complement (fixed)
\+ Haemolytic system
(sheep RBCs + Haemolysin)
Result = No haemolysis (Positive)

Antigen + Antibody (not specific) + Complement +
Haemolytic system
(free) Complement
Result = Haemolysis = Negative

When CFT is employed for the diagnosis of syphilis, it is called Wassermann test.

(d) **Agar gel precipitation technique :** In this test, the antigen and antibody diffuse in the gel and form a line of precipitation when they meet. When this basic principle is adopted in electrophoresis apparatus, it is known as Counterimmuno electrophoresis (CIEP).

(e) **Fluorescent antibody technique :** There are two main methods used in immunofluorescent work : the direct and indirect methods. The direct method consists of bringing fluorescein tagged antibodies in contact with antigens fixed on a slide, allowing them to react, washing off the excess of antibody and examining under the fluorescence microscopy. The site of union of the labelled antibody with the antigen can be determined by the apple green or orange yellow fluorescent area on the slide.

The indirect method is used to detect both specific antibody in sera and also, as a direct method, for identifying antigens. For the detection of antibody, a slide on which is a preparation of the antigen, is flooded with the specific serum, and after an interval, the excess serum is washed off. The localisation of the antibody on the antigen preparation is then visualised under fluorescent microscope by layering the slide with the fluorescein labelled antibody specific for the serum proteins of the serum under test. The most suitable type of labelled antibody is that directed primarily against the globulin fractions of the test serum i.e. fluorescein labelled antiglobulin serum.

(f) **Antinuclear factor test :** Sera that are able to induce the formation of Lupus Erythematosus (LE) cells contain the Antinuclear Antibody (ANF) which react with the nuclei of tissue cells. This factor present in the connective tissue diseases (Serum Lupus Erythematosus SLE) can be detected by the application of indirect fluorescent antibody technique.

(g) **Antitoxin-Toxin neutralisation test** is very useful to detect the toxigencity of certain strains of bacteria e.g. Clostridium tetani in mice. The control mouse, which has already been protected passively by Antitetanus Serum (ATS) against tetanus, will survive, as the toxin is neutralised by antitetanus serum; the mouse which receives the toxin of toxigenic strain of **Cl. tetani,** will show the symptoms and die of tetanus. The same principle is applicable in skin tests. Schick skin test is to diagnose diphtheria and Dick test to diagnose scarlet lever.

(h) **Anti-streptolysin-O (ASO)** titre is useful for the detection of clinically significant levels of Antistreptolysin-O antibodies found in the serum of persons following infection with a streptolysin-O producing strain of streptococci.

The ASO titre, expressed in Todd units, is the reciprocal of the serum dilution which completely neutralised the streptolysin-O. A serum with a titre of 166 Todd units should show no haemolysis.

(i) **Reverse passive hemagglutination (RPHA) test**

This test is an useful sensitive test to detect Hepatitis B surface antigen (HB_s Ag) in serum hepatitis patient. Besides, it is simple and specific.

A simple and convenient testing procedure to detect HB_S Ag :

25 µl diluent should be added into U or V cavity plates; then 7 µl test specimen (patient's serum) should be added into the same cavity and mixed; 25 µl of sensitised sheep erythrocytes should be added and mixed again. The test should be kept at room temperature for 2 hours. (Fig. 8.3)

Interpretation : Reactive screening test result. The cell setting pattern will appear as a large diffused pattern; non-reactive test result—a distinct compact bottom of cells (Fig. 8.3).

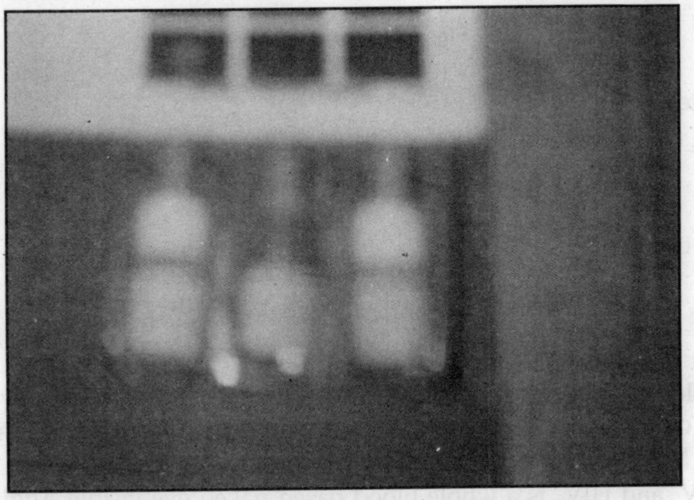

Fig. 8.3: Reverse Passive Haemagglutination (RPHA) test Kit

(j) **Enzyme Linked Immunosorbent Assay (ELISA) technique**

In the micro-ELISA for detection of antibody, the antigen is coated on to the surface of wells in microtitration plate. The patient serum is then added and time allowed for an antigen-antibody reaction to occur. An enzyme labelled specific antiglobulin is then added, which attaches to the antigen-antibody complexes. Any untreated antiglobulin is washed away. An enzyme substrate is then added which is acted upon by the attached **enzyme producing** colour which can be measured colourimetrically or interpreted visually. Incubation with enzyme substrate produces a yellow orange colour in the test well, if anti-HIV is present in the sample. Commonly used enzymes are Horse Radish Peri oxidase (HRP) or phosphatase. Penicillinase prepared in India is also useful and cheaper than other enzymes.

ELISA test is widely used to diagnose viral (AIDS, Hepatitis), bacterial and parasitic diseases (Fig. 8.4).

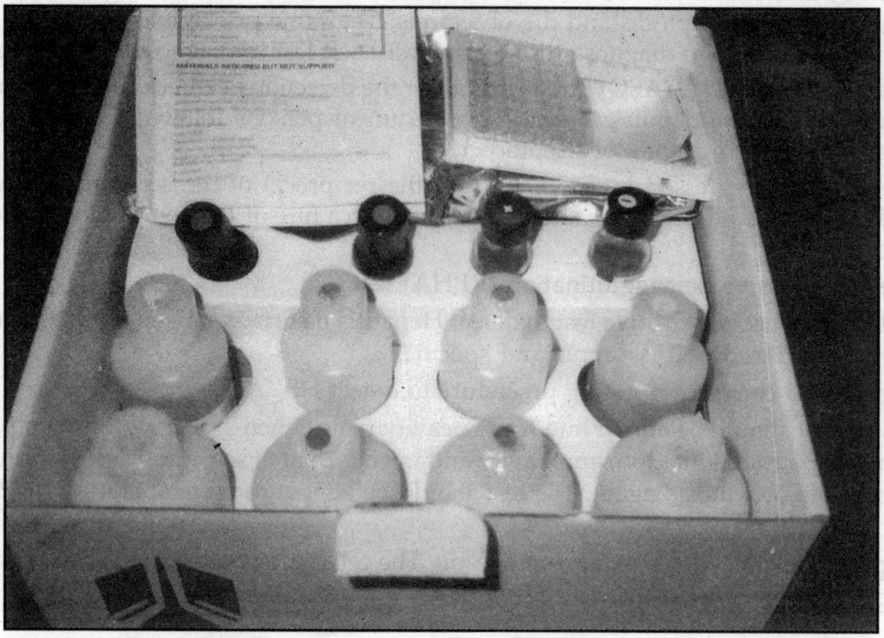

Fig. 8.4: Elisa Test Kit

Principle of the test

HIV Antigen → anti-HIV antibody (Positive sample)

+ Substrate

HIV Antigen → anti HIV labelled antibody

(k) **Western Blot** test is used to confirm HIV in patient sera screened positive for AIDS. This test is carried out only in AIDS Reference Laboratory (National Institute of Virology, Pune; All India Institute of Medical Sciences, New Delhi, India).

(l) **NEVA** HIV_1 and HIV_2 is a whole blood based naked eye visible Agglutination Assay (NEVA) for the detection of antibodies against HIV_1 and HIV_2 in a drop of blood.

SECTION II
IMMUNOLOGY

9
History—Antigen

The study of immune responses of the human body is known as **immunology.**

History

The inhabitants of East Africa have succeeded in vaccination against the bite of poisonous snakes from time immemorial, they could immunise artificially against tick borne relapsing fever and could protect their cattle from contagious pleuropneumonia by their old method of vaccination. In 2,000-3000 BC, children were vaccinated against small pox in South East Asia by the folk methods of direct contact of hands of the children. Only after 100 years of Jenner's work. Immunology was enriched with his own methods built on the scientific works of Louis Pasteur.

Antigen

Many substances (egg white, serum, milk, snake venom, dead and living bacteria, bacterial exotoxins and endotoxins, plant or animal tissue) containing proteins may act as antigen when introduced into the deeper tissues of the body. Protein taken in the gastrointestinal tract as food may not act as antigen under normal conditions because they are rapidly destroyed by the gastric juice. To act as antigen, a protein must gain entrance to the blood and other tissues in a chemically unaltered state. Entrance is commonly by **injection or infection** (i.e. by routes other than the gastrointestinal tract) or by **parenterally.**

An antigen (Gr. *anti*—against, *genos*—genus) is a foreign protein (organic substances of colloidal structure) which, when introduced parenterally (Gr. *para*—beyond or outside of; *enteron*—intestine), by route other than the gastrointestinal tract into the human body, will provoke the lymphoid tissue of the human to produce antibodies which will react specifically with the same antigen and not with other substances.

Antigens have the following main properties :

(a) **Antigenicity** (the ability to cause the production of antibodies); (b) antigenic **specificity** (the ability to enter into an interaction with the corresponding antibodies).

The small portion of a molecule may be called as unit of antigen. This unit is known as antigenic determinant. This determinant is a contour which locks one molecule of antibody. As antigenic determinants have three dimensional structures, the antibody molecule can approach or can get attached to any of the wide range of possible configurations in a single determinant (Fig. 9.1).

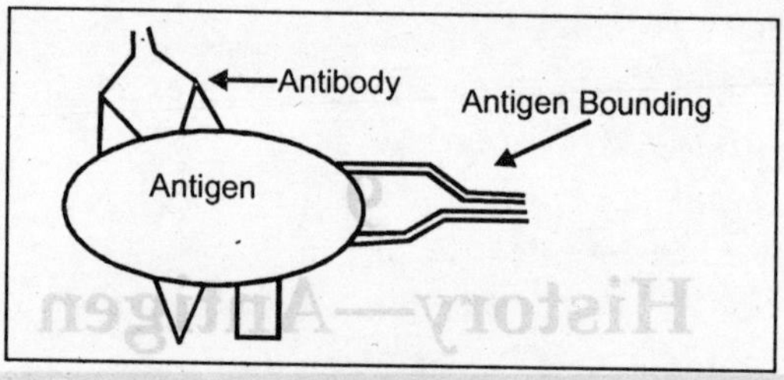

Fig. 9.1: Antigenic determinant site

The specificity of the antigen is dependent upon antigenic determinant (epitope) i.e. chemical groupings of the antigen molecules. When the antigen comes in contact, the animal reacts. This is known as "acquired immune response." The acquired immune response may be of two forms : (a) the humoral or circulating antibody response; (b) cell mediated response. An antibody directed against an antigenic determinant of a particular antigen molecule will react only with this determinant or another very similar structure. Even minor chemical changes in the determinant will reduce the ability of the original antibody to react with the altered determinant. Antigens which are capable of stimulating immune response are known as **immunogens.**

Antigens may be **complete** or **partial.**

Complete antigens are substances which cause the production of antibodies and react with them in **vivo** and in **vitro** (e.g. foreign proteins, bacteria, toxins, rickettsiae, viruses).

Partial antigens are known as **haptens.** They do not produce antibodies but react with the antibodies produced by another substance. They are lipids, complex carbohydrates and other substances of low molecular weight. The addition of protein to haptens in small quantity will convert the hapten into a complete antigen. In this case, the protein carries out the function of a conductor.

The antigenic function of bacteria, rickettsiae and viruses is characterised by species and type specificity. **Salmonella typhi** antigen induce immunity against typhoid and it will not produce immunity against paratyphoid fever. So this antigen is species and type specific. The type specificity is associated with the presence of special polysaccharide complexes in the bacterial cell.

In the laboratory, there is cross-reaction between antisera to certain bacterial antigens and antigens present in cells such as erythrocytes. These antigens are known as **heterophile antigens.** Antisera to such antigens will cross-react with cells of different species of animals and various microorganisms. Chemical groupings of **heterophile** antigens are not yet known. The best known of the heterophile antigens is the **Forssman** antigen which is present in the red cells of many species as well as in the bacteria such as pneumococci and salmonella. Another heterophile antigen is found in **Escherichia** and human red cells of Group B.

Semihaptens (iodine, bromine, quinine, antipyrin, colloidal iron, azoprotein) are not antigenic themselves, but, in combination with the protein of the body, they acquire the properties of complete antigen.

All natural proteins are inherited with the properties of chemical, structural and functional specificity. Proteins of different species of animals, plants, bacteria, rickettsiae and viruses can be differentiated by immunological reactions.

Chemical Nature of Antigens. Antigens may be proteins, polysaccharides or lipids. Antigens of cell wall of bacteria (streptococci, staphylococci, corynebacteria) are rather less well defined and appear to be complex mucopeptides, sometimes associated with lipids. Capsulated microorganisms (pneumococci) have complex high molecular weight polysaccharides in their capsules.

General Properties of Antigens

1. Antigen should be foreign, egg albumin is an excellent antigen in the rabbit, but fails to produce an antibody response in fowl;
2. More foreign—the more powerful antigen;
3. It should have a molecular weight of 5,000. Sometimes, some substances of low molecular weight (aspirin, penicillin, sulphonamides) can act as antigen when applied to the skin;
4. The ability of antibody to form a strong bond with an antigen depends on **intermolecular forces** which act strongly only when two molecules come in contact in a very precise manner. The better the fit the stronger the bond.

Isoantigens. Isoantigens are those substances which have antigenic properties and are contained in some individuals of a given species. They are found in erythrocytes of animals and man. At first it was established that there are two antigens (A and B) in the human erythrocytes and in the sera, there are two antibodies (anti-A and anti-B). Only heterogenic antigens and antibodies (agglutinins) are found in human blood. These combinations may be represented as:

Antigens of erythrocytes (Blood Groups)	Serum antibodies
0	Anti-A Anti-B
A	Anti-B
B	Anti-A
AB	0

On the basis of antigenic structure, the erythrocytes of all people can be divided mainly into four groups. Consequently, variants of antigens of erythrocytes in the second (A) and fourth (AB) groups were isolated. The Group-A consists of two sub-groups A_1 and A_2.

The AB groups containing A_1 B and A_2 B and the antigens M and N and M_2 and N_2 etc. have been revealed. At present 30 antigens are known. Besides, there is rhesus factor in the erythrocytes. All these groups are taken into account during blood transfusion.

Autoantigens are those substances (eye lens, spermatozoa, skin, kidney, lung) which do not, under normal condition, come in contact with the immune system of the body—then the antibodies are not produced against such cells and tissues. However, if these tissues are damaged, then the autoantigens may be released and may cause the production of antibodies which react with the corresponding autoantigens of the cells resulting in the development of glomerulonephritis, interstitial thyroiditis, orchitis, corneal opacity. The cooling, radiation, drugs (amidopyrine, sulphonamides), virus infection (virus pneumonia, infectious mononucleosis, bacterial proteins, toxins of streptococci, staphylococci, tubercle bacilli and other factors may release autoantigens from the tissues.

10
Antibodies (Immunoglobulins)

History : von Behring and Kitasato in Berlin in 19th century recognised antibodies in the blood stream of an immunised animal against tetanus and diphtheria. They observed clumping or agglutination of microorganisms and precipitation of soluble antigens by the serum of the immunised animal. They also practised the serotherapy method.

Serotherapy is the injection of antiserum, for the therapeutic use, from an immunised animal to non-immune patient. They also carried out the fragmentation of immunoglobulins by pepsin digestion.

Antibodies are synthesised under the influence of antigens which penetrate into the body and disturb the normal blood composition. Antibodies are specific substances in the bodies of the vertebrates secreted in the tissue fluids from the lymphoid cells that have been stimulated by foreign substances (antigens with which they react **specifically**).

Antibodies appear in the blood due to the infection or immunisation by live (attenuated) or dead bacteria, rickettsiae, viruses, toxins or toxoids etc. Antibodies which occur under the influence of active immunisation are named **Immune antibodies** in contrast to normal antibodies which are found in the sera of men and animals which had not been infected or exposed to immunisation. Normal and immune antibodies can render harmless the causal agents of infectious diseases.

The nature of antibodies

1. Antibodies are globulins which have been altered under the influence of antigens;
2. Molecules of antibodies, like normal serum globulins, are probably asymmetrical;
3. Antibodies are found in globulin fractions;
4. The transformation of normal globulin into immune globulins is due to alteration in the spatial configuration of active atomic groups of the protein molecules. A change in protein metabolism is responsible for this process. The mechanism of antibody production is not yet clear, though many theories are put forth;
5. Antibodies do not differ greatly from normal globulins;
6. They have almost similar isoelectric points, viscocity, molecular weight (from 100,000 to 1,000,000) and are sensitive to the temperature and to other denaturating agents.
7. Antibodies are thermolabile and denatured on heating at 70°C for one hour;
8. The pH of the medium and other factors affecting proteins can also affect the activity of antibodies;
9. Antibodies are not denatured by precipitation with ethyl alcohol at low temperature (from 0 to + 4°C) but are denatured by alcohol at high temperature. Natural salts (magnesium sulphate, ammonium sulphate and sodium sulphate) can cause the precipitation of proteins,

but do not denature antibodies. Ethyl alcohol at low temperature and natural salts can be used for fractionation of immune sera to obtain them in a pure state.

There are five types of human immunoglobulins : IgG; Ig M; Ig A; Ig D, and Ig E—on the basis of polypeptide chain structure consisting of heavy chains and light chains joined by disulphide bond.

Immunoglobulin G or IgG. Seventyfive per cent of total serum constitutes IgG. It is the major immunoglobulin component of serum and has a molecular weight of 150,000 in man. The molecule has two antibody combining sites (Fig. 10.1) which are called Fab (antibody binding) portions of the molecule. Fab fragment has both light and heavy chains. Light chains are of two types. They are known as K or L (k or l) chains. The heavy chain or γ chain exists in four forms : Ig G_1; Ig G_2; Ig G_3 and Ig G_4. The molecule has also Fc fragment for complement fixation.

Ig M, Ig A, Ig D, and Ig E

Like Ig G globulin, each of these classes of immunoglobulins in man contain k and l light chains. The heavy chains are unique for each of the types of immunoglobulins. Ig M contains μ chain, Ig A alpha chain, Ig D δ-chain and Ig E ε-chain.

Table 10.1: Human Immunoglobulins

Ig Class	Serum concentration mg/100 ml	Molecular weight	Light chain	Heavy chain	Properties
Ig G	900-1800	160,000	k & L	Y	Late antibody precipitation, complement fixation antibody
Ig M	67-145	960,000	k & L	μ	Early – Agglutination
Ig A	156-294	170,000	k & L	α	Surface protection
Ig D	0.3-40	184,000	K & L	δ	Not known
Ig E	10-130	188,000	k & L	ε	Reaginic antibody (hypersensitivity Intradermal)

Structure and Function of Immunoglobulins

In the fab portion, the heavy chain component (Fd portion) contains as much as 85 per cent of the antigen-binding ability. The light chain seems to act together with the heavy chain to form a stable antibody-combining site (Fig. 10.1). The Fc portion of the IgG molecule is responsible for activation of complement system. On combination with antigen, the IgG molecule springs open at the hinge region exposing the Fc portion which can activate the complement. If Ig G molecule has not combined with antigen, it will be unfolded. A single IgM molecule can get attached to a red cell by multiple combining sites and can bring about lysis; but for the same effect, 1000 IgG molecules are required.

Agglutination is due to linkage of a particulate antigen (red blood cell or bacterial) by two Fab fragments of IgM. The IgM is of large size, so it is confined in the blood stream and plays an important role in the protection against blood invasion by

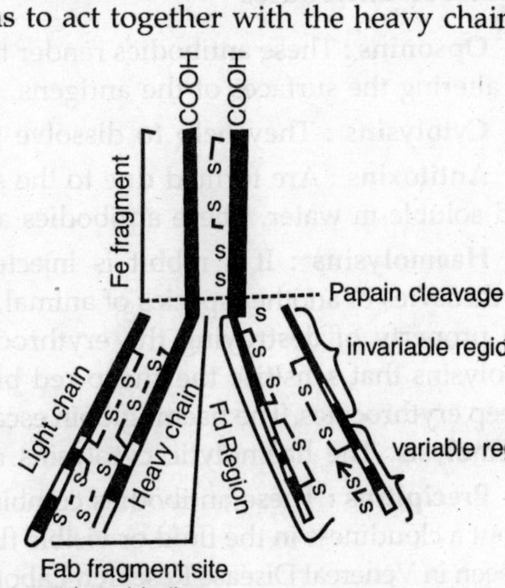

Fig. 10.1: Structure of Immunoglobulin

microorganisms. IgM deficiency may result into septicaemia. Diphtheria toxin, lysozyme or virus (polio virus) can be neutralised by IgG antibodies and IgG antibodies can neutralise more effectively than IgM antibodies. Fc fragment of IgG molecule may assist the Fab fragments in neutralisation of virus infectivity and also helps in the selective transport of IgG. The characteristic feature of IgE class immunoglobulin is responsible for the hypersensitivity reaction in man which is due to the activity of Fc portion of IgG molecule. IgM antibody specific for particulate antigen (bacteria) makes the antigen more susceptible to the phagocytosis by coating the surface of particulate antigen, so it is called as opsonising antibody (Opsonin).

Selective Transport of IgG

In pregnant women, IgG globulins can pass through the placenta and reach the foetal circulation; this process is not due to the mere filtration but due to the selective transfer of IgG molecules which is brought about by a part of Fc fragment of IgG heavy chains. This property is a characteristic feature only of the γ chain of IgG and is not found in the μ chain of I gM and α chain of IgA. This mechanism of selective transport is mainly observed in primates. Similarly, immunoglobulins are absorbed from the colostrum through the intestinal epithelium of the ruminants.

IgA globulins are selectively secreted into saliva, respiratory, intestinal mucous secretions and into the colostrum. This is another mechanism of selective transport. There are two types of IgA : Serum IgA and dimer secretory IgA.

Dimer form of IgA is manufactured locally and has an attached secretory transport piece which is not found in serum IgA. This transport piece is added to the IgA molecule during its passage into the mucous secretions from the lamina propria of the intestinal and respiratory tract. This secretory IgA would protect from the infection. The dimer form of IgA acquires the ability to fix the complement after attaching to Gram-negative organisms.

The monomeric form of IgA can also pass from the lamina propria to the blood stream via lymphatics so that the infection of the intestine may lead to increased serum IgA levels. Local application of vaccine may stimulate dimer IgA.

Kinds of antibodies

Opsonins : These antibodies render the microorganisms more susceptible to phagocytosis by altering the surfaces of the antigens.

Cytolysins : They help to dissolve the cells that stimulated their production.

Antitoxins : Are formed due to the stimulation of exotoxins which are protein in nature and soluble in water. These antibodies are inactivated or neutralised by the exotoxins.

Haemolysins : If a rabbit is injected several times with minute quantity of washed erythrocytes of another species of animal, e.g. sheep, the serum of the recipient rabbit acquires the property of destroying the erythrocytes of the sheep. This is due to the formation of cytolysins that sensitise the sheep red blood cells to complement and cause the lysis of the sheep erythrocytes. The haemoglobin escapes into the surrounding fluid. This process is called haemolysis. The haemolytic cytolysins are called **haemolysins.**

Precipitins : These antibodies combine with the molecules of soluble proteins and bring about a cloudiness in the fluid or visible flakes. This flocculent turbidity is known as precipitate as seen in Venereal Disease Research Laboratory (VDRL) test; they may form line of precipitation when they react with soluble antigens.

Agglutinins : They bring about the clumping of particulate antigens (bacteria, red blood cells)—hence agglutination (Fig. 8%). Many diagnostic tests are based on bacterial agglutinins. For example, Widal test is used to diagnose typhoid fever.

Haemagglutinins are responsible for the agglutination of red blood cells or haemagglutination; cold haemagglutins; viral haemagglutinins; and isohaemagglutinins:

(a) **Cold haemagglutinins** are substances that appear in the blood of person with certain respiratory diseases e.g. atypical pneumonia of unknown or viral origin and trypanosomiasis. The sera of the patient in dilution of 1 : 10,000 agglutinate their own erythrocytes (auto-agglutination) when cooled to 2°C, but not at 37°C. This agglutination at low temperature is known as cold haemagglutination.

(b) **Viral haemagglutinins :** Agglutination of red cells is brought about by several respiratory virus (influenza virus), **not by antibody.** The virus itself attaches to the red cells of the chick at 5°C and agglutinate them. It can be separated (eluted) from them by mixing with saline solution followed by an incubation at 37°C. The viral haemagglutination tests are useful in the study of viruses and the diagnosis of viral diseases. In some infections, antibodies may prevent the viral agglutination of erythrocytes. They are called as haemagglutination-inhibition (HI) antibodies.

Isohaemagglutinins. These antibodies are formed in response to one or more antigens (A, B, Rh, M) found in human erythrocytes. They do not agglutinate one's own red blood cells, but cause agglutination, at body temperature (37°C), of red blood cells of another person. They play an important role in blood transfusion. If the serum of the recipient agglutinates the red blood cells of a donor, or vice versa, then there is possibility of reaction or death of the recipient. It is not necessarily that the sera of all donors should agglutinate the erythrocytes of all the recipients, and vice versa, because there are numerous classes or groups of blood with respect to isohaemagglutinins, called **blood** groups.

Blood groups : One major system of blood groupings consist of A, B, AB and O groups. It detects the presence or absence of the agglutinogens (antigens) in the erythrocytes of the persons to be identified and grouped. For example, any one person may have antigen A (Group A) or B (Group B) or both (Group AB) or neither (Group O). A person's own serum never contains agglutinins against his own erythrocytes, but only against the absent agglutinogens (Fig. 8.2).

A person's blood group is a physiological constant determined by the basic Mendelian laws of inheritance. It is possible to avoid the haemagglutination, by properly selecting donors and recipients of compatible group. Blood banks collect citrated blood donations already grouped and store in the refrigerator until needed.

Blood grouping : A nurse should have the knowledge of grouping the blood. A drop of the patient's (recipient) blood should be added to a small amount of physiological saline (0.9 per cent sodium chloride) on a microscopic slide and then mixed with rabbit sera containing pure anti-A and anti-B antibodies. A readily visible agglutination will appear (Fig. 8.2) of the patient (recipient).

If the cells of the patient (recipient) are agglutinated by both anti-A and anti-B rabbit sera, then the cells of the patients are of group-AB.

If the cells are agglutinated by neither sera, they are of Group O. If anti-A serum agglutinates them and anti-B serum does not, then the blood cells are of Group A; if anti-B serum agglutinates them and anti-A serum does not, the cells are of Group B.

Certain irregularities in reaction can be eliminated and the blood groupings can be ascertained by testing the serum of the recipient against the red cells of the donor.

Table 10.2: Isohaemagglutination. International system of Blood Group

Sera from person of Group	Agglutinate the erythrocytes of patients of Group			
	AB	B	A	O
AB	–	–	–	–
B (anti-A)	+	–	+	–
A (anti-B)	+	+	–	–
O (anti-A and anti-B)	+	+	+	–

+ = agglutination; – e.g. no agglutination

Haemagglutination in blood grouping. Anti-B serum and anti-A serum have been mixed on a glass slide with erythrocytes of group O, A, B and AB. Anti-B serum agglutinates erythrocytes of persons of Groups B and AB; anti-A serum agglutinates erythrocytes of persons of Groups A and AB.

Universal donor : A person of Group O is sometimes called universal donor because his red blood cells are not usually agglutinated by serum of recipients of any other group; but he must receive only Group O blood because his serum agglutinates cells of all other groups in the A-B-O system.

Direct cross-matching between recipient and donor is necessary to have a "safe universal donor." There are several other antigen antibody systems in human bloods—e.g. Rh factor, M-N-s, p types which may cause serious transfusion reactions irrespective of A, B, O or AB groups.

Rh factor : When erythrocytes of Rhesus (Rh) monkeys are injected into rabbits, the serum of the rabbits contained anti-Rh agglutinins which agglutinate erythrocytes of 85 per cent or more human beings. The antigen in the human red cells which reacted with anti-Rh rabbit serum was designated as the Rh agglutinogen. The person having the Rh agglutinogen is called Rh positive (+). If the Rh agglutination is absent in red blood cells of the remaining 15 per cent whose red blood cells do not react with the anti-Rh rabbit serum, they are called Rh-negative. The Rh agglutinogen is complex and corresponds to several antibodies or blood factors—Hr, hr′, rh′, hr′, rh′. The most important is Rh factor.

Rh factor and transmission. If an Rh negative person receives a blood transfusion from a person who is Rh positive, the recipient develops in about two weeks antibodies that agglutinate the red cells of all Rh positive persons. Now, if a subsequent transfusion is given from an Rh positive donor and the Rh antibody titre (concentration) will rise to maximum, thereby all the red cells of the donor are agglutinated and, ultimately, haemolysis leading to severe transfusion reaction and death. Therefore, it is essential, before each blood transfusion, to evaluate the Rh factor and blood group.

Erythroblastosis foetalis (Haemolytic disease of the newborn). If Rh negative woman becomes pregnant by an Rh positive man, the child will most probably, inherit Rh antigen in its blood cells. During pregnancy, if the child is Rh-positive (i.e. Rh factor), foetal red blood cells with Rh antigen often cross the foetal barrier, pass into the mother's blood circulation and the foetal Rh factor stimulates the maternal tissue to produce Rh antibodies. These Rh antibodies diffuse back into the foetal blood circulation. In any initial pregnancy, since the mother's Rh antibody titre is too low, there will be no detrimental effects in the foetus; when Rh antibody concentration increases with subsequent pregnancies, the red cells of the foetus are destroyed by Rh antibodies. Hence, the child with Rh factor (i.e. Rh positive) and Rh antibodies may be born dead (uncommon) or with haemolytic disease of the newborn (erythroblastosis foetalis) which is common. This type of condition may prevail if Rh negative mother has received a blood transfusion from Rh positive donor.

The periodic check up of the maternal blood for rising titre of Rh agglutinins is of great importance as a precautionary measure.

11
Antigen Antibody Reaction

The interaction of the antigen and antibody is a chemical reaction and is specific. The molecules of the antigen and antibody bind with their terminal groups (Fig. 9) and form firm complexes. When molecules of antibody and antigen are brought together in solution, they interact with each other by the formation of a link between an **antigen** binding (a, b) site on the immunoglobulin molecule (part of the Fab fragment) and the particular chemical groupings which make up the **antigenic determinant** of the antigen molecule. The molecules are held together by intermolecular forces which are effective only when the antibody combining site and the antigenic determinant group are able to make close contact.

The study of the reaction between the antigen and antibody is known as "serology."

Serology is classified into :

(1) Precipitation; (2) Agglutination,
(3) Complement fixation; (4) Neutralisation;
(5) Immobilisation; (6) Intradermal reaction.

1. **Precipitation**—the reaction takes place between the antibody and antigen molecules which are **soluble** in nature; it is specific, sensitive and can detect even diluted antigen (1 : 1,000,000 – 1 : 10,000,000). VDRL, Kahn test for syphilis; gel diffusion test; counter immuno-electrophoresis.
2. **Agglutination**—there is reaction between antibody and **particulate** antigen (erythrocyte, bacteria) in the presence of electrolyte (0.85 per cent sodium chloride solution) in definite proportions—(Coombs' test; blood groupings; Widal test; Weil-Felix test, tube agglutination test for Brucellosis).

   Coombs' test : The Coombs' test (antiglobulin test) is used, in particular, to detect incomplete agglutinins in rhesus negative mothers. To determine the fixation of agglutinins by the patient's erythrocytes, antiglobulin serum is added which, in saline solution, is capable of causing marked agglutination of erythrocytes sensitised by incomplete agglutinins. A molecule of antiglobulin binds two molecules of incomplete agglutinins fixed to two different erythrocytes, due to which the agglutination reaction takes place.
3. **Complement fixation reaction,** in which the antibody molecule, after reaction with antigen, activate the serum complement which gets fixed with the antibody antigen complex – Wassermann test for syphilis.
4. **Neutralisation** test is used in virus identification;

   Antitoxin – toxin neutralisation test (in tetanus).
5. **Immobilisation** test for motile bacteria.
6. **Intradermal test** for the reaginic antibody characteristic of skin hypersensitivity.

12
Immunity

The term **immunity** (Lat. *immunis*—freed from homage, save from something) means resistance of the body to the pathogenic microbes, their toxins or to other kinds of foreign substances. In other words, it can be defined as the body's resistance power to infections.

Immunity (1) Natural (innate),
(2) Acquired.

(1) **Natural immunity (non-specific resistance)** is present from birth. The innate resistance mechanisms are non-specific in the sense that they are effective against a wide range of infective agents. The innate immunity is genetically controlled.

Determinants of natural immunity

(a) **Species and Strains**
Different species of animals are susceptible to different diseases. e.g. the guinea pig and man are not susceptible to diphtheria, whereas the rat is susceptible to diphtheria. Only man is susceptible to Syphilis, Gonorrhoea, Typhoid, Rabies and Brucellosis affect both man and animals. American Indian and the Negro are genetically more susceptible to tuberculosis than Caucasians.

(b) **Individual difference and influence of age.** Sickle cell anaemia (sickling) disease is genetically controlled. Sickle cell anaemia patients are resistant to malaria, as **Plasmodium falciparum** cannot parasitise red blood cells of sickle cell anaemia. Because of the immaturity of the immunological mechanisms affecting the lymphoid system, children and young animals are highly susceptible to infections, older persons have diminished resistance as a result of the probable waning of the activity of immune responses.

(c) **Hormonal influences, Sex**
Patients of diabetes mellitus, hypothyroidism, adrenal dysfunction have decreased resistance to infection. The reasons are not yet well propounded. Sexes will not show the marked differences.

(d) **Nutritional factors.** Inadequate diet may be associated with the increased susceptibility to various **bacterial diseases.** It has been experimentally proved that when a large number of animal species were undernourished, they become less susceptible than normal animals to a variety of viruses including vaccinia virus and certain neurotrophic viruses e.g. polio virus. The same condition may be observed in case of malaria. When the nutrition level is lowered, there may be deficiency of para-amino benzoic acid essential for the multiplication of malarial parasites.

Mechanism of natural immunity

(a) Mechanical barriers and surface secretion,

(b) Bactericidal substances of the tissues and body fluids :

(i) Lysozyme, (ii) Basic polypeptides.

(c) Phagocytosis and inflammation :

(i) Phagocytin,

(d) Temperature,

(e) Complement system

(a) **Mechanical barriers and surface secretions**

1. The intact skin and mucous membrane of the body give protection against non-pathogenic organisms and a high degree of protection against pathogens. Because of the horny layer of the skin consisting mainly of keratin, which is not digestible by most organisms and protects the living cells of the epidermis from the organisms and toxins, the skin is a most resistant barrier.
2. **Sebaceous secretions and sweat of skin** contain bactericidal and fungicidal fatty acids and have a protective mechanism. The microorganisms are trapped by the sticky, mucous secretion covering the mucous membrane of the respiratory tract. They are swept down by the cilia or hair-like processes of the mucosa alongwith the mucous secretion towards the oropharynx and are swallowed. In stomach, most of the microorganisms are destroyed by the acid secretion.

   Nasal secretion and saliva containing mucopolypeptide inactivate some viruses. The tear and mucous secretions of respiratory, alimentary and genitourinary tract contain lysozyme which is active against some Gram-positive bacteria.

(b) **Bactericidal substances and body fluids**

(i) **Lysozyme** is a basic protein present in leucocytes and body fluids except cerebrospinal fluid, sweat and urine. It splits the sugars of the cell wall of Gram-positive bacteria and causes lysis of bacteria. Egg white and human tear are rich source of lysozyme.

(ii) **Basic Polypeptide** is basic protein derived from the damaged tissue and blood cells. It has a bactericidal activity.

(c) **Phagocytosis and inflammation** : When the microorganisms invade into the blood stream or tissue fluids, they are engulfed rapidly by various circulating and tissue fixed phagocytic cells. These cells are of two types :

(a) Polymorphonuclear leucocytes or microphages of the blood;

(b) Mononuclear leucocytes or macrophages, distributed throughout the body. The cells fixed in the tissues are the cells of the reticuloendothelial layer lining liver sinuses (kupffer cells), red bone marrow, spleen and lymph node. Macrophages in the blood are known as monocytes, those in the connective tissue are known as histiocytes, those in spleen, lymph and thymus are known as the sinus lining macrophages (called littoral cells).

Inflammation is a defensive response of living body tissues to any irritating or injurious agent. The inflammatory reaction is a complex process involving several physiological process which 1. **removes** the cause of the irritation, and 2. repairs the damage i.e. to heal the wound or lesion.

The inflammation may be due to :

(a) Mechanical factors (trauma, cut),

(b) Chemical agents (acids, excessive application of mustard, gases, bee stings).

(c) Physical agents (excessive heat, cold, ultraviolet rays).

(d) Living agents (microorganisms, worms).

Four cardinal signs of inflammation are :

1. **rubor** (redness, hyperaemia);
2. **tumor** (swelling);
3. **calor** (heat); and
4. **dolor** (pain). They can be observed in a boil or in an inflamed area. The increased amount of blood in the dilated local blood vessels may cause the redness; the comparison and injury of the sensory nerve branches in the tissue may result into pain. The dilatation and increased permeability of the blood vessels resulting in the collection of fluid under slight pressure in the spaces between the tissue cells is responsible for swelling (often called **oedema**—inflammatory exudation of fluid).

Hyperaemia is due to increased amount of blood in an inflamed area. **Thrombi** or clots are formed in the tiny vessels all around the point of injury due to the slowing down of blood flow in that particular area and prevent the entry of microorganisms into the general circulation.

Pus formation. When the blood flow slows down or stops, the leucocytes begin to migrate in-between the cells of the vessel walls by amoeboid motion called **diapedesis.** The leucocytes become **pus cells.** In intense inflammation as in gonorrhoea, much pus is formed and discharged, but a mild inflammation may heal without pus formation.

Temperature changes. The inflamed area is usually hot compared to the temperature of the body surface which may be due to the warmth of the deep body blood brought rapidly to the body surface or warmth due to the chemical changes in the infected area.

Defensive fibrin. The inflammatory area is filled and surrounded by a continuous network of fibrin fibres. At the periphery of the infected area, connective tissue cells (fibroblasts) begin to grow among these fibres. The acute inflammatory area is therefore soon surrounded by a wall of fibrin that tends to continue the inflammatory process and prevent the spread.

A closed sac formed by pyogenic membrane is filled with pus, microorganisms and walled off forming abscess, pimple, boil, carbuncle. Several intercommunicable abscesses are called carbuncle.

Enzymes produced by various microorganisms digest the wall of the abscess nearest to the exterior finally making an opening through which the abscess drains. By this process, the boil heals.

Types of inflammation

(a) **Acute inflammation** is of short duration (for few days).

(b) **Chronic inflammation** is of long duration (weeks, months, years).

(c) **Catarrhal inflammation** is of mild type seen in the throat, nose in cold or influenza.

(d) In **serous inflammation,** the serum-like fluid is more and the fibrin is less. If pus formed is more, the process is described as **purulent** or **suppurative.** A fluid may be **sanguinopurulent** or **fibrinopurulent.**

Healing and scar formation. As soon as the infection or injury is brought under control by fibrin formation and other body defensive mechanisms, tissue cells (fibroblasts) and blood vessels start to grow into the area of healing from periphery and form new healthy tissues. This early healing process is known as **Organisation.** The tissue thus formed is a solid and tough connective tissue. This tissue constitutes **scar tissue** and this process is known as **Cicatrisation.**

When there is inflammation, there is a response, there is initial polymorph infiltration; bacteria are digested and disintegrated within one hour or two, probably due to acid and digestive enzyme of phagocytes.

Phagocytin. Polymorphs contain acid soluble protein (phagocytin) which is bactericidal to Gram-negative bacteria.

Temperature

Mycobacterium marinum, which infect cold blooded animals, cannot infect man. Anthrax bacilli cannot infect fowls because of fowl's high temperature, 107°C. If the temperature of the fowl is lowered, it can infect fowls. High temperature (above 40°C) can kill Gonococci and Treponema.

13
Complement System

Complement is a heat labile serum component which has the ability to lyse blood cells and destroy Gram-negative bacteria. It is an extremely complex group of serum proteins present in low concentration in normal serum. Components of complement are C_1, C_2, C_3, C_4, C_5, C_6, C_7, C_8, C_9. The complement is responsible for the biological activity of complement fixing antibodies.

Recently, a new pathway for complement activation has been described. C_1, C_4 and C_2 components are not involved. The activation starts at C3 and proceeds to the later components :

$C_3 - C_5, C_6, C_7 \rightarrow C_8$ Cell
C_9 lysis

Function

1. Complement action is of considerable importance because of its ability to get fixed with various types of cells such as Gram-negative bacteria or human red blood cells after they have been interacted with specific antibody
2. Renders bacteria susceptible to lysozyme by digesting holes in the polysaccharide which protect inner lysozyme sensitive layer of mucopeptide in the cell wall.
3. Complement also plays an important role in the attraction of polymorphonuclear phagocytes to the sites of antigen-antibody interaction. This chemotaxis appears to depend on the components of C_5, C_6, C_7 interacting with C_1, C_4, C_2, C_3 complex.

14

Acquired Specific Immunity
(Specific Resistance)

Microorganisms that overcome the innate non-specific resistance are faced, **after an interval,** by the host's second line of defense, i.e. specific immune response. Acquired **immunity is specific** in the same that it protects against a particular pathogen or its toxic product.

The specific immune response takes two forms :

(a) **Humoral immunity** depends on the appearance of globulins or **antibodies** in the blood. These antibodies combine specifically with antigens that stimulate their production. Examples—antigen molecule or particles of bacteria may be clumped, their toxins may be neutralised and, subsequently, they are ingested and digested by phagocytes. Cells are lysed by the activation of complement.

(b) **Cell mediated immunity** depends upon the development of lymphoid cells which are specifically sensitised to the inducing agents and which react directly with the **antigen** to bring about cytotoxic effects. The function of lymphoid tissue is not yet well understood.

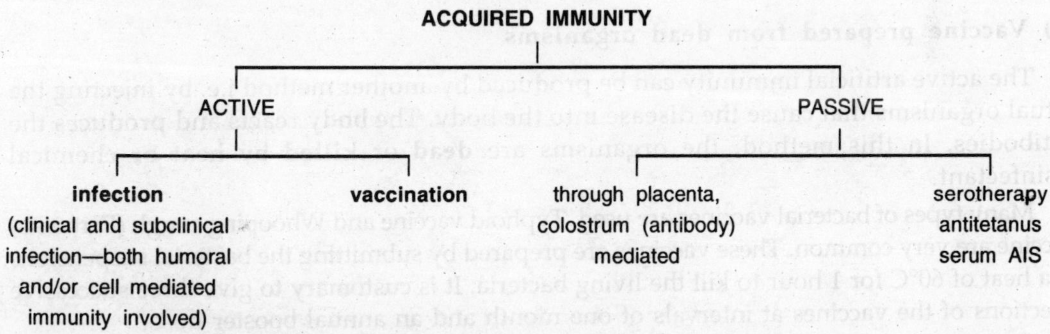

Actively acquired immunity is due to

(1) **Infectious agents** of two types :

(a) Some infections – diphtheria, whooping cough, small pox and mumps induce a long lasting immunity,

(b) Some infections like common cold and influenza confer immunity lasting for a short time.

(2) **Vaccination** is an artificial process which stimulates the lymphoid tissue and is adapted to meet practical requirement. It is under human control. Several such artificial

processes are used for artificial immunity, vaccines are cheapest and most effective means of controlling deadly, infectious diseases.

(A) Vaccine prepared from living attenuated organisms

Active specific immunity may be acquired artificially similar to subclinical infection, by means of injection of living attenuated (weakened) organisms in the human body which cannot cause a severe infection e.g. Bacille Calmette Guerin (BCG) vaccine; small pox vaccine; Anti-Rabies vaccine—*vacca,* Latin (for cow).

1. **BCG vaccination.** Calmette and Guerin, French scientists, developed a BCG vaccine consisting of live tubercle bacilli of low virulence for human being as an immunising agent against tuberculosis.
2. **Small pox vaccination** is carried out by inoculation of living cowpox virus into the human body which could give protection against small pox virus because of their antigenic relationship. The vaccine was available in freeze dried form, when small pox was in existence. In 1979, WHO declared the world free of smallpox.
3. **Anti-Rabies vaccine.** Sample vaccine is prepared from the brain of sheep infected with the fixed rabies virus. Infected sheep brain suspension inactivated by 0.5 per cent phenol vaccine may cause paralysis in small proportion (1 : 4,000 to 1 : 10,000) of human beings, because of the presence of nerve cell in the vaccine (allergic type of encephalitis).
4. **Avianised Rabies vaccine.** To avoid the nervous symptoms the vaccine is prepared from virus cultivated repeatedly in successive live embryonated avian eggs, inactivated by formalin, ultraviolet irradiation or phenol and, finally, the vaccine is dehydrated. This vaccine is reconstructed, used safely and effectively than sheep brain tissue vaccine.

(B) Vaccine prepared from dead organisms

The active artificial immunity can be produced by another method i.e. by injecting the actual organisms that cause the disease into the body. The body reacts and produces the antibodies. In this method, the organisms are **dead** or **killed** by heat or chemical disinfectant.

Many types of bacterial vaccines are used. Typhoid vaccine and Whooping cough (Pertussis) vaccine are very common. These vaccines are prepared by submitting the bacterial suspensions to a heat of 60°C for 1 hour to kill the living bacteria. It is customary to give three successive injections of the vaccines at intervals of one month and an annual booster dose.

1. **Mixed vaccines.** Vaccines containing **more than one** kind of organisms is known as mixed vaccines e.g. Triple vaccine (Diphtheria, Pertussis, Tetanus, DPT) vaccine is not only effective, but it saves many extra pricks.
2. **Sensitised vaccines.** Organisms meant for the preparation of vaccine are sometimes treated before use with the serum of a person or animal immune to the bacteria. These bacteria combine with the antibody in the serum, so that **they are acted upon quickly by the blood tissues or phagocytes of the person into whom they are infected** and, ultimately, immunity is produced rapidly and effectively. Such vaccines are called **sensitised vaccines.**
3. **Viral vaccines. Killed** viral vaccines are the vaccines against Influenza and Salk vaccine against Poliomyelitis.

(C) Injection of modified bacterial exotoxin

1. **Toxoid.** Certain bacteria damage the body tissue by elaborating the toxin. When these toxins are detoxified by formaldehyde, they can be used as immunising agents against the diseases e.g. Tetanus toxoid (TT) against tetanus, diphtheria toxoid against diphtheria.

Passively acquired immunity. Administration of immune serum from another species e.g. horse—diphtheria antiserum, tetanus antiserum (ATS) and gas gangrene antiserum were used therapeutically until the advent of antibiotics. Still now, it is used. Passive immunity due to maternal antibody across the placenta in some species, man and rabbit—where a particular part of immunoglobulin polypeptide chain has been found necessary for effecting the transfer. In other species, such as dogs and rats, antibodies are transmitted through the colostrum via the intestine and via placenta; the other animals, lamb and calf receive this form of immunity only by means of the colostrum. Pooled human immunoglobulin is also used as a source of antibody in a number of infections (measles, small pox and serum hepatitis) during the period of incubation to **modify** or prevent the infection.

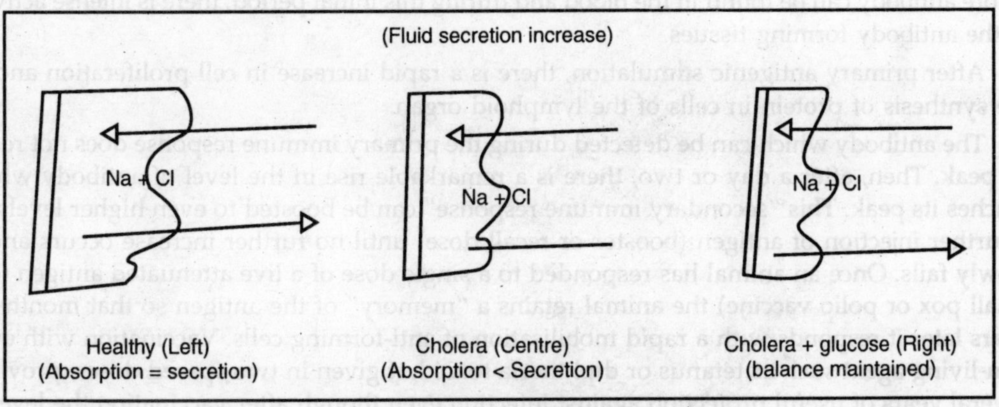

Fig. 14.1: Oral Rehydration Mechanism

15
The Immune Response

A. Humoral immune response

After first contact of the tissue with the antigen, there is an interval of about two weeks before antibody can be found in the blood and during this initial period, there is intense activity in the antibody forming tissues.

After primary antigenic stimulation, there is a rapid increase in cell proliferation and in the synthesis of protein in cells of the lymphoid organ.

The antibody which can be detected during the primary immune response does not reach its peak. Then, after a day or two, there is a remarkable rise in the level of antibody which reaches its peak. This "secondary immune response" can be boosted to even higher levels by a further injection of antigen (booster or recall dose) until no further increase occurs and it slowly fails. Once an animal has responded to a single dose of a live attenuated antigen (e.g. small pox or polio vaccine) the animal retains a "memory" of the antigen so that months or years later it responds with a rapid mobilisation of anti-forming cells. Vaccination with even non-living agent such as tetanus or diphtheria toxoid, if given in two spaced doses, provides several years of useful protection against infection even though after vaccination the level of antibodies falls to a low level, the "memory" is retained. To obtain a maximum response, the interval between the primary and secondary injections should not be too short and an interval of less than ten days is likely to reduce the level of the secondary response. This allows time for a maximal increase in the number of antibody forming cells which can be stimulated by subsequent injection.

Determinants of acquired specific immunity

1. **Form.** The natural ability of antigen to induce an immune response may be enhanced by altering or mixing it with another substance known as **adjuvant.** The antigen can be absorbed on a mineral gel such as aluminium hydroxide or aluminium phosphate—e.g. Alum precipitated antigen. Such particulate form of antigen seems to be able to initiate antibody production much more effectively than the same antigen in non-particulate form. The effect is not yet fully understood, but it may be due to the direct effect of the particulate antigen on the lymphoid cell membrane—leading to more effective transformation of the cell for antibody formation than that can be brought about by antigen in solution.

Another method has been developed to enhance antibody response i.e. preparation of a water-in-oil emulsion. The emulsion forms a depot of antigen in the tissues from which small quantities of antigen are released continuously, sometimes for a year or more. Example, Influenza vaccine.

Route. If an antigen is given intravenously, most of the antibody is produced by spleen, and some in lung, bone marrow, if given subcutaneously or intradermally—the antigen travels via lymphatics to local lymph nodes where antibody is produced initially.

Dose. The antibody response is proportionate to the dose of antigen. If the antigen dose is increased, the immune response is small, so if a particular level of antigen is increased then there will be specific paralysis of the antibody forming tissues—Immunological tolerance.

B. Cell mediated acquired immune response

Cell mediated immunity occurs particularly in infections by microorganisms that enter and grow within the tissue cells such as viruses, tubercle bacilli, brucella and some salmonella. It seems likely that the cell mediated immune response is involved in protection against infective agents—particularly those causing intracellular infection.

Cell mediated immunity is manifested by delayed hypersensitivity around the site of infection. The cell mediated response is initiated in different areas of spleen and lymph node (white pulp of spleen and paracortical areas of lymph). These areas are controlled by **thymus** —so these lymphocytes are called as T-cells.

Very recently a number of yet uncharacterised non-antibody lymphocytic factors (non-specific antibodies) are described and are called **lymphokines.** In 1969, Dudley Dumonde suggested the term lymphokine. They are released by sensitised lymphocytes, T-cells in contact with antigen.

Functions—Lymphokine has

(1) the property of inhibition of the **in vitro** migration of macrophages on glass slide;

(2) Macrophages can be grown in culture in capillary tube and will normally migrate out of the open end of the tube into the culture fluid.

(3) A factor released by lymphocytes exposed to antigen will prevent this migration by causing the macrophages to stick together. This factor is likely to be released also **in vivo** and may be responsible for the accumulation of macrophages in cell mediated immune reaction.

(4) Another factor released from sensitised lymphocytes after exposure to antigen causes stimulation and proliferation of normal unsensitised lymphocytes. This is known as mitogenic factor.

(5) Another lymphokine has a chemotactic effect on macrophages attracting them to the site of the inflammatory responses.

(6) A cytotoxic effect due to a lymphokine (lymphotoxin) has been demonstrated to damage the different types of cell.

(7) A factor which increased capillary permeability (skin reactive factor) can also be shown to be released by sensitised lymphocytes.

(8) It is generally thought that the lymphokines are the main effector mechanisms in the cell mediated response.

Tissue involved in immune response

Lymph nodes, spleen and bone marrow are mostly engaged in the immune response, while lung and, to some extent, the liver, can take part in immune response. The specialised lymphoid organs (spleen and lymph nodes) take up foreign antigen and initiate the immune response. The lymph nodes and spleen are made up of three types of cells which are involved in the initiation of the immune reaction, the three types of cells are lymphocytes, plasma cells and phagocytic cells of reticulo–endothelial system. The lymphoid tissues responsible for humoral antibody production are associated developmentally with the gut and consist of lymphocytes and plasma cells of the lymph nodes and spleen.

In the humoral immune response, immunoglobulins are secreted into the blood by the lymphoid cells, predominantly plasma cells situated in the spleen and lymph nodes.

In man, lymphoid tissues appear first in the thymus at about eight weeks gestation. Peyer's patches are distinguishable by the fifth month and immunoglobulin secreting cells appear in the spleen and lymph nodes at about 20 weeks. From this period onwards, both IgM and IgG globulins are sythesised by the foetus with IgM predominating. At birth, the infant has a blood concentration of IgG comparable to—or sometimes higher than that of maternal serum having received IgG but not IgM via placenta from the mother. The rate of synthesis of IgM in the infant increases rapidly within the first few days of life and does not reach adult levels until about a year. Cell mediated immune reactions can be stimulated at birth but these reactions may not be as powerful as in the adult.

Cells concerned in the antibody production

Cell cooperation between thymus dependent (T) lymphocytes and bone marrow derived (B) lymphocytes has been shown to occur. The (T) lymphocytes assist (B) lymphocytes in some as yet undefined way, possibly by concentrating antigen on their surface and presenting it to B cells or perhaps by releasing a **lymphocyte activation product** (lymphokine) to stimulate the B cells to respond to antigen.

In the spleen, the cells engaged in antibody production are found in the red pulp, whereas, in lymph nodes, they are found in germinal centres of the cortex.

Individual immunoglobulin producing cells synthesise the whole molecule of immunoglobulin—both heavy and light polypeptide chains. Individual cells make only one class of immunoglobulin and the light chains are restricted to one of the two types (K and L). T and B lymphocytes are morphologically similar.

Initially, B cells produce Ig M antibody and then switch over to IgG production. Antibody secreting "Russell body" is found in plasma cell. B cells are responsible for immunoglobulin (Ig) synthesis, and can either react to the direct contact with antigen or cooperate with T cells which are helper cells.

16
Protection and Immunity

A particular microorganism may become pathogenic, if it is capable to overcome the immune response system of the human host :

(1) Human host can be protected from the **bacterial** infections by

(a) Antibody mediated immunity, or

(b) Cell mediated immunity.

(a) Antibody Mediated Immunity in Bacterial Infections

Because of the production of the exotoxin, some microorganisms (i.e. **Corynebacterium diphtheriae, Clostridium tetani, Cl. welchii, Cl. botulinum)** are pathogenic. Antibodies acquired by immunisation or previous infection or given passively as antiserum are able to neutralise the bacterial toxins. Bacterial toxins are enzymatic in nature; most probably the antibody interacts with the active site of the enzyme and neutralises effectively the toxin.

When bacteria do not produce exotoxins, antibodies get attached to the surface of the bacteria. The most important effect of this attachment is to encourage phagocytosis by blood macrophages or polymorphs **(opsonisation).**

The mechanism is that the antibody alters the surface change of organisms and makes them more susceptible to phagocytosis. The phagocytes can also destroy the organisms by digesting by various enzymes produced in the intracellular lysosomes; but **Streptococcus pyogenes, Typhoid** bacillus, **Mycobacterium tuberculosis** are able to resist the digestion by enzymes. If immunity exists due to previous infection or artificial immunisation, streptococcus is susceptible to intracellular digestion, whilst the smooth strains are able to resist the digestion.

In case of enteric infections (typhoid and paratyphoid due to salmonella) antibodies are secreted into the intestinal lumen and attack these organisms before they invade the intestinal mucosa. These antibodies are known as "coproantibodies" and they are of IgA type which is selectively produced in mucous membrane of respiratory and intestinal tract.

Other effects of antibody attachment to the surface of the organism are :

(a) the lysis of Gram-negative bacteria brought about by the activation of complement system. The effect of the complement is to digest the cell wall of lipopolysaccharide so that the structural mucopeptide is exposed to the attack by lysozyme.

(b) Attachment of bacteria to red blood cells in presence of antibody and complement. This phenomenon, known as **"Immune adherence,"** may encourage the phagocytosis.

(c) Antibody precipitated on the surface of certain parasitic nematodes can block the excretory orifices of the nematodes.

(b) Cell mediated immunity in bacterial infections

Macrophages from animal immune to tubercle bacilli are more actively phagocytic than those taken from a normal animal. Similarly, macrophages from brucella infected animals show enhanced cellular immunity. The same was observed in **Listeria monocytogenes.**

(2) Immunity in viral infections

(a) Antibody mediated immunity

In virus infection, the antibody is mostly efficacious, if the virus passes through the blood stream to reach its target organ. For example, polio virus initially crosses the intestinal route, invades the blood stream and passes on rare occasions to the spinal cord and brain where it proliferates. Antibody present in the blood stream can neutralise the virus before it reaches its target cells in the nervous system.

A number of virus behave in the same way (e.g. virus of measles, small pox, mumps, rubella and chicken pox). In case of influenza and common cold, the viruses do not pass through the blood stream as their target organ is the respiratory mucous membrane. In this type of infection, a high level of antibody will be less effective against these viruses in comparison with its effect on blood borne viruses. Most of the antibody should pass through the mucous membrane into the respiratory secretion to act on such respiratory viruses. There is very little IgG and often no IgM in the content of mucous secretion, as this mucous membrane is not, most probably, very permeable to these classes of antibody. But IgA is manufactured by the plasma cells in the lamina propria of the mucous membrane and secreted in the nasal secretion. IgA has neutralising activity against common cold viruses. Intranasal administration of live attenuated Influenza virus can stimulate local production of IgA antibody in the mucous membrane of the nose. The high degree of immunity was provided by live attenuated oral polio virus may be due to locally produced antibody in the gut by neutralising the virus even before it reaches the blood stream. After oral vaccination, IgA against polio virus has been demonstrated in the faeces, in duodenal fluid and in saliva, whereas no antibody was demonstrated after injection of inactivated polio virus vaccine.

(b) Cell mediated immunity

The children with congenital hypogammaglobulinaemia can recover from virus infection without producing any demonstrable virus neutralising antibody, because of cell mediated immunity. The patients with Swiss type agammaglobulinaemia and an additional cell mediated deficiency are very much susceptible to virus infection and, ultimately, they may die.

(3) Immunity to protozoa and helminths

The life cycle of parasite is complicated and the immune response can be effective, if the life cycle is interrupted at a stage when the parasite is accessible to immune process. The antibody may, most probably, have the access to the parasite if the permeability of the red blood cell membrane is altered so that the immunoglobulin can enter and attack the parasite. In protozoal infection, immunoglobulin production is increased and all classes of immunoglobulins are involved.

Life cycle of helminths is also complex as in protozoa protective immuno-responses may act only at an early stage in the life cycle.

IgE (reaginic) antibody with pulmonary eosinophilia will appear in the parasitic infections and the immediate hypersensitivity reactions of anaphylactic type (type 1) is involved in the pathogenesis of helminth infections.

17
Allergy (Hypersensitivity)

von Pirquet coined originally the term allergy (*grallos*, altered, changed; *ergon*, action) to describe the altered reactivity of an animal after exposure to a foreign antigen. The allergy included both immunity and hypersensitivity. It is now restricted to refer only to **hypersensitivity.** There are two forms of hypersensitivity reactions :

(1) Immediate allergy; and

(2) Delayed allergy.

1. **The immediate form** appears rapidly after exposure of a sensitised person to further dose of antigen and usually depends upon the liberation of **histamine**—pharmacologically active mediator substance which is formed under the influence of antigen-antibody combination.
2. The **delayed form** appears more slowly (usually after 24 hours) and depends upon the immunologically activated lymphoid cells.

Various classifications of hypersensitivity reactions have been proposed, but the most widely accepted one is that of Coombs and Gell. The classification of Coombs and Cell recognises four types of hypersensitivity reactions, three of which come under the heading of immediate reaction:

Type I, **Anaphylactic** reactions;

Type II, **Cytotoxic** or cytolytic reactions; Type II reactions are intermediate, between hypersensitivity and autoimmunity. Combination with antibody, may cause stimulation instead of damage. Such antibody mediated cell stimulation has also been called Type V hypersensitivity.

Type III, **Toxic-complex** syndrome;

Type IV, **Cell-mediated** delayed hypersensitivity form of reaction.

HYPERSENSITIVITY (Disadvantageous reactions) →
- → **Immediate type** antibody mediated (Types I–III)
- → **Delayed type** cell mediated (Type IV)

(1) Anaphylactic reactions (anaphylaxis)—Type I.

If a guinea pig is injected with a small dose of a foreign antigen (egg albumin), no adverse effects are observed. When a second injection of egg albumin is given intravenously after an interval of ten days, a condition known as "anaphylactic shock" develops – the guinea pig becomes restless, starts to chew and rubs its nose with its own front paws. Its respiration is laboured; the animal becomes cyanosed, may develop convulsions and, ultimately, die.

The initial injection of antigen is termed "sensitising dose" and the second dose is known as "shocking dose." During the interval between the two injections, the animal has formed antibody which gets attached on the surface of cells; later, there will be interaction of shocking dose of antigen with the newly formed antibody on the surface of cells—ultimately leading to "anaphylaxis."

In anaphylactic reaction, four pharmacologically active substances have been implicated—the most important is histamine. The release of histamine can be demonstrated **in vitro** by exposing antibody sensitised piece of tissue to the contact of antigen. (Sensitisation may be induced by prior injection of antigen into the animal supplying the tissue which makes antibody as described above or tissue may be sensitised passively by the addition of antibody produced in other animal). The typical contractions induced in isolated strips of uterus and intestine are called **Schultz-Dale** reactions—after the discoverers.

In man, there are two types of reactions, **systemic** and **local,** which are related to the mode of entry of the shocking dose of antigen into the body. If the antigen is injected parenterally as in the case of serum (e.g. **horse** anti-tetanus serum), drug (penicillin) or perhaps by the bite of an insect, the systemic form of anaphylaxis is likely to develop, which is characterised by dyspnoea with bronchospasm, sometime skin rashes, a fall in blood pressure, and, occasionally, death.

On the other hand, if the antigen comes primarily in contact with the respiratory mucous membrane then, in a sensitised individual, the local form of anaphylaxis may develop i.e. hay fever, asthma. When the appropriate antigen (e.g. nuts, fish, strawberries) come in contact with the intestinal mucous membrane of a sensitised individual a mixed form of reactions may develop with the intestinal symptoms, urticaria, skin rashes and, sometimes, symptoms of asthma.

Antibodies in Anaphylactic reactions

In man, reaginic antibody is responsible for the sensitisation of the tissues for anaphylactic reactions. This antibody has an affinity for tissues and can readily be detected in the serum of a sensitised individual by injecting a small quantity of this serum into the skin of a normal recipient, which is followed by introduction of the appropriate antigen into the same site of injection, after an interval of 24-48 hours. A **wheal and flare** erythematous reaction develops within about 20 minutes at the site of injection, just like a response to an injection of histamine. This reaction is known as **Prausnitz-Kustner** (PK) test according to its originators.

(2) Cytotoxic or Cytolytic reactions—Type II

The antibody directed against a cell which is associated with an antigen brings about cytotoxic or cytolytic effect which involves participation of complement.

(a) In **incompatible blood transfusion,** the cytolytic effect of antibody on foreign red blood cells was observed.

(b) **Haemolytic disease** of newborn has a similar mechanism.

(c) **Sedormid purpura** is a cytotoxic reaction which is due to the union of the drug sedormid with platelets, as a result an antibody response against the platelet-absorbed drug brings about destruction of the platelets and thus cause purpura. Therefore, the drug sedormid was withdrawn from the market.

A variety of infectious diseases due to Salmonella and Mycobacteria are associated with haemolytic anaemia. Studies of salmonella infections revealed that the haemolysis is apparently due to an autoimmune reaction against a lipo-polysaccharide endotoxin which becomes coated on the erythrocytes. A detailed study has been conducted in **Salmonella gallinarum** infections in chickens.

(3) Toxic complex syndrome—Type III

This reaction is due to the combination of antigen with circulating antibody leading to formation of microprecipitates in and around small blood vessels with consequent inflammation and subsequent mechanical blockage of the vessels causing interference with the blood supply to surrounding tissues. There are two types of reactions:

(a) Systemic form – Serum sickness;

(b) Local form – Arthus phenomenon.

(a) **Serum sickness**—Develops in individuals given injection of foreign serum and it is described soon after the parenteral administration of horse antitetanus serum (ATS). Symptoms are asthma or laryngeal oedema. The organs affected are kidney, heart, and joints. Now-a-days the most likely causes of serum sickness are drugs (penicillin) which form drug-protein complexes in the host.

(b) **Arthus phenomenon**—Like serum sickness, Arthus phenomenon is brought about by the formation of antibody-antigen complexes, but, in this case, the phenomenon is local at the site of injection. Arthus reaction occurs in the walls of small blood vessels in the presence of large quantities of IgG antibody, which forms microprecipitates with antigen. This reaction may occur in diabetes patients who have received many injections of insulin and have developed high levels of IgG antibody to antigenic constituents in the insulin preparation. Similar reaction is also noted in case of anti-Rabies vaccination.

(4) Delayed hypersensitivity—Type IV

Cell mediated hypersensitivity. This type of reaction occurs after 24-48 hours after injection of antigen. The classical example of this type of reaction is **tuberculin** response which occurs when an individual previously or currently infected with tubercle bacilli is given an intradermal injection of 0.1 ml of 1 : 1,000 dilution of a protein extract of tubercle bacilli (purified protein derivative, PPD), 48-72 hours later an indurated inflammatory reaction of variable size can be seen on the skin. The injection site is infiltrated with large number of mononuclear cells-lymphocytes. The mechanism is not yet well understood.

Macrophages in delayed hypersensitivity reaction sites may contribute lysosomal enzymes from their intracellular granules and, thus, further inflammatory changes.

When macrophages come in contact with antigen, the sensitised lymphocytes release a number of non-antibody factors (i.e. lymphokines) which are

(a) a factor inhibiting macrophages migration;

(b) a chemotactic factor; and

(c) a cytotoxic factor. The role of these substances in delayed hypersensitivity is not clear.

Delayed hypersensitivity reactions are observed in brucella, salmonella, mycobacterium, pathogenic fungi and a wide range of viruses (herpes simplex, measles, small pox, vaccinia) infections. It can develop after sensitisation to a variety of metal (nickel and chromium) and dyes (hair dyes).

Skin sensitisation to penicillin is common after topical application of the antibiotic ointment or cream—clinical signs are redness, swelling, vesicles, scaling and exudation of fluid.

Types of allergy

Whether immediate or delayed allergy, the basic explanation of allergic manifestation is that a reaction between antigen and its specific antibody has occurred in the body. If this reaction occurs in the blood, it will not cause allergic response and is the normal defensive process. If antigen-antibody combination occurs in or **on the tissue cells,** there is **allergy.**

There are two types of allergy:

(1) **Immediate allergy** is due to **precipitin** reaction occurring **in** or **on** certain **tissue cells.** It is characterised by the painful itching wheals known as "hives." This type of allergy may occur after eating certain foods or after injections of therapeutic serum; other manifestations are : intense gastroenteritis appearing within few minutes after consuming certain foods to which the victim is allergic and asthma after contact with pollen or with certain animals.

Shock tissue. The signs, symptoms and appearance of immediate allergic reactions depend upon the tissue cells which suffer precipitin reaction. The tissues that suffer are known as "shock tissues."

If the tissues are smooth muscle fibres, the muscle contracts. If the muscle fibres of gastrointestinal tract contract, diarrhoea and cramps may result; if the gravid uterine muscle contracts, there is abortion; asthma may occur, if the bronchioles contract. Besides smooth muscle contraction, oedema and inflammation of mucosa are manifested in the allergy. 0.5 to 1 ml. of 1 : 1,000 epinephrine quickly reduces the swellings.

Anaphylaxis is one of the most dramatic manifestations of the immediate type of allergy.

(2) In **delayed allergy,** the tissue responses appears after 24 hours.

The tuberculin reaction is a best example of delayed allergy.

Histamine in allergy. In immediate allergy, an initial substance called **histamine** is released by tissue cells. The histamine causes many of the symptoms seen in hay fever, bee stings, serum reactions, antibiotic reactions and common colds. These discomforts can be relieved by **antihistaminics** which cause contractions of blood vessels.

Some common allergies

Pollen allergy. The pollen (sperm cells) of many plants—grasses, roses, rag weed—may cause allergy in some persons. When the proteins of the pollen come in contact with nasal and respiratory mucous membrane of the individuals, they are absorbed locally and set up a hypersensitivity condition of these tissues. When the individual inhales later more of the pollen proteins, the nose and throat become irritated, swollen and oedematous. Because of the severity of the reactions against pollen, there develop a symptom of severe "cold" which is commonly known as "hay fever" or nose fever. These conditions may be relieved by antihistaminics and nasal decongestants.

Food allergy. A person may become sensitised to certain foods (strawberries or cod fish). Due to a slight gastrointestinal irritation, lesion or disturbance, some of the food is absorbed **undigested** through the stomach or intestinal wall into the blood. The result is the same as if the protein has been injected. The next time—or perhaps every time—the same person eats strawberries or cod fish, he will react very violently. There will be allergic manifestation in the form of rash or blotches on the skin which itch persistently. These conditions are known as "hives." Some other victims may exhibit nausea, vomiting, gastrointestinal irritation and general symptoms. Antihistaminics are useful in these conditions.

Infection allergy. Due to the microbial proteins entering into the blood stream certain cells of the body may become sensitised to these microbial proteins resulting into the delayed allergy. A person suffering from tuberculosis may become allergic to tuberculosis. The relapses in rheumatic fever are due to repeated allergic responses (with damage to heart muscles) to reinfection with certain streptococci to which the patient is already allergic.

Allergy may also develop in viral, fungal, worm infections, such allergy is called as **Infection allergy.** Most of the damaging effect of infectious diseases is due to infection allergy.

Serum reactions. There are two forms of serum reactions : One is acute and serious form resembling anaphylaxis characterised by collapse, dyspnea, occurring after a few minutes after the injection of therapeutic serum (e.g., diphtheria antitoxin); the other one is milder, delayed form known as serum sickness. Both forms depend upon the precipitin in the patient. Either type of serum reaction is due to animal (horse) protein in the therapeutic serum, **not to the specific antitoxin.** Symptoms are chill, nausea, extensive painful itching hives or serum rash. Pain in the joints may occur later. If the patient is serious, there may be fatal end.

Delayed serum reactions. Serum sickness may appear after ten to fifteen days after a therapeutic use of horse serum. It is assumed that, during this period, the precipitin to horse serum protein may accumulate in the tissues. After reaching a certain concentration, the precipitins react with the proteins (even in residual portion) of the therapeutic **horse** serum which still remain in the body. If the therapeutic horse serum is to be given parenterally, a preliminary skin test for hypersensitiveness to horse serum may be performed as described below. If the test is positive, the patient should be **desensitised** by giving a number of a very small (0.1 to 1 ml) dose of the serum at intervals of an hour or so before the main injection. The possible shock to the patient is lessened. This process is called as "desensitisation."

Persons with previous injections of serum usually require desensitisation. Sometimes, even in the persons who have not had the previous injections of serum, the serum sickness may also occur.

Atopy. Some individuals inherit not allergy itself, but a certain increased tendency to form **reagins** and thereby to develop allergic reactions (i.e., asthma, hay fever) and perhaps certain forms of arthritis and rheumatic heart disease. These persons are called atopic (and are called 'unfortunate').

Drug idiosyncrasies. Certain plant perfumes, cosmetics, drugs, rubber goods, dyes etc. may also cause immediate allergy-like responses (hives, dermatitis, asthma) which may be previously dependent on specific antibodies at all. These allergy-like reactions restricted to only to certain individuals are known as drug **idiosyncrasies.** The mechanism is not yet well- understood.

Binding power of tissues : Because of natural infections or artificial injection of certain antigens (bacterial cells and exotoxins), cutaneous and mucosal tissue often acquire the property of combining with and holding fast to these specific antigens entering the body. This is a defense mechanism and is probably one manifestation of allergy. These tissues are said to be **sensitised** to the antigens. Once sensitised, the tissues tend to hold on and bind to these specific antigens, infections or toxins to prevent their further spread from the site of localisation whenever they gain entry into the body. The tissues may be damaged locally, but generalised infections or intoxication is prevented. The binding power of the tissues is the basis for the beneficial effect of several methods of artificial immunisation, as for example–Bacillus Calmette

Guerin (BCG) vaccine. This is also of great importance in resistance to brucellosis, syphilis, and other chronic diseases.

Skin tests for hypersensitiveness

When a very small dose of sensitising dose is injected or scratched into the skin of a person or animal hypersensitive to that particular antigen, a wheal (a large, red, swollen area) will develop after an interval of time. This allergic reaction persists for an hour or more. Hypersensitiveness to horse serum is tested in this way by injecting a very small quantity of the serum to be used therapeutically.

Similarly, for testing food or pollen allergy, alcoholic or aqueous extracts of various foods or pollens, likely to be involved, are introduced into (not under) the skin either by scarification or injection and the results are noted.

Application to nursing. The intelligent professional nurse, who acquired a sound knowledge about allergy during her training, will be able to understand and handle the untoward reactions encountered when certain sensitised individuals come into contact with that particular antigenic (allergic) substances – sera, antibiotics, some drug, vaccines, some foods. A severe allergic reaction may ensue following the injection of an antigenic substance. This reaction can be prevented and the patient's life can be saved by the perceptive nurse. For example, since the patient is under constant observation of the nurse on duty, the patient may narrate that he is allergic to eggs (foreign protein); if the physician, unware of this allergic reaction, prescribes a viral vaccine prepared from chick embryo, the nurse should inform immediately the physician about the allergy of the patient to the egg, so that a severe—possibly fatal—allergic reaction can be averted. If the patient who had a previous injection of horse serum, receives again a dose of antitoxic serum prepared in horse, he may have a severe and even fatal reaction to the serum, which, although given to provide the patient with immediate protection against a specific disease, becomes a very highly fatal dose to the patient, since the patient is allergic to horse serum. It is quite essential to understand that the patient reaction to the antitoxic serum is not due to antibodies present in it; but due to **animal** (horse) **proteins** in the serum. Thus, the proteins may react to any horse serum irrespective of presence of antibodies. The well- informed and trained nurse should keep in readiness epinephrine and antihistaminics to avoid such a fatal allergy which may occur due to the parenteral administration of horse serum for passive immunity and she should always be careful about immediate and delayed allergy to an allergenic substance and advise the patient to avoid in future the injections of this particular allergic substance.

18
Central Lymphoid Organs

1. **Thymus :** Thymus is a lymphoepitheial structure situated behind the upper part of sternum. It consists of two lobes. Each lobe contains several lobules. Each lobule is made of an outer **cortex** crowded with small lymphocytes and an inner **medulla** consisting of epithelial cells (thymocytes). The thymus develop into area of lymphoid cells and epithelial cells forming cortex and medulla, respectively. Maturation of lymphoid cells in thymus is most vigorous during foetal and neonatal development and proceeds till puberty.

Production of thymic lymphocytes is the primary function of thymus. During maturation process, the surface membrane of lymphocyte acquires new antigen (Thy antigen) from thymus and these thymus processed cells are called T-lymphocytes (thymus dependent). These **immunologically competent** T-cells, after release from thymus, circulate through blood and lymphatics and constitute 75% of the circulating lymphocytes in man. The life span of the T-cells is much longer than B-cells (i.e. months or years).

2. **Bone marrow :** Within the bone marrow some lymphoid stem cells develop into immunoglobulin (Ig) producing lymphocytes known as B-cells, because they mature into bone marrow. In chickens and birds, B-lymphocytes mature in the (lympho-epithelial organ). The bursal equivalent in mammals is bone marrow. It is the site for both stem cells proliferation and origin and maturation of pre B-cells into functionally mature B-lymphocytes.

The lymphoidal stem cells (pre B-cells) lack surface immunoglobulin but display intracytoplasmic mμ (μ) chains but no light chain. B-cells express IgM on their surface in early stage of their differentiation as the principal antigen receptor. They lack both C_3 and F_c receptors at this stage. At the next stage of differentiation B-cells bear either surface IgM alone or in combination with IgA or IgG depending upon the commitment to the production of a particular antibody class. Then IgD is also added to the surface of B-cells in addition to C_3 and F_c receptors required for the entrance of B-cells into mature phase. The cells now acquire receptors for immunoregulatory factors. These cells are called **virgin cells** as they have not yet been exposed to any antigen. Thus some virgin cells contain surface immunoglobulin of three different classes Ig M, IgG and IgD or IgM, IgA and IgD but all the immunoglobulin molecules on a single cell have the same idiotype. The virgin cells are now ready to respond to antigenic stimulus and migrate to lymph node and spleen.

Peripheral Lymphoid Organs

The peripheral lymphoid organs (lymph nodes, **spleen and mucosal associated** lymphoid tissues) are vascular filtration systems. These organs remove foreign antigens from the blood stream and lymph evoking immune response.

1. **Lymph nodes** are bean-shaped and arranged along the course of lymphatic vessels. They are surrounded by a capsule from which trabeculae penetrate into the nodes. A mature lymph node has (a) outer **cortex** (b) inner **medulla**, and (c) **paracortical zone** between the cortical follicles and base of medullary cords. Circulating lymphocytes of blood enter lymph node by penetration through specialised vessels.

The cortex contains lymphoid follicles which may be primary and/or secondary. **Primary follicles** consist of an accumulation of small lymphocytes. **Secondary follicles** develop during antigenic stimulation. They are large and possess germinal centres. Medullary cords are finger- like processes formed by lymphocytes.

The T and B-lymphocytes are largely separated into different anatomical components of lymph node:

1. **B-cell areas.** The cortical follicles contain B-cells.
2. **T-cell areas.** The paracortical area contains T-lymphocytes and constitutes thymus-dependent area.

Both T and B-lymphocytes migrate to sinusoidal spaces of medulla and pass into blood via different lymphatic vessels.

B lymphocytes are scattered in paracortical area, T lymphocytes are present in and around the germinal follicle. **Active cooperation** between the two types of lymphocytes and the antigen presenting cells in the production of an immunological response is indicated by the distribution of T and B-cells. The lymph node acts as filter for lymph draining the body tissues and foreign antigens which enter the subcapsular sinus by afferent lymphatic vessel. The dendrite macrophages capture and process the antigen. This helps the proliferation and circulation of T and B cells. The lymph passes via afferent lymphatics.

Spleen is the lymphovascular organ. It is without lymphatic supply. It processes material directly from the blood stream and it is divided into compartments by trabeculae extending from the capsule. It has two areas—**white** and **red pulp**. It has also (a) **Cortex** made up of densely packed B and T lymphocytes (b) loosely structured medulla. Unlike lymph node, medulla is external to cortex.

Spleen is an important organ of antibody production due to presence of large number of B cells.

Like lymph node, T and B cells areas are segregated.

B-cell area. Perifollicular region, germinal centre and marginal zone.

T-cell area. Thymus dependent area includes the lymphatic sheath and is adjacent to the central arterioles.

Mucosa Associated Lymphoid Tissue (MALT)

The subepithelial accumulations of lymphoid tissue guard immunologically the mucosa of alimentary, respiratory and genito-urinary tracts which are constantly exposed to numerous antigens.

The lymphoid tissue may be present as diffuse collection of lymphocytes, plasma cells and macrophages throughout the lung and lamina propria of the alimentary tract or as specialised aggregates with well-formed follicles (lingual, palatine, pharyngeal, tonsils, small intestinal peyer's patches and appendix. These are collectively called **mucosa associated lymphoid tissues.** MALT contains both B-cells and T-cells and phagocytes. It forms a separate inter-connected secondary system consisting of Ig A or Ig E producing cells.

In the alimentary canal, the antigen passing through the specialised epithelial cells enters Peyer's patches and stimulate the lymphocytes. These stimulated lymphocytes are drained into the lymph which ultimately reach the blood stream via thoracic duct. They pass into the lamina propria from the blood stream where they become Ig A forming cells, B-cells predominate in gut associated lymphoid tissue.

Lymphocytes in peripheral blood

In the circulating blood, about 75% lymphocytes are T-cells, 20% B-cells and 10% killer (K) cells.

Cells of Lymphoreticular system

Lymphocytes. They are small round cells in blood, lymphoid organs and other tissues. They may be small (5-8 μm), medium (8-12 μm) and large (12-15 μm). They have a thin rim of cytoplasm and spherical nucleus. The small lymphocytes are most numerous and devoid of endoplasmic reticulum. The life-span of short-lived lymphocytes is 10-20 days and that of long-lived lymphocyte is 100-200 days.

In the peripheral blood of an adult, lymphocytes constitute 25-45% of leucocytes, in lymph and lymphoid organs, they are predominant. Lymphocytes educated by central lymphoid organ become **Immunologically competent cells** (ICCS). Majority of long lived small lymphocytes are thymus derived. The short lived ones serve as effector cells in immune response, while long lived ones are store houses of immunological memory. Nucleus of lymphocyte is indented B-cell and similar to T-cell with more cytoplasm and rough surface endoplasmic reticulum.

Lymphocyte traffic is the process of lymphocyte circulation after lymphopoiesis in the central lymphoid organ and peripheral lymphoid tissues.

When an antigen encounters B-cells in spleen and on lymph nodes, B-cells are activated and transformed into plasma cells which synthesise **antibodies.** When T-cells encounter specific antigen, they produce certain activation products **(lymphokine)** and induce Cell Mediated Immunity (CMI).

Laboratory tests for detection of T and B-cells

(1) Sheep erythrocytes surface receptors bind around the T-cells forming rosette.
(2) B-cells rosette is developed by binding of IgG coated sheep erythrocytes in presence of C_3 forming a complex.
(3) B-cells have immunoglobulins on surface and surface receptors for Fc fragment of IgG which are absent on T-cells.

T-lymphocytes. Thymus derived lymphocytes (T-lymphocytes) have characteristic membrane bound markers or **receptors** which they acquire in the thymus during maturation from lymphoid stem cells. T-lymphocytes react only with antigen on the surface of an other cell, whereas B-cells react with antigen either in solution or on a cell surface.

Important T-cell receptors are (a) **enzyme receptor,** (b) **Ia protein receptor,** (c) **T-cell antigen receptor,** CD_4. T-cells serve as receptor for Immunodeficiency virus (HIV).

Differentiation of T-cells

Thymic lymphocytes acquire thymic antigens or markers (detectable by monoclonal antibodies) which were previously designed by the letters T_1-T_{11}. These markers or surface molecules of T-cells are now designed as CD **(clusters of differentiation)** proteins.

As T-cells migrate from cortex to medulla of thymus, they undergo a series of differentiation. As they mature they begin to express their characteristic cell membrane glycoprotein (gp).

The T-cell receptor is responsible for the recognition complexes and is different for every T-cell. So far more than fifty T-cell antigens are identified by monoclonal antibodies.

A brief outline of the relevant CD molecules is:

CD_1 : It is a cortical thymocyte marker associated with **beta globulin.** It is found in early stage of maturation, but disappears at later stage.

CD_2 (T_{11}): It is an early antigen and acts as a **receptor for sheep red blood cells.** It is involved in cell **adherence** and T-cell activation.

CD_3 (T_3) is CD_3 antigen is present in all T-cells and has a constant structure and associated with T-cells receptor cell membrane.

CD_4 (T_4) is present on 65% of the circulating T-lymphocytes and indicates **helper** function. It is also found on macrophages and monocytes. CD_4 recognises antigen by major histocompatibility complex (MHC) class II molecule.

Functional subset of T-cells : T helper (CD_4 cells). It has two subsets—Th_1; Th_2. Th_2 is the principal helper T-cells which interacts with B-lymphocytes and promote proliferation of resting B-cells and development of plasma cells that produce immunoglobulin.

Delayed type hypersensitivity T (Tdh cells)

T-cells are also responsible for delayed type of hypersensitivity. It is not possible to distinguish Th cells from Tdh cells on the basis of surface markers. It is believed that Tdh cells are one type of helper cell (Th_1). They bear CD_4 markers.

Th_1 cells secrete different lymphokines (eg. **gamma interferon)** which are responsible for inflammatory response of delayed hypersensitivity. Growth factors secreted by Th_1 are also believed to regulate lymphocyte activity.

3. **T suppression (CD_8) cells**

Some CD_8 cells block immune response of B-cells by secreting suppressor substances which are called T suppressor (Ts) cells. They block immune response by their action on Th or B-cells.

4. **Cytotoxic (Tc) cells and CD_8 cells** lyse specific target cells whose surface antigens can be recognised by them, eg. virus infected host cells, tumour cells and allogenic graft cells in transplanted tissues. Cytotoxic T-cells possess membrane glucoprotein (CD8). Ts cells can be differentiated from Tc cell **in vitro.**

Natural killer (NK) cells. Large lymphocytes containing azurophile granules in the cytoplasm are called large granule lymphocytes (LGL). NK cells are spontaneously cytotoxic for certain tumour lines, virally (herpes, mumps) transformed target cells and are involved in allograph rejection. They do not require antibody for activity and their action is now specific. They can recognise altered surface structure of target cells. Interferon and other agents that activate macrophages (like BCG vaccine) enhance the activity of NK cells. They are found in spleen and peripheral blood of men and animals. It is believed that NK cells play an important role in controlling the development of neoplastic cells (anti-tumour immunity) and viral replication (anti-viral immunity) in the body.

B-lymphocytes and plasma cells

The pre B-cell is programmed to produce only one class or subclass of immunoglobulin after a switchover from initial IgM production which occurs as a result of further series of gene rearrangement. B-lymphocytes can be subdivided into nine different isotypes or subsets—on the basis of Ig they are programmed to synthesise IgM, IgD, IgG_1, IgG_2, IgG_3, IgG_4, IgA, Ig A_2, Ig E.

The virgin B cells migrate to spleen and lymphoid tissues where a cognate Ag can trigger the second or Ag dependent stage.

Majority of resting tissues and blood B-lymphocytes are small with condensed chromatin and have IgM and only a small proportion (10%) of B cells have IgG on their surface. B-lymphocytes with IgA or IgE are abundant in association with exocrine gland of intestine, lungs where T helper cells also predominate. Each B lymphocyte carries about 10^5 antibody molecules on its surface.

B-cells in peripheral lymphoid organs are quiescent on resting cells and the immunoglobulin is an integral membrane protein. In eliciting a primary immune response. The antigen encounters innumerable lymphocytes all bearing different antibodies and recognition site. The antigen only binds to those Ig molecules on the surface of B-cells which it matches and can be recognised by the cell. The **antigen recognition** binding site is in **hypervariable region** of both heavy and light chains of Ig.

Macrophage presents the processed antigen to B-cells. The antigen binds to the receptor of B-cell. B-cell is stimulated to undergo blastoid transformation which divides rapidly becoming successfully plasma cell, blasts **(clone formation),** intermediate transitional cells and plasma cell. Mature plasma secretes antibody. In **plasma cell,** the nucleus is eccentric and contains coarse radially arranged chromatin (cart-wheel appearance). The cytoplasm contains conspicuous golgi apparatus and abundant endoplasmic reticulum. Immunoglobulin remains localised in the endoplasmic reticulum where it sometimes forms aggregates called Russell bodies. A plasma cell can only synthesise an antibody of a single specificity either IgM or IgG or Ig A. An exception is found in primary immune response, when a plasma cell producing IgM, initially, may later switch over to the synthesis of IgG antibody. Mature plasma cells are end cells and survive only a few weeks and die after a few (or no) cell division. Plasma cells are present in germinal centres of lymph nodes, spleen and diffuse lymphoid tissues of alimentary and respiratory tracts. Although plasma cell is the major antibody producing cell, lymphocytes, lymphoblasts and transitional cells may also produce antibody.

Macrophages may be: (1) **free** or **wandering macrophages** in tissues and monocytes in the blood stream; (2) **fixed** (literal) or **stationary** or **resident macrophages.**

Monocytes originate from monoblasts in the bone marrow, travel as monocytes in the blood stream and emigrate in tissues within two days where they enlarge and differentiate into macrophages and may live for months. In tissues, these mononuclear cells are distributed as **free macrophages** (in lung alveoli; peritoneum and inflammatory granuloma) or **fixed macrophages** integrated in tissues (cells lining sinusoids of liver, spleen and lymph nodes), central nervous system (microglia) and connective tissues (histiocytes). **Blood** macrophages (monocytes) and **tissue macrophages**—They may proliferate locally under certain inflammatory stimuli. **Multi-nucleated giant cells** and **epitheloid cells** in certain inflammatory processes originate from macrophages.

Monokines. Monocytes and macrophages produce a number of important soluble proteins called monokines (*cytokines*).

These monokines include *interleukin 1*, various colony stimulating factors—such as macrophage colony stimulating factor, M-CSF; granulocyte colony stimulating factor, G-CSF; and tumour necrosis factor (TNF):

1. *Interleukin 1 :* (IL-1) human interleukin-1 consists of two proteins IL-1a, IL-1b, produced by macrophages—it is mediator of inflammation, causes release of acute phage of proteins.

2. *Colony stimulating factor* (CSE) is produced by macrophages and stimulates division and differentiation of stem cell. Granulocyte colony stimulating factor promotes granulocyte differentiation process by binding to stem cell receptor. Granulocyte monocyte colony stimulating factor (GM-CSF) stimulate both granulocytes and monocyte cell differentiation.

3. *Tumour necrosing factor* (TNF) synthesised by macrophage is responsible for the tumoricidal activity of macrophages.

Function of macrophages

A. Active phagocytosis.

B. Role in acquired immune response.

A. *Active phagocytosis :* Engulfment of particles by macrophages is *phagocytosis;* engulfment of soluble material by phagocytes is *pinocytosis.*

The membrane of the pseudopod of macrophage fuses to form a pouch or *phagosome.* Lysosome containing hydrolytic enzyme migrates towards phagosome and fuses with the membrane of phagosome forming *phagolysosome.*

Microorganisms or particles sensitised by antibody are more readily phagocytosed. Most bacteria are *killed intracellularly* within few minutes by lysosomal enzyme, some salmonella, Brucella, Mycobacterium resist digestion and may grow *intracellularly* to other sites for transportation to other sites.

B. *Role in acquired immune response*

Macrophages play an important role in immune response. They trap and process bacterial antigens and present them in optimal concentration to the lymphocytes to induce specific immune response. It is a prerequisite for some antigens.

The activation of resting T-cells require Interleukin-1 (IL-1) and Interleukin-2 (IL-2). *Activated macrophages* secrete IL-1 which acts as *endogenous pyrogenes* and induces to T-cells to synthesise IL-2. IL-2 facilitates T-cell activation by rapid DNA synthesis, cell mitosis and T-cell clone formation.

Microphages

Microphages (granulocytes) include polymorphonuclear leucocytes (neutrophils, eosinophils, basophils).

Neutrophils play an important phagocytic role in acute inflammation by locating a foreign invader. Migrating towards it and finally engulfing the offending agent lysosome in their granules are discharged into the phagocytic vacuoles which hydrolyse red cells, many bacteria of low virulence.

Eosinophils are less pathogenic than neutrophils and their granular contents (various hydrolytic enzymes) can kill parasites which are too large to be phagocytosed by neutrophils. Their numbers are more in certain allergic inflammation, parasite infections and diseases with formation of antigen-antibody complex. Functions of eosinophils is not yet clear.

Basophils are found in very small numbers (0.2%) in blood and tissues (most cells). Basophilic granules contain certain heparin, histamine, serotonin and other hydrolytic enzymes. They possess plasma membrane receptors for the F_c portion of IgE and cross-linking of this immunoglobulin by antigen leads to release of pharmacological mediations in anaphylaxis and atopic allergy.

Immune phagocytosis. There are many antigens particularly capsulated bacteria which resist phagocytosis and for dealing with these organisms successfully phagocytic cells require to utilise the process of *immune phagocytosis.*

Mononuclear phagocytes, neutrophils and eosinophils have receptors for F_c portion of IgG and some activated components of C_3l and C_3 li. During the course of an immunological response the ability of neutrophils to phagocytosis is enhanced by *opsonisation*. Possibly, most of the pathogenic bacteria are disposed by *opsonic phagocytosis.* Once the bacteria are killed by lysosomal enzyme, their degradation products are released to the exterior.

Myco. tuberculosis, Listeria monocytogenes, Leishmania sp, *Trypanosoma cruzi, Toxoplasma gondii* can survive inside the macrophages and are able to evade the microbicidal system.

Major Histocompatibility (Complex) (MHC)

Transplants from one individual to another genetically non-identical individual of the same species are recognised as *foreign* by T-cells and rejected. The responsible antigens on the grafted cells are called *Transplantation* or *Histocompatibility* (or H) *antigens.* The major histocompatibility complex (MHC) antigens are those gene products that exhibit a strong (major) effect on the incompatibility of tissue between genetically non-identical individuals. In man—like mouse—some tissue antigens are very strong and others are very weak. The strong transplantation antigens of man include carbohydrate antigens of red blood cells (ABH) *blood group system* and glycoprotein of the cell membrane *(H L A system).* During experimental study of allograft rejection in mice, Groer (1930) observed two blood group antigen systems in mice —*Antigen 1* common to all strains of mice; *Antigen* 2 present in certain strains of mice only which is related to allograft rejection and tumour immunity. This was called H_2 antigen. In mice, H_2 antigen is *major histocompatibility* antigen coded for by a closely linked multi-allelic cluster of genes (H_2 complex) located in chromosome 17.

HLA Complex : The human counterpart of H2 antigen system of mouse are allo antigens present on surface of leucocytes and are called *human leucocyte antigens* (HLA); and cluster of genes encoding for them is termed as *HLA complex.*

The term histocompatibility refers to the degree of compatibility or lack of it between the given tissues. By histocompatibility antigen is meant *cell surface antigen* that can evoke immune response to an incompatible host terminating in allograft rejection.

The HLA complex of genesis located in three regions on short arms of chromosome 6 and consists of eight genetic foci grouped in three classes. They are termed class I (HLA—A, B, C), class II (HLA—DP DO DR) and class III genes and their products provide a system for intercellular communication. MHC antigens are essential for recognition of antigen by T-cells. They can only bind to antigen that are associated with these molecules. T helper cells with CD4 molecules on their surface recognise antigen in association with MHC class II molecules while T cells with CD8 molecules are restricted by MHC class I molecules.

2. MHC class III products are important complement system and responsible for many cellular events.

Indications of HLA typing : HLA antigens are widely distributed in tissues except red blood cells which contains only ABH antigens.

1. HLA system is very useful in tissue typing and matching prior to transplantation.

2. It can be also used in paternity determination, anthropological survey and in establishing association between HLA and disease susceptibility.

3. HLA-B27 is associated with ankylosing spondylitis, more frequently seen among the Caucasians (0.2%).

4. Other diseases showing strong association with HLA include *Reiter's syndrome, juvenile rheumatoid arthritis, acute anterior uveitis, Coeliac disease* and *Grave's disease.*

HLA typing

1. *Class I loci, HLA-A, B,* C are detected by complement dependent cytotoxic reactions. Non-specific antiserum is collected from patients with whole blood transfusion and multi-parous women who are often sensitised by foetal antigens. Monoclonal antibodies are now available. Lymphocytes of donor is typed against a panel of standard and recipient sera in presence of complement.
2. *Class II antigens* are identified by mixed leucocyte reaction (M.L.R.). This is done by cocultivation of donor and recipient lymphocyte to permit DNA synthesis. Enhanced DNA synthesis in the responder cells indicates more foreignness of class I MHC antigen.
3. *Preformed cytotoxic* antibodies in patient's sera is measured by mixing with donor's lymphocytes and complement. Cytotoxic or cytolytic effect on donor's lymphocytes indicates that recipient's serum is reactive against the graft.

19
Autoimmunity

Immune response of an animal does not, under normal circumstances, react against its own body constituents. It is a fundamental characteristic. However, there is a mechanism that makes the cells of the immune system to recognise what is "foreign" and what is "self."

Ehrlich and Morgenroth (1900)—after immunising a goat with red blood cells or other goats—found that the animal readily made antibody against the red blood cells of other goats, but this antibody failed to react with the animal's immunological response to self-antigen was prevented.

Coombs et al (1946) developed a technique to detect the presence of antibody globulin on red blood cells by adding an antiglobulin serum which, after reacting with the globulin coating the cells, linked the cells together and agglutinated them. This technique is known as "Coombs" or "antiglobulin" test and could detect a variety of human and animal diseases in which the antibody was capable of reacting with a number of different antigens of the individual's own tissue.

Haemolytic anaemia in man, in which red blood cells are coated with antibody globulin, was first discovered with Coombs' test. *Systemic lupus erythematosus* (SLE), in which antinuclear factor (ANF), an antibody to nucleus of the cell, is involved. This autoantibody serum factor is present in the blood of patients suffering from connective tissue disease. This (SLE) disease was the second discovered by adopting Coombs' technique. *Interstitial thyroiditis*, (known as Hashimoto's disease) in which an antibody to thyroglobulin is involved, was the third discovery.

The control mechanism for autoimmunity tolerance could be overcome by two days :

(1) The first category is the evasion circumvention of a normal functioning mechanism; and

(2) The second one is the failure of the mechanism itself in the first category, evasion may occur in two ways :

(a) a particular body antigen is not normally accessible to the cells of the immune system as the antigen is *hidden* within a cell or tissue; in the second category, a tissue antigen is *altered* in some way by a chemical, a drug, or an infective agent. The sperm antigen and lens antigen of the eye are *equestered* (hidden) antigens; whereas antigen in the human colon is altered antigen.

(1) In the human colon, there is an antigen which can be extracted. This antigen is similar to a polysaccharide antigen present in *Escherchia coli* O14. So, it is believed that the inflammatory conditions of the colon known as "ulcerative colitis" in which anti-colon antibodies are involved and produced as a result of the immune response initiated by the cross-reacting bacterial antigen.

(2) Group A streptococci causing rheumatic fever have an antigen common with that of human heart. Antibody to the antigen of streptococci may cross-react with the antigen of human heart causing heart lesions.

(3) Streptococci carry surface antigen similar to that found in human glomeruli and so streptococal infection is associated with the development of acute glomerulonephritis.

(4) The association of *Mycoplasma pneumoniae* with primary atypical pneumonia may cause the development of IgM agglutinins which in the cold react with the patient's own red blood cells and may produce haemolytic anaemia.

Studies on the effect of herpes or rabies viruses on tissue culture cells suggested that the viruses are able to bring about alterations of cell membrane. The association of virus with lymphocyte membrane may possibly interfere with normal lymphocyte reaction to antigen.

Pathogenesis of Autoimmune diseases

Three types of hypersensitivity reactions are involved in autoimmune diseases:

(i) *Cytotoxic reaction* : Autoimmune haemolytic anaemia is an example of the cytotoxic reaction in which two types of antibodies are involved.

(1) *IgM antibodies* which agglutinate the patient's own red cells in the cold.

(2) IgG type antibodies which do not cause direct agglutination of the red cells, can be detected by Coombs' test with antiglobulin serum.

In mycoplasma infections, the IgM cold agglutinins react with a common red cell antigen known as the I antigen.

(ii) *Toxic Complex type reaction* : Complex of antibody and tissue antigens, particularly nuclear antigens, are the cause of glomerulonephritis and systemic lupus erythematosis (SLE) where a wide variety of anti-tissue antibodies are found.

(iii) *Cell mediated reaction* : In both man and animal the development of a number of autoimmune states is paralleled by the existence of cell mediated reaction of the delayed hypersensitivity type demonstrated by skin test with tissue antigens.

There is an association between the reactions of cell mediated immunity and humoral antibody in induced autoimmune orchitis in guinea pigs.

Other diseases associated with autoimmune states is rheumatoid arthritis in which IgM antibody called rheumatoid factor is present in the patient's serum. This factor can be detected in vitro by its ability to agglutinate the red blood cells or latex particles coated with IgG globulin.

20
Immunisation
(Prevention is better than cure)

Over 200 years after Edward Jenner's discovery (1798) of small pox vaccination, mankind benefits from this process more than ever before. Several new vaccines were evolved and are now made available to eradicate many diseases e.g. Jenner's own first small pox vaccine has finally banished, in our time (1979), small pox from the earth.

The basic principle of vaccination remains quite the same as in Edward Jenner's day; Jenner noticed that milkmaids who suffered from cow pox—a relatively harmless but contagious disease in cattle—did not contact the small pox. So, Jenner took some cow pox germs from Sarah Nelmes, a young milkmaid, who had fresh cow pox lesions on her fingers, and inoculated an eight year old boy with it. Later, he inoculated the boy again with the small pox germs and proved that the disease could not develop in the boy as the immune system of the boy started to act against small pox germs.

Louis Pasteur, almost hundred years later, discovered that a deadly germ could also offer protection against the disease it caused, if the germ is altered or killed and then injected. This provided a basis for developing at least 20 good vaccines. But recent advances in molecular biology and genetic engineering have led to a new era in vaccinology.

The first genetically engineered vaccine approved in 1986, was designed to prevent hepatitis B which affects an estimated 200 million people around the world. This vaccine was produced by using simple yeast cells into which was inserted the gene for the production of the disease causing virus's outer-coating. The outer coat itself is not infectious but on recognising the outer coat, an immune response can trigger a protective reaction against the whole virus.

Though there was already a vaccine against hepatitis B virus made by altering live viruses extracted from the blood plasma of patients infected with the disease, it is suspected that all vaccines derived from blood products may carry the Acquired Immuno Deficiency Syndrome (AIDS) virus or Human Immunodeficiency virus (HIV). There will be no such risk in the new genetically engineered vaccine.

Recently, when a vaccine of bacterial meningitis was found to be the only partially effective for babies under two, it was reengineered and an improved vaccine was produced.

Yet all these new findings and techniques have not made vaccine production easier in some cases. e.g., the common cold has no vaccine, because more than a hundred known viruses cause common cold. So, it is not possible to have a vaccine for each virus. And the influenza virus can change its form in every season. Therefore, any vaccine can become useless in a year.

Even worst is the HIV virus which changes its form at least twice as fast as influenza virus. Besides, AIDS itself is a disease of immune system. However, a vaccine was produced which prevented AIDS in monkey using inactivated monkey AIDS virus. This vaccine cannot protect human beings against AIDS, as this monkey AIDS virus shares only 40 per cent of the genetic make-up with the human AIDS virus. Most experts believe that a human AIDS vaccine may take at least another five to ten years. Antiviral therapy against AIDS is under experimentation.

In Mumbai (India), since 1950 work was carried out for a leprosy vaccine. In 1965, the researchers could grow in the laboratory artificial medium a bacterium which seems similar to a close cousin of *Mycobacterium leprae.* They studied every characteristic of these new bacteria, treated them with radiation, experimented on animals injected into the first human subject in 1979. The first human subject had a single white patch on the skin. In a short time, the single white patch disappeared. Today, some 30,000 persons have been injected with this vaccine as a part of field trials in Maharashtra (India). None of these persons living in close contact with leprosy patients had any sign of leprosy infection. Yet this vaccine must await more trials before it is sold.

During an epidemic of infectious diseases, a great significance is given to specific immunoprophylaxis and immune therapy. Prophylaxis (Greek *pro*—before, *phylasein*—to guard or protect), is generally thought of being used in advance to prevent disease or infection. *Vaccine* (Lat. *vacca*—cow) received its name from the anti small pox preparation from the virus of cow pox. Vaccines are preparations consisting of attenuated or dead causative agents or products of their life activity, while the method of inoculation is known as *vaccination* or *immunisation.*

Vaccines are introduced parenterally or orally or intranasally within a definite period of time (from several days to several weeks). Vaccines give active immunity. Vaccines should be highly immunogenic (capable of causing sound and long immunity) and should not be toxigenic.

Modern vaccines which are under routine use :

1. Vaccines from live causative agents with a decreased (attenuated) virulence;
2. Vaccines from dead cultures of pathogenic microorganisms (bacteria, rickettsiae, viruses).
3. Vaccines from the products of chemical cleavage of some bacteria (chemical vaccines);
4. Antitoxin (detoxified toxin by formalin at a temperature of 38°C to 40°C).
5. *Associated* vaccines (diphtheria, pertussis, and tetanus – DPT) vaccine.

Serotherapy : Sera are employed for treatment and prophylaxis of tetanus, gas gangrene, botulism. The length of protective action of sera by serotherapy (Passive immunity) is from eight to twenty days. *Gamma globulins* obtained by the method of fractionation of serum protein by means of alcoholic solution of at temperature lower than 0°C, are used for prophylactic purposes against measles, poliomyelitis, whooping cough, serum hepatitis, small pox and are completely harmless as they do not contain hepatitis-B virus and causative agents of other diseases.

Immunisation is an answer to the life saving protection against childhood diseases.

Five gentle pricks for life saving protection against childhood diseases. An infant has to be immunised five times before he completes first year of life:

1. Soon after birth	one BCG injection against tuberculosis, OPV-O dose. [OPV = Oral polio vaccine]
2. At the age of 1½ months	one DPT injection against Diphtheria, Pertussis, Tetanus and first dose of polio drops.
3. At the age 2½ months	Second dose as above.
4. At the age of 3½ months	Third dose as above.
5. At the age of 9 months	One injection against measles.

Three in One (3 in 1)

For protection against three killer diseases : Diphtheria, Pertussis—Whooping cough and Tetanus, three vaccines are given together in a single injection called DPT. Dose of polio drops are also given alongwith DPT to avoid repeated visits. For the complete protection of the child, DPT injections should be given at the interval of 1½, 2½ and 3½ months.

To be borne in mind

(i) If, due to some reason, the child is not immunised in time, it is vital to have the child immunised at the earliest possible thereafter,

(ii) There should be at least a gap of one month between two doses of immunisation,

(iii) It is essential for the infants to complete full course of immunisation. If the prescribed repeat doses of immunisation are not taken the child will not have full protection from the killer diseases;

(iv) Vaccination against measles is recommended at nine months of age, because for the first few months of the life, the child has natural protection against it inherited from the mother. After about 9 months the natural protection comes to an end and the child must be immunised against the risk of measles as soon as the child attains the age of 9 months.

Is it safe to immunise a sick child?

Yes, it is safe to immunise a child suffering from any minor illness or malnutrition. All efforts should be made to get the child immunised even if he has mild fever, cough, cold, moderate diarrhoea or some other mild illness on that day. No time should be lost in having him protected from the dangerous diseases before it is too late.

Protection of women against tetanus

(a) In many parts of our country, mothers give birth in unhygienic conditions. Hence, the mother and newborn are at risk of tetanus;

(b) Tetanus bacilli grow in dirty wounds made by an unclean knife used to cut the umbilical cord during delivery. The knife to be used should be first cleaned, boiled or heated in flame and allowed to cool before use;

(c) If the mother is not protected against the tetanus, the exotoxin liberated by tetanus bacilli in the infected wound may be absorbed into the mother's body and endanger the life of both mother and child;

(d) Tetanus toxoid (TT) injections at one month's interval are necessary as soon as the mother becomes pregnant. If she is already immunised, then one injection is enough;

(e) As a rule, every woman between the age of 15 and 44 years should be fully immunised against tetanus. Every woman who becomes pregnant should make sure that she is immunised. All infants should be immunised against tetanus during the first year of life.

Where to get the immunisation services : Immunisation services can be obtained free of cost from all health, family welfare, primary health centre and public hospitals throughout the country.

Adverse effects of vaccines : Vaccines for immunisation have no side-effects. A child may cry after an injection, develop slight fever, rash or small sore. As with other illnesses, the child may be given plenty of fluid and food and it may be alright soon. If the problem is serious and the child has vomiting, diarrhoea, high fever, a paediatrician may be consulted.

Breast feeding is important : Breast feeding is a kind of natural immunisation against several diseases. Mother's resistance to disease is transferred to the child through her milk i.e. the thick yellow milk (colostrum) which is a rich source of antibodies and is produced in the breast during the first few days after the birth.

1. *Immunisation* protects the pregnant woman against tetanus and the children against several dangerous childhood diseases i.e. three killer diseases (diphtheria, pertussis, tetanus (DPT), tuberculosis and measles;
2. Immunisation is provided through vaccines which are given orally or parenterally;
3. The child's body defence mechanism against diseases is built up by vaccination. If the diseases strikes before the child is immunised, then the immunisation is too late;
4. Children who survive the diseases are weakened and may die later from nutritional deficiency and other illness. The diseases may hamper the child's growth and development.

Why Immunisation is of great necessity

If the child is not immunised:

(a) he is more likely to become undernourished, disabled or to die;

(b) The child is likely to get measles and whooping cough. These diseases can kill the child. Measles is also an important cause of mental retardation and blindness.

(c) The child may be infected with polio virus which can cripple him for life.

(d) The child is exposed to the danger of tetanus which kills most of the people who become infected.

It is the right of every parent to ask for immunisation for the protection of their children.

Immunisation when

- Protection of the child has to begin right after a woman becomes pregnant. This is done by injection of TT to the mother to be at one month interval at the earliest possible after conception.
- Immunisation is urgent. It is very important to immunise a child early in life.
- All immunisations should be completed within the first year of a child's life.
- Half of all deaths from whooping cough, one-third of all cases of polio and one-fourth of all deaths from measles occur before the age of one year.

Adverse reactions following vaccines

Some instructions to field workers

The reactions that follow vaccination are generally mild and of short duration. Serious reactions are known to occur but they are extremely rare and form a small fraction of similar type of complications that occur as a result of disease itself. Neurological syndromes can also occur spontaneously in infant and vaccination may only be coincidentally related.

The common reactions are mild fever, redness, tenderness and pain at the site of injection. Fever and rash on the sixth or seventh day after measles vaccination have also been reported. The number of severe reactions and deaths following vaccination are rare.

Measures to minimise risks

The following measures are to be followed to minimise risks of adverse events following vaccination :

(1) Vaccination sessions should be held on fixed days. The children should be collected at the sub-centre at a central point of a village. Door to door vaccination should not be practised as such a strategy carries a high risk of break in the cold chain and contamination of the syringes and needles.

(2) Procedures for sterilisation of syringes and needles should be scrupulously followed and monitored whenever feasible, steam sterilisation should be preferred to boiling.

- Single sterile syringe and a single sterile needle are used for each injection.
- Issue of the vaccine to the field staff should be strictly monitored. Only required quantities of the vaccine should be taken from the primary health centre on the day of the session.
- Vaccines may be taken on the previous day only if these are carried in vaccine carrier with fully frozen icepacks.
- Supervision should include measures to ensure that vaccine vials are not stored in the periphery and reused subsequently. Batch number and expiry date should be recorded before issue.
- Vaccine should be discarded at the end of the session. Opened vials of vaccine should not be reused under any circumstances.
- Potentially harmful injectible drugs should be kept separate from vaccine vials and diluent.
- Field monitoring of the services must be regular so that any deficiency could be noted and corrected in time. Reporting of abscesses by the health workers in their areas should be made compulsory.
- Measles vaccine should be reconstituted with the diluent provided with the vaccine. The diluent should be cooled before use. The vaccine should be kept on ice while in use. The children should be administrated 0.5 ml of the vaccine in the arm subcutaneously. A separate sterile syringe and needle should be used for each injection. (Extract from "National Immunisation Mission." Ministry of Health and Family Welfare – 1989, New Delhi, India).

Remember

- An unimmunised child is more likely to become disabled, undernourished and to die.
- Immunisation is no less important than the mother's love for a baby. It is urgent. It has to begin soon after birth and completed within the first year of a child's life.
- The last dose of Tetanus Toxoid (TT) injection during pregnancy for protection against tetanus must be had at least thirty days before the expected date of delivery and also for protecting the child to be born against neonatal tetanus.
- For protection against three killer diseases, three vaccines are given together in a single injection called DPT.

Cold Chain for Vaccine

Vaccines are thermolabile products, hence they require special storage and transportation arrangement to retain their efficiency.

If vaccines are kept at the recommended minimum temperature, they will remain potent for a longer period of time. All vaccines retain their potency at temperature +2 to +8 degree C. The vaccines must be transported and stored at these temperature at district and primary health centres.

For long term storage, measles and polio vaccines are kept at sub-zero temperature. If freezers are available these vaccines should be kept in a freezer. DPT, DT and TT vaccines should not be frozen. Vaccines should not be exposed to direct sunlight. The cold chain for vaccines consists of three vital elements – the cold storage equipment, transportation, and motivated and trained manpower for operating the vital link.

The importance of people in the cold chain cannot be overemphasised. Often the cold chain is thought to refer only to the refrigeration of the vaccine. Even if the finest and most modern equipment and transportation are available the cold chain will not be effective, if the people do not handle the vaccine properly. Several steps have been taken over the last few years to strengthen the cold chain for vaccines. The activities have been directed both at improving the storage and transportation facilities as well as in training manpower in logistics of vaccines and handling of the refrigeration.

(Excerpts from the publication – "National Immunisation Programme" published by National Institute of Health and Family Welfare, New Delhi, India).

Preventable Pediatric Diseases

Tetanus

Symptoms

- For the first two days of life, the newborn does normal suckling but keeps crying;
- The infant is unable to suckle between the 3rd and 21st day;
- The child cannot open the mouth fully;
- Facial, neck and trunk muscles of the child get stiff and the child gets convulsions;
- His body bends like a bow due to contraction of neck and trunk muscles.

Danger : The survival rate is very low.

Diphtheria

Symptoms

- Sore throat with or without difficulties in swallowing;
- Mild fever, no appetite;
- The child looks ill;
- Neck is swollen;
- Whitish membrane in the throat;
- The child has difficulty in breathing due to obstruction in airways.

Danger

- The toxin can affect the heart muscle and nerves;
- Diphtheria has high rate of fatality;
- It is highly infectious, painful and dangerous for the children.

Pertussis (Whooping cough)

Symptoms

- To begin with, the child has slight fever, running nose, cold and cough;
- Gradually, cough gets worse, child gets fits of cough and struggles for breath;
- Breath is with a long in rush of air into the almost empty lung with a characteristic whoop;
- Spasms are common during cough, the eyes bulge and bleed;
- The child often vomits after or during cough.

Poliomyelitis

Symptoms

- The child has fever and headache;
- Feels sudden onset of weakness and paralysis—generally of one leg or arm or trunk;
- Muscle pain with touch sense remaining normal;
- Wasting of the affected muscles later.

Danger

- Paralysis of one of the limbs leading to lameness;
- May even lead to paralysis of muscles of respiration.

Measles

- The disease starts with fever, running nose, and cough;
- The child's eyes become red and watery;
- Rash appears on the face between the third and seventh day,

  It appears over the whole body.

Danger

- The child gets weak, becomes prone to secondary infections of lungs, ears, eyes, and gastrointestinal tract. It can be fatal due to complications like pneumonia.

Tuberculosis (Childhood)

Symptoms

- Low grade fever;
- Swelling of lymph glands;
- Loss of weight; cough and weakness; high fever;
- Severe headache, stiffness of the neck and convulsion in the case of tuberculosis meningitis;
- The child becomes hunch-backed;
- If not cared, the disease becomes fatal.

Recommended age for BCG vaccination against tuberculosis is just after birth; only one dose is given.

SCHEDULE OF IMMUNISATION

For whom/when	What	Why
To pregnant woman at the earliest possible after conception	Two injections of Tetanus Toxoid (TT) at an interval of one month (if already vaccinated, only one injection of TT in pregnancy)	Protects the mother and new-born from the tetanus
To the infant after birth	One injection of BCG Zero dose of polio drops	Protects the infant from tuberculosis
When the child is 1½ months old	One injection of DPT and first dose of polio drops	Protects the child from diphtheria, pertussis, tetanus and polio
When the child is 2½ months	Second dose as above	—
When the child is 3½ months	Third dose as above	—
When the child is 9 months old	One injection of measles	Protects the child from measles
When the child is 1½ years	One booster dose of polio drops, and DPT injection	Protects the child from diphtheria, pertussis, tetanus and poliomyelitis

- At the age of five years, an injection of DT and one injection of TT at the age of ten, and again at sixteen years, particularly in the case of girls;
- Interval between two doses of vaccination should not be less than one month;
- Vaccination for immunisation can be done without hesitation even in the case of minor cough, fever, diarrhoea, in consultation with a physician or health worker;
- For the health of the child, it is essential to have the child vaccinated at the right time;
- Polio drops are given orally when the child is brought for DPT. These drops are to be given when the child is 1½, 2½ and 3½ month of age;
- BCG injection is given for protection against tuberculosis to the infant at birth—only one injection is enough.

So little care, so big a protection

Application to Nursing

The knowledge of immunology is extremely essential for the professional nurse in her day-to-day practice and is of great importance, particularly, for the public health nurse. Public health nursing can be very effective, if the nurse could teach about the basic facts of immunology – why the administration of specific antigens are important to the health of the children, and how the epidemics are controlled, and how the susceptible individuals can be protected against the dreadful diseases. One of the frequent responsibilities of the nurse is the administration of antigens and antibodies (immune sera). While shouldering this responsibility she should be able to intelligently understand what are to be administrated with precaution, their adverse reactions, and the expected results of the immunisation.

In conducting the field trial programme of a newly developed vaccine, the nurse is one of the important members of the team to find out the efficacy of the administration of the antigens. Besides this, the nurse has a great role to collect data and to convince the people to participate in the full programme by explaining them in explicit clear local language. Because of her sound knowledge of immunology and immunisation schedule, she will be able to communicate the parents the importance and necessity of repeated childhood vaccination at fixed time interval and about the blood collection for the evaluation of antibody titres in the blood after vaccination.

In public health nursing; since the nurse is always in touch with the public; she will be the first person to recognise the necessity of active and passive immunisation in an individual, family, community. For this important and quick decision, she should be well equipped with the essential knowledge of immunity and she can transmit this information to the higher authority who will be responsible for the immunisation of the public living in that situation.

The nurse is always on the *frontline* and comes in close contact with the patients because of the nature of her work and she is always at the risk of getting infected with the communicable diseases during epidemics. Therefore, she should maintain the highest degree of protection against all these diseases for her own good health and life—by regular immunisation.

21
Transplantation, Tumour Immunology and Graft Rejection

Transplantation is a useful procedure in surgical repair on replacement of diseased tissues or organs.

It has been well-established that an animal accepts grafts of its own tissue or that of an identical twin, while a graft from another animal of the same species is rejected. The immune response induced by the *transplantation* (HLA) *antigens* present in all mammalian cells is the reason for the rejection of exogenous grafts. The first record of plastic surgery is found in Sushrut Sanhita (800 BC). The first Indian surgeon Sushruta reconstructed a severed nose of a patient with the patient's own skin flap. Transplantation may be fresh organs or stored organs in *orthotopic* grafts, the transplant is applied in anastomosed normal site (eg. skin graft), whereas *heterotopic* grafts are placed in anatomically abnormal sites (eg. thyroid transplanted in subcutaneous tissue).

Types of transplant

1. *Autograft* (Autogenic graft). It is a tissue of one site engrafted to another site in the same individual.
2. *Isograft* (Syngenetic graft). It is a graft placed in another individual of the same genetic constitution (e.g. monozygous twins or members of inbred strains).
3. *Allograft* (Homograft or allogeneic graft). It is a graft transfer between two genetically different members of the same species.
4. *Xeno graft* (Xenogeneic graft). Grafts between members of different species are called xenograft. It was formerly known as heterograft.

   Autograft and isograft are usually accepted and survives causing a minimum inflammatory reaction. Allografts and xenografts usually undergo necrosis and are rejected due to genetic and antigenic incompatibility.

Allograft reaction

Rejection of the *graft* by *recipient* is called *allograft reaction.* The most successful organ transplant is that of kidney. Other organ transplants such as bone marrow has been tried but with little success.

Mechanism of transplant rejection

Changes observed in human renal allograft rejection is almost similar to that observed in mice:

1. The graft becomes *vascularised* within a few days and appears to be accepted initially.
2. Between 3-9 days, there is increasing infiltration of the graft by *lymphocytes* and *monocytes* with *marked reduction in circulation*. At this stage, very few plasma cells invade the graft.
3. Between 10-11 days, the necrosis begins to be visible to the naked eye.
4. On 12th or 13th day, the graft *sloughs* off completely.

Cell mediated reaction is almost responsible for the rejection. Rejection is brought by helper T cells which activate cytotoxic T cells, macrophages and B cells when *second allograft* from the same donor is applied on a sensitised recipient, it will be rejected in 5-6 days. In this accelerated rejection of second graft second set reaction, antibodies play an important role along with cell-mediated immunity. Antibodies are formed abundantly from the 11th day onward of transplantation.

Thus a graft is rejected either by sensitised T cells or by circulating antibodies. Antibody induces platelet aggregation or type II hypersensitivity reaction (ADCC), Antibody Dependent cell mediated cytotoxicity.

Tissue typing and matching

ABO compatibility is essential in all tissue transplantation. Survival of an allograft depends on *HLA compatibility*. HLA antigens are expressed on the surface of leucocytes (especially lymphoid cells). A full HLA type of an individual contains two haplotypes (*haplotype*—one strand of chromosome pair), inherited from each parent. There is reasonable opportunity for genetic matching of siblings of a patient, 25% chance for both haplotypes and 50% chance of one haplotype. With many HLA antigens discovered, there is possibility of thousand halotypes. There is a remote chance that two random individuals will have completely identical haplotypes. The best HLA compatible donors are selected from the family members.

1. *Leucocytes grouping* : The HLA antigens of class I type on leucocytes are identified by sera obtained from

   (i) multiparous women who usually possess antibodies to HLA antigens of their husbands

   (ii) recipient of multiple blood transfusion

   (iii) volunteers who are repeatedly skin grafted

   (iv) monoclonal antibodies prepared against HLA antigens.

   Cytotoxic test: A purified suspension of blood lymphocytes of donor is mixed with the recipient's serum and a panel of standard sera for HLA antigens in presence of complement.

   When lymphocytes carry the appropriate antigens, the cytotoxic antiserum will combine with the lymphocytes (target cell). The antigen-antibody complex will activate the complement and damage the cell membrane and the permeability of cell membrane is increased and the same is detected by dye (trypan blue) uptake into the cell, i.e. the dead cells are stained by the dye.

2. *Mixed leucocyte culture test:* The test detects class II antigens of HLA complex and cell mediated immunity. Lymphocytes from both donors and recipients are cultured together (co-cultivation). The test is based on the principle that T-lymphocytes—when exposed

to incompatible HLA antigen—undergo blastoid transformation, take up thymidine and divide.

3. *Lymphocyte transfer test :* Peripheral blood lymphocytes of recipient is injected intradermally into several prospective donors. Delayed hypersensitivity reaction at the injection site is indicative of immune response of recipient leucocytes against the donor tissue. Persons showing no response against recipient's leucocytes is chosen as donor.
4. *Detection of preformed antibody :* Donor's lymphocytes are matched with recipient's serum. If preformed antibodies are present in patient's serum, the lymphocytes of the donor undergo lysis.

Prevention of graft rejection

1. *Immuno-suppression :* When HLA typing of the recipient and donor is well-matched, a state of immuno-suppression is produced in the recipient so that the transplant tissue survives for a long time.
   By irradiation, corticosteroids and anti lymphocytic serum (ALS) the immunological reactivity may be non-specifically depressed. Such patients are susceptible to infections and prone to development of lymphomas.
2. *Transplantation in anatomically protected sites:* There are certain anatomically protected sites where allografts are permitted to survive, eg. cornea, cartilage and testicle grafting. The avascularity of cornea limits the entry of lymphocytes into the graft.
3. *Immunological enhancement:* The circulating antibody produced against graft antigens can—under circumstances—protect the graft from cell mediated immune response. This phenomenon is known as *"Immunological enhancement"*. If the recipient animal is previously immunised with one or more injections of tissue from the prospective donor and transplant applied subsequently, the transplant survives for longer duration. Following transplantation of kidney in rats by this method, the graft maintains normal function for a year or more. The immunological enhancement phenomenon can be passively transferred from immunised animal to a normal animal. In certain human kidney transplantations, the method has been used with some success.

22
Tumour Immunity
(Immune Response to Tumours)

With malignant transformation, cancer cells express a range of antigens, some of which are found in normal cells while others are tumour associated antigens which are immunologically distinct from normal tissue antigens (histocompatibility antigens) of the host—which the host recognises as "nonself". A cancer, therefore, behaves as an allograft and induces an immune response. However, immune response against cancer cells is weak. Immune response to tumour antigens offers some degree of resistance to the patient which may result in partial regression of the tumour.

Evidence of immune mechanism in malignancy

1. Patients with certain immuno-deficiency disorder (e.g. congenital immuno-deficiency states) and patients undergoing chronic immuno-suppressive therapy seem to be more prone to increased incidence of cancer—particularly of the mononuclear phagocyte (i.e. lymphomas).
2. Spontaneous regression metastases after surgical removal of the primary tumour or recovery that sometimes follow chemotherapy of choriocarcinoma and Burkitt's lymphoma—they suggest the role of tumour immunity. Spontaneous regression of tumour has been observed with neuroblastoma and malignant melanoma.
3. The phenomenon of immunological enhancement in tumour transplants.
4. Evidence of anti-tumour reactions are found in certain cancers by the presence of lymphocytes, plasma cells and macrophages after infiltrating the stroma simulating the cellular response of allograft reactions.

Tumour antigens

Tumour specific antigens are present on the membrane of cancer cells. When syngenic animal is injected with such tumour specific antigens which reject the human transplant in immunised hosts, it is referred to as *Tumour Specific Transplantation Antigen* (TSTA).

In human beings, few tumours are caused by viruses. It is now evident that, in most cases of tumours, there is genetic alterations such as mutation, gene amplification, chromosomal deletion or translocation. Some of these genetic alterations lead to expression of altered proteins in tumour cells which probably serve as antigenic targets for mounting immune responses by the host.

Viruses causing human tumours

Virus	Tumour
Hepatitis B	Liver cancer
Human papilloma viruses (HPV 16 and 18)	Cervical cancer
Epstein-Barr virus	Burkitt's lymphoma and lymphomas in immuno-suppression
Epstein-Barr virus	Nasopharyngeal Carcinoma—Adult
Human T-cell leukemia virus (HTLV-1)	T-cell Leukaemia

Tumour associated transplantation antigens (TATAS)

There are two types of TATAS

1. *Shared tumour antigens.* These antigens are shared by many tumours. They are found on tumours induced by viruses e.g. small DNA of polyoma viruses, SY 40 viruses and the papilloma viruses.

2. *Tumour specific transplantation antigens* (TSTA)

These antigens specific to an individual tumour can provoke an immune response to injected tumour cells, but only if the animal has been previously immunised with the same tumour.

The following are considered as the immunological expression of tumours:

Virally induced antigens: virus induced tumour cells express three types of antigens:

(a) "V" antigen is associated with the virion.

(b) Tumour (T) or nuclear antigen is located in the nucleus of infected tumour cells and are specific for inducing virus and not the tumour.

(c) TSTA antigen or cytoplasmic membrane antigens are important as these come in contact with immune system. All tumours induced by specific virus contain the same TSTA even when the tumours are in different animal species. This is in contrast to the case with chemically induced tumours in which TSTA is private (tumour specific) to a particular neoplasm, i.e. different tumours produced by a single chemical possess different antigens.

(II) *Embryonic antigens :* Certain tumours in adults contain antigen found in foetal or embryonic cells but not corresponding normal adult cells, e.g. Carcino Embryonic Antigen (CEA) detected in serum of patients with neoplasm of gut (colonic cancers) and *alpha feto-proteins* present in serum of patients with hepatoma and testicular embryonic carcinoma. The *carcinoembryonic antigen* (CEA) is a *glycoprotein.* In some malignancies, a metabolic shift of the cancerous cell from an adult to immature pathway of protein synthesis occurs leading to rise of embryonic Ag in serum. As CEA also appears in serum of patients with alcoholic cirrhosis, its detection has limited diagnostic value. *Alpha feto-protein* (alphaglobulin) is produced by normal foetal (embryonic) hepatocytes and its serum level sharply declines after birth and is virtually absent in normal adult blood. It appears in blood in high concentration in hepatic carcinoma.

(III) *Idiotypic antigen :* As already mentioned, tumours induced by chemical agents (e.g. benzopyrene) possess tumour specific (provate) own idiotypic antigen. For example, two anatomically distinct tumours induced on a single animal (mouse) by one chemical carcinoma will contain two antigenically distinct TSTA.

Mechanism of immune response to tumours

Resistance to tumour growth is offered primarily by cell mediated immunity. Specific tumour resistance can be passively transferred to normal animal using lymphoid cells from immunised animals. The sensitised T-cells attack the foreign tumour cells and tend to limit their growth. The transferred natural killer cells can also kill some of the tumour cells in absence of antibody.

The tumour antigens also induce humoral antibody production and some of these antibodies may be cytotoxic while others may facilitate the tumour growth by interfering with recognition and disposal of tumour cells by cell-mediated immunity of the host. Such interfering antibodies may produce an enhancement of tumour growth.

Immune surveillance

It is held that malignant cells arise by mutation of somatic cells that occur frequently in the body. The concept of *immune surveillance*—first proposed by Ehrlich (1909) and by Burnet (1970)—stated that the immune system keeps a constant vigilance on each type of malignant mutation of somatic cells of individuals and destroy them on the spot. Accordingly, the development of tumours represent an escape from this surveillance. This is perhaps an over-simplication of a complicated issue. If this view was fully true there would have been higher incidence of tumours on patients receiving immuno-suppressive therapy.

SYSTEMATIC BACTERIOLOGY

According to the morphology and staining reaction, lower bacteria can be divided into :

(1) **LOWER BACTERIA** (2) HIGHER BACTERIA Actinomyces israelii

- **COCCI**
  - Gram-positive
    - Staphylococcus aureus
    - Staph. albus
    - Staph. citreus
    - Streptococcus pyogenes
    - Strep. viridans
    - Streptococcus pneumoniae
    - Gaffkya tetragena
    - Sarcina lutea
  - Gram-negative
    - Neisseria meningitidis
    - Neisseria gonorrhoeae
- (A) **NON SPORULATING BACILLI**
  - Gram-positive
    - Corynebacterium diphtheriae
    - Listeria monocytogenes
    - Mycobacterium tuberculosis (Acid fast bacilli)
  - Gram-negative
    - Bordetella pertussis
    - Salmonella typhi
    - Salmonella paratyphi
    - Shigella dysenteriae
    - Escherichia coli
    - Proteus vulgaris
    - Klebsiella pneumoniae
    - Pseudomonas pyocyanea
    - Vibrio cholerae
    - Yersinia pestis
    - Brucella abortus
    - Bacteroides fragilis
- **SPIROCHAETES, VIBRIOS SPIRILLA** (Gram-negative)
  - Treponema pallidum
  - Borrelia recurrentis
  - Leptospira

(B) **SPORE FORMING BACILLI**

- **AEROBIC**
  - Bacillus anthracis
- **ANAEROBIC**
  - Clostridium welchii
  - Clostridium tetani
  - Clostridium botulinum

SECTION III
SYSTEMATIC BACTERIOLOGY

23
Staphylococci, Streptococci
(Dental abscess) (Localised abscess)

The Staphylococci are Gram-positive cells arranged in grape like clusters, cause suppuration, abscess formation, pyogenic infection, osteomyelitis, septicaemia, Toxic Shock Syndrome (TSS), food poisoning. There are about 20 species of Staphylococci.

Morphology and Staining : Staphylococci (Fig. 23.1) are spherical, 1 μ in diameter, arranged in clusters. Single cocci, pairs, tetrads and chains are also seen in liquid cultures. Young cocci are stained strongly Gram-positive, old ones may become Gram-negative. They are non-motile and do not form spores.

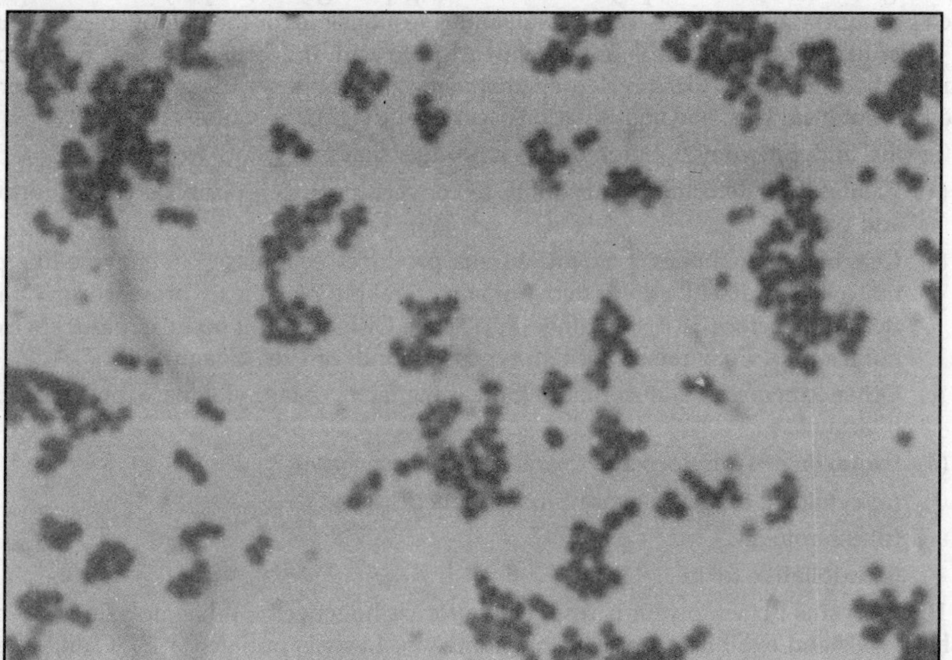

Fig. 23.1: Staphylococci (1000X) in cluster

Cultural characteristics : They grow readily on most of the bacteriological media under aerobic or microaerophilic condition at 37°C but form pigment at room temperature (20-25°C). The pigment is believed to be a liporprotein allied to carotene. **Staph**. **aureus** forms deep golden-yellow colonies; **Staph. albus** colonies are white, and those of **Staph. citreus** are lemon-yellow. On milk agar the pigment is intense. No pigment is produced anaerobically or in broth. On nutrient agar slant, their growth presents "oil paint" appearance. On blood agar, most strains are haemolytic and produce B type haemolysis. Similar pink colonies are seen on

MacConkey's medium (Fig. 5.14) due to lactose fermentation. For primary isolation, sheep blood agar is recommended rather than human blood agar as human blood contains antibodies of inhibitors.

Biochemical reactions: Staphylococci ferment a number of sugars with acid only. **Staph aureus** ferments mannitol which is of diagnostic value to differentiate from **Staph. albus.** It is catalase positive unlike Streptococci, hydrolyses urea, reduces nitrate to nitrite, liquefies gelatin and Methyl Red (MR) and Voges Proskauer (VP) positive but Indole (I) negative. When grown on media containing egg yolk, **Staph. aureus** produces dense opaque colonies as they are proteolytic. By culturing on nutrient agar containing phenolphthalein diphosphate, the production of phosphatase can be demonstrated by exposing this culture to ammonia vapour. The colonies assume a bright pink colour due to presence of free phenolphthalein. This phosphatase test can distinguish **Staph. aureus** from **Staph. albus** in mixed culture.

Pathogenic **Staph. aureus** (1) coagulase positive, (2) ferments mannitol, (3) produces phosphatase, (4) liquefies gelatin, (5) produces β-haemolysis on blood agar, (6) produces golden-yellow pigment on nutrient agar, (7) produces black colonies on medium containing potassium tellurite by reducing potassium tellurite.

Antigenic structure : Staphylococci contain peptidoglycan, a polysaccharide polymer, which produces the rigidity to the cell wall and is responsible for the pathogenesis of infection and when this peptidoglycan is linked with teichoic acid, it is antigenic. Cell wall protein A with attached IgG molecule directed against a specific antigen will agglutinate bacteria that have that antigen. This "Coagglutination" test is of diagnostic value.

Toxins and Enzymes : Staphylococci produce enzymes and toxins.

(a) **Catalase :** is detected by its ability to convert hydrogen peroxide (H_2O_2) into water and oxygen.

(b) **Coagulase :** Pathogenic **Staph. aureus** produces coagulase, an enzyme-like protein that clots oxalated or citrated human or rabbit plasma in presence of Coagulase Reacting Factor (CRF) contained in plasma. CRF does not occur in other species (e.g. guinea pig). Coagulase is of two types—Bound, or Free Coagulase.

(c) **Other enzymes :** Hyaluronidase (Spreading factor), staphylokinase, proteinase, lipase, β-lactamase.

(d) **Exotoxin :** Staphylococcal toxins are of three types:

(a) cytotoxic toxins (haemolysin and leucocidin);

(b) enterotoxin;

(c) exfoliative toxin.

Haemolysins : Haemolysin is responsible for pathogenecity; β-haemolysin is haemolytic to sheep cells and exhibits a hot cold phenomenon; Lysis is initiated at 37°C and is evident only on chilling; gamma lysin—the weakest—acts on human, sheep, rabbit erythrocytes; delta lysin is lytic to human cells; alpha and delta lysin are found in human strains of Staphylococci; while beta lysin is from strain of bovine origin.

Leucocidin is lethal to white blood cells.

Enterotoxin : There are six soluble enterotoxins (A-F)—produced by **Staph. aureus.** Ingestion of 25 μg of preformed enterotoxin B causes food poisoning-nausea, vomiting, diarrhoea within six hours. Toxic shock syndrome toxin 1 (TSST-1)—which is same as enterotoxin F and pyrogenic exotoxin C—is associated with fever, shock, and multisystem involvement including a desquamative skin rash.

Exfoliative toxin produces generalised desquamation of the staphylococcal scaled skin syndrome.

Pathogenicity and clinical features : Staphylococci cause pyogenic lesions in man; furuncles, stye, boils, abscess, carbuncle, impetigo, pemphigus, neonatorum, sepsis in wound, burn, breast abscess, nosocomial infection, deep infection (osteomyelitis, tonsillitis) pharyngitis, sinusitis, pneumonia). Staphylococcal food poisoning results due to consumption of preformed toxin elaborated by Staph. aureus on contaminated food-nausea, vomiting, diarrhoea. In bullous impetigo, pemphigus neonatorum, Ritter's disease, toxic epidermal necrolysis, there is stripping of superficial layers of skin. In TSS, there is multisystem/illness characterised by acute onset of high fever, hypotension, vomiting, diarrhoea and rash with desquamation. Severe cases may lead to acute renal failure. It is associated with the use of tampon of menstruating women.

Table 23.1. Infections caused by Staph. aureus

Group	Lesions
Superficial infection	
Skin infection	Pustules, boil, carbuncle, abscess, styes, impetigo, pemphigus, neonatorum, sepsis in wounds and burns
Deep infection	
Bone and joint	Osteomyelitis, septic arthritis,
Respiratory tract	Tonsillitis, pharyngitis, pneumonia, lung abscess, empyema, suppurative mouth lesions (dental abscess) localised oral abscess,
Intestinal	Enterocolitis
Cardiac	Endocarditis, pericarditis
Central nervous system	Meningitis, brain abscess
Blood stream	Septicaemia, pyaemic abscess
Toxin associated infection	
Toxin food poisoning	Ingestion of preformed toxin in food
Skin exfoliation	Stripping of superficial layer of skin from underlying tissue by exfoliative (epidermolytic) toxin
Toxic shock syndrome	TSS is a syndrome caused by enterotoxin E produced by Staph. aureus

Laboratory diagnosis

(a) **Specimens :** Surface swab, blood, tracheal aspirate or spinal fluid for culture depending upon the localisation of the process.

(b) **Smear :** Typical staphylococci are seen in stained smears of pus or sputum. It is not possible to distinguish morphologically Staph. aureus from other Staphylococci.

(c) **Culture :** Specimens planted on blood agar plates give rise to typical colonies in 18 hours at 37°C, but haemolysis and pigment production may not occur until several days later and are optimal at room temperature. Specimens contaminated with bacterial flora can be cultured on media containing 10% NaCl; the salt inhibits most other normal flora but not Staph. aureus.

(d) **Catalase test** is carried out by placing one drop of H_2O_2 solution on a slide and mixing it with a small amount of bacterial growth. The formation of bubbles (the release of O_2) indicates positive test.

(e) **Coagulase test** may be of two types : (1) Slide test; (2) Tube test.

(1) **Slide test :** detects "bound" coagulase. From an agar plate, the organism is emulsified in two drops of saline placed on a slide. If no spontaneous agglutination,

a drop of undiluted human or rabbit plasma is added to one of the emulsions and mixed gently. Prompt clumping indicates the presence of bound coagulase. False positive results are caused by citrate utilising bacteria, enterococci, pseudomonas.

(2) **Tube test,** citrated rabbit (or human) plasma diluted 1 : 5 is mixed with an equal amount of broth culture and incubated at 37°C. A tube of plasma mixed with sterile broth is included as a control. If clots form in 1-4 hours, the test is positive and detects free coagulase liberated by pathogenic **Staph. aureus.**

(f) **Serological and phage typing tests.** The serology has little practical value; the phage typing is used for epidemiological study.

Bacteriophage typing. Staph. aureus strains are distinguished by their susceptibility pattern to lysis by different phages. A set of over 28 bacteriophages are employed, most strains are lysed by more than one phage. Thus, several hundred phages of *Staph. aureus* can be identified. The phages are divided into five groups :

Group I 29, 52, 52 A, 79, 80

Group II 3A, 3B, 3C, 55, 71

Group III 6, 7, 42E, 47, 53, 54, 75, 77, 83A, 84, 85

Group IV 42D

Group V 94, 96

Phage typing technique : The strain of *staph. aureus* to be tested is inoculated on a nutrient agar plate to produce a "Lawn" culture by a four hour growth and the plate is dried. Then a set of over 28 phages are applied over marked areas in a routine dilution (RTD) in a quantity of 0.2 ml each. The plate is incubated overnight. The culture will be seen to be lysed by a phage or a number of phages denoting the phage type of the particular strain of *staph. aureus.* Phage types are designated according to the phages capable of lysing the bacterial strain. The phage types prevalent in most parts of India are 52/52 A/80/81. (Staphylococcal Phage Reference Laboratory, Department of Microbiology, Maulana Azad Medical College, New Delhi).

Control measures

1. Source isolation.
2. Detection of staphylococcal lesion and carriage among doctor, nurses and other staff and their isolation and treatment.
3. Sterilisation of instruments and disinfection of the environment.
4. Regular use of antiseptics of skin and wounds of patients and the hands of nursing staff.
5. Judicious use of antibiotics.

Staph. aureus is usually sensitive to flucloxacillin, erythromycin, lincomycin, vancomycin and cephalosporins and many develop rapidly drug resistance. Eighty per cent of the hospital strains are at present pencillin resistant. It also shows multiple drug resistance and chronic infection should be treated by more than one drug.

Penicillin resistance is due to *beta lactamase* production which is plasmid-coded and transmitted by transduction.

Multiple drug resistance. Several drug resistance *genes* present in a single plasmid are responsible.

Treatment. As drug resistance is so common among Staphylococci, the appropriate antibiotic should be chosen by antibiotic sensitivity test.

24

Streptococcus Pyogenes

CLASSIFICATION OF STREPTOCOCCI

STREPTOCOCCUS

O_2 requirement

↓

Aerobes and **facultative anaerobes** | **Obligate anaerobes** Peptostreptococci

↓

Haemolysis

↓

Alpha-haemolytic
(The viridans group)
classified into species by
physiological and biochemical properties

3. Gamma-haemolytic
The enterococcus group
classified into species by physiological
and biochemical properties

2. Beta-haemolytic
(The haemolytic streptococci)
Serological Grouping (Polysaccharide C)
20 Lancefield groups (ABCDEFGHKLMNOPQRSTUV)
Group A – **Streptococcus pyogenes**
↓
Serological typing (M protein)
Griffith types (1, 2, 3 etc. up to 80)

The streptococci are Gram-positive spherical or oval bacteria that form short or long chains. They are associated with important human diseases (tonsllitis, respiratory infection, skin infection, genital, suppurative and non-suppurative infections (rheumatic fever, glomerulonephritis).

Morphology and staining : Individual cocci are spherical (0.5-1 μ in diameter) and arranged in chains (Fig. 24.1). The lengths of chains are variable. The chains are longer in liquid than in solid media. Streptococci are Gram-positive. As the culture ages, they loose their Gram-positivity and appear to be Gram-negative. They are non-motile non-sporulating. Some strain of group A and C have capsules composed of hyaluronic acid. Hair-like pili project through the capsule of group A Streptococci and are important in the attachment of streptococci to epithelial cells.

Cultural characteristics : They grow on solid media as discoid colonies—usually 1-2 mm

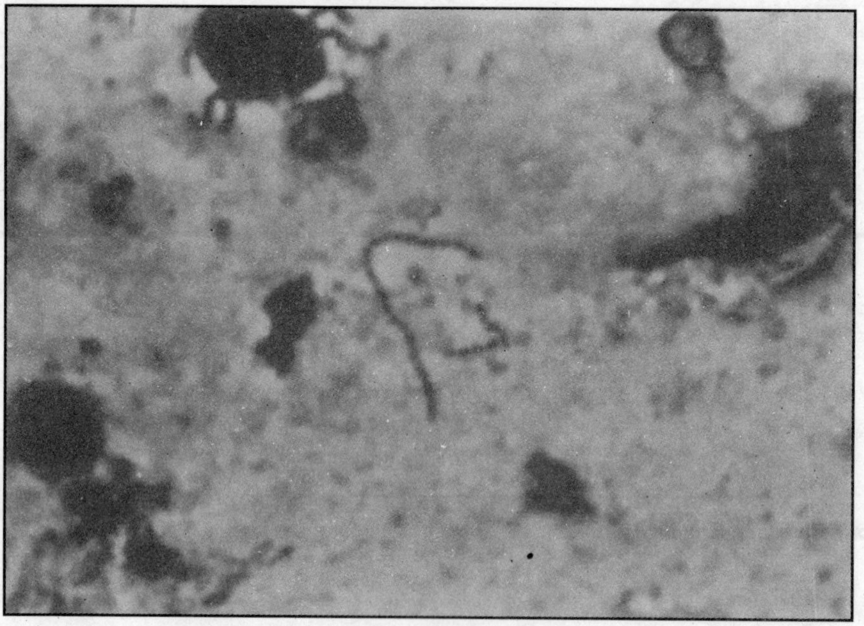

Fig. 24.1: Streptococcus pyogenes (1000X) in chain

in diameter. Group A strains that produce capsular material often given rise to mucoid colonies. They are aerobic; and facultative anaerobic grow best at 37°C. They grow only in media enriched with blood or serum. On blood agar, after 24 hours incubation at 10% CO_2, colonies are small (0.5-1 mm), circular, semi-transparent, low convex discs with an area of clear haemolysis around them. Virulent strains, strains isolated from lesions produce a "matt" (finest granular) colony, while avirulent strains form "glossy" colonies. In liquid media (glucose or serum broth) growth occurs as a granular turbidity with a powdery deposit. No pellicle is formed.

Biochemical reaction : Streptococci ferment several sugars producing an acid but no gas. Fermentation of sugars has been replaced by serological grouping. They are catalase negative and not soluble in 10% bile, unlike pneumococci.

Antigenic structure : Streptococci are grouped into alpha (**Str. viridans),** beta (**Str. pyogenes),** and gamma (**Str. faecalis)** haemolytic streptococci : Haemolytic streptococci can be classified into 20 serological groups (A-V except I, J) on the basis of the nature of carbohydrate 'C' antigen. The majority of haemolytic streptococci that produce human infection belong to group A—known as **Str. pyogenes.** Streptococci from primary isolation plates can be grouped by a recent Reverse Passive Haemagglutination (RPHA) technique.

Toxins and enzymes : More than 20 extra-cellular products that are produced by group A streptococci include streptokinase, streptodornase, hyaluronidase, erythrogenic toxin, diphosphopyridine nucleotidase, haemolysin.

Erythrogenic toxin is soluble and destroyed by boiling for 1 hour. It causes rash in scarlet fever. Only lysogenic strains elaborating this toxin cause scarlet fever. This toxin is antigenic and is neutralised by antibody found in convalescent sera. This property has been used in the diagnosis of scarlet fever (Dick test and Schultz Charlton reaction) which is no longer a common disease.

Haemolysin : Beta haemolytic streptococci of group A elaborate two haemolysins (Streptolysins).

Streptolysin O is a protein which combines with antistreptolysin O, an antibody that appears in human following infection with any streptococci. This antibody blocks haemolysis by streptolysin O and form a basis of a quantitative test for the antibody. An anti-streptolysin O (ASO) serum titre in excess of 160-200 units is considered high and suggests recent infection.

Streptolysin S is responsible for haemolysis on blood agar medium and is not antigenic.

Table 24.1. Group classification of beta haemolytic and other antigenically related streptococci — Pathogenesis and clinical features

Group	Haemolytic	Specific name	Main habitat	Pathogenicity
A	β	Str. pyogenes	Man	Many human diseases
B	β (NH, α)	Str. agalactiae	Man	Neonatal meningitis
C	β	Str. equi	Cattle Horse	Mastitis
	β	Str. equisimilis	Many animals	Respiratory infection
	β		Man	
	β	Str. dysgalactiae	Cattle	Bacteriaemia
		Str. zooepidemicus	Many animals	Endocarditis
D	(Enterococci)			
	NH, β	Str. faecalis	Man, animal	UTI wound infection
	α NH	Str. faecium	plant	Endocarditis
	NH, α, β	Str. durans	Milk, dairy product	Endocarditis
D	(Non-enterococci)			
	β (NH, α)	Str. ruis	Pig	Pyogenic lesion
	NH α	Str. bovis	Animal gut	
	α	Str. equinus	Horse	
N	NH, β	Lactic streptococci	Milk, dairy	
EFGH (KU) mainly β			products primarily occur in animals	

NH-Non-haemolytic

(1) **Erysipelas :** When haemolytic group A streptococci enter the skin, erysipelas results with massive brawny oedema and a rapidly advancing margin of infection.

(2) **Puerperal fever :** If they enter the uterus after delivery, puerperal fever develops, which is essentially septicaemia.

(3) **Sepsis :** Infection of surgical wound results in surgical scarlet fever.

(4) **Sore throat :** When they adhere to the pharyngeal epithelium by means of their pili, the sore throat occurs.

(5) **Pyoderma :** Local infection of superficial layers of skin in children is called impetigo. It consists of superficial blisters that break down and erode areas whose denuded surface is covered with pus and or crust.

Infective endocarditis : In course of acute bacteriaemia, beta haemolytic streptococci and pneumococci may settle on normal or previously deformed heart valve and produce acute endocarditis. Rapid destruction of the valve leads to fatal cardiac failure.

Subacute endocarditis involves abnormal valves (congenital deformities and rheumatic lesions).

Post-streptococcal disease (Rheumatic fever, glomerulonephritis) Following an acute infection, there is a latent period of 1-4 weeks after which nephritis or rheumatic fever occasionally develops. Nephritis is more commonly preceded by the infection of the skin; rheumatic fever, by infection of the respiratory tract.

Table 24.1. Streptococcal diseases

Group	Lesions
1. Str.pyogenes	
(a) **Suppurative lesions**	
Respiratory tract	Sore throat and tonsillitis
	Scarlet fever
Skin and soft tissue infections	Impetigo, erysipelas
	Infections of wound, burns and chronic skin lesions (eczema, psoriasis)
Genital infection	Puerperal sepsis
Deep infection	Bone and joint infections
	Lymphadenitis
	Septicaemia, acute endocarditis
	Abscess in internal organs, Localised dental abscess
(b) **Non-suppurative complications**	
Heart	Rheumatic fever
Kidney	Acute glomerulonephritis
2. Str. faecalis (enterococci)	Endocarditis
	Urinary tract infection
3. Viridans streptococci (Str. mitis, sanguis, mutans, salivarius)	Endocarditis
4. Group B Streptococci	Neonatal infection (pneumonia, meningitis, respiratory disease).

(1) **Acute Glomerulonephritis** may be initiated by antigen antibody complexes on the glomerular basement membrane. In acute nephritis, there is blood, protein in the urine, oedema, high blood pressure and urea nitrogen retention; serum complements are low. Some patients develop chronic glomerulonephritis with ultimate kidney failure.

(2) **Rheumatic fever** : Certain strains of group A streptococci contain cell membrane antigens that react with human heart tissue antigens, thereby heart muscle and valves are damaged. Typical symptoms and signs of rheumatic fever include fever, malaise, polyarthritis and carditis.

Table 24.3 Differential characteristics of glomerulonephritis and rheumatic fever

	Actue rheumatic fever	Actue nephritis
Primary infection	Throat	Skin or throat
Latent period	Longer (2-5 weeks)	Shorter (1-3 weeks)
Prior sensitisation	Essential	Not necessary
Str. pyogenes serotypes	Types 5, 18 and 24 are notable	Pyoderma types types 49, 52, 53, 54 and 57-61. Throat infection types, types 12, 21, 25, 4 and 3
Repeated attacks	Common	Absent
Manifestation Pathology	Swelling of joints and pericarditis	Haematuria, albuminuria, oedema,
	Connective tissue disease typical lesion in "Aschoff nodule"	Increased cellularity of glomeruli with larger deposits on outer and smaller deposit on inner surface, deposit on inner surface of basement membrane

Pathogenesis (immune mechanism)	Antibodies produced against protein and polysaccharide cross react with myocardial and heart valve tissue	It may be due to antigenic cross-reaction between glomerular membrane antigen and some component of nephritogenic streptococci or more often due to immune complexes formed by combination of antistreptococcal antigens already present on basement membrane or in circulating blood to be deposited later on basement membrane often formation of immune complex
Immune response (ASO titre)	Marked (ASO titre 200 or more is significant	Moderate, ASO titre may be low
Complement level course	Unaffected	Lowered
Prognosis	Progressive	Spontaneous resolution
Penicillin	Variable	Good
Prophylaxis	Essential	Not indicative

Laboratory diagnosis

A. **Specimens :** Throat swab, pus or blood is obtained for culture and serum for serology.

B. **Smears :** Smears from pus show Gram-positive cocci in chains; cocci which are no longer viable are sometimes Gram-negative.

C. **Culture :** They are grown on Blood agar medium. Incubation in 10% CO_2 often speeds haemolysis. Blood cultures in cases of suspected endocarditis may turn positive after a week or longer as alpha haemolytic streptococci and enterococci may grow slowly.

Serological tests : Several commercial kits are available for rapid detection of group A streptococci antigen from throat swab. ELISA and agglutination tests can demonstrate the presence of antigen. These tests can be completed in 1-4 hours after the specimen is obtained. They are more sensitive and specific when compared to culture test.

In respiratory disease, a rise in titre of antibodies can be estimated by ASO titre which is most widely used. In skin infection, antihyaluronidase test is useful.

The streptozyme test is passive slide haemagglutination test using erythrocytes sensitised with a crude preparation of extracellular antigen of streptococci. It is a sensitive specific screening test for skin or throat infection.

Treatment : They are sensitive to penicillin, erythromycin. Antimicrobial drugs have no effect on glomerulonephritis and rheumatic fever.

25

Streptococcus Pneumoniae (Pneumococcus)

The pneumococci are Gram-positive diplococci, often lancet shaped, cause lobar pneumonia, sinusitis, otitis, bronchitis, bacteriaemia, meningitis.

Morphology and staining : They are Gram-positive lancet shaped diplococci, often seen in young cultures. Also in sputum, pus, single cocci or chains. With age, the organisms become Gram-negative and tend to lyse spontaneously.

Cultural characteristics : They are aerobic and facultative anaerobic. They grow best in enriched media at 37°C. Growth is improved by 5-10% CO_2. On blood agar, after incubation for 18 hours, the colonies are small (0.5-1 mm) dome shaped and glistening with an area of alpha haemolysis which causes confusion with *Str. viridans*. The colonies are at first plateau shaped, later develop elevated margins and concentric ridges—draughtsman colony. Green pigmentation is more obvious when the organism is growing on heated blood agar.

Biochemical reaction : They ferment various sugars, differ from *Str. viridans* by frequently fermenting inulin. They are catalase- and oxidase-negative.

Bile solubility : Pneumococci are soluble in bile. The test consists of adding 1 part of sterilised 10% solution of sodium taurocholate in normal saline to 10 parts of broth culture and incubating at 37°C. Pneumococci are lysed within 15 minutes.

Optochin sensitivity : Pneumococci are sensitive to optochin (hydrocuprein hydrochloride). They are tested by making radial stock cultures on a blood agar plate and by placing in the centre of the plate a sterile disk of filter paper impregnated in optochin. Pneumococci are inhibited in a zone of at least 5 mm from the circumference of the disk.

Antigenic structure : At least 80 specific serotypes have been recognised by "capsular swelling reaction or Quellung reaction." In this technique a loopful of broth culture is mixed with a loopful of diagnostic antiserum and the mixture is covered with a coverslip and examined under oil immersion lens, the substage condenser is lowered and diaphagm partially closed. The capsule swells markedly and the sharpness of the capsule is more significant.

Pathogenicity and clinical features : Pneumococci produce no toxin and the disease onsets through its ability to multiply in the tissues. Their virulence is a function of its capsule. The onset of pneumococcal pneumonia is usually sudden with fever, chill and sharp pleural pain. The sputum is bloody or rusty. Empyema (pus in the pleural cavity) is a significant complication.

Table 25.1 Distinguishing features of Pneumococcus and Viridans Streptococci

Properties	Pneumococcus	Viridans streptococci
Morphology	Capsulated, Lanceolate diplococci	Non-capsulated oval or round cells in short chain
Colony on blood organ	Raised and circular initially, later "draughtsman" colonies	Dome shaped
Bile solubility	Lysis of pneumococci	Negative
Optochin sensitivity	Sensitive	Resistant
Inulin fermentation	Ferments	Does not ferment
Animal pathogenecity (Intraperitoneal inoculation in mice)	Fatal infection	Non-pathogenic
Human infection	Lobar pneumonia	**Caries teeth** (common), in **dental pulp** and periapical infection (as major congenital or valvular cardiac defects—patients should be protected by penicillin before **dental attention**).

Lactobacillus acidophilus Bacillus acidophilus odontolyticeus : Dental caries This destructive condition is noted in earlier stages of discolouration of the **enamel of the tooth** and loss of translucency, cavity formation follows and, at the **dentino-enamel junction,** there is always lateral extension of the process with progressive softening of the **dentine.**

For many years, there have been differing opinions on the part played by bacteria, particularly lactobacillin **providing caries.** Their role has been confused with that of cariogenic food; even with such a diet, **caries** does not apparently occur in the absence of bacteria. Thus germ free rats do not develop caries with a cariogenic diet **unless streptococci, lactobacilli are added to the diet, then caries develops rapidly in the molar teeth.**

Lactobacilli count. It is known that there is quantitative difference in the number of lactobacilli in the mouths of those prone to caries in comparison with those who are apparently immune. The estimation of lactobacilli is of increasing importance in dentistry.

The saliva flow is activated by the person chewing a small piece of paraffin wax for ten minutes, saliva is collected in a sterile container as it is produced and the volume is made up to 10 ml. with sterile saline. Then Lactobacilli count is the numbers of lactobacilli present in 1 ml. of this standard specimen of the sample which is serially diluted in broth of peptone water and distributed in 0.1 ml. quantities on a selective medium for lactobacilli, eg. in Kulp's tomato peptone agar plates. After three or four days incubation at 37°C counts of more than 10^5 lactobacilli per ml of saliva are often taken as indicative of caries activity. In the same individual, significant reductions in this count are noted when a non-carcinogenic diet is taken.

Laboratory diagnosis : Blood is drawn for culture and sputum collection for demonstration of pneumococci by smear and culture. Serum antibody tests are impracticable.

The sputums may be examined in several ways:

(1) **Stained smears :** A Gram stained film of rusty red sputum shows typical organism.

(2) **Capsule swelling test :** Fresh emulsified sputum mixed with anti-serum gives capsule swelling reaction for identification of Pneumococci.

(3) **Culture :** Sputum cultures on blood agar and incubated in CO_2 or candle jar. Blood culture is also done.

(4) Animal (mouse) inoculation. Sputum is injected intra-peritoneally into the mouse. Animal dies in 18-48 hours. Heart blood gives pure culture of pneumococci.

(5) **Pneumolysin Polymerase Chain Reaction** (PCR) is sensitive; it is a specific new method to study pneumococcal acute otitis media.

(6) **Pneumococcal meningitis** is diagnosed by prompt examination and cultures of CSF.

Treatment : Pneumococci are sensitive to many antimicrobial drugs. Penicillin is the drug of choice.

Demonstration

1. A smear from culture (Gram stain) showing Gram-positive cocci in grape-like clusters (Fig. 23.1).
2. Growth of staphylococci on nutrient agar.
   (i) Staph. aureus produces golden yellow pigmented colonies;
   (ii) Staph. albus gives rise to white pigmented colonies;
   (iii) Staph. citreus gives rise to lemon yellow colonies.
3. Clear zone (B) haemolysis is produced by Staph. aureus in blood agar; haemolysis of rabbit red cell suspension can also be observed after addition of broth culture filtrate of Staph. aureus to rabbit red blood cells.
4. Tube and plate coagulase tests are to be observed.
5. Common staphylococcal lesions should be studied.
6. A smear from pus (Gram stain) showing Gram-positive cocci in long chains. (Fig. 24.1).
7. Haemolysis in blood agar medium:
   (a) Beta haemolysis (Clear zone) is produced by haemolytic streptococci;
   (b) Alpha haemolysis (Greenish discolouration around the colonies) by alpha haemolytic streptococci;
   (c) No change around the colonies by non-haemolytic streptococci.
8. Alpha haemolytic streptococcus is insoluble in 10% bile solution.
9. Common streptococcal lesions should be observed.
10. Smear showing Pneumococci with capsule.
11. Candle jar.

Practical Work : The pus smear should be stained by Gram method and the morphology of the organisms should be studied.

Questions

1. What is the importance of coagulase and bile solubility tests?
2. What is the chemical nature of pigment produced by *Staph.* aureus and why is it confined to the colony?
3. Describe the relationship of different staphyloccal toxins with lesions.

26
Neisseria

Neisseria is Gram-negative coccus arranged in pairs with long axes parallel and is strictly a human parasite. Neisseria gonorrhoeae (gonococcus) and N. meningitidis (meningococcus) are the two principal human pathogens.

Classification

I. Pathogenic 1. **N. gonorrhoeae** – causes gonorrhoea Greek word *gonos* (reed) and *rhoia* (flow)

2. **N. meningitidis** – causes pyogenic meningitis.

II. Non-pathogenic (commensals)

N. pharyngitidis (includes **N. flavo, N. sicca, N. perflava, N. subflava,** and other species.

Neisseria Gonorrhoeae (Gonococcus)

It is a causal agent of gonorrhoea, a venereal disease. **Morphology and Staining. N. gonorrhoeae** are Gram-negative non-motile diplococci, about 0.8 μ in diameter, and are intracellular—so pus cells are almost filled with gonococci (Fig. 26.1).

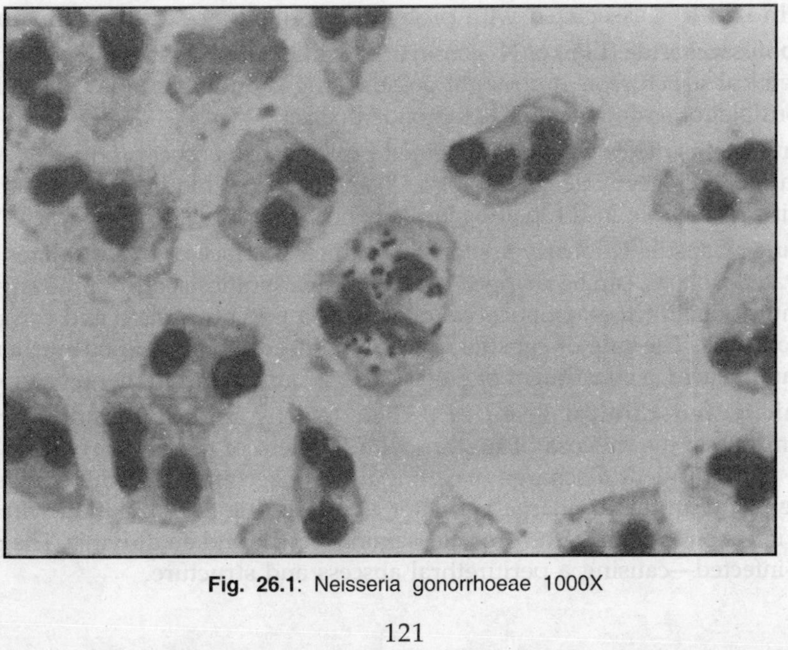

Fig. 26.1: Neisseria gonorrhoeae 1000X

Cultural Characteristics : They are aerobe and grow well at optimum temperature of 37°C on chocolate agar (Fig. 5.4). Thayer Martin, New York City, Chacko Nair egg, Mueller Hinton media under 5-10% CO_2 (Candle jar) and produce five types of colonies (T_1-T_5). T_1 and T_2 are usually seen in primary isolates, whereas T_3 and T_4 in subcultures, and they differ in certain properties.

Colonies are transparent disks of about pinhead, discrete, circular or with crenated margin.

Biochemically, they are oxidase positive, ferment glucose and not maltose.

Viability : They die at 55°C in 5 minutes, are fragile and cannot resist an adverse conditions.

Antigenic structure : N. gonorrhoeae is antigenically heterogenous and its surface structures include the following : (a) Pili; (b) Protein I (Porin); (c) Protein II; (d) Protein III; (e) Lipopolysaccharides; (f) other proteins.

(a) **Pili :** These are hairlike structures extending from the surface and measures about 7 mm in diameter. They are seen on the surface of fresh isolates. The piliated organisms produce altered appearance of colonies on culture media with sharply defined borders. Pili help the attachment of organisms to the host cells and can recognise specific receptors on the surface of host cells.

Though pilin proteins of almost all strains are antigenically different, a single strain can produce several antigenically distinct pilins.

(b) **Protein I (Por) :** Extends through the cell membrane and forms pores on the surface. Each strain of gonococcus possesses only one type of protein I; 18 serovars of Type I A and 28 servoars of type I B have been demonstrated by serotyping of protein I. Through the pores, some nutrients enter the cell. Molecular weight of por protein is 34,00 to 37,000 daltons.

(c) **Protein II (Opa) :** A portion of protein II is in the outer membrane and the rest is exposed on the surface of gonococci, which is responsible for their adhesion, within colonies and attachment to host cells. Opaque colonies formation by gonococci is due to Type II protein, molecular weight of Opa is 24,000 to 32,000 daltons. Not more than 3 Opa are expressed by one strain of **N. gonorrhoeae,** though every strain has about 10 genes for the expression.

(d) **Protein III :** It is associated with protein I in cell surface in the formation of pores.

(e) **Lipopolysaccharide** (LPS) of **N. gonorrhoeae** differs from that of Gram-negative bacilli in chemical structure as it does not possess long O-antigenic side chains. It is mainly responsible for endotoxic effects in gonorrhoeae.

(f) **Other proteins :** They are poorly defined proteins. Gonococci produce Ig AI proteases which split and inactivate Ig AI. Lip (1-18) and Fbp (iron binding protein) are two other proteins. Their role in the pathogenesis is not yet established.

(g) **Capsule :** Capsule is loosely associated with cell surface of fresh isolates on **in vitro** cultivated isolates, can be stripped off and can be synthesised from the environmental and nutritional factors. Gonococcal capsule is a polyphosphate and can prevent the phagocytosis. The role of capsule in infection needs to be studied further. **N. acetyl neuramine acid,** a constituent of eukaryotes, is only found in meningococcal capsule.

Pathogenicity and Clinical Features : Their toxicity is due to endotoxin. In **male,** these organisms infect the mucosa of urethra with the help of pili and produce suppurative inflammation with purulent discharge (morning drop of secretion). At the early stage, these organisms are plenty in the discharge and later diminish due to association with secondary infection. The infection spreads to the prostate, seminal vesicle and epididymis. The periurethral tissue is also infected—causing a periurethral abscess and structure.

In adult **female,** the urethra and cervix uteri are infected, not the vagina—as the vaginal mucosa of married women is stratified and acidic vaginal secretion—hence gonococci cannot get attached to the vaginal mucosa by their pili. Endometritis, salpingitis, peritonitis may occur.

In **female** infants and children, they may produce vulvovaginitis, but in newborn infants, ophthalmia neonatorum may ensure. Arthritis, tenosynovitis, ulcerative endocarditis, purulent conjunctivitis are the complications due to blood invasion.

Laboratory diagnosis : Specimens : In **male,** the meatus should be cleansed with sterile gauze soaked with sterile normal saline and the specimens are taken with the help of sterile wire loop or directly on slides.

In **female,** from the urethra or the cervix uteri with the wire loop or swabs are transported in Stuart's transport medium.

Smears are stained with (a) Methylene blue, and (b) **Gram's stain; the presence of Gram-negative intracellular diplococci** is suggestive of gonorrhoea.

In **chronic infection,** they are scanty; in **male** the "morning drop" of secretion should be examined.

Culture : The diagnosis should be confirmed by the cultivation selective media and identification by oxidase and other biochemical tests.

A coaglutination test is currently available which uses monoclonal antibody reactive with protein I (Porin) of **N. gonorrhoeae.** This test is sensitive (99.7%) and specific (100%) to identify this organism.

ELISA is sensitive and specific to detect gonococcal antigen in the urethral discharge. A biotinylated DNA probe can identify it in 10 minutes.

A liquid probe system with chemiluminescent detection system for direct detection of gonococci in the general specimens is equally sensitive as that of ELISA system.

Production of enzyme beta lactamase (Penicillinase) should also be ascertained for an effective therapy.

Treatment : For penicillin resistant gonococci, spectinomycin, tetracycline, doxycycline and ceftriaxone are used. Resistance to spectinomycin and tetracycline has been reported.

Prevention and control

Gonorrhoea can be controlled by identification of cases, tracing of contacts, educating about spread of this disease through sexual contact and other general measures which will improve the health condition.

Non-specific (non-gonococcal) urethritis or cervicitis

Now the non-specific infection of urethra is considered as the most common sexually transmitted disease. It constitutes about 50% of all cases of urethritis and is predominant in males; but is symptomless in females.

The infection is caused by :

(1) **Bacteria – Chlamydia trachomatis (TRIC)** is the most important causal agent. **Urea-plasma urealyticum, Mycoplasma hominis, Gardnerella vaginalis** and **Acinetobacter** are also included.

(2) **Virus – Herpes** and **Cytomegalovirus**

(3) **Fungus – Candida albicans**

(4) **Protozoa – Trichomonas vaginalis.**

27
Neisseria Meningitidis (Meningococcus)

It causes meningitis in man.

Morphology and staining : Under microscope, meningococci resemble gonococci morphologically, but biochemically they differ by their maltose fermentation reaction only (Fig. 27.1).

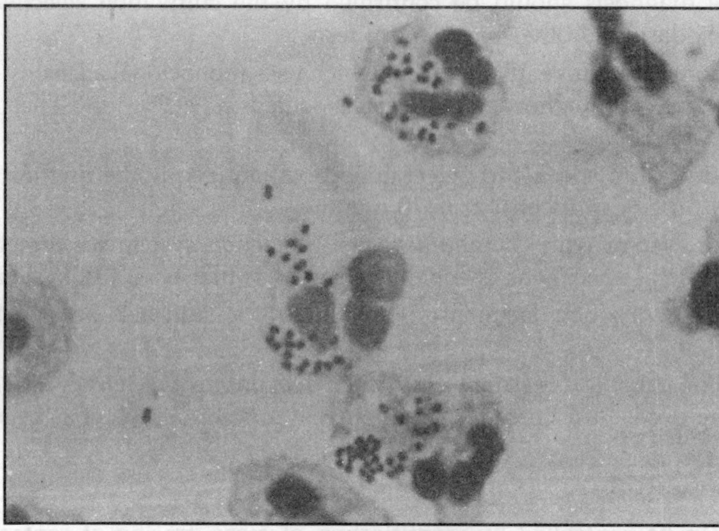

Fig. 27.1: Neisseria meningitidis 1000X

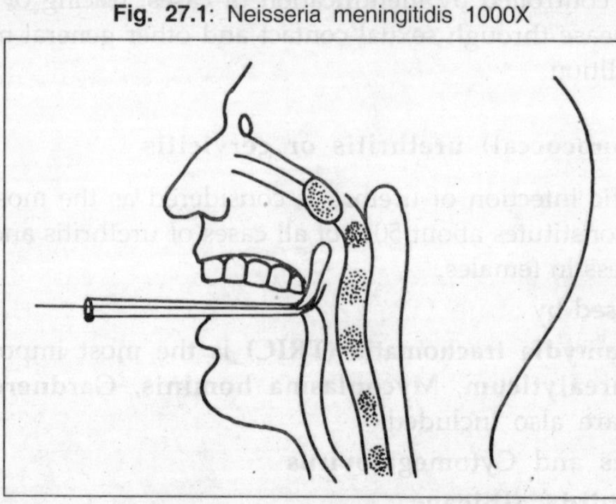

Fig. 27.2: Post-nasal swab in situ

Antigenic structure : On the basis of capsular polysaccharide, 13 serogroups of meningococci have been identified. The most important serogroups associated with human disease are A, B, C, Y and W-135.

Table 27.1 Comparison of surface components of N. gonorrhoeae, N. meningitidis

Properties	Gonococcus	Meningococcus	Function
Capsule	Not chemically defined	Polysaccharide	Antiphagocytic basis for serogrouping of meningococci
Polyphosphate	+	+	Unknown
Pili	+	+	Adhesion, Antiphagocytosis serogrouping of meningococci
Other membrane proteins (OM)	Not described	Class I	Probably porins; defined meningococcal serotypes
	Por (Protein I)	Class 2	N. gonorrhoeae; Por I A with 18 subtypes
	Por (Protein II)	Class 3	Por 1B with 28 subtypes
	Rmp (Protein III)	Class 4	Only one type, function not known
	Opa (Protein II)	Class 5	Attachment to human cells, antigenically variable
Lipopolysaccharide	6 serotypes	12 serotypes	Endotoxic Components of cells
Fbp (Iron binding protein)	One	—	
Lip (1-18)	One	—	
IgA I phase	One	—	

Pathogenicity and Clinical Features : They may spread through the cribriform plate to the subarachnoid space by the olfactory nerve or they may attach to the submucosa of nasopharynx with the aid of pili, then reach the blood stream-bacteriaemia. Fulminant meningococcaemia is more severe with high fever and haemorrhagic rash; there may be disseminated intravascular coagulation and circulatory collapse.

Pyogenic meningitis in all ages including children and young adults are mainly caused by **N. meningitidis.** Other bacteria responsible for pyogenic meningitis are **Haemophilus influenzae, Pneumococcus, Listeria monocytogenes; Leptospira interrogans** can rarely causes this infection.

Serogroups A, B and C of **N. meningitidis** are common cause of **meningococcal meninigitis** but in carriers other serogroups are often identified. Serogroups A causes epidemic meningitis in most countries.

Since human nasopharynx harbours **N. meningitidis,** the infection is mostly via droplet spray of infected respiratory secretions from the patients on carriers. In normal population, the incidence of carrier rate is about 10-20%, in household contacts of sporadic cases and during epidemics, it may rise to 40%. The incubation period is about 3 days. The organisms may spread from nasopharynx to the meninges via blood stream; it may also spread along the perineural sheath of olfactory nerve. There is acute fever with petechial rash in skin and mucosa. Probably the pathogenicity is due to bacterial endotoxin during fulminating meningococcal septicaemia the adrenal insufficiency may occur.

Meningococcal meningitis is very common in children and infants. Asymptomatic carriage of avirulent strain may most probably produce bacterial antibodies to invasive strain.

Meningitis usually begins suddenly with intense headache, vomiting, stiff neck and progresses to coma within few hours.

Laboratory diagnosis : Specimens. Blood for culture; punctured material from petechiae and CSF for smear and culture.

Smear : Gram stained smear from all specimens will show polymorphonuclear leucocytes with meningococci.

Culture : Specimens are plated on Mueller Hinton, Chocolate or Thayer Martin medium and the growth is identified by oxidase test and fermentation reaction. Gonococci and meningococci form convex, glistening, elevated, mucoid colonies, 1-5 mm in diameter. Colonies are transparent or opaque, non-pigmented and haemolytic. Identification of serogroup can be done in a smear by using fluorescein isothiocynate containing antisera.

The Limulus test for endotoxin is useful for detection of meningitis caused by meningococci—if the organisms are present at more than $10^3/cm^3$.

ELISA test is not useful for the rapid diagnosis of meningitis. The availability of rapid immunodiagnostic tests (coagglutination, CIEP and latex agglutination test) has made the diagnosis easier and sensitive. Latex agglutination test is now widely available and produces result within minutes of the testing of supernatant of CSF.

Treatment : Penicillin is the drug of choice—Cefotaxime or Ceftriaxone. Chloramphenicol can be used in persons allergic to penicillin.

Prevention and Control

Immunoprophylaxis can be done by meningococcal vaccines prepared from surface polysaccharides of a number of serogroups A, C, W 135 and Y.

The eradication of the bacteria from nasopharynx of close contacts of patients can be conducted by **Chemoprophylaxis** (Rifampicin, ciprofloxacin, minocycline).

Avoidance of over-crowding in living and working environment is an important control measure.

Neonatal meningitis

Coliform bacilli **(Escherchia coli, Klebsiella, Proteus)** are most common aetiological agents of neonatal meningitis; **Streptococcus pyogenes** may sometimes cause this infection. During delivery, the neonates may acquire the infection through infected mother's vagina. Premature babies may also get infected.

(i) Gentamicin and penicillin
(ii) Chloramphenicol
(iii) Cefotaxime are administrated.

Other Neisseriae

Neisseria lactaemia, N. sicca, N. subflava, N. cinera, N. mucosa, N. flavescens are the normal flora of respiratory tract and are important as they grow on selective media (Muller Hinton, Thayer Martin etc.).

Cultural Character

Neisseria flava, N. perflava, N, sicca and **N subflava** are commensals and can be differentiated from the pathogenic **Neisseriae** by following method :

(a) Their primary isolation does not require CO_2.

(b) They produce pigmented (yellow to greenish) colonies and most of them ferment a variety of carbohydrates.

Branhamella

In 1970, a **new genus Branhamella** has been proposed on the basis of fatty acid content and it is now called as **B. catarrhalis.** Earlier, it was classified as a species of **Neisseria** which shared many characters with commensal **Neisseria** and it was named **N. catarrhalis.** It is normal flora of the upper respiratory and genital tract. Though this genus was later shifted genus **Moraxella,** it is still included in the genus **Branhamella.**

Morphology. They are Gram-negative diplococci measuring 0.6-1 µm, oval, with adjacent sides flattened or rounded.

Culture

On nutrient agar (ordinary medium) they form colonies with a smooth and glistening surface.

Biochemical reaction

This organism does not ferment carbohydrate but hydrolyses tributyrin—a test for its identification. It produces catalase and oxidase.

Pathogenicity. B. catarrhalis is now recognised as a cause of lower respiratory tract infection, though it is normal flora of nasopharynx. It has been encountered in otitis media, meningitis, sinusitis, endocarditis. About 50% strains of **B. catarrhalis** produce **beta-lactamase** which are resistant to penicillin and ampicillin.

These commensal Gram-negative diplococci (Neisseria) occur on various mucous surfaces of the body and are found regularly in the mucous secretions of the throat, nose and mouth.

Organisms of Genus Veillonella, Gram-negative cocci (.3 µ) occurring in masses as commensals in natural cavities of man—particularly the mouth and alimentary tract. They do not prove pathogenic though sometimes isolated from cases of appendicitis (pyorrhoea) and pulmonary lesions and regarded as potentially pathogenic.

Demonstration

1. A smear from acute urethritis showing pus cells and Gram-negative intra or extracellular cocci arranged in pairs (Fig. 26.1).
2. Oxidase test in detail is given in V. cholerae.
3. A smear of CSF from meningococcal meningitis showing Gram-negative intra and extra cellular diplococci (Fig. 27.1).
4. West post-nasal swab to collect specimens from nasopharynx of carriers (Fig. 27.2).

Practical work

Stain the given smear by Gram's method.

Questions

1. What is morning drop?
2. What is the importance of oxidase test in the identification of Neisseria?

3. Why the vagina of married women is not infected by gonococci?
4. How can you differentiate gonococci from meningococci in the laboratory?
5. Why the meatus should be cleansed with gauze soaked in sterile normal saline instead of antiseptics?

   Why Stuart transport medium is used?
6. Why non-pathogenic Neisseriae are important during identification of gonococci and meningococci?
7. Describe the mode of entry of meningococci from nasopharynx to brain.
8. Describe the recent serological techniques used to identify meningococci and gonococci.

Answers should be written in the practical note book. Must be drawn in the practical notebook.

Enteric Gram-negative Bacilli

The family enterobacteriaceae is composed of numerous Gram-negative bacilli (enteric bacilli) which may be non-motile or motile with peritrichous flagellae. They do not form spores, may or may not be capsulated, are aerobes or facultatively anaerobes, grow on ordinary media, ferment glucose rapidly producing acid and gas or acid only, and reduce nitrates into nitrites. Many species are intestinal pathogens or commensals. Very recently, **Yersinia (Pasteurella) pestis** is included in this family, though it is not an intestinal pathogen of man.

Once these enteric bacilli were classified into three groups based on their lactose fermentation activity—though this classification was not taxonomically accepted, it has practical value in the diagnostic bacteriology:

A.	Lactose	(1) Escherichia coli
		(2) Klebsiella
B.	Non-lactose fermenters	(1) Salmonella
		(2) Shigella
C.	Late lactose fermenter	(1) **Shigella sonnei**

28
Escherichia Coli

Table 28.1. Properties of Escherichia species

Properties	Esch. coli	Esch. blattac	Esch. fergusonii	Esch. hermanii	Esch. vulneris
Motility	+	–	+	+	+
Christensen's citrate	+	V	+	V	–
Growth in KCN medium	–	–	–	+	–
Malonate fermentation	–	+	–	–	+
β-Galactosidase	+	–	+	+	+
Arginine dihydrolase	V	–	V	–	+
Ornithine decarboxylase	V	+	+	+	–
Adonitol : acid production	–	–	+	–	–
Cellulose : acid production	V	–	–	+	–
Dulcitol : acid production	V	–	–	+	–
Glycerol : acid production	+	+	–	–	–
Mannitol : acid production	+	–	+	+	+
Raffinose : acid production	V	–	–	–	+
Salicin : acid production	V	–	+	V	+
Sorbitol : acid production	+	–	–	–	–
Indole : production	+	–	V	+	–

+ most stains positive; – most stains negative; V, variable (some positive)

E. coli is an intestinal pathogen or commensal of the human or animal intestine and is voided in the faeces remaining viable in the environment only for some days. Detection of **E. coli** in drinking water is an indication of pollution with faeces.

Morphology and Staining : E. coli is Gram-negative straight rod, 1-3 μ × 0.4-0.7 μ, arranged singly or in pairs (Fig. 28.1). It is motile by peritrichous flagellae, though some strains are non-motile. Spores are not formed. Capsules and fimbriae are found in some strains.

Cultural characteristics : It is an aerobe and a facultative anaerobe. The optimum growth temperature is 37°C. On Nutrient agar (Fig. 5.4), colonies are large, thick, greyish white, moist, smooth, opaque or translucent discs. The smooth (s) form seen in fresh isolation is easily emulsified in saline, whereas the rough (R) form often autoagglutinates in saline. Some strains may form "mucoid " colonies. On MacConkey agar (Fig. 5.3) medium, colonies are bright pink due to lactose fermentation. On selective media (Desoxycholate citrate agar-DCA; salmonella shigella-SS medium) used for the isolation of salmonella, their growth is inhibited, however their colonies are pink on DCA as it contains lactose and neutral red. In broth, there is generalised turbidity and deposit which disperses on shaking.

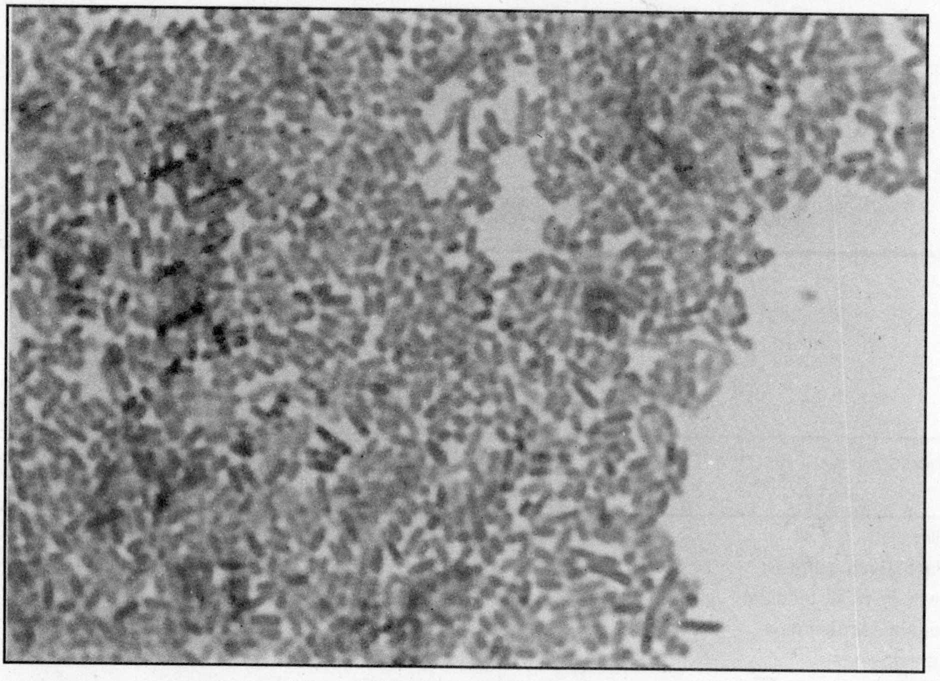

Fig. 28.1: Escherichia coli 1000X

Biochemical reaction : Glucose, lactose, mannitol, maltose are fermented with acid and gas production, but sucrose is not fermented by typical strain of E. coli. In Triple sugar iron (TSI), acid and gas are produced. The four biochemical tests widely used for enterobacteriaceae classification are Indole (I), Methyl Red (MR), Voges Proskauer (VP) and Citrate (C) utilisation which are referred to by the mnemonic $IMV_{(1)}$ C.E. coli is Indole and MR positive VP and citrate negative ($IMV_{(1)}$ C++ --), H_2 S is not formed and urea is not hydrolysed.

Antigenic structure : E. coli has three antigens : O Somatic, Greek Ohne Hauch—without flagella; H—flagella; Greek Hauch—flagella and K (Kapsular) antigens. K antigen is an envelope antigen, which encloses the O antigen, renders the strain inagglutinable by the O antiserum and contributes to virulence by inhibiting phagocytosis. It may be of three types —L, A and B. Though L type is common, the B antigen is medically important as it is found on enteropathogenic **E. coli.**

F (Fimbrial) antigen. The F antigen has no significance in antigenic classification of **E. coli.** Type I fimbriae mediates adhesion of bacterium to human and animal cells. Such adhesion enhances bacterial pathogenicity e.g. urinary tract infection in which type I fimbriae has some possible role to play.

Several fibrin structures resembling fimbriae have been demonstrated. They, most probably, play a very important role in pathogenesis of diarrhoeal diseases and urinary tract infection.

Toxin

Besides the endotoxin associated with O antigen, some strains produce two types of exotoxin—enterotoxin and haemolysin.

Enterotoxins responsible for diarrhoea are of two types—heat labile (LT); heat stable (ST). LT is similar to cholera enterotoxin antigenically and in its mechanism of action—by stimulating the adenyl cyclase—cyclic adenosine monophosphate (cAMP) system to produce fluid accumulation in the intestinal lumen. ST appears to stimulate fluid secretion into the gut through the mediation of cyclic guanosine monophosphate (cGMP) resulting into dehydration.

Haemolysin : Three types of haemolysins produced by E. coli are not related to pathogenesis.

E. coli forms a part of normal intestinal flora of man and animal and the commensal strains belong to several O groups. There are many strains of **E. coli** which include commensal strains as well as strains with virulence determinants that cause a wide variety of infections of all age groups of men and animals. The virulent strains of **E. coli** are specific pathogens in the gut (enteritis) and of extra-intestinal sites (urinary tract infection, wound infection).

Clinical infections caused by **Esch. coli** are :

1. Urinary tract infection (UTI)
2. Septic infections of wound
3. Diarrhoea
4. Dysentery
5. Septicaemia
6. Pneumonia
7. Neonatal meningitis
8. Abscess in various organs.

Other pathogens of the family **Entero-bacteriaceae** causing UTI are **Klebsiella, Proteus (P. mirabilis), Providence** and **Citrobacter.** Gram-positive organisms **(Staph. aureus, Enterococcus, Str. pyogenes)** are also frequent pathogens of UTI. The hospital acquired infections following instrumentation and catheterisation are mostly due to **Pseudomonas** and **Proteus.** Pregnant women (6-8%) do suffer from asymptomatic bacteriuria, if undetected and untreated, which may terminate into symptomatic infection later in pregnancy resulting to pyelonephritis and hypertension.

Calculi, enlarged prostate, pregnancy are predisposing factors in UTI. The reservoir of infection is the bacterial flora of colon. Urinary tract infection is usually from the perineum in ascending order via urethra. A prerequisite for UTI is the colonisation of peri-urethral area by the pathogens. Due to shortness of urethra, the females are more prone to this infection. The haematogenous spread of this infection may be possible in newborn.

Infection : E . coli causes : (1) Infantile acute diarrhoea or gastroenteritis; (2) Urinary tract infection in pregnant women and men with prostatitis; (3) Wound and burn infection, and (4) Septicaemia.

1. **Diarrhoea :** Four groups of **E. coli** responsible for diarrhoea in infants, children and adults are : Enteropathogenic **E. coli** (EPEC); Enterotoxigenic E. coli (ETEC); Enteroinvasive **E. coli** (EIEC); Enterohaemorrhagic E. coli (EHEC).

   EPEC is responsible for infantile diarrhoea. The pathogenic mechanism of EPEC has only recently been developed. They adhere to the intestinal mucosa, cause the loss of microvilli and prevent the entry of bacteria into the mucosa. They also produce a shigella-like toxin.

   ETEC : The enterotoxins are now known to produce diarrhoea in children with dehydration, traveller's diarrhoea in adults, and sometimes cholera infantum similar to cholera. ETEC also possess colonisation factors (pili, K antigen) to enhance their virulence.

   EIEC do not produce enterotoxin but invade the intestinal mucosa like dysentery bacilli. They cause keratoconjunctivitis on instillation into the eyes of guinea pig (Sereny test) which is a diagnostic method for EIEC. Another diagnostic method is their invasion of HeLa cells in tissue culture. EIEC is late lactose fermenter and may be anaerogenic. They have antigenic relationship with shigella.

EHEC has been very recently identified and is found to cause colitis with marked haemorrhage and absence of fever, produces Verotoxin (Cytotoxin) which affects the vero cells in tissue culture.

Table 28.2 Serogroups of E. coli causing Diarrhoea

Pathogenic	Common serogroups
Entero-pathogenic **E. coli** (EPEC)	026, 055, 086, 0111, 0114, 0119, 0125, 0126, 0127, 0128, 0142
Entero-toxigenic **E. coli** (ETEC)	06, 08, 015, 025, 027, 063, 078, 0115, 0148, 0153, 0159, 0167
Entero-invasive **E. coli** (EIEC)	028 ac, 0124, 0136, 0143, 0144, 0152, 0164
Verotoxin producing **E. coli** (VTEC)	0157

Antigenic typing of E. coli

Each **E. coli** has been primarily subdivided into a number of O groups which have been subdivided into subgroups with different K antigens. Each subgroup includes strains with different H antigens; separate numbers were previously allotted for B antigens, but afterwards these numbers have been included in the same consecutive series as the rest of K antigens. Thus, a strain is recorded as 0111; K58; H12. The B number is no more in use, or, when used, the old number of B is written within brackets e.g. 0111; K58 (B4); H12.

2. **Urinary tract infection** is caused by **E. coli** during catheterisation or pregnancy or due to urinary obstruction by prostitis. Pyelonephritis is produced due to haematogenous infection.
3. **Pyogenic infection :** Superficial infections (wound or burn) or deep infections (peritonitis, cholecystitis, meningitis in children) are caused by E. coli.
4. **Septicaemia : E. coli, Pseudomonas aeruginosa** or Gram-negative bacilli septicaemia is characterised by fever, hypotension, endotoxic shock (intravascular coagulation).

Laboratory Diagnosis

1. Diarrhoea

For the detection of EPEC, fresh diarrhoeal stool is plated directly on blood agar (Fig. 5.12) and MacConkey agar (Fig. 5.3) medium. After overnight incubation, **E. coli** colonies are emulsified in saline on a slide and tested by agglutination with polyvalent and monovalent O antiserum against entero-pathogenic serotypes and further identified by biochemical tests. Enzyme linked immuno-sorbent assay (ELISA) test is simplest and used to detect LT of ETEC. LT and cholera entero-toxin are antigenically similar. Sereney test is the only method available recently to demonstrate EIEC.

2. Urinary tract infection

Catheterisation for urine collection is not advisable for diagnosis as it leads to urinary tract infection. Hence, in male, after cleaning the retracted prepuce and glans penis, with sterile cotton soaked in sterile normal saline, the first portion of urine that flushes out commensal bacteria from the anterior urether is discarded. The next portion (midstream) of urine is collected in a sterile wide-mouthed container and despatched immediately to the laboratory as the urine is an ideal medium for the growth of bacteria. If there is a delay of 2-3 hours, it should be refrigerated.

Quantitative culture is done by pour plate or surface culture methods using ten-fold diluted urine. In the active urinary tract infection, the urine will contain 100,000 bacteria or more per ml. which is referred to as "significant bacteriuria," counts of 10,000 bacteria or less are indicative of contamination.

The most commonly used "standard loop method" can transfer a fixed small volume of urine on non-inhibitory medium (Blood agar) for estimation of bacteria and on an indicative medium (MacConkey medium) for presumptive diagnosis of bacteriuria. The isolates are further identified and tested for antibiotic sensitivity. Antibiotic sensitivity may also be done directly using the urine samples.

Other screening techniques for the presumptive diagnosis of significant bacteriuria are: (1) Griess nitrite test – The presence of nitrite indicates the presence of nitrate reducing bacteria in urine but nitrite is absent in normal urine. (2) Catalase test – The frothing on addition of hydrogen peroxide due to catalase is an indication of bacteriuria. (3) Triphenyl tetrazolium chloride test is based on the production of pink red precipitate in the reagent due to the respiratory activity of growing bacteria. (4) Microscopic demonstration of bacteria in Gram stained film of urine. (5) Glucose test paper is based on the utilisation of minute amount of glucose present in normal urine by bacteria causing the infection. (6) Dip slide culture method – Agar coated slides are immersed in the urine or exposed to the stream of urine are incubated and the colonies are estimated by colony counter. These screening tests are not sensitive and reliable as cultural test.

The antibody coated bacteria test has been employed for localisation of the site of urinary infection. Pyogenic infection and septicaemia diagnosis depends on the isolation of bacteria on culture.

Treatment : Infantile diarrhoea can be treated by Oral Rehydration Solution (ORS) as per World Health Organisation (WHO recommendation).

Medical importance : E. coli is medically important because it

(a) is used to produce insulin by adopting the genetic engineering technique,

(b) produces certain vitamins in the intestine,

(c) is used as parameter to determine the faecal contamination of drinking water,

(d) is used for the plasmid study in the bacterial genetics.

29
Klebsiella

Klebsiella are widely distributed in nature, occurring as commensals in intestine and as saprophytes in soil and water. They are non-motile, capsulated rods. They grow on ordinary media. On MacConkey Agar medium, their colonies are large dome shaped, mucoid and pink (Fig. 11.8). Mucoid colonies can be identified by string formation, when they are touched and lifted up with platinum wire. They ferment glucose, lactose, sucrose, mannitol with acid and gas production. They are Indole and MR negative, VP and citrate positive Fig. 11.9 ($MV_{(1)}$ C - - + +); they produce urease and are differentiated from Enterobacter which are motile.

Klebsiella have been classified into three species (**K. pneumoniae, K. ozaenae** and **K. rhinoscleromatis**) and over 80 serotypes based on biochemical and on the capsular (K) antigenic reactions, respectively.

Table 29.1 Biochemical reactions of Klebsiella

Property	K. aerogenes	K. ozaenae	K. pneumoniae	K. oxytoca	K. rhinoscleromatis
Gas in glucose	+	+/–	+	+	–
Acid in lactose	+	–	+	+	–
MR	–	+	+	V	+
VP	+	–	–	V	–
Citrate	+	+/–	+	+	–
Urease	+	+/–	+	+	–
Malonate	+	–	+	+	+
Lysine	+	+/–	+	+	–
Indole	–		–	+	–

Klebsiella pneumonia is characterised by massive mucoid inflammatory exudate **K. pneumoniae** which causes diarrhoea, urinary, pyogenic (abscess, meningitis), nosocomial infections and septicaemia. Some strains of **K. pneumoniae** produce enterotoxin (similar to heat stable toxin of **E. coli**) which is determined by plasmid.

Pathogenicity

K. pneumoniae is the second-most common bacterial flora of intestine of man and animals. It is next to **E. coli** and is also common in hospitalised patients. The hospital acquired intestinal strains are resistant to a wide spectrum of antibiotics, however, they are sensitive to few drugs (cefoxitin, cefotaxime and ceftazidime).

Through certain respiratory strains **K. pneumoniae** (Friedlander bacillus) causes severe pneumonia with fatality rate of 80% if untreated. Middle-aged and elderly persons are more susceptible to **K. pneumoniae,** if they are already suffering from diabetes mellitus, chronic bronchopneumonia or other underlying medical problems.

Capsular serotypes 1-6 are most common in the respiratory tract infection in man, capsular swelling reaction, agglutination, complement fixation, fluorescent antibody, counter immuno-electrophoresis can be performed for the identification of capsular antigen.

Other methods of typing. Bacteriocins known as **Klebocins** or **pneumocins** are produced by many klebsiella strains. In **Klebocin typing,** a liquid preparation of bacteriocins obtained after induction with mitocin C was used.

The combination of klebocin typing and capsular serotyping can be used for epidemiological study. Besides, phage typing with temperate phages derived from other **Klebsiella** strains can also be adopted for epidemiological investigation.

Diagnosis is done by culture and identification by biochemical reactions. Since many strains carry plasmids determining multiple drug resistance, antibiotic sensitivity test should be invariably undertaken.

K. ozaenae and **K. rhinoscleromatis**—certain subspecies of **K. pneumoniae**—derived their names from the disease with which they are associated e.g. **K. ozaenae** was isolated from the nasal mucosa in oezena, a disease characterised by foul smelling nasal discharge with progressive atrophy of mucous membranes; and **K. rhinoscleromatis** from rhinoscleroma, a chronic granulomatous disease of the nose and pharynx.

30
Proteus

Proteus are saprophytic, widely distributed in nature and also occur as commensals in the intestine and on the moist skin. They cause urinary or respiratory tract or ear wound, burn infections, infantile diarrhoea as opportunistic pathogen. There are five species: **Proteus vulgaris, Pr. mirabilis, Pr. morganii, Pr. rettgeri,** and **Pr. inconstans.** They are Gram-negative pleomorphic motile rods (0.5-1-3 μ). They are aerobic and facultative anaerobic.

Their colonies emit a characteristic 'fishy' or "seminal" odour. **Pr. vulgaris,** and **Pr. mirabilis** produce "swarming" (concentric circles) growth on nutrient agar medium at 37°C as they are motile; but other species do not. The swarming is inhibited by increasing the concentration of agar (6%) or incorporation of chloral hydrate, sodium azide, alcohol etc. On MacConkey agar, the swarming does not occur, but smooth, pale colonies are formed. The swarming mechanism is yet to be understood.

In broth, an uniform turbidity with a slight powdery deposit is produced by proteus with ammoniacal odour.

Proteus transforms phenyl alanine to phenyl pyruvic acid (PPA), other members of the family enterobacteriaceae do not. Urea is hydrolysed by all Proteus species as they produce urease (Fig. 30.1) except **Pr. inconstans** (Providencia). They are MR +ve and VP –ve, ferment glucose with acid and gas production. They are further classified into species on the basis of Indole and H_2 S, citrate utilisation:

Table 30.1 Biotypes of the genus Proteus

	Pr. vulgaris	Pr. mirabilis	Pr. morganii	Pr. rettgeri	Pr. inconstans
Gas from glucose	+	+	+	d	d
Acid from sucrose	+	d	–	d	d
Acid from mannitol	–	–	–	+	–
Acid from maltose	+	–	–	–	–
Indole	+	–	+	+	+
H_2S	+	+	–	–	–
Citrate	d	d	–	+	+
Gelatinase	+	+	–	–	–
Ornithine decarboxylase	–	+	+	–	–
Urease	+	+	+	+	–

d = variable

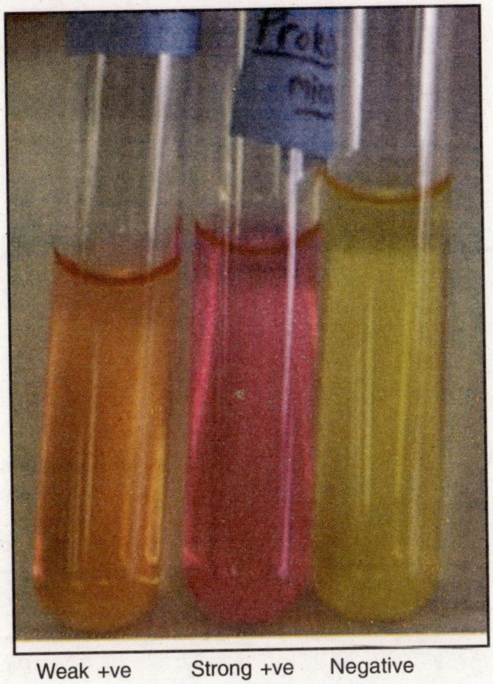

Fig. 30.1: Urease test

Antigenic structure

Motile stains of proteus possess thermostable 'O' (somatic) and thermolabile H (flagellar) antigen and all strains have distinct "O" antigens.

The "O" antigen has got alkali labile and alkali stable fractions. The alkali stable fraction of "O" antigen (polysaccharide) is common to OX19, OXK and OX2 strains with **rickettsia prowazeki** (causing typhus fever) which are agglutinated by sera of typhus patients (**Weil Felix reaction**).

Pathogenicity

Proteus are opportunistic pathogens and are responsible for the production of :

1. Urinary tract infection.
2. Pyogenic infection (abscess, bedsore, infection of wound, ear and respiratory tract).
3. Summer diarrhoea in children (mainly caused by **Pr. morganii**).
4. Exogenous infection in patients having obstructive lesions of urinary tract which may be due to prolonged catheterisation or diagnostic instrumentation.
5. Endogenous infection by their dissemination through blood (haematogenous spread). However the human infection is mostly caused by **Pr. mirabilis.**

Proteus can be isolated on MacConkey agar, blood agar with 6% agar which inhibit swarming so that other bacteria are not overgrown and identified by biochemical reaction. Many strains are sensitive to nitrofurantoin, tetracycline and kanamycin.

31
Pseudomonas

Classification

On the basis of r RNA/DNA homology, the genus **Pseudomonas** has been mainly classified into 2 groups.

Table 31.1: Medically important species of Pseudomonas

r RNA group	Species
1. Fluorescent pseudomonas	**Ps. aerugenosa**
	Ps. putida
	Ps. fluorescens
Non-fluorescent pseudomonads	**Ps. alcaligenes**
	Ps. pseudoalcaligenes
	Ps. stutzeri
2. Pseudomallei group	**Ps. pseudomallei**
	Ps. mallei
	Ps. cepacia
3. Other pseudomonads	**Ps. acidovorans**
	Ps. maltophilia
	Ps. diminuta
	Ps. vesicularis

Pseudomonas aeruginosa (P. pyocyanea) is the only one human pathogen. It is slender Gram-negative bacillus, 1.5-3 μ × 0.5 μ, actively motile by a polar flagellum, is non- capsulated and non-spore forming. Strains from clinical specimens do possess pili.

It is an obligate aerobe, grows well on ordinary media at 37°C forming large opaque, irregular colonies with a distinctive earthy or fruity smell (Fig. 31.1). On MacConkey and DCA media, it forms non-lactose fermenting (pale) colonies, whereas on blood agar some strains are haemolytic. Selective medium (Cetrimide agar) can be used for the isolation from the clinical specimens. In broth, it forms a dense turbidity with surface pellicle.

It produces various pigments (pyocyanin, fluorescein). Pyocyanin (Fig. 31.1) is bluish green phenazine pigment soluble in water and chloroform, which is produced by **Ps. aeruginosa,** fluorescein is greenish yellow pigment soluble in water but not in chloroform, but it is produced by many other species also. In older culture, it may be oxidised to a yellowish brown pigment. Other pigments are pyoverdin, pyorubrin, and pyomelanin. The role of pigment in the pathogenesis is not yet well-established. **Ps. aeruginosa** emerges as the dominant bacterium in the mixed infection.

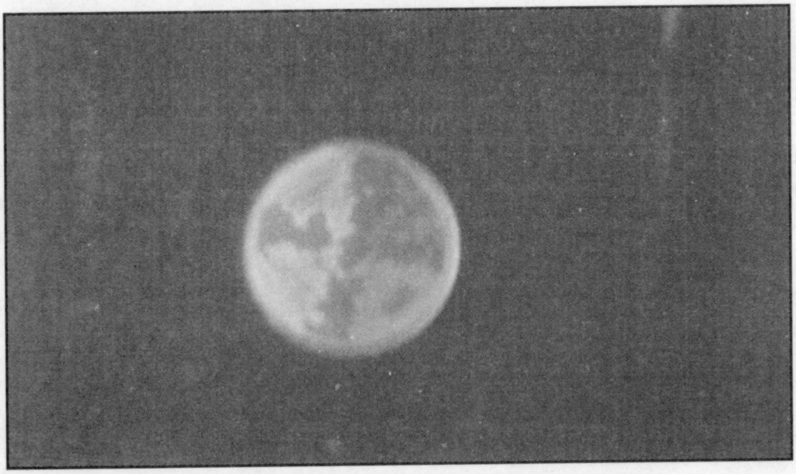

Fig. 31.1: Pseudomonas (Colony pyocin in pigment)

Toxins and Enzymes

Ps. aeruginosa produces toxins and enzymes responsible for its virulence:

(a) **Extracellular products :** Mitochondrial enzyme in mammalian tissue are inhibited by pyocyanin. Besides, pyocyanin is responsible for the description and cessation of ciliary beat on ciliated nasal epithelium that clears the respiratory mucosa of offending agents, thus the colonisation of organism in the nasal mucosa is favoured.

(b) **Extracellular enzymes and haemolysins** : Proteolytic enzymes (protease, elastase), haemolysins (phospholipase C, heat stable rhammolipid) and lipase play an important role in the formation of local lesions.

(c) **Exotoxins :** The exotoxins are two extra-cellular ADP-ribosyl transferase, exotoxins A and S. Toxin A is a polypeptide of MW 68000, inhibits protein synthesis.

(d) **Endotoxins :** It is a lipopolysaccharide with many biological properties of enterobacterial lipopolysaccharide.

Resistance : Since **Ps. aeruginosa** is not heat resistant, it is easily killed at 55 C in one hour. It grows in antiseptic lotions used in hospital as they are resistant to most antiseptics and disinfectants (chloroxylenol and hexachlorophane). It is also resistant to many antimicrobial agents due to production of potent chromosomally mediated β-lactamase classification of **Ps. aeruginosa.** It can be done by three methods of typing :

1. **Serotypes Ps aeruginosa** has been divided into 29 serotypes by O agglutination test, though it is not of much use.
2. **Phagetypes** : It has been proposed that phage typing can be carried out by using specific bacteriophages lysing a particular strain of **Ps. aeruginosa,** but it is not yet accepted.
3. **Pyocin typing** : **Ps. aeruginosa** is differentiated into 105 types by 13 indicator strains, based on production of particular type of pyocins (bacteriocins).

Metabolism is oxidative but not fermentative. Glucose is utilised oxidatively forming acid only, Indole MR, VP andd H_2S are negative. Catalase and oxidase are positive.

Though **Ps. aeruginosa** is not heat resistant, it is resistant to common antiseptics (dettol, cetrimide), lotions kept for use in hospitals.

Pathogenicity : This bacillus is responsible for nosocomial infection, wound infection, suppurative otitis, bed sore, eye infection, urinary tract infection, infantile diarrhoea.

When body resistance is lowered and body tissue is damaged, **Ps. aeruginosa** produces human infection as opportunistic pathogen, since it is prevalent in water, sewage, soil, air and also as commensals in human intestine. In the hospital the wound infection is very common due to mixed infection of **Ps. aeruginosa** and **Pyogenic cocci.**

The infection takes place from the environment and by **cross-infection** in the hospital by the use of contaminated syringes, needles, cystoscope, catheters. The **hospital acquired infections** are mostly due to **Ps. aeruginosa** (aeruginosa, pyocyanea means **"blue pus"**). Pathogenic lesion (wound) is covered with blue pus.

Patients with severe burns, malignancy and who have undergone catheterisation of the urinary tract are often infected.

Laboratory diagnosis can be done by subjecting the specimens (pus, wound swabs, mid-stream urine, CSF, sputum, blood) to the Cultural test, Biochemical test, Animal pathogenicity test and Typing.

Epidermiology

Cross-infection : Ps. aeruginosa has the ability to resist and multiply in most environment of hospital wards, bathrooms, kitchens, equipment, antiseptics or disinfectants solution. This ability has a great importance in **cross-infection.**

Though exogenous or endogenous sources may be responsible for many **cross-infections,** it may also occur in patients with urinary tract infection. Healthy carriers (10%) may harbour **Ps. aeruginosa.**

Epidemics

In newborns in nurseries and young infants in paediatric wards, epidemics and out-breaks of **Ps. aeruginosa** have been reported. Sometimes milk-fed babies were infected due to drinking of **Ps. aeruginosa** contaminated milk. This has been confirmed by further investigation that rubber lungs used to close feeding bottles have been stored in antiseptic solutions.

Risk group

(1) Burned patients are most vulnerable to **Ps. aeruginosa** super-infection.
(2) Patients with immuno-suppression, and
(3) Individuals who have undergone cardiac and renal surgery.

Vaccine

It has been claimed that the polyvalent vaccine prepared from the cell surface of 17 internationally recognised serotypes of **Ps. aeruginosa** stimulated active immunity in man. It is not commercially available at present.

Control and prevention

By constant vigilance and by the use of combined drug therapy, the **hospital cross-infection** can be prevented.

Treatment: Polymyxin B, colistin, gentamicin, amikacin, carbenicillin and cefuroxine are effective against most strains.

Demonstration

(1) A smear from pure culture stained by Gram's method to show Gram-negative bacilli (1-3 μ 0.4 0.7μ).
(2) Study of the motility of **E. coli** by hanging drop method (Fig. 2.2).
(3) Large, thick, greyish white, moist, smooth, opaque or translucent disc-like colonies of **E. coli** on nutrient agar.
(4) Pink colonies of **E. coli** on MacConkey agar (Fig. 5.3).
(5) Glucose, lactose, mannitol, maltose fermentation by **E. coli** with acid and gas production but sucrose is not fermented in Triple Sugar Iron (TSI) medium gas and acid produced.
(6) $IMV_{(1)}$ C ++ - - for **E. coli.**
(7) Heavily capsulated diplobacilli (**K. pneumoniae**) in a smear from pure culture.
(8) Large, pink and mucoid colonies of **K. pneumoniae** on MacConkey agar medium. (Fig. 5.14)
(9) $IMV_{(1)}$ C - - ++ for **K. pneumoniae,** Citrate utilisation positive test.
(10) Swarming growth of **Pr. vulgaris** on nutrient agar with 'fishy' or seminal odour.
(11) Hydrolysis of urea by Proteus (urease test).
(12) Diffusion of pyocyanin or fluorescin pigment of **Pr. aeruginosa** into the nutrient agar medium with fruity smell.

Practical work

Given smear should be stained by Gram's method. Answers to the following questions should be entered in the journal :

(1) Why **E. coli** produces pink colonies on MacConkey agar; why butt of TSI is yellow in case of **E. coli**?
(2) How **E. coli** is identified biochemically?
(3) Enumerate the infections caused by **E. coli.**
(4) How many groups of **E. coli** are responsible for diarrhoea?
(5) Describe briefly physiopathology of infantile diarrhoea with dehydration by **E. coli;** what is Verotoxin Sereny test?
(6) What is the significance of the presence of E. coli in the drinking water?
(7) What is the medical importance of **E. coli**?
(8) Why ORS is recommended for infantile diarrhoea?
(9) Why mucoid colonies are produced by **K. pneumoniae** and how will you confirm them?
(10) How is swarming growth of Proteus on nutrient agar inhibited?
(11) Enumerate the infections by Proteus, as well as the tests used to identify Proteus.
(12) What are the pigments produced by **P. aeruginosa**?
(13) Why lotions or antiseptics used in the hospital contain **Ps. aeruginosa**?
(14) Define nosocomial infection and enumerate the infections caused by **Ps. aeruginosa.**

32

Salmonella (Enteric Fever, Food Poisoning)

Currently there are about 2,000 serotypes of Salmonellae which are essentially human pathogens. Practically, they may be divided into two groups on the basis of the common clinical symptoms :

(1) ENTERIC FEVER GROUP

- S. typhi causes typhoid
- S. paratyphi A, B, C, cause paratyphoid similar to typhoid, but are of shorter duration

(2) FOOD POISONING GROUP

(S. typhimurium, most common species; S. enteritidis; S. heidelberg; S. agona, S. indiana, S. newport; S. anatum), which is mainly animal parasite, may cause gastroenteritis, septicaemia, localised infection in man

Morphology and Staining : Salmonellae are Gram-negative non-sporing, non-capsulated bacilli, 2-4 μ* 0.5 μ in size, fimbriate and actively motile with peritrichate flagella except **S. pullorum** causing "white diarrhoea" in chick and **S. gallinarum** fowl typhoid.

Cultural characteristics : Aerobe and facultative anaerobe, optimum temperature 37°C, grow well on ordinary media, also on Salmonella Shigella (SS) selective medium. Colonies on nutrient agar are moderately large, thick, greyish white, moist, circular disks, dome shaped and smooth; but on MacConkey agar and DCA medium, similar pale or colourless colonies are observed, since salmonellae do not ferment lactose. On Wilson and Blair bismuth sulphite medium, **S. typhi** produces jet black colonies with a metallic sheen due to H_2S production, whereas **S. paratyphi** A and other species that do not form H_2S, produce green colonies. Selenite F and tetrathionate broth are used as enrichment media. Triple Sugar iron (TSI) agar medium can be used for identification. On XLD, Salmonellae result in pink colonies with black centres produced by H_2S.

Biochemical reaction : Glucose and mannitol are fermented without gas production; lactose and sucrose are not fermented nor is indole produced (Table 32.1)

	Glucose	Mannitol	Lactose	Sucrose	Xylose	d-tartarate	Mucate
S. typhi	1	1	-	-	V	1	V
S. paratyphi A	+	+	-	-	-	-	-
S. paratyphi B	+	+	-	-	+	+	+
S. paratyphi C	+	+	-	-	+	+	-

1 = acid, no gas; + = acid and gas; V = variable reaction; - = no reaction.

Antigenic structure : Salmonellae possess the following antigens based on which they are classified and identified : (1) Somatic antigen O, (2) flagellar antigen H; (3) surface antigen Vi found in **S. typhi** and **S. paratyphi** C; but fimbrial antigen is not important for identification.

H. antigen is heat labile protein, destroyed by boiling or treatment with alcohol, but not formaldehyde; when mixed with specific antiserum. H suspensions agglutinate rapidly producing loose, large fluffy clumps. The H antigen is strongly immunogenic and induces antibody formation rapidly to a high titre following infection and immunisation. It occurs in two phases—phase I and phase II.

O antigen is a phospholipid polysaccharide complex of cell wall, identical with endotoxin, can be extracted from the bacterial cell wall by trichloracetic acid treatment. When mixed with antisera, O antigen suspensions forms compact, chalky, granular clumps.

O agglutination takes place more slowly at higher temperature (50-55°C) than H agglutination (37°C).

O antigen is less immunogenic than H antigen;

O antigen titre is generally less than that of H antibody.

V_i antigen interfers the O agglutination, is related to the virulence. The development of the carrier state is indicated by the persistence of V_i antibody in the blood.

Pathogenesis and clinical features : Infection is by ingestion; from the small intestine, the organisms pass via the lymphatics to mesenteric glands, whence—after a period of multiplication—they invade the blood stream via the thoracic duct; the liver, gall bladder, spleen, kidney and bone marrow become infected during this bacteriaemic phase in the first seven to ten days of the disease-positive for blood culture. From the gall bladder, further invasion of the intestine results—Peyer's patches involved in an acute inflammatory reaction followed by necrosis, sloughing, characteristic typhoid ulcers and—less frequently—by intestinal perforation.

The incubation period of typhoid is usually 14 days. The onset is gradual with headache, malaise, anorexia, a coated tongue, abdominal discomfort with either constipation and diarrhoea. The typical feature is of a step-ladder pyrexia. "Rose spots" that fade on pressure appear on the skin during the second or third week. Some develop deafness and meningitis.

Laboratory diagnosis – Direct (blood, faeces, urine culture),
Indirect (Widal test, demonstration of circulating antigen)

Blood culture : About 5-10 ml of blood is collected by venepuncture and inoculated into a culture bottle containing 50-100 ml. of 0.5% Bile broth or Hartley's broth (Fig. 32.1). After overnight incubation at 37°C the Bile broth is subcultured on MacConkey's medium. Pale colonies are picked up for biochemical and motility studies. A loopful of the growth from the agar slant is emulsified in two drops of saline on a slide, then a loopful of O antiserum is added to a drop of bacterial emulsion; after rocking the slide gently there will be agglutination.

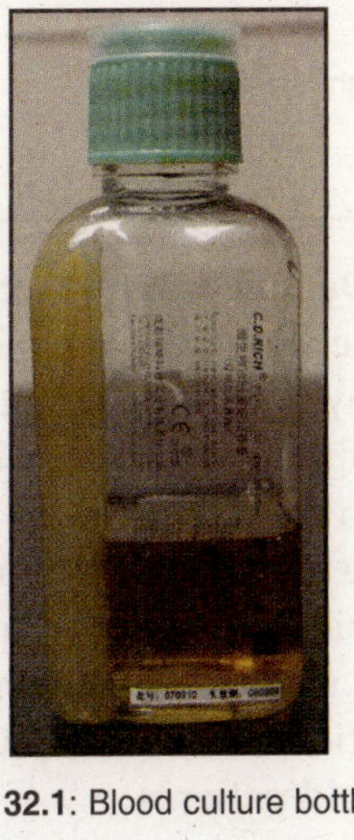

Fig. 32.1: Blood culture bottle

Clot culture is an alternative to blood culture. 5 ml of blood is allowed to clot in a sterile plain test tube, the serum is pipetted off for Widal test. The clot is broken with sterile glass rod and added to Bile broth medium containing Streptokinase (100 units per ml) which causes lysis of the clot which may yield higher rate of isolation then blood culture.

Faeces culture : Salmonellae can be isolated from the faeces throughout the illness, most frequently during second and third weeks. Wilson and Blair medium is highly selective than MacConkey's agar, SS and DCA media.

Urine culture : Clean mid-stream urine is collected and centrifuged. The deposit is inoculated into the enrichment media and then in selective media. Urine culture is less useful.

Culture of other materials (bile, rose spots, pus, CSF, sputum) can also be done.

(2) **Widal test** (Fig. 8.1) is used to diagnose typhoid and paratyphoid by determining O and H agglutinin titres in patient's sera. Two types of tubes (Felix tube with round bottom, Dreyer's tube with narrow bottom) are used for O and H agglutination, respectively. The serially diluted serum (1 : 10 to 1 : 640) is mixed with equal quantity of H and O antigens. After overnight incubation at 37°C, the agglutination was observed. O agglutination is caused by both **S. typhi** and **S. paratyphi,** whereas H agglutination is specific to each species of salmonella.

Relapse

It is mostly observed in typhoid fever and rarely in paratyphoid C due to presence of V_i-antigen on **Salmonella** typhi. Some organisms escape the effects of chemotherapeutic agents and remain viable in gall bladder. On withdrawal of drug, **S. typhi** reappears and in the blood causes relapse. In **Relapse,** V_i-antigen masks "O" antigen of **S. typhi** and only V_i-antibody is produced in patient's serum and "O" antibody production is inhibited. V_i-antigen is not routinely included Widal test. In relapse, diagnosis is made by detection of V_i-antibody by agglutination (1 : 10 or more) test.

Interpretation : If O and H agglutinations are positive with a significant titre, then it is paratyphoid due to S paratyphi A, B or C. Plate Widal test can also detect enteric fever (Fig.8.1) but not the agglutinin titres.

Table 32.1. Examination of samples at different phases of enteric fever

Stage	Examination	Result (% positive)
Ist stage	Blood culture	95
	Blood picture	Leucopenia with lymphocytosis
2nd week	Blood culture	40-50
	Widal test	Low titre antibody
3rd week	Widal test	100
	Blood culture	15-20
	Stool and urine culture	80
4th week	Widal test	100
	Stool and urine culture	90
	Blood culture	5-10

Demonstration of circulating antigen : Typhoid bacillus antigen is consistently present in the blood in the early phase of the disease, and also in the urine. The sensitised staphylococcal coagglutination test can detect this antigen; **Staph. aureus** (Cowan 1 strain) containing protein A is is established with formaldehyde and coated with S. typhi antibody. When a 1% suspension of this sensitised cells is mixed on a slide with serum from patients in the first week of typhoid, there will be visible agglutination within two minutes. The test is rapid, sensitive and specific. Counter electro-immunoelectrophoresis and ELISA have also been used to detect typhoid antigen in blood and urine. The nested Polymerase Chain Reaction (PCR) technique is sensitive and specific to detect S. typhi in blood of polymerase typhoid patients.

Prophylaxis can be done by TAB vaccination. The vaccine is given in two doses of 0.5 ml subcutaneously at an interval of 4-6 weeks. Recent oral Ty 21 a typhoid vaccine can be used more than once in the expectation that they would stimulate an immune response.

Epidemiology

The faeces of convalescent and healthy carriers are a more important source of contamination of food and drink than the frank clinical cases. Several typhoid out-break may be water-borne or food borne:

1. **Water-borne.** Sewage contaminated by a carrier is responsible for drinking water pollution (typhoid outbreak in Croydon, 1937, and in Zermatt, 1963).
2. **Food-borne.** Polluted water or the hands of carriers may contaminate the food (e.g. **"Typhoid Mary"**, a cook in United States of America, was a first carrier in the world and was responsible for several outbreaks of Typhoid fever.

(a) **Public health.** Sanitary measures for clean water supply, proper disposal of sewage. Both **S. typhi** and **S. paratyphi** multiply very quickly in food. Tinned food may get contaminated during canning. Infected poultry, meat, contaminated tinned food should be properly cooked.

(b) **Carriers.** They should not be allowed to prepare food and should follow strict personal hygiene.

(c) **Immunisation.** Vaccination is essential for those who live or travel in endemic areas of Typhoid fever.

(1) **Killed whole cell vaccines.** The bacterial cultures of **S. typhi**—1,000 millions, **S. paratyphi** A and B, 750 millions each per ml, are killed by heating at 50-60°C and preserved in 0.5% phenol. This killed vaccine is injected subcutaneously in two doses of 0.5% ml each at an interval of 4-6 weeks followed by booster dose every 3-7 years. In India a divalent vaccine containing **S. typhi** and **S. paratyphi** A are now in use. Local and general reactions are common after vaccination which vanish in 36 hours.

(2) **Live oral (Ty 21 a) typhoid vaccine.** It is a recent vaccine prepared by using a live avirulent mutant strain of **S. typhi** (Ty 21 a), lacking UDP-galactose-4-epimerase (Gal E mutant). It is administrated orally and has given encouraging results in Egypt. The mutants intiate the infection in the intestine but "self destructs" after four to five cell divisions and cannot produce any illness.

This oral vaccine is available in enteric coated capsule or in liquid form. It is safe and gives 65-96% protection for 3-5 years. Three doses of the vaccine are given to children on alternate days.

(3) **Purified Vi polysaccharide vaccine.** It contains purified Vi antigen and it is injected intramuscularly in a single dose of 25 μg. Its efficiency is about 75%.

Treatment : Chloramphenicol is the drug of choice. Ampicillin, amoxycillin, furazolidone and cotrimoxazole are useful. Multi-drug resistant salmonellae or salmonella resistant to chloramphenicol can respond to norfloxacin, ciprofloxacin therapy.

Drug resistance. Multiple drug resistance transmitted genetically by plasmids among the strains of **S. typhi** had been reported for the first time in 1972 from Mexico. The transmissible plasmids carry **R. determinants** to chloramphenicol, streptomycin, sulphonamide and tetracycline. Multiple drug resistance has become a problem in India and South East Asia

Chloramphenicol resistant typhoid fever had appeared first in epidemic form in Kerala (Calicut) India in 1972. The drug resistant strains of **S. typhi** that had been reported from India were originally confined to include phage D_1-N, but later to types C_5, A and O.

Phage types which are most prevalent throughout the world are E_1, A, B_2, C_1, D_1 and F_1 phage types prevalent in India are N, D1-N and O.

Salmonella food poisoning

Human infection is due to the ingestion of food contaminated by salmonellae from poultry, meat, milk, cream and eggs. Clinically the food poisoning is characterised by diarrhoea, vomiting, abdominal pain and fever.

Laboratory diagnosis is made by isolating the salmonellae from the faeces, article of food.

Treatment is symptomatic, antibiotics should not be used. Prevention of ingestion of contaminated food can be a measure to control the food poisoning.

Demonstration

1. Motility of **S. typhi** by hanging drop method.
2. Pale colonies of **S. typhi** on MacConkey agar of DCA medium; jet black colonies witn metallic sheen of **S. typhi** on Wilson Blair medium.
3. Biochemical reaction of **S. typhi** on T.S. I. Glucose and mannitol are fermented with acid only.
4. TAB vaccine is heat killed suspension of S. typhi (1,000 million/ml) and **S. paratyphi** A and B (each 500 million/ml) 0.2 and 0.5 ml are injected weekly interval). Immunity is for 18 months. Recent oral Ty 21, a Typhoid vaccine can also be used.

The following are to be entered briefly in the journal:

(a) Salient features of **S. typhi.**

(b) Laboratory diagnosis of typhoid.

(Must be drawn in the practical notebook)

33
Shigella

There are four species of Shigella **(Sh. dysenteriae, Sh. flexneri, Sh. boydii, Sh. sonnei)** which cause bacillary dysentery which is characterised by the passage of loose motion with blood and mucus, abdominal pain, tenesmus, pyrexia and prostration.

Morphology : They are short Gram-negative bacilli, 0.5 μ × 1-3 μ in size, fimbriate, non-motile, non-sporing and non-capsulated.

Cultural characteristics : They are aerobes and facultative anaerobes, grow best at 37°, pH 7.4 on ordinary media. Colonies are small, about 2 mm in diameter, circular, convex, smooth and transparent; on MacConkey's agar medium they are pale or colourless except **Sh. sonnei** which is late lactose fermenter. DCA and Salmonella and Shigella (SS) agar medium are useful selective media, but their growth is inhibited on Wilson and Blair medium. On XLD, Shigella produce pink colonies without black centres.

Biochemical reaction

Sub-Groups	Species	Serotypes	Glucose	Lactose	Sucrose	Mannitol	Dulcitol	Indole	Ornithine
A	Sh. dysenteriae	12	1	-	-	-	-	V	-
B	Sh. flexneri	8	1	-	-	1	-	V	-
C	Sh. boydii	18	1	-	-	1	V	V	-
D	Sh. sonnei	1	1	(1)	(1)	1	-	-	+

Key : 1 = acid; no gas; () = delayed reaction; V = variable; + = positive

Pathogenicity : Infection is by ingestion of a much lower dose of shigellae than that of salmonellae (except **S. typhi**). After reaching the large intestine, shigellae multiply locally with resultant inflammation of the mucosa which, in severe cases, may progress to ulcer formation and sloughing of larger areas of mucosa; bacteriaemia is very rare as their invasion is usually restricted to mucosa membrane.

Laboratory diagnosis can be done by immediate isolation of the bacillus from faeces obtained by rectal swab or fresh stool. The specimens should be transported in glycerol saline (Fig. 5.2(a)) never in highly alkaline transport Cary Blair medium used for vibrio. Mucus flakes are preferred and can be inoculated on MacConkey agar and DCA media. After incubating overnight at 37°C, pale colonies are tested for motility and biochemical reactions. The identification is confirmed by slide agglutination with polyvalent or monovalent sera.

Identification of shigellae in faeces can also be done by fluorescent antibody technique. Serodiagnosis is of no value.

Colicin typing

Bacteriophage typing of Shigella is cumbersome, therefore colicin typing is adopted in many centres. **Sh. sonnei** and **Sh. boydii** produce **Colicin** bacteriocins which have wide range of activity against enteric bacilli and, on this basis, **Sh. sonnei** strains (Group D) are subdivide into 17 **Colicin types** against 15 **indicator strains** and each type is characterised by the production of specific colicin.

Treatment : Oral rehydration therapy (ORT) is adequate in all uncomplicated shigellosis cases.

Routine antibacterial treatment is not indicated in dysentery because of the multiple drug resistance of shigellae. However, antibodies are reserved for the severe toxic cases.

Prevention and Control

Man is the main source of infection (bacillary dysentery). He may transmit dysentery bacilli by touching door handle of latrine with the contaminated fingers. The disease may also be transmitted by contaminated food through faeces and flies from person to person. The infection can be controlled by satisfactory sanitation along with the detection and treatment of patients and carriers.

Demonstration

1. Absence of motility by hanging drop method.
2. Pale colonies on MacConkey agar and DCA media.
3. Biochemical reactions of all four species of shigella.
4. Glycerol saline transport medium (Fig. 5.2(a)).

Questions

1. Why shigellae produce pale colonies on MacConkey agar or DCA media except **Sh. sonnei**?
2. Why is there no bacteriaemia in shigellosis; why shigellae are more in mucus flakes?
3. Why are antibiotics avoided in dysentery except in severe toxic cases?

Answers to the questions should be entered in the journal.

34
Vibrio Cholerae

Vibrio cholerae causes cholera which is characterised by acute profuse "rice water" diarrhoea of sudden onset and often running a rapid course, the patient becoming acutely dehydrated, acidotic and shocked within few hours.

Table 34.1. Differential character of V. cholerae and allied genera

Character	Vibrio	Aeromonas	Piesiomonas	Pseudomonas	Campylobacter
1. O_2 requirement	Aerobic	Aerobic	Aerobic	Aerobic	Micro-aerobic
2. No. of flagella	1+	1+	> 1	1 or > 1	1
3. Fermentation without gas					
(a) Glucose	+	+	+	+*	–
(b) Mannitol	+	+	–	–	–
(c) Inositol	–	–	+	–	–
4. Indole	+	+	+	–	–
5. Hydrolysis					
Gelatin					
Starch	+	+	–	V	–
6. Oxidase test	+	+	+	+	V
7. Sensitivity to O/129 @	+	–	+	–	–

V = Variable

\+ = some halophilic vibrios and aeromonas strains have also 1 at equal flagella

@ = zone of inhibition around 150 my disc

= oxidative breakdown

O/129 = 2, 4-diamino - 6, 7-di-isopropylpteridine (all vibrios are sensitive to this compound)

Morphology and Staining : Vibrio cholerae are short, curved, comma shaped gram-negative bacilli which can be readily stained by aniline dyes. They measure about 1.5 µ 0.2-0.4 µ in size, have rounded or slightly pointed ends. On subculture, the comma shape is lost. In stained films of fresh mucus from acute cholera case, they appear as "fish in stream" (Fig. 34.1). Because of single polar flagellum, they are actively motile. This type of motility is called as "darting motility" and suggests a "swarm of gnats". They do not form spores and capsules.

Cultural Characteristics : Vibrio cholerae are predominantly aerobic and their growth is best at an optimum pH 8.6 and temperature 37°C and.is inhibited by 7 percent sodium chloride. They grow very well on ordinary alkaline media. On alkaline nutrient agar, the colonies are moist, translucent, round disks (1-2 mm in diameter) with a bluish tinge in transmitted light and a distinctive odour. On MacConkey's agar, their colonies become reddish on prolonged incubation as **V. cholerae** are late lactose fermenters. On blood agar, the greenish zone initially

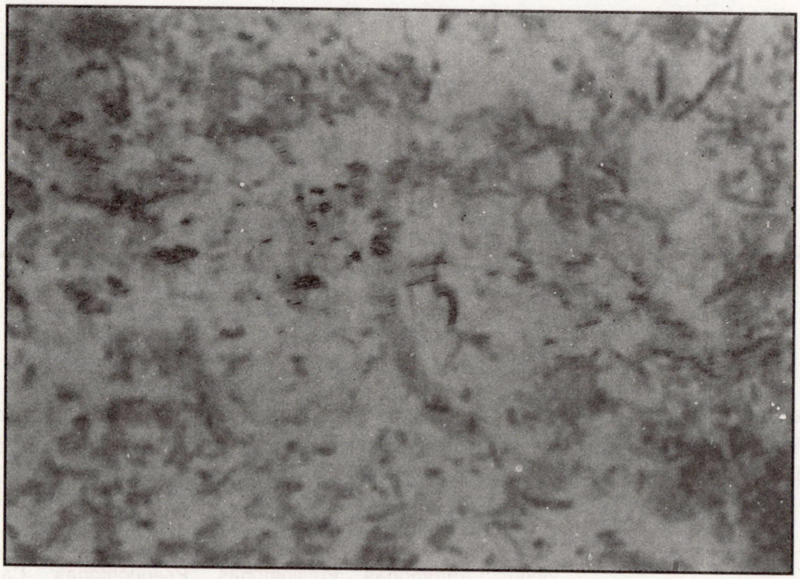

Fig. 34.1: Vibrio cholerae 1000X

appears around the colonies and later becomes clear due to haemodigestion. In gelatin stab culture, napi-form or funnel shaped liquefaction occurs in 3 days at 22 C. In alkaline peptone water, a fine surface pellicle appears within 6 hours and breaks on shaking.

On alkaline bile salt agar (BSA), Colonies are similar to those on nutrient agar. On Monsur's gelatin taurocholate trypticase tellurite agar (GTTA) medium the colonies are small translucent with a greyish black centre (due to tellurite reduction) and a turbid halo due to gelatin liquefaction.Thiosulphate citrate bile and sucrose (TCBS) medium can be used though it is not cost effective. On this medium, colonies convex yellow; because of the acid, from fermented sucrose, which turns the indicator, bromothymol blue of this medium into yellow. These yellow colonies may become green on prolonged incubation.

"String" test can be used to identify **V. cholerae** colonies. A loopful of the growth is mixed with a drop of 0.5% sodium desoxycholate on a slide. If the mixture looses its turbidity, becomes mucoid and forms a string when the loop is drawn away slowly, the test is positive.

Transport and enrichment media: Venkatraman and Ramakrishnan (VR) medium (crude sea salt 20 g; peptone 5 g in 1000 ml distilled water, pH 8.6); Cary Blair medium (sodium chloride, sodium thioglycollate, disodium phosphate and calcium chloride) are suitable transport media whereas alkaline peptone water and Monsur's taurocholate tellurite peptone water are good transport and enrichment media.

Biochemical reaction : V. cholerae ferment glucose, mannitol, maltose, mannose and sucrose, but lactose is fermented late. Indole is formed and nitrate is reduced to nitrite. These two properties can be demonstrated by "Cholera Red Reaction" which is tested by adding a few drops of sulphuric acid to a 24 hours peptone water culture. A reddish pink colour develops due to the formation of nitroso-indole. This reaction is not specific as other non-pathogenic vibrios share this reaction.

A positive oxidase test is a key step in the preliminary identification of **V. cholerae.** A small strip of filter paper, soaked in the oxidase reagent (freshly prepared 1 per cent tetramethyl-p-phenylenediamine hydrochloride solution), is placed on a microscopic slide. The colony to be tested is fished out with a platinum loop and is smeared on this paper. In a positive reaction, the smeared area turns purple in 10-60 seconds.

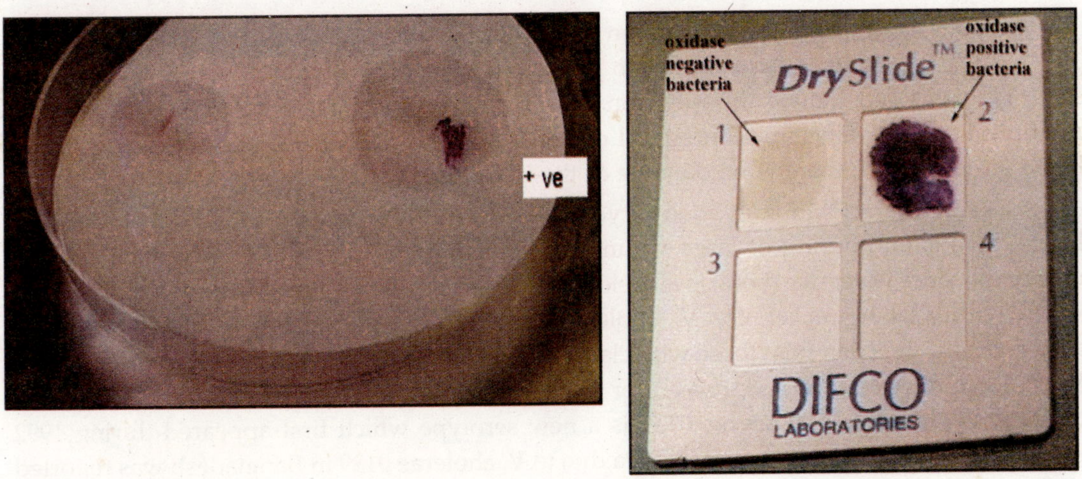

Fig. 34.2: Oxidase test

The classical **V. cholerae** are Voges-Proskauer (VP) negative and non-haemolytic while el tor vibrio is VP positive haemolytic. Equal volume (0.5 ml) of 24 hours heart infusion broth culture and 1 per cent sheep erythrocyte suspension are mixed and incubated at 37°C for 24 hours and examined for haemolysis after holding at 4°C overnight. The classical **V. cholerae** are agglutinated by O serogroup 1 antiserum but other vibrios, similar to **V. cholerae,** which do not agglutinate with O serogroup 1 antiserum are called as non-agglutinating (NAG) Vibrio or non-cholera vibrio (NCV) which are not of much medical importance. The main serotypes are Ogawa, Inaba and Hikojima. Recent pulsed field get electrophoresis (PFGE) is more discriminating serotyping of **Vibrio cholerae.**

Differences between classical and el´ tor V. cholerae (biotype)

Test	Classical V. cholerae	el´ tor V. cholerae
Haemolysis	-	+
Voges-Proskauer	-	+
Chick red cell agglutination	-	+
Polymyxin B sensitivity	+	-
Group IV phage sensitivity	+	-

Chick red cell agglutination test : A loopful culture is emulsified in a drop of saline on a slide and a drop of 2.5% chick erythrocyte suspension is added, erythrocytes will clump if test is positive. All el´ tor V. cholerae are positive, but classical V. cholerae are negative.

Sensitivity to Polymyxin B is done by disk diffusion method using antibiotic disks. All classical **V. cholerae** are sensitive to Polymyxin but el´ tor **V. cholerae** are not.

Sensitivity to Cholera phage group IV is a now available test to differentiate between classical and el´ tor V. cholerae. Only classical **V. cholerae** lysed Mukherjee's group IV phage at routine test solution.

Cholerae enterotoxin (exotoxin) is a protein which is composed of two subunits—A (active) B (binding). Single subunit is not toxic; but mixture of these 2 subunits is toxic. Subunit B binds to the receptor of the intestinal mucosa. Subunit A can be dissociated into A_1 and A_2. A_1 subunit activates adenyl cyclase in the intestinal mucosa.

Pathophysiology of Cholera : Human infection is by ingestion of food or water containing 10^{-5} to 10^{-10} **V. cholerae,** in contrast to Salmonella Shigella in which ingestion of 10^{-2} to 10^{-5} organisms can induce the infection. Those **V. cholerae,** which escape gastric acidity, multiply in the alkaline small intestinal content. They do not invade into the gut wall and blood stream, hence there is no damage of the intestinal mucosa.

As a result of activation of adenyl cyclase cAMP levels are raised in the gut epithelium, hence there is outpouring of large volume of fluid into the lumen of the intestine causing dehydration, rice water diarrhoea, loss of electrolytes. The death may ensure due to hypovolaemic shock within 24 hours. el′ tor V. cholerae, though highly infectious, causes mild and asymptomatic infection than those with classical **V. cholerae.** In the seventh pandemic classical **V. cholerae** has been replaced by el′ tor **V. cholerae;** the previous pandemics were due to classical **V. cholerae, V. cholerae** 0139 is a new serotype which first appeared during 1992 in Southern India. An outbreak of cholera due to **V. cholerae** 0139 in Bangladesh was reported in December 1992. The same serotype was isolated in April 1993 from Cholera cases in Thailand indicating that it has the potential for extensive geographical spread.

Laboratory Diagnosis

Stool can be collected in the acute stage by rubber catheter, rectal swab; on a clean paper of leaf; it should never be collected from the bed-pan which may still contain disinfectants, used for disinfection, that may destroy **V. cholerae.** For rapid diagnosis, the darting motility of **V. cholerae** is inhibited by the addition of the specific antiserum. This immobilisation test can be done under dark ground illumination. Specimens, media, colonies suggestive of **V. cholerae** can be tested by slide agglutination with **V. cholerae** subgroup 01 antiserum; this agglutination test can be repeated by using monospecific Ogawa and Inaba antisera for serotyping. If positive, the isolates should be differentiated from el′ tor **V. cholerae.** A novel rapid, colorimetric immunodiagnostic kit, Cholera SMART can detect directly **V. cholerae** in clinical specimens similar to recent coagglutination test and PCR.

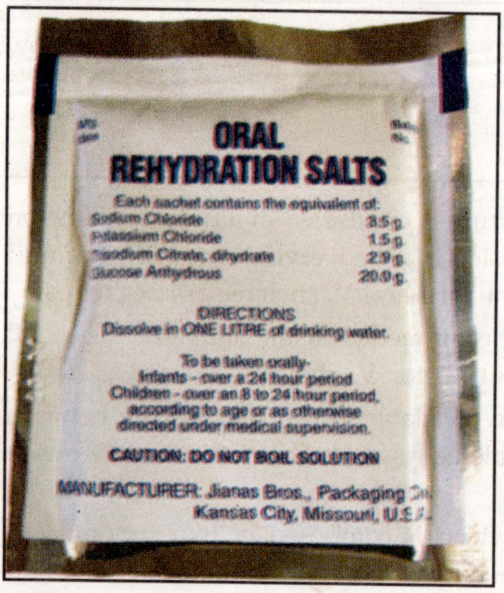

Fig. 34.3: ORS packet

Treatment : The dehydration should be compensated immediately by Oral Rehydration Therapy (ORT) (Fig. 34.3). In resting healthy gut (left) absorption roughly equals secretion. As a result of action of cholera endotoxin (centre) secretion greatly exceeds the absorption with net loss of a large quantity of isotonic fluid. When glucose electrolyte solution is administrated orally (right) glucose facilitates fluid absorption and counter-balances toxin induced fluid secretion and fluid balance is maintained. Antibacterial therapy is of secondary importance.

(i) **Prophylaxis-Killed Vaccine :** The initial trials were with parenteral, killed whole cell vaccines. These vaccines showed protective efficiency ranging 30-80% lasting several months to one year.

(ii) **Oral Vaccine :** As only A subunit is responsible for toxin mediated pathophysiology,

A subunit gene has been deleted from a classical Inaba strain retaining B subunit. This modified strain provides important protective efficiency with minimal side-effects.

Whole cell/B subunit (WC/BS) Oral vaccine is a mixture of killed classical and el′ tor biotypes and purified B subunit and has shown in Bangladesh a high level of protective efficiency with few side effects, although protection only lasts for six months.

(iii) **Live vaccine :** Recombinant DNA vaccine with expression of **V. cholerae** O1 in attenuated strain of **Salmonella typhi** Ty21 has been developed. Ty21 a as a carrier bacteria does cause significant side effects. It colonises Peyer's patch induces Ig response by local immune system.

(II) **Chemoprophylaxis :** It is useful when attendants in endemic areas are administrated with antibiotics.

Prevention and control

(A) **General measures :** For the prevention of cholera, like enteric fever, it is necessary to introduce (a) large-scale **purification of water supplies;** (b) better sanitary methods for the disposal of sewage; (c) an **isolation ward for all infected patients** with the facility for the disinfection of their excreta; besides, the carriers and contacts should be followed up.

(B) **Specific measures**

(I) **Active artificial immunisation**

(i) For active immunisation, a **killed vaccine,** containing 8,000 million **V. cholerae** per ml with equal numbers of **Inaba** and **Ogawa** strains, is widely used. Two injections are given at an interval of one month each. 50-60 per cent inoculated persons are protected against clinical attack and the immunity lasts for 3-6 months. In mass immunisation programme only one injection is possible and protects adults due to its action as a booster on top of prior natural immunisation, but in children below 5 years of age, it is not effective.

The aluminium hydroxide and phosphate adjuvant vaccine induces a high degree of immunity in young children. The use of cholera toxoid as vaccine was not successful.

(ii) **A non-living oral B. subunit-whole cell** (BS-WC) **vaccine** has undergone field trial in Bangladesh, conducted by the International Centre for Diarrhoeal Diseases, Dacca, in 1985. This vaccine was prepared by Institute Merienix, France, and National Bacteriological Laboratory, Sweden and contains :

(1) Oral cholera toxin B subunit
(2) Heat killed classical vibrio : Ogawa – 2.5×10^{10}
(3) Heat killed classical vibrio : Inaba – 2.5×10^{10}
(4) Formalin killed el′ tor vibrio : Ogawa – 2.5×10^{10}
(5) Formalin killed el′ tor vibrio : Inaba – 2.5×10^{10} cells

Protection was 85% for 1 year and 60% for 2 years. BS-WC vaccine conferred significant protection against diarrhoea due to **E. coli** (LT-ETEC).

Demonstration

1. A smear of **V. cholerae** stained with carbol fuchsin showing comma shaped or curved organisms.
2. Hanging drop preparation showing typical darting motility.

3. Yellow colonies on TCBS medium (Fig. 34.4).
4. Funnel shaped liquefaction in gelatin stab culture.
5. String test to identify **V. cholerae** colonies.
6. Table showing biochemical reactions of **V. cholerae.**
7. Cholerae red reaction.
8. Haemolysis test el′ tor **V. cholerae** is positive.
9. VR medium (Fig. 5.2d)
10. Cary Blair medium (Fig. 5.2b).

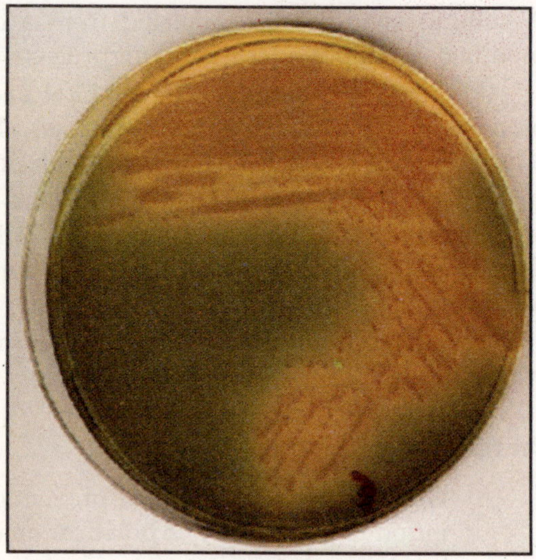

Fig. 34.4: V. Cholerae on TCBS Agar

Practical work

1. Stain the given smear with dilute carbol fuchsin for 1 minute and study the morphology of the organisms.
2. Perform the immobilisation test of **V. cholerae** with specific antiserum.

Questions

1. Why **V. cholerae** show darting motility and why the immobilisation test is required?
2. What is the utility of oxidase, string tests and cholera red reaction and why cholera red reaction is not specific?
3. How will you differentiate classical and el′ tor **V. cholerae**? What is NAG Vibrio?
4. Why are **V. cholerae** colonies yellow on TCBS medium? What is the use of VR medium?
5. On GTTA medium, why is there turbid halo around the colony?
6. Why gelatin liquefaction is of funnel shape?
7. What subunit of cholera enterotoxin is responsible for pathophysiology?
8. Why is there no damage in the intestinal mucosa in cholera case?
9. Why is ORT is given in cholera?
10. Why is A subunit gene excluded from the classical Inaba strain for the preparation of oral vaccine?
11. In which country **V. cholerae** 0139, very recent new serotype, first appeared and became responsible for a very recent (April 1999) endemic in Thailand?

Answers to the questions should be entered in the notebook.

35
Campylobacter

Campylobacter (Greek, curved rod) is distributed world-wide has now emerged as new recent pathogen causing campylobacter enteritis in children (acute infantile diarrhoea) and consists of **C. jejuni** and **C. coli.** They are urease negative.

Small, flagellate, Gram-negative curved, coccoid, degenerate bacilli and exhibit the rapid darting type of motility of **Vibrio cholerae.** They grow best at 42°C under 5-10% CO_2 on Skirrow or Butzler blood agar medium or on blood free medium—Charcoal Cefazolin Sodium Desoxycholate Agar (CCDA) medium of Bolton and produce typical grey, flat spreading moist colonies, which form an important identification characteristic of Campylobacter. They produce oxidase, catalase, H_2S biochemically. **C. jejuni** biotype 1 do not produce H_2S.

Table 35.1 Biochemical properties of Campylobacters

Properties	C. fetus	C. Jejuni	C. coli	C. lari
Growth at 42°C	–	+	+	+
Flagellum	+	+	+	+
Catalase	+	+/w	+	+
Nitrate reduction	+	+	+	+
Hippurate hydrolysis	–	+	–	–
Urease	–	–	–	+/–
H_2S production	–	+	+	+
Nalidixic acid	R	S	S	R

W = weak, R = resistant, S = sensitive

The incubation period of Campylobacter enteritis is 1-13 days. It is an acute self-limiting diarrhoeal disease mostly affecting children. It is a zoonosis (disease transmitted from animal to man through contaminated milk, food or water with cowdung). There is general malaise, headache, backache, aching limbs, dizziness, abdominal pain and seldom vomiting. First report in children in India (Panjarathinam, 1993) at Ahmedabad.

Table 35.2 Campylobacter biotypes

Species	Biotype	DNA se	H_2S
C. jejuni	I	–	–
	II	+	–
	III	–	+
	IV	+	+
C. coli	I	–	–
	II	+	–
C. lari	I	–	+
	II	+	+

Laboratory diagnosis : Rectal swabs should be carried to the laboratory in transport medium, Cary-Blair medium. Rapid bacteriological diagnosis can be made by direct dark ground microscopy by characteristic darting motility and by colony characteristics, isolation of Campylobacter on selective media.

Treatment: Erythromycin, furazolidone, tetracycline, gentamicin are used.

Prophylaxis—Avoidance of contamination of food or drink with cow dung from animals.

Helicobacter pylori (originally **Campylobacter pyloridis)** is spiral or curved organism. **H. pylori** on gastric mucosa can be demonstrated by Cresyl violet stain. It can be cultivated on Campylobacter medium in 3-5 days.

It is the major cause of gastritis, peptic ulcer with subsequent development into gastric cancer. The symptoms are abdominal pain, nocturnal awakening, vomiting, the presence or absence of epigastric tenderness.

Laboratory diagnosis : During each examination, two biopsy specimens can be obtained from the first part of duodenum. In addition, two biopsy specimens were taken from the antral mucosa. One specimen for rapid urease test and the second for the histological assessment. Children can be considered to be infected with **H. pylori** if both the rapid urease test is positive and Cresyl violet stain revealed spiral organisms on gastric mucosa.

Treatment : Famotidine; combination of Colloidal bismuth subcitrate and metronidazole is effective. The resolution of infection can be confirmed by the negative urease test and absence of **H. pylori** after treatment.

Table 35.4 Campylobacters of medical importance

Species	Habitat	Diseases in man
C. jejuni	Domestic animals, poultry	Diarrhoea
C. coli	Pigs	Diarrhoea
C. lari	Animals and birds	Diarrhoea
C. fetus	Cattle and sheep	Septicaemia in patients
C. sputorum	Man (mouth)	Non-pathogenic

36
Yersinia Pestis

Yersina (Pasteurella pestis) causes plague in man, which is characterised by a sudden onset with a high fever, great prostration, delirium and septicaemia and plague is a zoonotic disease.

Table 36.1 Genera species of Yersinia Pasteurella, Francisella

Genera	Species	Diseases
A. **Yersinia**	1. Y. **pestis**	Plague in man, rodents
	2. Y. **pseudo** tuberculosis	Pseudo-tuberculosis of guinea pigs, animals
	3. **Y. enterocolitica**	Enteritis, mesenteric lymphadenitis in animal,
B. **Pasteurella**	**P. multocida**	Haemorrhagic septi-caemia in animals
C. **Francisella**	**F. tularensis**	Tularaemia

Table 36.2 Differentiating features of Yersinia, Pasteurella, Francisella species

	Growth on nutrient broth	Growth on MacConkey's agar	Motility at		Acid from		Indole production	Urease activity
			22°C	37°C	Maltose	Sucrose		
Y. pestis	+	+	–	–	+	–	–	–
Y. pseudo-tuberculosis	+	+	+	–	+	–	–	+
Y. entero-colitica	+	+	+	–	+[a]	+	–	+
P. multocida	+	–	–	–	–	+	+	–
P. haemolytica	+	+/–	–	–	–	+	–	–
P. pneumotropica	+	–	–	–	+	+	+	+
P. ureae	+	–	–	–	+	+	–	+
P. tularensis	–	–	–	–	+	–	–	–
a Late			(22°C)	(37°C)	Maltose	Sucrose		

Morphology and staining : Y. pestis is short oval bacillus with rounded ends—i.e. coccobacillary—1.5 μ * 0.7 μ, occurring singly and in pairs. In the tissue, a capsule may be formed; in cultures grown at 37°C capsule may be demonstrated by India Ink method. It is Gram-negative and, when stained with Wayson's stain or methylene blue, it shows typical bipolar staining which is an important feature of metachromatic granules. It is highly pleomorphic, non-motile and non-sporing.

Cultural characteristics : Y. pestis grows aerobically and anaerobically on ordinary media (blood agar, MacConkey's agar) at an optimum temperature of 27°C. Colonies on agar are at first very small, transparent, white, circular disks (1 mm or less) later becoming larger (3-4 mm) and opaque. If cultured in a flask of broth with drops of sterile oil or ghee on the surface without shaking the flask, a characteristic growth develops like stalactites hanging down in the fluid from the oil-drop. On Cary Blair transport medium (Fig. 5.2(b)), **Y. pestis** can survive for at least 75 days. Sunlight drying kills **Y. pestis** quickly.

Biochemical reaction

Y. pestis is a non-lactose fermenter and ferments glucose, maltose, mannitol, with production of acid and no gas (Table 36.2). MR is positive, and catalase activity is more prominent in virulent than the avirulent strains. Indole is negative. On the basis of glycerol fermentation and nitrate reduction, **Y. pestis** is grouped in three epidemiological types, each one has a specific geographical distribution (Table 36.3).

Table 36.3 Biotypes of Y. pestis

Variety	Glycerol fermentation	Nitrate reduction	Geographical distribution
Y. pestis var orientalis	–	+	Primary foci in Burma (Myanmar), India, China, Western USA, South Africa
Y. pestis var. antiqua	+	+	Transbaikalia, Mongolia Manchuria
Y. pestis var medievalis	+	–	South East Russia

Resistance

The thermal death point for **Y. pestis** is 55°C for 15 minutes. It is destroyed by heat, sunlight, drying and chemical disinfectants (0.5% phenol in 15 minutes). It can survive in the soil of rodent (rat) burrow and is sensitive to gentamycin, streptomycin, tetracycline, chloramphenicol.

Antigenic structure and toxins

Y. pestis recovered from man and rodents from different parts of the world are biologically identical and serotypes do not exist. They have a complex antigenic structure and some 30 different antigens have been identified which include:

1. A heat labile **envelope antigen (protein)** produced at 37°C, **inhibits the phagocytosis** and is usually found in virulent strains. It is F1 (fraction 1) glycoprotein antigen complex virulent strains carry plasmid. The virulent or wild type **Y. pestis** produce VW antigen (somatic antigens) which are encoded by genes of plasmid.
2. **Virulent** strains of **Y. pestis** produce a **bacteriocin (pesticin)**, coagulase and fibrinolysin. Coagulase is produced by **Y. pestis** at 28°C (body temperature of rat flea).
3. **Exotoxins** are of many types, one is lethal for mice in a dose of 1 microgram. This **lethal toxin** (protein in nature, M.W. 74,000) produce beta-adrenergic block and is cardiotoxic in animal.
4. Plague toxins found in culture filtrates are both **exotoxins** and **endotoxins.**

Bacteriocins and Bacteriophages

Y. pestis liberate two types of **bacteriocins (pesticin I and pesticin II).** The production of pesticin I is plasmid mediated and inhibits the growth of **Y. pseudo-tuberculosis, Y. enterocolitica** and **E. coli. Pesticin II** is also produced by **Y. pseudotuberculosis** and is active against certain strains of **Y. pestis.** Bacteriophage typing of **Y. pestis** is useful for identification.

Pathogenicity and Clinical Features : Plague may occur mainly in two forms : 1. Pestis major (bubonic, septicaemic, pneumonic plague); 2. Pestis minor (ambulatory form with mild pyrexia and lymphadenitis).

Sylvatic Plague : *Occurs in wild rats.*

When a host specific rat flea **(Xenopsylla cheopis)** (Fig. 110.18) attracted towards rat bites an infected rat, it ingests **Y. pestis** which multiply in the gut of the flea and produce a coagulase enzyme at 28°C (normal temperature of the flea) which helps the blocking of the proventriculus (stomach) so that the food cannot pass through. The coagulase is not produced at 35°C. Hence the transmission via flea is low or absent in very hot weather. The low temperature of rat burrows is congenial for the survival of **Y. pestis** in the absence of fleas and rats. The blocked, hungry flea becomes angry and bites the exposed parts (leg or hand) of the human body. The inoculated organisms are phagocytosed, carried to inguinal or axial lymph nodes. An intense haemorrhagic inflammation develops into enlarged lymph nodes which may necrose and become fluctuant. The resultant mass is the primary "bubo" (1) Bubonic plague. Secondary buboes may develop in other lymph nodes. **Y. pestis** reach the blood stream and become widely disseminated. Haemorrhagic and necrotic lesions may develop in all organs, resulting into 2) Septicaemic, and 3) Pneumonic plague. The last report of Plague in India (Karnataka) was in 1966. In 1994, there was an epidemic of pneumonic plague in Gujarat (Surat) and bubonic plague in Maharashtra (Mamala, Beed, Majalgaon), India.

An incubation period of 2-7 days is followed by high fever, painful lymphadenopathy (greatly enlarged tender lymph nodes—"buboes" in the groin and axilla), vomiting, diarrhoea, hypotension, altered mental status, renal and cardiac failure. Signs of pneumonia and meningitis can appear terminally and **Y. pestis** can be seen in blood smear. Massive involvement of blood vessels may result into purpuric lesions in the skin—known as "black death."

Laboratory diagnosis : Blood is taken for culture and lymph node aspirate for smear and culture. Sputum culture for pneumonic plague, Cerebrospinal fluid (CSF) for culture and smear in possible meningitis, stained smear will show **Y. pestis** with bipolar deep staining. **Y. pestis** can be grown on blood agar and MacConkey's agar. All cultures are highly infectious and must be handled with care. Experimental animals should be deeply buried with lime. The disease can be contracted if the infected material comes in contact with broken skin (bite or scratch).

A presumptive diagnosis can be confirmed in about 80% of cases by fluorescent antibody staining. Microscopical examination of buffy coat smear of peripheral blood may show **Y. pestis** in septicaemic cases.

Antigen detection

F 1 glycoprotein antigen complex may be detected in sputum and aspirated fluid from bubo by immunofluorescence and ELISA test.

Serological tests

Antibodies to F1 antigen appear towards the end of first week of the illness and may be detected by haemagglutination or complement fixation tests which are useful to identify plague foci as the test remains positive for several years after recovery from plague. It has a limited use in the laboratory diagnosis as the antibody levels (1 : 16 or more) reach only after 2-3 weeks following onset of disease.

Treatment and Prophylaxis : Tetracycline is the drug of choice, which is followed by streptomycin, sulphonamides. Haffkine killed plague vaccine is recommended and is available at Haffkine Institute, Parel, Mumbai, its immunity lasts for 6 months; live attenuated vaccine may provoke unacceptable reactions. Rat fleas can be killed by insecticides, though there is the possibility to develop the resistance to the insecticides. The rat hole/burrows may be fumigated by formaldehyde gas to destroy **Y. pestis** which survive at low temperature of rat holes, as well as rats and fleas by suffocation due to fumigation.

Epidemiology

Eradication of plague is never possible as it is disease of the earth, of creatures that run and burrow and of the fleas that live on them.

The disease persists in natural foci because of latent infection in resistant hosts during hibernation, by prolonged survival of **Y. pestis** in soil of rodent burrows and by survival of infected fleas.

When sylvatic rodents spread the infection into urban, rats via rat flea, the domestic plague may occur. This is the basic cycle of epidemic bubonic plague. Because of his occupation, man may get accidently infected when he comes in close contact with wild rodents.

Plague persisted in urban areas of different parts of the world during 1980-87.

Table 15.4 Countries with plague (1980-87)

Country	Number of cases
Africa, (Madagaskar, Tanzania, Uganda, Zaire)	1412
America, (Bolivia, Brazil, Ecuador, USA)	1555
Asia (Burma-Myanmar, China, Vietnam, India)	1302

Yersinia pseudo-tuberculosis and Yersinia entero-colitica

These two organisms differ from **Y. pestis** morphologically; rodents, birds, wild and domestic animals are reservoirs of infection. They sometimes cause gastroenteritis with abdominal pain and fever in man. They differ from **Y. pestis** in the following aspects—they are non-capsulated, motile at 22°C (not at 37°C), urease positive, oxidase negative and are not lysed by **Y. pestis** bacteriophage (Table 15.2).

Y. Pseudo-tuberculosis

On the basis of **somatic** and flagella antigens they are distinguished into serological groups and nine serotypes **have been distinguished**. Antigenically they cross-react with **Y. pestis** and **Salmonella.** Infection occurs in animals through alimentary tract in **enzootic** and **epizootic** forms. Multiple tubercle like lesions are seen in liver, spleen and lungs of infected animals, hence it is named as **Y. pseudotuberculosis.** Most probably, man gets infected via ingestion of water contaminated with animal faeces.

Y. enterocolitica

On the basis of cultural and biochemical characters, they are distinguished into five serotypes and they are antigenically distinct : 50 O serotypes and 19 H factors have been identified. Serotypes O3, O8 and O9 are mostly responsible for human infection. There is serological cross-reaction between O9 and **Brucella** contaminated food may probably cause human infection.

Pathogenicity

The roots of infection is by alimentary tract. The bacteria multiply in the mucosa of the intestine during the incubation period of 5-10 days. The symptoms are fever, abdominal pain and diarrhoea. The severe watery to bloody stool is probably due to an enterotoxin or invasion of mucosa by bacteria which may progress to septicaemia in individuals with lowered body resistance.

Y. enterocolitica are susceptible to antibiotics. Systemic infection has high mortality. They can be isolated from faeces, blood, mesenteric lymph nodes. There is a rise of antibody titre.

Epidemiology occurs through contaminated food or water or via faeco-oral route.

Pasteurella multocida (P. septica)

They are non-motile, Gram-negative (0.7 × 0.4 μ m) with bipolar staining resembling **Y. pestis.** They fail to grow on MacConkey's agar medium. They are **Oxidase** and **Indole positive.** They cause chicken cholera and haemorrhagic septicaemia (very common in India) in various animals. They are usually normal inhabitants of the respiratory tract of animals. Similarly, they occur in the throat of humans. Human infection is rare causing septic wound after cat or dog bite, meningitis after head injury. Penicillin is effective.

Other pasteurella species **(P. haemolytica, P. pneumotropica, P. ureae)** differ from **P. multocida** in several aspects. Their pathogenic role in man is yet to be known.

Francisella tularensis

It causes tularaemia, a zoonotic disease, in **rabbits** (mainly) in USA. Human infection is by handling or eating infected rabbits or drinking contaminated water. They enter the host via skin or mucous membrane through the arthropod bite or via respiratory or gastrointestinal tract. After an incubation periodof 3-5 days, an ulcerating papule develops at the primary site of penetration on finger or hand. The regional lymph node enlarges and suppurates like bubos of plague. There is bacteriaemia with headache, chills and high fever. The organisms are seeded in various organs with granulomatous lesions which ultimately undergo necrosis.

Laboratory Diagnosis

Examination of smear from blood, pus, sputum will reveal Gram-negative cocco-bacillus (0.7 × 0.2 μ m) with capsule which can be demonstrated by India Ink method.

The isolated **cultures** in blood-glucose-cysteine can be tested by (a) biochemical reactions (b) specific agglutination test (c) fluorescent antibody staining.

Intraperitoneal injection of bacilli into guinea pig may cause **death of animal**.

Serology : A titre of 1 : 80 or above can be considered positive, provided there is no brucella agglutinins since this organisms shares somatic antigen with **Br. abortus** and **Br meltensis.** The skin test is specific.

Epidemiology. Tularaemia is worldwide in distribution.

Prophylaxis and **Chemotherapy.** A live vaccine prepared from avirulent strain can be used. Streptomycin is the drug of choice.

Demonstration

1. A smear stained with Gram stain showing Gram-negative bacilli.
2. A smear stained with methylene blue to show bipolar appearance of metachromatic granules in Y. Pestis.
3. Stalactite growth in broth culture.
4. **Rattus norvegicus** (brown sewer rat) and **R. rattus** (black house rat). As a result of infection in sewer rats, house rats are attacked by fleas and the plague spreads to man.
5. **Xenopsylla cheopis** (rat flea) is an Indian Vector of plague (Fig. 110(A).1-18).
6. Haffkine plague vaccine is prepared by culturing **Y. pestis** in case in hydrolysate broth for 2 weeks at 37°C and killed by formalin. Two doses—1 ml and 2 ml.

Questions

1. Why **Y. pestis** shows bipolar staining with methylene blue?
2. What is blocked flea? When and where the last out-break of plague occurred in India?
3. How the stomach of flea is blocked?
4. Which enzyme of **Y. pestis** helps the blocking of the stomach of the flea? Why the temperature of rat hole favours the survival of Y. pestis?
5. Why blocked flea bites; why the plague transmission is absent in very hot weather?
6. Where is Haffkine plague vaccine available in India?

Answers to the questions should be entered in the practical notebook.

Must be entered in the practical notebook.

37

Brucellae (Brucellosis)

Brucella melitensis – infects man, goats; **Br. suis** — Swine; **Br. abortus** — cattle.

Human brucellosis is characterised by an acute bacteriaemic phase followed by a chronic stage lasting for many years involving many organs.

Morphology and Staining : Brucellae are obligate, intracellular parasites, are Gram-negative coccobacillary forms, non-motile, non-sporing; some variants are capsulated.

Cultural characteristics : They are aerobic, grow at 37°C on Brucella agar, Albumin agar, Trypticase soy agar media. Only **Br. abortus** requires 5-10% CO_2. Biochemically, carbohydrates are fermented without gas and acid. Some strains produce oxidases, catalase, H_2S.

Table 37.1 : Characteristics of Brucellae

Species	CO_2 requirement	H_2S production	Growth in Thionin (1 : 25,000)	Presence of Basic fuchsin (1 : 50,000)
Br. abortus	+	++	-	+
Br. melitensis	-	-	-	+
Br. suis	-	-	+	-
Br. canis	-	-	+	-

Pathogenecity and Clinical Features : Human infection is commonly by ingestion of infected milk or by skin (contact) or by mucous membrane (droplets). Brucellae progress from the portal of entry via lymphatics, blood stream and are seeded into various organs (liver, spleen, bones); osteomyelitis, meningitis, cholecystitis, orchitis may occur. Histologically, there is proliferation of mononuclear cells, exudation of fibrin, coagulation necrosis and peripheral fibrosis. The incubation period is 1-6 weeks. In acute stage, there is insidious onset with malaise, fever, weakness, ache, sweat; the fever rises in the afternoon, fails during night, is followed by drenching sweats. There may be gastrointestinal or nervous symptoms. Spleen is palpable, hepatitis with jaundice. In chronic stage there is weakness, pain, low grade fever, nervousness.

Laboratory diagnosis : Blood, lymph nodes biopsy for culture and serum for serology are used. Blood can be cultured in diphasic trypticase soy agar medium in 10% CO_2. Serology Tube agglutination test — 80 International units (IU) and above is positive and sensitive; 2-Mercaptoethanol test is not so sensitive; Skin test is unreliable.

Brucellosis is a systemic febrile disease with varied clinical manifestation. Clinical diagnosis is often difficult. Hence, Laboratory Diagnosis is of great necessity.

Specimen. The most definite method of diagnosis is blood culture during **acute phase** of the disease. Urine, sputum, and milk may yield positive culture as the organisms are excreted intermittently in these specimens. In **chronic stage,** biopsied lymph node or bone marrow will become culturally positive.

(A) **Blood culture** can be done by **Castaneda method** using diphasic medium (both liquid—liver infusion broth; and solid medium—3% nutrient agar slope) in one Castaneda blood culture bottle. In this medium, the broth flows over the surface of agar slant when the bottle is tilted resulting in automatic subculture and incubated at 37°C under 5-10% CO_2 for about 3-5 days to six weeks. Blood culture becomes positive in 30-50 cases. **Br. melitensis** is more easily cultured than **Br. abortus.**

Identification : Isolated organism is identified by dye test, biochemical tests, agglutination with monospecific serum and lysis by bacteriophage.

(B) **Serology :** When cultures are negative, serological tests are very useful in laboratory diagnosis. Antibodies against **Br. melitensis** and **Br. abortus** are detected. Ig M antibodies appear first and decrease in chronic stage, whereas Ig G appears later and persists longer. Ig M is mainly responsible for agglutination reaction and Ig G for complement fixation. Incomplete (blocking) of Ig G and Ig A may prevent agglutination which can be detected by Coombs' test.

(a) **Direct agglutination test.** Diluted serum of patients is tested by slide or tube method against a brucella suspension. A titre of 80 IU or more is an indication of **infection,** latent active or past infection (Table) : **"Prozone phenomenon"** (absence of agglutination in low dilution of serum due to high concentration of antibodies is common and hence a serial dilutes of serum is to be tested.

(b) **Indirect agglutination test.** The agglutination can be prevented by blocking antibodies, therefore antibodies to brucella organisms can be detected by **Coombs' test.** In this test, organisms are exposed to patient's serum, incubated for half an hour and then centrifuged, washed and resuspended in normal saline. The washed cells are treated with anti-human gobulin which will cause agglutination.

(c) **Screening test :** A loopful of patient's serum is placed on a dried spot of stained brucella antigen. Antibody fixes the antigen **(Castaneda strip test).**

(d) **Complement fixation test** can detect blocking antibodies and is easier to perform than Coombs' test.

(e) **ELISA** and **RIA** are valuable and very sensitive and can distinguish Ig M, Ig G and Ig A brucella specific antibodies and helpful to distinguish acute and chronic brucellosis.

Brucellin test (skin test) is an intradermal test carried out by using the extract of brucella for the detection of delayed hypersensitivity. An area of erythema and induration of 6 mm diameter within 24 hours indicates a positive reaction. It is not always reliable.

Antibody levels

1. **Acute brucellosis :** Agglutination titres of 1,000 or more are seen. Both Ig M and Ig G are raised and antibody titres slowly decreased to low levels or zero with recovery.
2. **Chronic brucellosis :** Ig G and Ig A are raised but not Ig M. Coombs' test and CFT may be positive and direct agglutination test may become negative.
3. **Healthy carriers.** In persons with occupational risk who separately come in contact with brucella organisms, the serological test for Ig G and Ig A becomes positive.

Table 37.2 : Serological test in brucellosis

Type of infection	(FT Agglutination test)		Anti-human globulin test (Coombs' test)
Acute	+	+	
Chronic	+	W/–	+
Past infection	–	W/–	W/–

CFT = complement fixation test, W = weak

Detection of animal infection

Direct agglutination (tube agglutination, plate agglutination test), Coombs' test, CFT and skin test are useful in the diagnosis of brucellosis in animals. Milk and urine culture may give positive results. **Milk Ring Test** (MRT) can detect antibodies in milk.

Milk Ring Test

It can detect brucella agglutinins in the milk of infected dairy cattle and is sensitive for testing the bulked milk supply from a herd :

1. One ml. of pooled milk is taken in a 3 × 3/8 inch test tube.
2. A drop of concentrated suspension of **Br. abortus** or **Br. melitensis** stained with haematoxylin is added to the column of milk and mixed thoroughly by shaking.
3. The test tube with milk and stained bacterial suspension is incubated in a water bath at 37°C for 40-45 minutes till the cream rises.

Result

In a positive test, the bacteria are agglutinated and rise with cream to form a blue line above the white skimmed milk, but if it is negative i.e. when brucella agglutinins are absent, the cream-line will be white and lies above a blue milk column.

Treatment, Prophylaxis : Tetracycline or ampicillin is effective though combined treatment with streptomycin and tetracycline is more effective as brucellae are intracellular. **Prophylaxis :** Pasteurised milk should be used.

38

Corynebacterium Diphtheriae

C. diphtheriae causes diphtheria which consists of a localised inflammation in the throat with adherent exudate (Pseudomembrane) and a toxaemia due to the absorption of highly potent exotoxin.

Morphology and Staining : C. diphtheriae are slender, slightly curved bacilli measuring 3μ x 0.3 μ with club or dumbell-shaped appearance. In culture, involution forms can be seen. They are Gram-positive bacilli arranged in palisades or Chinese letter; stained with methylene blue, they show beaded or barred appearance, which is characteristic of **C. diphtheriae intermedius** type, because of the presence of metachromatic or volutin granules. Diphtheroid bacilli which are non-toxigenic, do not have volutin granules.

By Neisser's method, volutin granules are stained blue black and the cytoplasm is brown; by Albert's stain, volutin granules are blue black and the cytoplasm is greenish.

Cultural characterisitcs : Aerobe, optimum temperature 37°C; On Loeffler's serum medium, the colonies are small, granular, grey with irregular edges.

Based on their characteristic growth **C. diphtheriae** are classified into C. diphtheriae, gravis type, intermedius type and **mitis** type.

Table 38.1 : Characteristics of C. diphtheriae types

Type	Gravis	Intermedius	Mitis
Microscopic	Short evenly stained	Usually barred appearance granules club shaped	Usually long with many volutin granules
Morphology		**On Potassium Tellurite Chocolate Agar**	
Colonial	Large irregular, dull, grey raised centre radial striations like "daisy head"	Small, dull grey dorned centre; flat; irregular margin-like "Frog's egg"	Small, round, smooth, convex black with greyish periphery 'Poached egg' colony
		In broth	
Growth	Granular flakes, pellicle variable	Uniform turbidity sometimes slightly granular soft pellicle	Finely granular turbidity
Biochemical			
Fermentation	–	–	–
Glycogen	+	–	–
Starch	+	–	–

Toxin : C. diphtheriae produces a powerful exotoxin (Protein) which consists of two fragments — A and B. Both fragments are necessary for toxic effect, Fragment A has an enzymatic activity of the toxin. Fragment B is responsible for binding the toxin to the cells.

Toxoid : A filtrate (toxin) of broth culture of a toxigenic strain is treated with 0.3% formalin and incubated at 37°C until toxigenicity has disappeared.This toxoid is purified and standardised in flocculating units (Lf doses).

Pathogenicity : Diphtheria toxin is absorbed into the faucial mucous membrane and causes the destruction of the epithelium; the necrosed epithelium becomes embedded in exuding fibrin, red and white cells so that greyish "pseudomembrane" is formed. An effort to remove this false membrane may result into severe bleeding. This toxin has an affinity for cardiac muscle causing endocarditis, cardiac failure, may damage liver, kidneys, adrenals with haemorrhage.

Clinical features : In respiratory tract, sore throat, fever usually develops. Prostration and dyspnoea soon follow because of the obstruction which may even cause suffocation. Irregular cardiac rhythm indicates damage to the heart. Later there may be difficulty in vision, speech, swallowing or movement of legs or arms.

In general, **C. diphtheriae gravis, intermedius** types tend to produce more severe disease than **mitis** type.

Laboratory Diagnosis : Note : Specific treatment must never be delayed for want of laboratory reports, if the clinical feature is suggestive of diphtheria.

A. **Specimens :** The nasal, throat swabs must be obtained.
B. **Smears :** Smears stained with methylene blue show beaded rods in typical arrangement.
C. **Culture :** Loeffler serum and potassium tellurite chocolate agar media should be inoculated. Colonies on tellurite medium are sufficient to recognise the types of **C. diphtheriae.**

Any diphtheroid like organisms should be submitted to the toxigenicity test, as only toxigenic strains of **C. diphtheriae** can cause diphtheria. Tests for toxigenicity can be done in three ways :

Production of toxin

The pathogenicity is due to elaboration of powerful exotoxin by lysogenic C. diphtheriae. The toxigenic property depends on the presence of a **tox** gene determinant controlling toxin production. The tox gene can be transferred from one bacterium to another by lysogenic phages of which beta phage is most important. The beta phage is transmitted to daughter cells from generation to generation. The pathogenicity is maintained as long as the bacteria is lysogenic when bacteria is freed of its phage, such as culture in medium containing antiphage serum, the toxigenic strain gets transformed into non-toxic. About 90-95% gravis and intermedius strains are toxigenic and only 80-85% mitis strains are toxin producing.

The structural gene for diphtheria toxin for diphtheria toxin **(tox)** forms part of the phage genome. It is a temperate phage. In addition to beta phage (β-phage), other phages (α, p, L r) are also known to carry **tox** genes. **Tox** phages (β) of C. diphtheriae can lysogenize **C. pseudotuberculosis** and **C. ulcerans** and cause them to secrete toxin.

1. **In vivo test :** An emulsified culture is inoculated into two guinea pigs, one of which has received 250 units of diphtheria antitoxin intraperitoneally two hours previously. The unprotected animal dies within 2-3 days and the protected one will survive.

2. **In vitro (Elek's agar gel precipitation) test :** A strip of filter paper soaked with antitoxin is placed on an agar plate containing horse serum. The cultures to be tested for toxigenicity are streaked across the plate at right angles to the filter paper. After 48 hours' incubation, the antitoxin diffuses from the filter paper and toxin from the toxigenic cultures resulting into the line of precipitation.
3. **Tissue culture test :** The toxigenicity of **C. diphtheriae** can be shown by incorporation of culture into an agar overlay of cell culture monolayer. Toxin produced diffuses into the cells and kills them.

Schick test is a skin test to diagnose diphtheria. Diphtheria toxin is very irritating and results into a marked local reaction when injected intradermally unless it is neutralised by circulating antitoxin. One Schick test dose of unheated toxin is injected into the skin of one forearm and an identical dose of heated toxin is injected into another forearm as a control. The test should be read at 24, 48 hours and 6 days and interpreted as :

1. **Positive reaction** (susceptibility to diphtheria toxin i.e. absence of adequate amount of antitoxin). Toxin produces rednesss and swelling that increases for several days and then slowly fades leaving a brownish pigmentation. The•control site shows no sign.
2. **Negative reaction** (adequate amount of antitoxin present). Neither injection site shows no reaction.
3. **Pseudoreaction :** Schick test may be complicated by hypersensitivity to materials other than the toxin contained in the injection. A pseudoreaction shows redness and swelling on both arms, these signs disappear simultaneously on the second or third day. It constitutes a negative reaction.
4. **Combined reaction** begins like a pseudoreaction with redness and swelling at both injection sites; the toxin later continues to exert its effects; however, whereas the reaction at the control site subsides rapidly. This denotes hypersensitivity and susceptibility to toxin.

Treatment and Prophylaxis

Diphtheria antitoxin is obtained from animal immunised with repeated injection of concentrate toxoid. The antitoxin (20,000 to 100,000 units) is injected intramuscularly or intravenously after skin test on the day the diphtheriae is diagnosed clinically.

The treatment must be guided by antimicrobial drug susceptibility test. Antimicrobial drugs inhibit the growth of diphtheria bacilli in the throat and, hence, they arrest the toxin production.

Fluid toxoid : A filtrate (toxin) of broth culture of a toxigenic strain is treated with 0.3% formalin and incubated at 37°C until toxigenicity has disappeared. This toxin is purified and standardised in flocculating units (L.F. doses). Fluid toxoid is not used as such but it is absorbed on aluminium hydroxide for delayed absorption. It is the better antigen. Such toxoid is commonly combined with tetanus, toxoid and pertussis vaccine as a single injection of "Triple vaccine" and diphtheria, pertussis and tetanus in immunisation of children. Three doses are given intramuscularly at 4-8 weeks intervals from 2 months of age (i.e. 2, 4, 6, 15-19 months; 4-6 years) as per manufacturer's directions.

Table 38.2 : Diseases caused by medically important non-diphtheriae corynebacteria

Disease	Organisms
Acute pharyngitis	**C. ulcerans**
	C. haemolyticum
Cutaneous infections	**C. minutissimum**
	C. jeikeium
Granulomatous lymphadenitis	**C. pseudo-tuberculosis (C. ovis)**
Infective endocarditis	**C. jeikeium**
	C. xerosis
	C. pseudo-diphtheriticum
	C. bovis
Line, shunt, or Cannula infections	**C. jeikeum**
	C. xerosis
	C. bovis
Necrotizing pneumonia	**C. equi**
Urinary tract infection	CDE group D-2

Demonstration

1. A smear from a fresh throat swab stained with methylene blue showing club shaped with barred appearance volutin granules, bacilli arranged in Chinese letter.
2. A similar smear stained with Neisser stain showing bacilli with blue black metachromatic granules and brown cytoplasm.
3. Similar smear stained by Albert's stain showing blue black granules and greenish cytoplasm.
4. Small, dull grey, domed centre, flat irregular margin-like "frog's egg" — colonies of **C. diphtheriae intermedius** type.
5. Gel precipitation (Elek) test to show toxin production.
6. Toxigenicity test in guinea pigs, showing marked congestion and haemorrhage in the suprarenal in the guinea pig died following subcutaneous inoculation of C. **diphtheriae.**
7. Schick test—reactions following intradermal injection of test dose and control.
8. Triple vaccine (DPT) used for active immunisation.
9. Throat swab used for the collection of specimens.
10. Chart showing the difference between **C. diphtheriae** and diphtheroid bacilli.

Practical work

Stain given smear by Gram's method.

Questions

1. How will you differentiate **C. diphtheriae** from diphtheroid bacilli?
2. Why **C. diphtheriae** showed barred appearance after Albert, Neisser of methylene blue stain?
3. Why are **C. diphtheriae** black in potassium tellurite chocolate agar medium?
4. Which type of **C. diphtheriae** shows "daisy head" appearance?
5. What fragment of toxin is toxic? Describe pseudomembrane of diphtheria?
6. How will you demonstrate the toxigenicity of **C. diphtheriae in vivo and in vitro?**

7. Why should not specific treatment be delayed if diphtheria is clinically diagnosed?
8. Describe the underlying principle in Schick test.
9. Why pseudoreaction should be interpreted carefully in Schick test?
10. What is toxoid? Why should it be absorbed on aluminium hydroxide?
11. Why Triple vaccine (DPT) is used? Describe the schedule for active immunisation of children with DPT.
12. Why skin test should be performed before administrating antitoxin?

Answers to the questions must be written in the Journal.

Must be entered in the Journal.

39

Mycobacteria

Classification

MYCOBACTERIA

CULTIVABLE

(A) **Typical tubercle bacilli** (mammalian)

1. Human type — **M. tuberculosis**
2. Bovine type — **M. bovis**
3. Vole type — **M. microti**
4. Human type — **M. africanum**

(B) **Atypical mycobacteria**

Group I — **Photochromogens**

Group II — **Scotochromogens**

Group III — **Non-chromogens**

Group IV — **Rapid growers**

(C) **Saprophytic mycobacteria** (non-pathogenic)

1. **M. smegmatis** — Present in smegma, thermophile (grow at 52°C)
2. **M. phlei** — Present in grass
3. **M. stercoris** — Present in dung
4. **M. thermo** — Resistible

NON-CULTIVABLE

M. Leprae—Leprosy in man

They cause generalised tuberculosis (TB) in man

Sometimes pathogenic to man

Causes tuberculosis in man

Table 39.1 Comparison between M. tuberculosis and M. bovis

Test	M. tuberculosis	M. bovis
1. Morphology	Slender, long, curved	Short, stout, straight
2. Staining	Barred, beaded	Uniform
3. Growth	Eugonic	Dysgonic
4. Action of glycerol	Growth enhanced	Growth inhibited
5. Colony	Dry, rough, wrinkled, consistency, rough, tenacious difficult to emulsify, colour creamy white, buff coloured	Moist smooth flat consistency friable, white
6. Biochemical reaction		
(i) Niacin production	+	–
(ii) Nitrate reduction	+	–
7. Animal pathogenicity		
(i) Progressive disease in rabbit	– or mild lesion	+ (generalised lesion)
(ii) In guinea pig	+ (progressive, fatal disease)	+ (similar action)

Mycobacterium tuberculosis (Human type) causes tuberculosis in man.

Morphology and Staining : M. tuberculosis are thin straight acid fast bacilli (AFB) Stained by Ziehl Neelsen method; measuring 3 × 0.3 µm. In smears of sputum and sections of tissue, they can be demonstrated by yellow orange fluorescence after staining with fluorescence dye (e.g. auramine, rhodamine), non-motile, non-sporing, non-capsulated.

Cultural Characteristics : They are aerobes, grow slowly at 37°C. On Lowenstein-Jensen medium, their growth is more luxuriant (i.e. "eugonic") than bovine type (dysgonic) they form thin, white, smooth, slightly moist, wrinkled, granular and easily broken up growth. Glycerol favours the growth of human type. Biochemical activities are not characteristic.

Pathogenicity : The most common forms of primary infection is a pulmonary lesion which may be due to inhalation of organisms in very small particles into the alveoli, then it is carried by lymphatic drainage to the regional lymph nodes which are enlarged and followed by caseation and calcification.

Clinical features : The clinical manifestations are different as the tubercle bacilli involve every organ system. Fatigue, weakness, weight loss and fever are main signs. Pulmonary involvement may give rise to chronic cough and splitting of blood in advanced cases. Meningitis or urinary tract infection may occur.

Laboratory Diagnosis

A. **Specimens :** Sputum, urine, pleural, spinal, joint, fluid, biopsy materials.
B. **Smears :** Sputum and other specimens are examined for acid fast bacilli by Z-N method or by fluorescence microscopy with auramine rhodamine stain. If AFB are present, it is suggestive of mycobacterial infection.
C. **Concentration for stained smears :** If the dried smear is negative, sputum may be liquefied by addition of 20% chlorine bleach (1% hypochlorite solution) and then centrifuged. The sediment is stained and examined microscopically. The "digested material" should not be used for culture.
D. **Culture :** Specimens are first treated with 2% sodium hydroxide, neutralised and centrifuged. The sediment is inoculated into the approximate medium and incubated up to 4-8 weeks. Isolated mycobacteria should be identified and tested for drug sensitivity.
E. **Serology :** DNA probes and Polymerase Chain Reaction (PCR) can detect even single **Mycobacterium tuberculosis** in clinical specimens with 100% sensitivity. ELISA is the method of choice compared to CFT agar gel diffusion. HA, Radioimmunossay gives promising result. Active infection cannot be proved by tuberculin or serological test.

Biochemical reactions : Though the biochemical activities are not characteristic, they can distinguish different species of Mycobacteria:

1. **Niacin test :** Only **M. tuberculosis** produces **niacin,** a nicotinic acid, in sufficient quantity during their growth in egg medium to give positive test.

   When a freshly prepared reagent (containing 10% cyanogen bromide and 40% aniline in ethanol) is added to a suspension of bacterial culture, a canary yellow colour develops showing positive reaction. Cultures of **M. cheloneii** and **M. simiae** also give positive niacin test.
2. **Aryl sulphatase test :** The test becomes positive in culture of atypical mycobacteria as they produce the enzyme aryl suphatase.

   The atypical mycobacteria are first grown in media containing tripotassium phenolphthalein disulphate (0.001 M) for 2-4 weeks, when 0.2 N NaOH is added drop by drop, a pink colour develops in positive reaction due to the liberation of free phenolphthalein.

3. **Catalase test :** Most atypical mycobacteria are strongly catalase positive and peroxidase negative. The tubercle bacilli **(M. tuberculosis, M. bovis)** are peroxidase positive and weakly catalase positive. They loose peroxidase and catalase activity when they become isoniazid (INH) resistant. Strains are avirluent to guinea pigs.

The reagent is prepared by mixing equal volume of 30% vol. H_2O_2 and 0.2% catechol in distilled water. This reagent is added to a 5 ml test culture in phosphate buffer (pH 7) at 68°C in a water bath and left for a few minutes for the reaction to occur. Catalase production is indicated by the effervescence and peroxidase activity by growing of colonies.

Identification of Pathogenic Mycobacteria

If AFB are present

A. Growth in less than 7 days (rapid growers):
   1. Positive aryl sulfatase test (3 days), growth on MacConkey's agar
      (a) Nitrate reduction positive—**M. fortuitum**
      (b) Nitrate reduction negative—**M. cheloneii**
   2. Negative aryl sulphatase test—various non-pathogenic Mycobacteria.

B. Growth in more than 7 days (Slow growers) — if non-pigmented expose to light for 2 hours, then reincubate for 18 hours.
   1. Non-pigmented growth:
      (a) Niacin test positive, nitrate reduction positive—**M. tuberculosis.**
      (b) Niacin test negative, nitrate reduction variable—Mycobacteria other than **M. avium intracellulare.**
   2. Pigmented growth:
      (a) Pigmented when grown in light, non-pigmented in dark—Photochromogen-**M. kansasii.**
      (b) Pigmented when grow in light or dark—Scotochromogen—**M. scrofulaceum.**

Acid fast bacilli—which are neither human or bovine type—cause human diseases, they are called anonymous or atypical mycobacteria.

"Atypical mycobacteria" were initially grouped as :

(a) Photochromogen **M. kansasii.**

(b) Scotochromogen—**M. scrofulaceum**

(c) Non-photochromogen—**M. avium intra-cellulare**

(d) Rapid growers

Treatment : In addition to physical, mental rest, nutritional build up, the specific chemotherapy (isoniazid, rifampin, pyrazinamide) is supplanted.

Time-old triple therapy

The prolonged treatment of tuberculosis with streptomycin, isoniazid (INH) and para-aminosalicylic acid (PAS) extending for two years or more was widely and successfully used.

Present recommended therapy

The above mentioned regimen is nowadays replaced by less toxic but equally effective drugs (in combination) with short course of therapy. The combined therapy consists of INH, rifampicin, pyrazinamide and ethambutol. These are given orally and the duration of treatment is for 6 months. Pyrazinamide and ethambutol is stopped after 8 weeks. The treatment is continued for 8 months in non-respiratory tuberculosis. Direct observed treatment short course (DOTs) is conducted in India.

Alternative or second line anti-tuberculosis drugs widely used in developed countries are streptomycin, PAS, cycloserine and capreomycin. These drugs are both effective and cheap. When there is no improvement with therapy, sensitivity test for the infecting strain to a range of anti-tuberculous drugs is to be carried out.

Immunoprophylaxis (by BCG vaccine)

Albert Calmette and Camittee Guerin (1921) prepared an attenuated strain of **M. bovis** by growing it on potato medium. The same strain was rendered completely avirulent by repeated subcultures, every 3 weeks for 231 times in glycerine potato medium in the course of 13 years. When this strain found to be incapable to cause tuberculosis in susceptible guinea pigs, it was named as **Bacille Calmette Guerin.** (BCG) All BCG strains now used all over the world are derived from the original Bacille Calmette Guerin strain maintained at Pasteur Institute, Paris (France). Any strain to be used for vaccine preparation has to be documented and approved by World Health Organisation (WHO). Pasteur 1173 P_2, Tokyo—172, Copenhagen 1331 and Glaxo—1077 are four widely used strains.

The characteristics of the present strains of the BCG vaccine are :

(i) BCG strains grow well on glycerol contanining medium

(ii) They are aerobic

(iii) They are resistant to cycloserine.

Dose and administration

BCG vaccine is available in (1) Liquid form, and (2) Freeze-dried (lyophilised) form. The freeze-dried vaccine supplied by BCG vaccine Laboratory, Chennai, is reconstituted by sterile physiological saline to make a final concentration of 0.1 mg (moist weight) in 0.1 ml of the vaccine; once reconstituted the vaccine should be readily used. The vaccine has become almost mandatory in developing countries.

Administration of the vaccine. The vaccine is given **intradermally** in a dose of 0.1 ml reconstituted BCG vaccine.

Age at vaccination. BCG vaccine should be administrated soon after birth, failing which it should be given at any time during the first year of life. WHO recommended routine use of BCG vaccine to all children below 15 years of age.

Observation of the reaction. At the site of vaccination a papule develops 2-3 weeks after intradermal injection of BCG, increases slowly in size and by about five weeks attains a diameter of 4 to 8 mm. Then the papule subsides and breaks into a shallow ulcer which heals up spontaneously leaving a 4 to 8 mm diameter permanent round ulcer. Such individual becomes tuberculin positive after 4 to 6 weeks. The cell-mediated immune response lasts for 7-10 years.

Prophylactic chemotherapy involves use of Isoniazid (INH) alone assuming that the bacillary load is very small and no chance of emergence of a drug-resistant mutant.

40
Atypical Mycobacteria

Acid fast bacilli—which are neither human nor bovine types—cause human diseases, they are called **anonymous** or **atypical** or **unclassified** mycobacteria. Their pathogenic role was recognised in 1950 because of their repeated isolation from clinical specimens in the absence of typical mycobacteria.

Classification

Atypical mycobacteria were first classified into four groups by Runyon (1959) on the basis of production of pigment and rate of growth with include group I—**Photochromogens;** group II—**Scotochromogens,** group III—**Non-photochromogens** and group IV—**Rapid growers.** Runyon's classification is widely accepted.

Culture

Atypical mycobacteria grow in Lowenstein-Jensen (LJ) medium, sometimes at lower (25°C) or higher (41°C) temperatures than normal. Colonies appear in 2 to 3 weeks except rapid growers which produce colonies in 4 to 5 days.

Photo-chromogens produce pigment when colonies are exposed for one hour in under light and reincubated for 24 to 48 hours. The pigment is chemically **beta-carotene** and yellow orange in colour. The **scotochromogens** produce pigmented growth in the dark and **non-photochromogens (or non-chromogens)** produce **pigmentation** not related to exposure to light. The **rapid growers** produce colonies within 4 to 5 days after incubation **M. Kansasii** and **M. intracellulare** are the common atypical mycobacteria which are the common atypical mycobacteria which are responsible for the production of the disease (Table 40.1).

Biochemical test

Different species of atypical mycobacteria can be distinguished by their growth at 20°, 25°, 35°, 42° or 45° Celsius; aryl sulphatase test; pigment production, catalase test; nitrate test; Tween hydrolysis; urease test; iron up take; growth rate and agglutination test.

Table 40.1. Atypical mycobacteria

Runyon group	Name	Species	Disease in man
I	Photochromogens	**M. kansasii**	Pulmonary disease
		M. simiae	
		M. balnei	
		M. marinum	Swimming pool granuloma

Runyon group	Name	Species	Disease in man
II	Scotochromogens	**M. scrofulaceum**	
		M. gordonae	Lymphadenitis in children
		M. szulgai	
III	Non-photochromogens	**M. avium**	
		M. intracellulare	Pulmonary disease in immuno-compromised
		M. xenopi	
		M. ulcerans	Buruli ulcer Pulmonary disease
		M. malmoense	Lymphadenitis
IV	Rapid growers	**M. cheloneii**	
		M. fortuitum	Superficial and epidemic disease

Group I—Photochromogens

M. kansaii

In patients with preexisting lung disease and with impaired immune response, **M. kansasii** causes pulmonary and systemic disease. The lesions are similar to tuberculosis. Transmission from man to man is not yet known; however, the bacilli are distributed in soil, water and milk. Their pigment is yellow-orange in colour in air under light. **M. kansasii** are sensitive to rifampicin and other antitubercular drugs.

M. simiae

They are orginally isolated from pulmonary lesions of monkeys, grow well at 37°C, synthesise niacin like **M. tuberculosis,** thus they may be falsely identified as **M. tuberculosis.**

M. marinum (M. balnei)

They are the causative agents of a superficial granulomatous skin disease of man known as **swimming pool granuloma** or **fish tank granuloma** which is acquired through contaminated water. They grow at 33°C but not at 37°C, they are nitrate negative, hydrolyse pyrazinamide and show α-L-fucosidase activity.

Group II—Scotochromogens

M. scrofulaceum

It is a common cause of chronic cervical lymphadenitis (scrofula) in children. In the dark, it produces yellow, orange, red pigmented colonies. It also occurs in the environment as saprophyte.

M. Szulgai

In 1972, Szulga of Poland discovered **M. szulgai** causing pulmonary disease and bursitis. At 37°C incubation, it is a scotochromogen; but at 25-27°C, it is photochromogenic. Hence it is an unusual scotochromogen.

M. gordonae

Though this bacterium was known formerly as **M. aquae** Paa it was named in honour of Dr. Ruth Gordon, a pioneer of mycobacterial taxonomy, as **M. gordonae.** It was also called tap water scotochromogen as it is very frequently found in water and is a common contaminant of the clinical material. It rarely causes pulmonary disease in man.

Group III—Non-photochromogens

The medically important non-photochromogens are **M. intracellulare, M. avium**, and **M. xenopi.**

M. intracellulare

This organism was first detected in the Battey State Hospital for tuberculosis, USA. Hence it was called as **Battey bacillus.** It causes chronic pulmonary disease in man, indistinguisable from tuberculosis, which is common in soil and water and about 50% population show positive skin reaction to PPD.

M. avium

Mostly fowls and sometimes pigs suffer from tuberculosis due to **M. avium.** In man, the infection due to **M. avium** is not common; however, in immuno-compromised patients and in children, this organism may cause overt pulmonary disease and cervical lymphadenitis, respectively. The infection occurs commonly in farmers and their children and also in man with silicosis. These bacteria are thermophiles and grow best at 41°C.

M. avium-intracellulare complex

M. intracellulare is closely similar to **M. avium** and these two are considered to be variants of a single group named **M. avium-intracellulare** (MAI) **complex.** They are commonly found in soil. Though they are resistant to antituberculosis drugs, they respond to the combined therapy of rifampicin and streptomycin.

M. xenopi

Though they are originally recovered from xeno pus toads, they produce chronic lung disease in man. They have been also isolated in hot water taps of hospital and they have a limited geographical distribution. In London, South-East England and France, cases of pulmonary lesions due to **M. xenopi** have been reported. These organisms are thermophiles and grow best at 45°C.

M. ulcerans

These organisms were isolated from skin lesions of man in Australia and Uganda and are identical to **M. buruli.** Hence the name of the disease is buruli ulcer. They are saprophytes in the environment and grow **in vitro** at a temperature of 31-34°C.

M. malmoense

In 1977, they were isolated in Malmo (Sweden) from patients suffering from pulmonary disease and lymphadenitis. On primary isolation their colonies appear only 10-11 weeks after inoculation.

Group IV—Rapid growers

M. fortuitum and **M. cheloneii** were originally identified as the frog tubercle bacilli and the turtle tubercle bacilli, respectively. Both of them were found in water and soil, grow rapidly at 37°C or 45°C and their colonies appear in 4-6 days and are medically important as they are principally responsible for post-injection abscesses and wound infections. Pulmonary lesions are sometimes produced by **M. fortuitum** and are indistinguishable from tuberculosis. **M. smegmatis** and **M. phlei** are saprophytes and chromogenic rapid grower.

Saprophytic mycobacteria

M. phlei and **M. gordonae** are saprophytes found in soil, water and plants. Whereas **M. smegmatis** is found in smegma and sebaceous secretion. These organisms are chromogenic rapid growers and may be confused with pathogenic acid fast bacilli.

Ecology and epidemiology

(A) **Distribution :** The **atypical** mycobacteria are commonly distributed in the environment (soil, marshland, streams, rivers and estuaries). Hence they are also called environmental mycobacteria.

False positve sputum findings may be due Ziehl-Neelsen staining reagents prepared by water contaminated with **M. terrae, M. marinum,** M. gordonae, M. kansasii and **M. xenopi.**

(B) **Environment and man :** Human beings are often exposed to environmental mycobacteria by drinking contaminated water, washing, showering and inhalation of aerosols. Repeated exposure to these atypical mycobacteria may cause subclinical infection in man that may

(1) induce the sensitisation to tuberculin and other mycobacterial skin testing reagents;

(2) affect the subsequent ability of BCG vaccine to induce protective immunity.

Pathogenicity

Though the transmission of atypical mycobacteria from man to man is very rare, its transmission from environment is common. Due to their low virulence, the incidence of overt disease is very low in countries where there is growing number of immuno-compromised patients with AIDS infection. In several European countries, **M. malmoense** infection is very high.

Clinical features

Though **atypical mycobacteria** are saprophytes from the environment, they sometimes cause disease in man and animals. The diseases are : **localised lymphadenitis, tuberculosis-like pulmonary lesions** and **skin lesions (Buruli ulcer, swimming pool granuloma** (Table).

Localised cervical lymphdenitis

It commonly occurs from the tonsillar infection (tonsillitis) in children under 5 years of age. It is a self-limiting disease and can be diagnosed by histological examination of lymph node biopsy. **M. scrofulaceum** is causal agent in USA; whereas **M. avium-intracellulare** and **M. scrofulaceum** are responsible for **cervical lymphadenitis** in Great Britain.

Pulmonary disease

Cystic fibrosis, malignant disease, damage acquired and congenital immune deficiencies are the predisposing factors for pulmonary disease. Sometimes, persons without underlying disorder may also be affected. This infection, which is indistinguishable from tuberculosis, is caused by **M. avium-intracellulare** and **M. kansasii.** These causative organisms must be isolated repeatedly from the sputum over a period of at least one week for the conformative diagnosis in the laboratory and they should also be differentiated from **M. tuberculosis.**

Skin lesions

Post Injection Abscesses

M. cheloneii and **M. fortuitum,** rapid growers, cause abscesses following injection of drugs contaminated by these bacteria, abscesses appear within a week. They are 8-10 cm in diameter, painful, and last for many months. Farmers may get infected due to **M. terrae** when their wounds get contaminated with soil while farming.

Buruli ulcer

M. ulcerans is the causal agent of Buruli ulcer which was first described in Buruli district of Uganda where there was a large outbreak. Hence, its name was derived. This infection is common in marshy land with surface water of pH 6.1-6.9 and thorns of prickly grass. These contaminated thorns may introduce these organisms into the skin of the body. The leg is vulnerable to this infection.

A painful hard subcutaneous itchy nodule is first formed. This nodule enlarges, becomes soft at its centre, breaks down due to necrosis of the underlying tissue, discharges caseous material and, ultimately, forms a deep ulcer containing many acid fast bacilli.

M. ulcerans elaborates a toxin which cause necrosis of the skin of the experimental guinea pigs. The role of the toxin in Buruli ulcer formation is not yet clear.

During the healing stage, acid fast bacilli disappear; cellular infiltration and granuloma formation ensue and the patient becomes immuno-reactive to **burulin**—a specific skin testing reagent.

Swimming pool granuloma

M. marinum, previously known as **M. balnei (balneum** meaning bath) is a natural pathogen of cold blooded animals (fish) causing tuberculosis in fish and may also cause swimming pool granuloma in man due to the use of contaminated swimming pools or fish tanks. The abrasions on the skin of the elbow, knees, ankles, fingers, toe or nose may get infected. The lesions are single or multiple and appear as wart. Though the disease is self-limiting, its resolution is hastened by the use of minocycline, rifampicin or cotrimoxazole.

Laboratory Diagnosis

Microscopy : It can be done by repeated microscopic examination of Ziehl Neelsen staining of sputum, pus or exudate. Positive smear will show acid fast bacilli.

Culture

In Lowenstein-Jensen (LJ) and Dubo's media, atypical mycobacteria grow well; but in ordinary laboratory media, some rapid growers will grow. For distinguishing species, several LJ media should be inoculated with the specimen and incubated in dark and light. When heavy growth of the atypical mycobacteria is repeatedly isolated, then only it should be separated as positive culture.

Allergy and Immunity

Hypersensitivity (allergy) and immunity (resistance to infection) are two different manifestations of the same mechanism in tuberculosis as both are mediated by T-cells sensitised to bacterial antigen. Humoral antibodies have no influence in the course of the disease.

(1) In the **non-immune host, M. tuberculosis** are readily phagocytosed, but inside the mononuclear cells, they multiply and resist digestion. The intracellular parasitism is associated with the development of **delayed hypersensitivity** and of activated macrophages (within 10 days after infection) with an increased ability to destroy the ingested bacilli.

(2) After first infection, the host acquires some resistance against reinfection as evident from quick healing of local ulcer following **reinfection** of the guinea pig **(Koch's phenomenon).** This is due to cell mediated acquired immunity that has led to localisation of tubercle bacilli, inhibition of their multiplication and prevention of their dissemination.

In the immune host the sensitised T-cells (developed during primary infection) proliferate and release lymphokines that make the macrophages bactericidal.

Delayed hypersensitivity can be induced by live, attenuated and killed **M. tuberculosis,** their products and tuberculo-protein with a purified wax extract-protein **(tuberculin)** injection can detect the **hypersensitivity** status mycosides. Agglutination test can identify mycobacteria that form stable smooth suspensions. **M. avium-intracellulare** group has been extensively studied by agglutination test. The original claim that **cord factor** was a major determinant of virulence is not accepted. The **cord factor** consists of two mycolic acids linked to **trehalose.**

(2) **Cytoplasmic or soluble antigens**

These are proteins used to type the mycobacteria by precipitation test and are divided into four groups:

(a) Group I antigens present in all mycobacteria

(b) Group II antigens occur in slow growing mycobacteria

(c) Group III antigens in rapidly growing mycobacteria

(d) Group IV antigens in individual species of mycobacteria

Group I antigens can also be detected in **Nocardia, Listeria** and **Corynebacterium.** All these antigens are obtained from ruptured bacterial cells. When the protein antigen binds with a wax fraction, it elicits the tuberculosis reaction.

Bacteriophage

Some tubercle bacilli are infected with temperate phage. Unlike true lysogenic bacteria, the phage genome appears like a plasmid in many mycobacteria. There are four main phage types of **M. tuberculosis**—types I, A, B and C; type I is intermediate between A and B. In India and in neighbouring countries, the infection due to type I is very frequent. But the infection due to phage type A is distributed worldwide and is very common. Phage 33 D recovered from a lysogenic bacterium can kill strains of mycobacteria except Bacilli Calmette Guerin (BCG) mycobacterium.

Antigenic structure

Antigens of mycobacteria are :

(1) Cell wall (insoluble), and

(2) Cytoplasmic (soluble) antigens

(1) **Cell wall :** Its structure is complex and is made of lipids, proteins and polysaccharides. A particular characteristic cell wall is the lipid content (about 60% of cell wall weight). Lipids of cell wall—particularly the **mycolic acid** fraction—are responsible for **acid-fastness** of mycobacteria and also for cellular tissue reactions of the body. The **phosphatide** fraction is responsible for tubercle-like cellular responses and caseation necrosis.

Cell wall has four layers :

(a) **Peptidoglycan (murcin) layer** is the innermost layer that maintains the shape and rigidity of the mycobacterial cell wall.

(b) **Arabinogalactan layer** is external to murin.

(c) **Mycolic acid layer** is a dense band of characteristic long chain of α-alkyl and β-hydroxy fatty acids attached by ester bonds to the terminal arabinose units of arabino-galacton. Mycolic acid is important constituent of cell wall.

(d) **Mycosides** (peptidoglycolipids or phenolic glycolipids) constitute the outermost layer of cell wall. In some mycobacteria, the mycoside layer is thin; whereas in intracellular bacteria (M. avium, **M. leprae, M. leprae murium)** this layer is thick like a capsule.

(2) **Insoluble agglutination antigens :** These antigens are located as sugar moieties.

(3) **Neutral red :** The virulent strains of tubercle bacilli can bind neutral red in alkaline buffer solution whereas avirulent strains fail to do so. **M. tuberculosis, M. bovis, M. avium** and **M. ulcerans** give positive neutral red test.

(4) **Amidase test :** Acetamide, benzamide, carbamide, nicotinamide and pyrazinamide are commonly used amides in this amidase test. A typical mycobacteria can be differentiated by their ability to split the amides **M. tuberculosis** splits the amides by its nicotinamidase and pyrazinamidase production.

(5) **Nitrate reduction test : M. tuberculosis** can reduce nitrate but **M. bovis** cannot. The test organism is suspended in a buffer solution containing nitrate and incubated at 37°C for 2 hours. Then sulphanilamide and N-naphthylethylene diamine dihydrochloride solution is added. Positive reaction is indicated by development of pink or red colour.

(6) **Susceptibility to pyrazinamide : M. tuberculosis** is sensitive to 50 μg/ml pyrazinamide whereas other mycobacteria including **M. bovis** are resistant.

(7) **Susceptibility to thiopen-2-carboxylic acid hydrazide (TCH) :** The addition of 10 μg/ml TCH will not inhibit the growth of **M. tuberculosis,** but the growth of South Indian strains of **M. tuberculosis** and **M. bovis** are inhibited by this TCH.

Treatment : Though the atypical mycobacteria are resistant to various anti-tubercular drugs **in vitro** there is a good clinical response to the combination of these drugs.

(1) A triple therapy of rifampicin, isoniazid and ethambutol can cure pulmonary disease caused by **M. avium intracellulare** and **M. kansasii.**

(2) **M. malmoense** and **M. xenopi** are sensitive to the standard triple drug regimen for a period of 18 months.

(3) A simple excision of the ulcerative lesions due to **M. ulcerans** is beneficial along with clofazimine therapy.

(4) **M. cheloneii** and **M. fortuitum** are sensitive to the combination of erythromycin and trimethoprim therapy.

(5) **M. kansasii, M. xenopi** and **M. fortuitum** infections respond very well to ciprofloxacin and ofloxacin.

(6) The combination of rifabutin (ensamycin) and clofazimine (antileprosy drug) is effective in **M. avium-intracellulare** infection in immuno-compromised hosts including AIDS.

Mycobacterium leprae : Causes Leprosy in man. It was discovered in 1873—9 years before the discovery of tubercle bacilli in 1882. These bacilli occur singly, in parallel bundles. They are stained by Z-N method by substituting 5% sulphuric acid for 20%. They are found in skin, mucous membrane, endothelial cells of blood vessels and mononuclear cells. They have limited growth in living animals (footpads of mice or armadillos). **M. leprae** from armadillo or human tissue contains a unique O-diphenoloxidase, enzyme. The lesions are confined to cooler tissue of the human body. Leprosy is divided into 2 types, lepromatous (skin nodule) tuberculoid (skin nodule, nerve involvement).

Laboratory diagnosis : Skin or nasal mucosal scrapings or biopsy of ear lobe, skin are smeared on a slide and stained by Z-N technique to demonstrate **M. leprae.** No serological tests are of value and are in experimental stage.

Treatment : Dapsone, DDS, and rifampin suppress the growth, clofazimine is an oral drug used in sulfone resistant leprosy.

Recent vaccine (Leprovac) stimulates immune system to kill **M. leprae** and accelerates Bacterial clearance which enables the patient to get cured.

Demonstration

1. A smear stained by Ziehl-Neelsen method showing red, pink bacilli within blue background (Fig. 40.1).

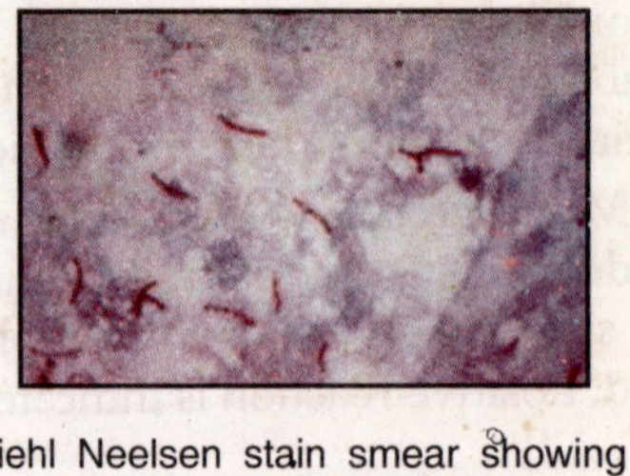

Fig. 40.1: Ziehl Neelsen stain smear showing pink or red stained acid fast bacilli and blue stained non acid-fast bacilli.

2. Lowenstein-Jensen medium.
3. Tuberculin syringe with needle.
4. Chart showing identification of pathogenic mycobacteria.

Questions

1. Why should **M. tuberculosis** be incubated up to 4-8 weeks?
2. What is eugonic and dysgonic growth?
3. What is a typical Mycobacteria. How can you differentiate it from **M. tuberculosis**?
4. When is the concentration of sputum required to show **M. tuberculosis** in stained smears?
5. What are the recent serological methods used to diagnose tuberculosis?
6. Where can you demonstrate **M. leprae** in the human body?

Answers to the questions should be written in the practical notebook?

Must be entered in the Journal.

41
Mycobacterium Leprae

Leprosy was known since antiquity and millions of world human population (mainly in Asia and Africa) are infected till today by this scourage. It is caused by **Mycobacterium leprae** (Lepra bacilli) which was discovered by Hansen (1873) nine years before demonstration of tubercle bacilli.

Morphology

M. leprae occur singly in parallel bundles (like cigarettes in a packet). They are slender, slightly curved or straight rods, measuring 1-8 μm × 0.2-0.5 μm, with considerable variation in size. The fragmented, granular bacteria are seen in smears from skin, mucous membrane scrapings of nasal septum of patients under treatment. Though they are Gram-positive, they cannot be easily stained by Gram stain as they contain wax like substance (mycolic acid) in their cell wall; but they can be stained by Z-N method by substituting 5% sulphuric acid (H_2SO_4) for 20% which is used for decolourisation after staining with steamed carbol fuchsin. They are uniformly stained solid rods in smears from patients without treatment in endothelial cells of blood vessels or in mononuclear cells.

Cultivation

M. leprae cannot be grown on artificial media and tissue culture which are still under controversy. Their generation time in experimental animals is about 12-13 days.

They can be cultivated in experimental animals : (1) mouse (2) armadillo, (3) monkey of west Africa or chimpanzee which were found to suffer from natural disease (Leprosy). The relationship of this natural disease with human infection is yet to be established.

Antigenic structure

M. leprae contain carbohydrate and a characteristic surface lipid, phenolic glyco lipid I (PGL I). This lipid has been extracted from **M. leprae** and a carbohydrate antigenic determinant has also been synthesised from its carbohydrate and used to prepare a monoclonal antibody. This antibody can be used to detect and identify **M. leprae** in tissues.

Besides, they also contain a unique O-diphenoloxidase, an enzyme characteristic of Lepra bacilli from armadillo or human tissue.

Resistance : Lepra bacilli can survive in ultraviolet light for 30 minutes, in warm humid environment for 9-16 days, and in moist soil for 96 days.

Pathogenesis clinical features : Leprosy is a chronic progressive disease of man. Lepra bacilli prefer lower temperature, therefore they localise in superficial cooler tissue, i.e. skin, ears, nasal mucosa and peripheral nerves, lungs, liver, testes, eyes and bones are also affected.

The incubation period is 3-15 years. Nasal discharge and skin lesion are the sources of infection. Lepra bacilli enter through damaged skin, cut, wound and nasal mucosa. The transmission of the disease is mostly by prolonged contact with infective patients. Schwann nerve cell is the target for these bacilli; thereby the nerve is damaged and ultimate manifestations of Leprosy are anaesthesia and muscle paralysis. Visible lesions are due to infiltration of **M. leprae** into skin and cutaneous nerve. The first sign of Leprosy that heals spontaneously is a non-specific or inflammatory or indeterminate skin lesion.

Clinical features : Clinically there are four types of Leprosy: (1) **Lepromatous** or **nodular type**; (2) **Tuberculoid type**; (3) **Dimorphous** or **borderline type**; (4) **Indeterminate type**.

Delayed type hypersensitivity plays a great role in determining the response of the host to infection and production of clinical type : **Tuberculoid** type of Leprosy is very common in patients with high degree of Cell-Mediated Immunity (CMI); whereas in **lepromatous type** leprosy the cell-mediated type immunity is either absent on deficient. The **indeterminate form** occupies a position between the two extreme forms (tuberculoid and lepromatous type). According to alteration of immune status of the host and chemotherapy clinical type of Leprosy may change.

(1) Lepromatous or nodular type

It is a generalised form of Leprosy and is encountered in individuals where the **host resistance is low.** The course of the disease is progressive and severe with nodular skin lesions (**lepromata**) on face, ear lobes, hands, feet and trunk. There is slow thickening of peripheral nerves and anaesthesia. Large number of **M. leprae** present in skin lesions and in mucosa of nose, mouth and upper respiratory tract are shed in sweat, nasal and oral secretions.

The granulation tissue with a large aggregation of vacuolated mononuclear cells containing lepra bacilli is a characteristic feature of lepromatous to repeated trauma and may get secondary infected resulting to distortion and **mutilation** of extremities.

Lepromatous leprosy is more infectious than other types. It is severe and its prognosis is poor due to deficient MI (Table) humoral antibodies against mycobacterial antigens are not protective. **Lepromatous leprosy** patients give false positive reaction in standard serological tests for syphilis.

(2) Tuberculoid type

It is a localised form of the disease and found in patients with high degree of CMI and the skin is infiltrated with helper T-cells. The course of the disease is benign, non-progressive and is self-healing. The skin lesions are few and consist of non-elevated hypo- or hyper-pigmented macular anaesthetic patches on the face, trunks, and limbs. The deformities of hands and feet are due to thickened, hard, tender nerve trunks. Lepromin test is positive due to high degree of CMI. Anti-mycobacterial and autoimmune antibodies are rarely produced.

(3) Dimorphous or borderline type

In this type, the lesions clinically resemble tuberculoid leprosy, but bacteriologically and immunologically resemble lepromatous type. Depending on chemotherapy and alterations in resistance of the host, this clinical form may shift to any of the two extreme types.

(4) Indeterminate type

In this type, there is a mild transient tissue lesion, resembling maculo-anaesthetic patches, due to an early unstable tissue reaction. This is either characteristic of tuberculoid nor lepromatous type. Skin scraping for **M. leprae** examination and lepromin test are either negative or positive. The lesion heals spontaneously in many persons and in others it may progress to tuberculoid or lepromatous type.

Ridley and Jopling's classification

For therapeutic purpose, they classified Leprosy into 5 groups : (a) Tuberculoid; (b) Borderline tuberculoid; (c) Mid-borderline; (d) Borderline lepromatous; (e) Lepromatous.

According to World Health Organisation (WHO), Leprosy is divided into two groups :

Paucibacillary which includes all tuberculoid types and **multibacillary** which includes all lepromatous types and some borderline type.

Table 41.1. Difference between lepromatous leprosy and tuberculoid leprosy

Character	Lepromatous leprosy	Tuberculoid leprosy
1. Lesion	Patches on nodules of 1-2 cm appear first on face, ear lobes; located in skin, subcutaneous tissue, mucous membrane of nose. Later on extends into extremities	Asymmetrical patches with well defined margin. Anaesthesia present in patches if involves face, gluteal region and limbs.
2. Nerve involvement	Mild, asymmetrical anaesthesia is a late sign	Thickened peripheral nerves are features
3. Lepra bacilli in lesion	Numerous	Scanty
4. Infectivity	Highly infective	Usually non-infective
5. Cell-mediated immunity	Deficient/absent	Adequate
6. Lepromin test	Negative	Positive
7. Prognosis	Bad	Good

Table 41.2. Characteristics of the five points on the spectrum of Leprosy Tuberculoid Borderline, Mid-Borderline, Borderline Lepromatous

	Tuberculoid			Lepromatous	
Bacilli seen in skin	–	+/–	+	++	+++
Bacilli in nasal secretions	–	–	–	+	+++
Granuloma formation	+++	++	+	–	–
Reaction of lepromin	+++	+	+/–	–	–
Antibodies to M. leprae	+/–	+/–	+	++	+++
Main phagocytic cells	Mature epitheloid	Immature epitheloid	Immature epitheloid	Macrophage +/–	Macrophage –
In vitro correlates of CMI	+++	++	+	+	–
Type 1 reaction	–	+	+	+/–	++
Type 2 reaction	–	–	–		

CMI, Cell mediated immunity

Table 41.3. WHO study Group's recommendations for multi-drug therapy

Type of Leprosy	Drug	Dose	Frequency	Total duration
Paucibcillary	Rifampicin	600 mg	Monthly, supervised	6 months
	Dapsone	100 mg	Daily, unsupervised	
Multi-bacillary	Rifampicin	600 mg	Monthly, supervised	2 years or more
	Dapsone	100 mg	Daily, unsupervised	
	Clofazimine	300 mg	Monthly, supervised	
		+50 mg	Daily, unsupervised	

Complications of therapy

I. Lepromatous type

There may be suddenly acute exacerbation, testicular atrophy, necrosis of bone and cartilage, loss of upper incisor teeth, diffuse thickening of the face.

II. Tuberculoid type

Peripheral neuropathy may occur due to delayed hypersensitivity reaction to degenerated lepra bacilli. Corneal ulcer may occur due to damage of Vth and VIIth cranial nerves, foot drop in lateral popliteal nerve damage; loss of digits due to absorption of phalanges from base or due to osteomyelitis resulting from trauma to the insensitive area followed by secondary bacterial infection.

Immune reaction

Immune reactions in leprosy cause additional tissue damage. They are due to delayed hypersensitivity reaction (Jopling type I reactions) or to formation of antigen antibody complexes (Jopling type 2 reactions, erythema nodosum). Jopling type I reaction is observed in borderline cases which may lead to permanent nerve damage while Jopling type 2 reaction in borderline lepromatous and lepromatous leprosy (Table 41.1).

Immunity

A high degree of innate immunity exists in man for this disease, but only few contacts develop clinical diseases. The infection induces both humoral and cell mediated immunity; the circulating antibodies have no effect but the cell mediated immunity plays an important role for the response of the host for this infection. Tuberculoid type develops in patients with hypersensitivity. Lepromatous type may develop in those with deficient cell mediated immunity.

Lepromin test

Lepromin is a boiled (sterilised) extract of Lepromatous tissue in isotonic saline. When 0.1 ml of lepromin (containing 40 millions dead lepra bacilli) is injected intradermally to an individual, it produces at the site of injection an area of nodular infiltration in skin which reaches its maximum size in 3 to 5 weeks. The lepromin test can detect the hypersensitivity in a leper. There are two types of reactions : (1) Early reaction, (2) Delayed reaction.

There is also another type of skin testing reagent known as **Leprosins** which are ultrasonates of tissue-free bacilli from lesion. They are designated as **Leprosin H** if it is from human origin and **Leprosin A** if from Armadillo origin. Type of reaction elicited by **Leprosins** is similar to that of Lepromin:

1. **Early or Fernandez reaction**
   Erythema and induration of 10-30 mm in diameter is observed after 24-48 hours after injection.
2. **Delayed Mitsuda reaction**
   Similar nodular lesion of 3-5 mm in diameter appears in 3 to 5 weeks after injection. This test is negative in lepromatous leprosy and is positive in tuberculoid leprosy. The positive reaction is an indication of resistance to leprosy.

Significance of Lepromin test

1. **Classification of Leprosy :** On the basis of Lepromin test, Leprosy can be classified into (a) lepromatous leprosy, if this test is negative; (b) tuerculoid type, if it is positive; (c) borderline and indeterminate leprosy, if lepromin test is either negative or weakly positive.
2. **Prognosis of Leprosy :** If the test is positive, the prognosis is better, if negative reaction converts into positive during treatment, it shows an improvement by therapy.
3. **Assessment of resistance** to leprosy is preferable for field workers. They should be lepromin positive.

Laboratory diagnosis

A. Direct skin smear examination

Smear made from the scraping of skin, ear lobes, patches, nodules etc. can be stained by modified Z-N method using 5% sulphuric acid and examined. The living bacilli stain uniformly as a strong rod; whereas dead bacilli are fragment and granular. Demonstration of bacilli under microscope is a direct evidence of Leprosy:

1. **Bacteriological index :** It is associated from stained smear by oil immersion lens (× 100) of microscope. International bacteriological index is from 1 to 6+ :
   1-10 bacilli in 100 fields = 1 +
   1-10 bacilli in 10 fields = 2 +
   1-10 bacilli per field = 3 +
   10-100 bacilli per field = 4 +
   100-1,000 bacilli per field = 5 +
   More than 1,000 bacilli per field = 6 +
2. **Morphological index :** It is the percentage of uniformly stained bacilli in a lesion out of the total bacteria present in the lesion and it can assess the prognosis and response of the disease to the drug.

B. Histological examination of skin nerve biopsy : When lepra bacilli cannot be demonstrated by direct smear the histological examination of the biopsy material can be undertaken to confirm tuberculoid leprosy.

C. Animal inoculation : Injection of ground tissue from the lesion into foot pad of mouse may produce typical granuloma in six months. This test is also useful to confirm doubtful diagnosis, to test drug resistance and to evaluate antimicrobial activity of newer drugs.

D. Indirect method

1. **Lepromin test :** Though it is useful to assess the prognosis of leprosy, it has a limited diagnostic value.
2. **Serological test :** Various serological tests were aimed at the detection of antiphenolic glycolipid I (anti-PGL I) antibodies. They are latex agglutination, Mycobacterium leprae Particle Agglutination (MLPA) test and ELISA.

In MLPA test, gelatin particles coated with natural. Trisaccharide phenyl propionate Bovine serum Albumen (NTPBSA) has a stable hydrophilic substance that exhibits stronger sero reactivity than the natural PGL I antigen used to detect anti-PGL I antibodies. Anti-PGL-I antibody titres are very high in new untreated lepromatous cases as compared to old treated patients. The Tuberculoid cases show low titres. The positivity rate is as follows : lepromatous (78-80%); borderline (45-50%) and tuberculoid (20-22%). The antibody titres decrease following effective chemotherapy. Standard Serological Test (STS) gives false positive reaction in lepromatous leprosy.

Treatment

Dapsone (4.4′ diamino diphenyl sulphone) (DDS) monotherapy was standard drug for all types of Leprosy till 1982. Later WHO recommended multi-drug therapy (MDT) for all types of Leprosy by the use of rimfapicin, dapsone and clofazimine (Table 41.3).

Epidemiology : Man is the main source of infection. Nasal secretions and discharges from nodular lesions are infectious materials for family contacts by inhalation and through the skin. Transmission of Leprosy occurs in children exposed to heavy shedders of bacilli for long period. Blood of lepromatous leprosy patients may have adequate number of bacilli which may be transmitted by blood-sucking insects.

Leprosy is endemic and widespread in the underdeveloped countries—mainly Asia and Africa. Out of 11 million world-wide cases, four million are in India.

Prevention and control : BCG vaccine seems to give some protection against leprosy in children of 0-15 years in countries where BCG vaccine was used against tuberculosis. Similar trial in children in Myanmar (Burma) claimed 82% protection where lepromatous leprosy is prevented. Recent vaccine (LEPROVAC) stimulates immune system to kill **M. leprae** and accelerates bacterial clearance which enables the patient to be cured under experimentation.

42
Spore Forming Bacilli

(Anthrax, tetanus, gas gangrene, botulism)
↓

Aerobic, Central spore within bacilli, (Bacillus anthracis)	Anaerobic, spore bulging from bacilli, Clostridium tetani, Cl. welchii, Cl. botulinum

Table 42.1. Important sporogenous aerobic bacilli (Differential characteristics)

Property	B. anthracis	B. cereus	B. subtilis	B. stearothermophilus
Size (μm)	Large (6 × 1.5)	Large	Small (3 × 0.6)	Small
Motility	–	+	+	+
Capsule	+	–	–	–
Optimal growth temperature (°C)	37	30	37	55
Pathogenicity in mouse	+++	+	–	–

Bacillus anthracis : causes anthrax, a zoonotic disease, in animals and malignant pustules or Wool sorter disease in man.

Morphology and Staining : Gram-positive, straight, rectangular (4-8 × 1-1.4μ) bacilli arranged in long chains with square ends and central spores (Fig. 42.1), they are non-motile. In blood and tissue, they exhibit a distinct capsule composed of D-glutamic acid which, when stained with polychrome methylene blue, is purplish and the bacillus is blue — this is known of Methylene blue reaction of Mc Fadyean.

Table 43.1. Differentiating features of B. anthracis and anthracoid Bacilli

Chapter	B. anthracis	Anthracoid bacilli
1. Motility	Non-motile	Motile
2. Capsule	Present	Absent
3. Chain formation	Grow in long chains	Grow in short chains
4. Turbidity in broth	No turbidity	Uniform turbidity
5. Colony on N. agar	Medusa head	No such colony
6. Gelatin stab culture	Inverted "fir tree" appearance	Liquefication (rapid)
7. Haemolysis on blood agar	Absent or weak	Well-marked
8. Growth in penicillin agar—10 units (ml)	No growth	Usually grow
9. Growth at 45°C	No growth	Usually grow

	Chapter	B. anthracis	Anthracoid bacilli
10.	Ascoli's precipitin test	Strongly positive	Negative
11.	Fluorescent Antibody Test with anthrax antiserum	Positive	Negative
12.	Susceptibility to gammaphage	Susceptible	Not susceptible
13.	Pathogenicity test in guinea pig	Pathogenic	Not pathogenic
13.	McFaydean reaction	Positive	Negative

Cultural Characteristics ; Bacillus anthracis is aerobe and facultative anaerobe, optimum temperature 37 C, grows well on all ordinary media; on nutrient agar, colonies are white, granular, circular disks which—under the low power of the microscope—show a wavy margin like locks of hair — "medusa head" appearance; On agar stroke, the growth is of ground glass appearance; in gelatin stab, "inverted fir-tree" growth appears haemolysis on blood agar medium is uncommon with **Bacillus anthracis,** but common with the saprophyte bacilli.

Biochemical reaction

It has little value. Glucose, sucrose and maltose and fermented with acid production only. B. anthracis are catalase positive and reduce nitrates to nitrites.

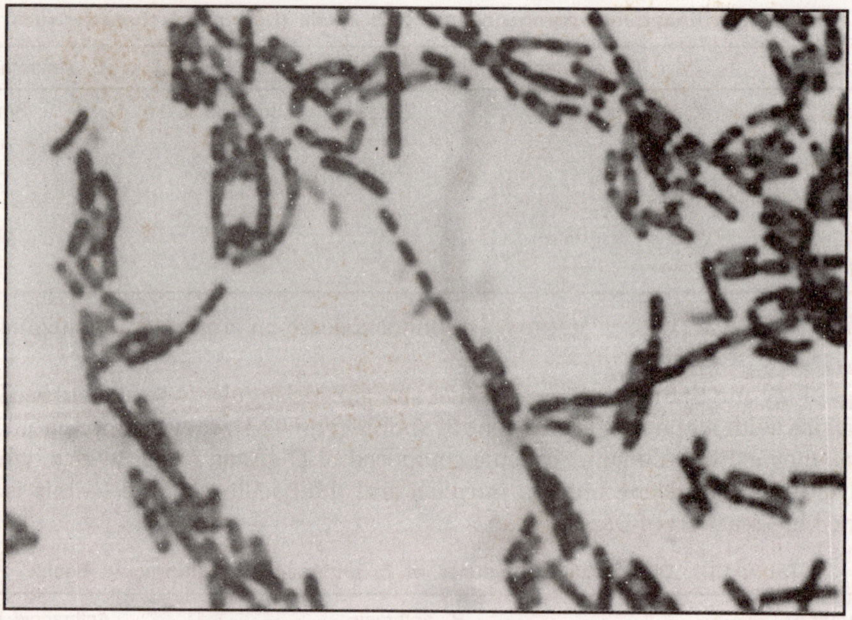

Fig. 42.1: Bacillus anthracis 1000X in chain

Resistance

(a) **Vegetative forms** are killed at 56 C in 30 minutes.

(b) **Spore forms** (Figs. 42.1, 2) resist dry heat at 140 C for 1-3 hour and boiling and steaming at 100 C for 5-10 min. They remain viable in environment in dry state for years.

Spores are destroyed by

1. Chemicals (mercuric chloride, 1 in 1,000); potassium permanganate solution, 4%; formaldehyde, 10%) in half an hour.

2. Autoclaving at 121 C (15 lbs/in^2) for 15 minutes.

B. anithracis are sensitive to several antibiotics penicillin, streptomycin, erythromycin, tetracycline and chloramphenicol. Since these antibiotics have no effect on "Anthrax toxin complex", it is necessary to administrate immuno serum alongwith antibiotics.

Antigenic structure

B. anthracis have three main antigens:

A. **Capsular antigen.** It is present in virulent strains and consists of a polypeptide D-glutamic acid which acts as a hapten.
B. **Cell wall antigen** is a polysaccharide.
C. **Somatic antigen** is present in tissue or oedema fluid of anthrax lesion; it is heat labile protein. It is protective antigen, it stimulates immunity, the antibody thus produced is protective.

Toxin : From culture filtrate (anthrax toxin), three substrates have been separated by glass filtration and chromatography:

1. Protective antigen (a protein), 2. oedema factor; 3. toxic factor; Mixture of 1, 2 and 3 is more toxic in animals and more immunogenic than single substances. It is known as "Anthrax toxin complex".

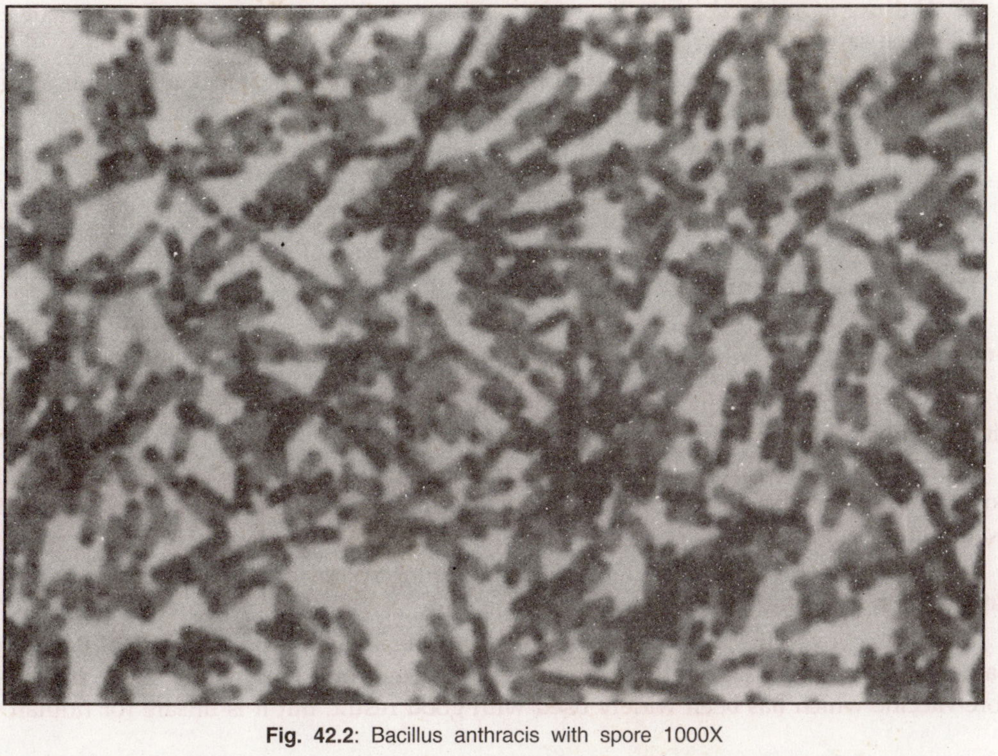

Fig. 42.2: Bacillus anthracis with spore 1000X

The toxic complex is lethal and produces intensive vascular permeability and oedema which results into death of infected animal. Besides, this toxin has, probably, an affinity for cells of mononuclear phagocytic system. The capsular antigen inhibits opsonisation and phagocytosis. The production of toxin by **B. anthracis** is controlled by a plasmid, loss of which renders the strain avirulent.

Pathogenicity and Clinical features

The infection is usually acquired by the entry of spores through injured skin and mucous membrane, rarely by inhalation of spores in the lung. The spores germinate in the tissue at the site of entry and the growth of the vegetative organism results in the formation of a gelatinous oedema and congestion. Men (farmers, veterinarians) acquire the infection from contact of the infected animals. The resulting lesion is malignant pustule in which the papule changes into vesicle, then pustule and, finally, into a necrotic ulcer which is responsible for the dissemination of infection resulting into septicaemia.

Another type of anthrax is inhalation anthrax (Wool sorter disease). The inhalation of anthrax spores from the dust of wool, hair or hides results in the germination of spores in the lungs and the production of pneumonia, meningitis and sepsis which are rapidly fatal. In anthrax sepsis, the number of organisms in the blood is more than 10^7/ml just before the death.

Laboratory diagnosis

A. **Specimens :** Fluid or pus from local lesion, blood sputum.

B. **Smears :** Anthrax bacilli occur in long chains of large Gram-positive bacilli and can be identified by immunofluorescence staining technique.

C. **Culture :** On blood agar, they are non-haemolytic, grey colonies. On nutrient agar, medusa head appearance colonies.

   In semi-solid meidum, they are non-motile but saprophytic bacilli are motile. Virulent anthrax culture kills mice or guinea pig upon intraperitoneal injection.

D. **Ascoli test :** Extract of infected tissues show a ring of precipitate when layered over immune serum.

E. **Serological tests :** Precipitating or haemagglutinating antibodies can be demonstrated in the patient serum.

Treatment : Many antibiotics are effective.

Immunity

Immunity is produced and the "**toxigenic complex**" acts as immunogen when susceptible animals are vaccinated with the attenuated **B. anthracis.**

Alum precipitated toxoid prepared from the protective antigen has been successfully used in occupational 'risk groups'. It is administrated intramuscularly in three doses at intervals of 6 weeks and 6 months. After one year a booster may be given.

A "**Sterne vaccine**" has been developed containing spores of a non-capsulated avirulent mutant strain of **B. anthracis.**

A "**Mazucchi vaccine**" contains spores of stable attenuated Carbazoo strain of **B. anthracis** in a preservative of 2% saponin. The animal is protected for a year with a single injection of spore vaccine which has been widely used with good result. But it is unsafe for human use.

Treatment

Penicillin is the drug of choice. The case fatality of **malignant pustule** has been brought down from 20% to 5% by the treatment with penicillin and streptomycin. Antibodies are of no use when the toxin is formed.

Scalvo immune serum—prepared in ass by active immunisation—can neutralise toxin septicaemia; can be treated with antibiotics and together with immune serum.

Epidemiology

Anthrax is primarily a disease of animals transmitted secondarily to human beings (**Zoonosis**). WHO reported in Asia and African many agricultural anthrax which were contacted by the animals after grazing the pasture contaminated with the anthrax spores. These spores may enter the oral mucosa damaged by dry sharp grass and germinate in the wound into vegetative forms liberating toxin thus causing Anthrax **(enzootic anthrax).** In 1980, in Zimbabwe, during **epizootie** of anthrax, about 9,000 human cases were reported.

Industrial anthrax is due to contaminated imported hides, hairs, bone meals which can be diagnosed by **Ascoli's test**.

Prophylaxis

1. Animal died of Anthrax should be disposed off by burning or deep burial in a lime pit at a depth of 6 feet (2 meters).
2. During epizootie, all animals should be protected by live attenuated vaccine.
3. Animal products (wool, horse, hair etc.) should be disinfected.
4. During outbreak, antibiotics along with immune serum should be administrated to person at risk.

43
Clostridium Tetani

The genus **Clostridium** is anaerobic sporing, Gram-positive bacilli. The diameter of spore is wider than that of bacterial body giving the bacillus a swollen appearance resembling a spindle. The name **Clostridium** is derived from the word *'Kloster'*, meaning spindle. (Fig. 43.1).

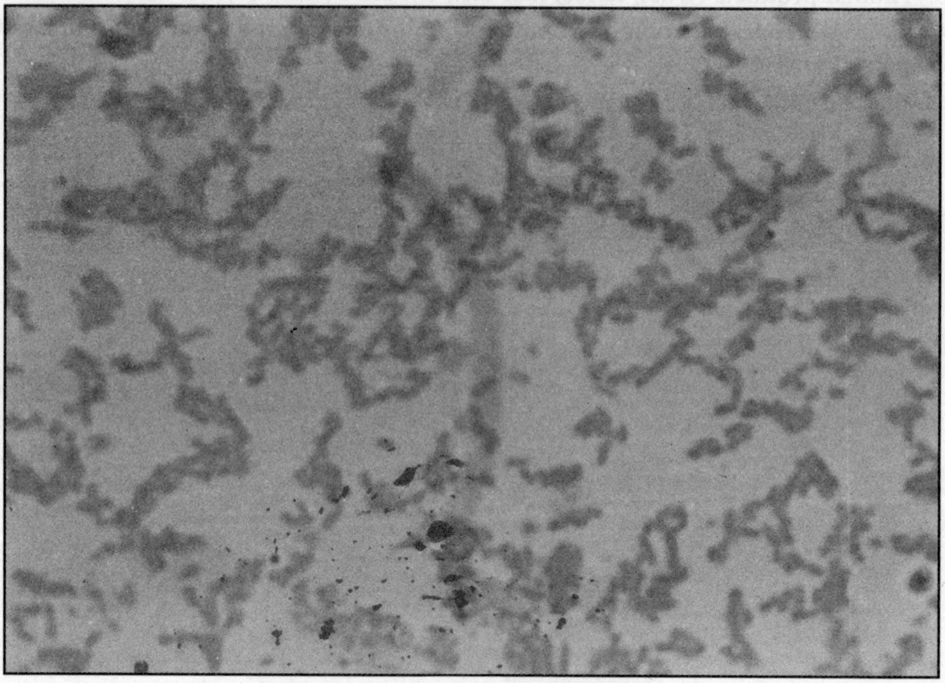

Fig. 43.1: Clostridium tetani 1000X

Classification

The clostridia can be classified on the basis of diseases produced by them:

A. Tetanus	**Cl. tetani**
B. Gas gangrene	
1. Established pathogens	**Cl. welchii**
	Cl. septicum
	Cl. novyi (Cl. odematiens)

2. Less pathogenic	**Cl. histolyticum** **Cl. fallax**
3. Doubtful pathogens	**Cl. bifermentans** **Cl. sporogenes**
C. Food poisoning	
1. Gastroenteritis	**Cl. welchii** (a subgroup of type A)
2. Botulism	**Cl. botulinum**
D. Acute colitis	**Cl. difficile**

Table 43.1. Important properties of Clostridia

Diseases and Causal agents	Aerobic growth	Spores	Motility	Lecinithase	Toxicity (mice)	Milk	Gelatinase	Lactose	Glucose	Maltose	Sucrose	Indole	Toxin neutralisation	for specific identification	Organic acid detected by GLC
A. Tetanus	–	T	+	–	+	NC	+	–	–	–	–	V	+	+	A P B
Cl. tetani															
B. Gas gangrene															
Cl. welchii	–	ST	–	+	V	CG	–	A	A	A	A	–	–		A B
Cl. novyi	–	ST	+	+	V	V	+	–	A	V	–	–		+	A, P, B
Cl. septicum	–	ST	+	–	+	NC	+	A	A	A	–	–			A B
Cl. histolyticum	+	ST	+	–	V	CD	+	–	–	–	–	–			A, L
Cl. tertium	+	T	+	–	–	V	–	A	A	A	A	–			A, B, L
Cl. bifermentans	–	ST	+	+	–	D	+	–	A	A	–	+			A,P, Ib, IV, IC
C. sporogenes	–	ST	+	–	–	CD	+	–	A	A	A	–			A, IV, B
C. Botulism															
Cl. botulinum	–	ST	+	–	+	V	+	–	A	V	–	–		+	
D. **Pseudo-membranous** Enterocolitis															
Cl. difficile	–	ST	+	–	V	NC	V	–	A	A	–	–		+	A P, IB, B IV, V, Ie

A, Acid; C, Coagulated; D, Digested; G, gas; NC, No coagulation; ST, Subterminal; T, Terminal; V, Variable * Gas Liquid chromatography; A, Acetic acid; B, Butyric acid; IB, Isobutryic acid; IV, Isovaleric acid. Ie, Isocoproic acid; L, Lactic acid; P, Probinic acid; V, Valeric acid; + spores not found in direct; smears from wound or culture but can be seen when grown on special medium

Clostridium tetani : Causes tetanus characterised by hyperexcitability of voluntary musculature and responses to trivial stimuli. When the muscles of jaw are affected, the trismus occurs as an early sign of tetanus in man, ultimately lockjaw occurs.

Morphology and Staining : Straight, slender rod shaped Gram-positive organisms, 2-3 × 0.4 - 0.5 u. There are ten types of Cl. tetani which are motile except type 6. Spore is terminal and spherical, 2-4 times the diameter of the bacillus producing drum stick appearance (Fig. 43.1).

Cultural Characteristics : Cl. tetani is an obligatory anaerobe, optimum temperature 37°C, grows on nutrient agar medium under anaerobic condition (Fildes or McIntosh jar,) Agar plates or culture tubes are placed in an airtight jar from which air is removed and replaced by nitrogen with 10% CO_2 or oxygen must be replaced by "Gaspack." On solid media, smaller colonies that extend (more than 1 mm in diameter) in a meshwork of the fine filaments are formed. **Cl. tetani** forms haemolysis on blood agar medium. Robertson's cooked meat medium (RCM) shows slight digestion and blackening of meat due to sulphur containing amino acid. Cultures have an unpleasant slightly pungent smell. Biochemically, **Cl. tetani** are inert.

Resistance

Majority of **Cl. tetani** strains are killed by boiling for 15 minutes but **some** withstand boiling for 3 hours and dry heat at 160°C for one hour. The spores can survive in soil for years, but they are killed by autoclaving at 121°C; Iodine (1% aqueous) solution) and hydrogen peroxide (10 volumes) kill the spores within few hours.

Antigenic structure

All strains of **Cl. tetani** share a common somatic (O) antigen. On the basis of specific flagellar (H) antigens, ten types (I-X) of **Cl. tetani** are recognised by agglutination test. Type VI of **Cl. tetani** is a non-flagellar strain which is only one non-motile strain.

All types produce the same toxin which is pharmacologically and antigenically identical. Toxin production seems to be **plasmid** mediated, Exotoxin of **Cl. tetani** has two components.

Toxin : The potent exotoxin consists of (a) tetanospasmin, and (b) tetanolysin; tetanospasmin, essential pathogenic constituent, acts in several ways upon central nervous system (CNS). It inhibits the release of acetylcholine, thus interfering with neuromuscular transmission, which results into generalised muscular spasms, hyperreflexia and seizures. This toxin has been separated as a pure crystalline protein which is lethal to a mouse in 0.000001 mg dose. Thus it is a powerful poison second in potency only to the exotoxin of **C. botulinum** and its production is favoured by (1) necrotic tissue, (2) calcium salts, (3) pyogenic infection. The toxin culture filtrate is absorbed by motor end plates and is spread up the spaces between the nerve fibres and reach the CNS or via blood stream. When tetanus toxin is injected into guinea pigs or mice, the animals die within a day or two with typical signs of tetanus. Tetanic spasms may start in the muscles related to the site of injection.

Tetanolysin. It is heat and oxygen labile and causes lysis of red blood cells of many species of animals (horse, rabbit). It may act as leucocidin and its pathogenic role is still unclear.

Antitoxin : Tetanus antitoxin, called Anti-Tetanus Serum (ATS) can be obtained by immunising horses with toxoid and is of value in the prophylaxis of tetanus when given as passive immunisation.

Clinical features : The incubation period is 4-5 days to weeks. The disease is characterised by convulsive tonic contraction of voluntary muscles. Muscular spasms often involve first the area of injury and infection and then the muscles of jaw (trismus, lockjaw) which contract so that the mouth cannot be opened. Gradually, other voluntary muscles become involved—resulting in tonic spasm.

Tetanus

It is characterised by severe and painful muscle spasms. Masseter muscles are first affected causing "Lockjaw"; when extensor muscles of the body are affected by the progressive spasm the body becomes arched in opisthotonus patients. Usually the wound is infected by **Cl. tetani** and its spores—which ultimately produce toxin responsible for tetanus. Wounds of face, neck and upper extremities are greater risk.

Mode of infection

1. Exogenous infection

Cl. tetani are usually found in the intestine of man and animals and are excreted out alongwith faeces which contaminate the soil. The spores of **Cl. tetani** in soil and dust may infect the deep penetrating wound or street accident wound. The growth of tetanus bacilli is promoted by the anaerobic condition and also by the presence of dead tissue and effused blood. The contaminated surgical equipments may infect surgical wound and umbilical stump thorn prick may cause tetanus.

2. Endogenous infection

Tetanus may result from septic abortion and puerperal sepsis in a person harbouring **Cl. tetani** in intestine. The spores of tetanus bacilli germinate in wound under a favourable condition (low oxygen tension, presence favourable) of necrotic tissue, effused blood and associated pyogenic infection of the wound. Tetanus neonatorum, post-abortal and puerperal tetanus may cause high fatality (15-50%). The warm climate, unhygienic conditions and poor medical services are the factors responsible for higher incidence of tetanus in developing countries.

Laboratory diagnosis : Diagnosis rests on clinical picture and history of injury. Anaerobic culture of contaminated tissue may yield **Cl. tetani.** However, the preventive and therapeutic use of antitoxin should never be withdrawn pending the cultural test. Proof of isolation of **Cl. tetani** must rest on production of toxin and its neutralisation by specific antitoxin.

Wound swab, exudate, in tissue from wound should constitute as specimens.

1. Direct smear after Gram's staining shows Gram-positive bacilli with drum-stick appearance, morphologically similar to other non-pathogenic bacilli. Hence, they should be distinguished by their specific toxigenic property in mice.
2. **Culture :** If the tissue is heavily contamined, the specimen should be heated at 80°C for 10 minutes before culture, because it destroys non-sporing organisms. **Cl. tetani** grow in blood agar and aminoglycoside blood agar under anaerobic condition or in Robertson's cooked meat medium. The medium is made in one selective by addition of polymyxin B which inhibit all aerobes but not clostridia. **Cl. tetani** produce swarming growth after 1-2 days of incubation.
3. **Animal inoculation :** It is carried out to demonstrate the toxigenicity of isolated **Cl. tetani** which establishes the pathogenicity.

Two mice were used, in one mouse, 0.2 ml of 2 to 10 days old cooked meat broth culture filtrate is injected subcutaneously into the right side of the base of the tail of the mouse (test animal), same quantity of toxin filtrate is injected into the other animal (control) which has already received 1,000 units of tetanus antitoxin one hour prior to testing.

In positive case, the test animal shows the symptoms of tetanus (stiffness, spasm of the tail, hindlimb) within 24 hours and death.

The control animal shows no symptoms due to neutralisation of toxin by antitoxin.

Immunisation

Tetanus is a fatal disease and can be prevented by immunisation:

1. Active immunisation can be done by Tetanus Toxoid (TT) which is prepared by detoxifying the toxin with formal (formal toxin) and by absorbing the toxoid into aluminium hydroxide or phosphate (API).

Dose : Two doses of toxoid (API) of 0.5 ml each are injected intramuscularly at initial stage at an interval of 6 weeks. After 6 to 12 months a third dose (0.5 ml) of toxoid is administrated. During the first year of life all children are immunised by DPT vaccine which contains diphtheria toxoid, pertussis vaccine and tetanus toxoid in which vaccine acts as an adjuvant. Thus immunity is conferred for 7 to 10 years. After 5 years, on entry into school, a booster dose of toxoid is given and thereafter booster dose is given every 7 to 10 years.

2. Passive immunisation is carried by anti-tetanus serum (ATS). This ATS is obtained by immunising horses with toxoid and is used as **prophylaxis** in a dose of 1,500 International Units (IU) by intramuscular injection immediately after injury for systemic protection against toxin. ATS is repeated at weekly intervals till the risk of tetanus persists. The dose is same for adults and children. The ATS has a risk of hypersensitivity reaction. Before administrating ATS, a skin test (subcutaneous injection of 0.1 ml ATS) is performed.

The risk of heterologous serum (ATS) can be avoided by using human tetanus immunoglobulin (HTIG) which is a homologous serum prepared from humans and used in advanced countries in prophylaxis and treatment of tetanus. A single dose of 250 units is used in prophylaxis.

3. Combined immunisation : After an injury, in emergency it is advisable to immunise an individual with tetanus toxoid in one arm alongwith the administration of 1,500 IU of ATS or 250 units of HTIG in another arm. The other doses of toxoid are given at appropriate intervals. In prophylaxis, penicillin is also recommended.

Prevention and Treatment

Prevention depends upon 1. active immunisation with toxoid, 2. Proper care of wound contaminated with soil, 3. Prophylactic use of antitoxin, 4. Administration of penicillin.

Antitoxin : Tetanus antitoxin can neutralise the toxin, but only before it becomes fixed in nervous tissue. Because of hypersensitvity to foreign serum, the administration of human antitoxin is preferable.

Patients who develop symptoms of tetanus should receive muscle relaxants, sedation and assisted ventilation. Surgical removal of necrotic tissue. Pencillin inhibits the growth of **Cl. tetani** and stops further toxin production. **Booster shot,** when a previously immunised individual sustains a potentially dangerous wound, an additional dose of toxoid should be injected to restimulate the antitoxin production.

Control : Three injections of alum adsorbed tetanus toxoid (TT) comprise the initial course of immunisation followed by another dose of about one year later. Initial immunisation should be carried out in all children during the first year of age. A booster dose is given upon the entry into school. The immunisation by triple vaccine can also cover tetanus.

44
Clostridium Welchii

Clostridium welchii (Cl. perfringens) causes gas gangrene and food poisoning in man. There are five types—A-E.

Table 44.1. Characteristics of other gas gangrene producing bacilli

Species	Cl. septicum	Cl. oedematiens	Cl. histolyticum
1. Morphology, size	3 × 1.6 μ	3-10 × 1-2 μ	3-5 × 0.6 μ
Spore (ova, subterminal)	Yes	Yes	Yes
Motile by peri-trichous flagella	Yes	Yes	Yes
2. Lecithinase	Negative	Positive in egg yolk	–
3. Oxygen requirement	Anerobe	Anaerobe	Anaerobe; some aerotolerant
4. Haemolysis (Horse blood) agar	+	+	+
5. Toxins, enzymes	Four toxins α,β,y,d	Antigenically 4 types A-D, only type A is medically important Toxins s, β,y,d,e,e,n	Five toxins : α, β, y, d, E
6. Pathogenesis	Associated with gas gangrene in man; braxy in sheep; malignant oedema in cattle. It escapes intestine of man and invades tissues	Gas gangrene	Associated with gas gangrene in man, pathogenic role yet to be evaluated

Morphology and staining : Relatively large Gram-positive bacilli, 4-6 × 1 u, with square or rounded ends, **capsulated** in the tissue and are non-motile. Their spores are oval and subterminal.

The spores of **Cl. welchii** are not readily produced in artificial culture and in animal tissues and their absence is a characteristic of **Cl. welchii.** Spore formation can be induced only on special medium (Ellner medium). It appears that more toxin producing strains of **Cl. welchii** produce few spores, and vice versa.

Cultural Characteristics : Cl. welchii are obligate anaerobes, optimum temperature 37°C, grow best on glucose agar or glucose blood agar medium. On nutrient agar medium, the colonies are large, round, smooth, regular and slightly opaque disks. On blood agar medium, **Cl. welchii** typically produces multiple zone of haemolysis arround the colonies.

In selective medium containing polymyxin B, neomycin and iron citrate **(Marshal's medium), Cl. welchii** produce black colonies.

Boichemically, **Cl. welchii** is actively saccharolytic, ferments many sugars with gas and acid production. In litmus milk medium, lactose of milk is fermented, gas and acid are produced, and casein is formed as clot which is broken up by gas producing "stormy clot" appearance. In RMC medium, the meat is reddened and no digestion occurs.

Resistance

Spores of **Cl. welchii** are destroyed by autoclaving at 121°C for 15 minutes; the effects of disinfectants as spores are similar to that of **Cl. tetani.**

Antigenic structure

The different strains of **Cl. welchii** produce 12 distinct toxins (Table 44.1). These toxins are four (4) major lethal toxins and 8 minor lethal or non-lethal toxins. On the basis of production of the 4 major toxins **(alpha, beta, epsilon and iota), Cl. welchii** are differentiated into 5 types—A, B, C, D and E:

1. Type A strains produce **alpha** toxin.
2. Type B strains produce **alpha beta** and **epsilon** toxins.
3. Type C strains produce **alpha** and **epsilon** toxins.
4. Type D strains produce **alpha** and **epsilon** toxins.
5. Type E strains produce **alpha** and **iota** toxins.

Thus all strains produce **alpha** toxin and type A in particular produces only **alpha** toxin. **Cl. welchii** type A causes gas gangrene in man while other types (B, C, D, E) are mostly related to diseases in animals. Some strains of type A of **Cl. welchii** produce enterotoxin causing food poisoning.

(A) **Alpha (α) toxin and Gas gangrene**

It is produced by all strains of **Cl. welchii** but **more abundantly** by **Cl. welchii** type A of gas gangrene. Chemically, it is phospholipidase (Lecithinase C) and most fatal of all clostridial toxins and is responsible for profound toxaemia in gas gangrene patients. It is relatively heat stable, necrotising, cytotoxic or membranolytic. The α toxin **splits lecithin** which is an important constituent of the cell membrane. The specific effect of toxin is utilised in the rapid detection of **Cl. welchii** in clinical specimens and is confirmed in **Nagler reaction.** This toxin also causes haemolysis of erythrocytes of animals (except horse and goat).

Toxin, Cl. welchii produces 12 different exotoxins. Of these, alpha, beta, epsilon and iota are the major lethal toxins which are lethal, necrotising, haemolytic. The alpha toxin of **Cl. welchii** type A is a lecithinase enzyme which is lethal as it splits lecithin (an important constituent of cell membrane) to phosphorylcholine and diglyceride, and it can be demonstrated by production of opalescent colonies on egg yolk agar which is known as "Nagler reaction." In this reaction, the cholesterol of egg yolk is split by lecithinase and precipitated on the colonies. DNase, hyaluronidase, and collagenase that digest collagen of subcutaneous tissue and muscle are also produced. The theta toxin has similar effects but it is not lecithinase.

Nagler reaction

In presence of Ca++ and Mg++ ions, **alpha toxin** (Lecithinase C) splits lipoprotein of complexes in serum or egg yolk of the agar and produces **opalescent** colony of neutralisation of **alpha toxin** by specific antitoxin can be demonstrated by incorporating the antitoxin in egg yolk agar medium. If neutralised there will be no lipid deposit around the colony i.e. no opalescent colony.

Certain lecithinase producing bacteria **(Cl. oedematiens),** some vibrios and spore bearers may produce opalescence in egg yolk medium but it is not neutralised by specific anti-toxin of **Cl. welchii** except **Cl. bifermentans** which produces a lecithinase serologically related to that of **Cl. welchii.**

Other soluble substances

1. **Haemagglutinins** variety of RBCs (man, sheep, cattle, pigs) are produced by **Cl. welchii** type A and D.
2. **Neuraminidase** produced by **Cl. welchii** destroys Myxovirus receptors on red blood cells.
3. Histamine, haemolysin, fibrinolysin are also produced.

Table 44.1. Toxins produced by different types of Cl. welchii

Type	Occurence	Major lethal toxins				Minor lethal or non lethal toxins							
		α	β	ε	ι	γ	δ	η	Θ	κ	λ	μ	Ω
A	Gas gangrene, puerperal infection, septicaemia,	+++	–	–	–	–	–	(+)	(+)	(+)	–	+	– –
	Food poisoning	+++	–	–	–	–	–	(+)	+	–	+	+	++
B	Lamb dysentery,	+++	+++	++	–	++	–	++	(+)	++	–	+++	++
	Haemorrhagic enteritis of goat and sheep	+++	+++	+++	–	?	–	–	+++	+++	–	–	+ –
C	Slinek of sheep	+++	+++	–	–	++	+++ –	+++	–	–	–	–	
	Enteritis in animals				–	–	?	–	–	+++	+++ –	–	+ –
	Necrotic enteritis of man in Germany	+++	+++	–	–	+++	–	?	–	–	–	–	+++
D	Enterotoxaemia in sheep, goat, cattle	+++	–	+++	–	–	–	–	++	++	–		++ –
E	Doubtful pathogen of sheep, cattle	+++	–	–	+++	–	–	–	++	++	(+)		++ –

Some strains of **Cl. welchii** type A produces a powerful enterotoxin that induces "Food poisoning" with its characteristic intense diarrhoea, abdominal cramps, fever, vomiting in 6-18 hours after ingestion of toxin. This illness is self-limited.

Pathogenecity and Clinical Features : Spores of **Cl. welchii** which contaminated the wounds with free Ca and Mg ions germinate, multiply, ferment carbohydrates of the tissue and produce gas. The spread of infection is favoured by the distension of tissue and interference with blood supply together with the toxin causing tissue necrosis suitable for bacterial growth—haemolytic anaemia, severe toxaemia and death may ensue finally.

When a wound gets contaminated by soil with faecal matter containing spores of **Cl. welchii,** there may be 3 types of anaerobic wound infection:

1. Simple contamination of wound : There are some clostridia of low virulence which cannot multiply due to lack of proper anaerobic environment. They do not invade the tissue but their presence delays healing of wound.

2. Anaerobic cellulitis : This type of lesion is caused by clostridia of low virulence and poor toxigenicity. The spores germinate in necrotic tissue and invade fascial plane with minimal toxin production without invasion of muscle tissue. There is gas production but little toxaemia and prognosis is good. It tends to be a self-limiting lesion which is common in war casualities.

3. Anaerobic myelitis (Gas gangrene) : Cl. welchii type A is the predominant causal agent of anaerobic myelitis (gas gangrene). The condition is always associated with the formation of excessive amount of exotoxin (alpha toxin) and is very serious. Clinically, it is a spreading gangrene of the muscles with profound toxaemia and shock. There is increasing pain, tenderness; oedema with blackening of tissues and foul smelling of serous exudate. Crepitus due to accumulation of gas bubbles is mostly detected under the skin. Its incubation period is from 6 hours to 6 weeks. The spores of **Cl. welchii** germinate and thrive in dead tissue; oxygen tension is low. The infection may complicate wound with extensive destruction of tissue (accidental injury), pelvic infection of women. The gas bubbles may cause distension of sarcolemmal sheath of muscle cells and ischemia. Destruction of cell membrane of muscle fibre and alteration of vascular permeability caused by the **alpha toxin** of **Cl. welchii** may result into necrosis of muscle tissue which favours the bacterial growth. Other toxins and enzymes **(hyaluronidase, collagenase, leucocidin, fibrinolysin)** and **haemolytic toxins** may help the spread of infection. There is rapid development of anaemia and, in terminal stage, the bacterial dissemination may lead to **bacteriaemia,** shock and death.

B. Food poisoning

It is caused by some streams of **Cl. welchii** type A. When meat is cooked in bulk, heat resistant spores survive due to slow penetration of heat (100°C for 30 minutes). These spores germinate into vegetative forms during cooling after cooking in anaerobic condition. After consumption of large dose of organism along with contaminated cooked meat or poultry, a heat labile **enterotoxin** is liberated in the small intestine. This toxin acts on the intestinal mucosa like enterotoxin of **E. coli** causing dehydration and symptoms of food poisoning (abdominal pain, diarrhoea and nausea for 1-2 days). The incubation period is 8-12 hours. It is self-limited disease.

C. Other diseases

Gangrenous appendicitis, urogenital infection, puerperal infection, brain abscess, meningitis and panophthalmitis are also due to incrimination of **Cl. welchii.**

D. Necrotising enteritis

It is a severe and often fatal necrotising jejunitis caused by type C of **Cl. welchii** reported in New Guinea, Germany, Thailand, Nepal and East Africa. Protection against this disease is offered by active immunisation with toxoid of **Cl. welchii** type C.

Laboratory Diagnosis

A. **Specimens :** Wound, pus, tissue.

B. **Smears :** The presence of large Gram-positive, spore forming bacillus suggests gas gangrene, they may be capsulated in the tissue, but the spores are present in culture.

C. **Cuture :** Material is inoculated into RCM and on blood agar medium and incubated anerobically. The growth is inoculated into litmus milk medium and if stormy clot appears it is identified as **Cl. welchii** and its lecithinase activity is shown by Nagler reaction. Final identification rests on toxin production and neutralisation of toxin by specific antitoxin in mice and guinea pigs.

Treatment is by surgical removal of all devitalised tissue with administration of penicillin. Hyperbaric oxygen may help to detoxify patients rapidly. Polyvalent antitoxin may be used. Toxoids are not in practical use. Food poisoning due to **Cl. welchii** requires only symptomatic care.

45
Clostridium Botulinum

Causes botulism due to the ingestion of its "preformed" toxin. This form of food poisoning is characterised by oculomotor paralysis, pharyngeal paralysis, aphonia. Eight antigenic types of toxin (A-H) are known. Of these, types A, B and E are mostly responsible for the illness.

Morphology and Staining : Spore forming Gram-positive bacilli, with rounded ends, 4-6 ××0.9-1.2μ, occur singly or in pairs. Spores are oval, subterminal and bulging. This bacillus is motile.

Cultural Characteristics : They are strict anaerobes and grow on ordinary media anaerobically at 37°C. RCM yields abundant growth. Surface colonies are large, greyish, irregular, semitransparent with a central nucleus, haemolytic on horse blood agar. Meat is digested and usually blackened by toxigenic types A, B and F. All types produce lecithinase.

Resistance

Though the spores of **Cl. botulinum** are destroyed by autoclaving at 121°C for 15 minutes, they are resistant to 100°C for 4 to 5 hours. Spores of type A of Cl. botulinum are more resistant to heat and may survive up to 30 minutes at 120°C, whereas types B, C, D and E are resistant to heat. The resistance of the spores of **Cl. botulinum** to radiation is of great significance in food processing factory.

Antigenic structure

On the basis of their antigenically distinct toxins, eight serotypes – A, B, C, D, E, F, G and H—of **Cl. botulinum** have been distinguished.

Toxins liberated by different strains have identical pharmacological action, but they are neutralised by their specific antitoxin.

Haemagglutinin, haemolysin and haemolytic lecithinase are also produce in little quantity by some strains.

Toxin : Cl. botulinum produces a powerful exotoxin which can be destroyed at a temperature of 80°C for 30-40 minutes. The toxin of type A has been purified as a pure crystalline protein which is lethal to a mouse in a dose of 0.00000033 mg.

One mg of toxin can kill more than 200 million mice. The lethal dose of toxin for human being is not yet well known and it may be less than one microgram since it is the most toxic substance so far known. Only 1 kg of botulinum toxin can kill one billion people.

The toxigenicity of **Cl. botulinum** is most probably under control of temperate phage.

Botulism may be of three types (a) food borne botulism; (b) infant botulism; (c) wound botulism.

(a) Food borne botulism

It is a rare disease of intoxication caused by ingestion of **preformed toxin** in food contaminated with **Cl. botulinum.** Sometimes bacteria may also produce toxin in the intestine. Human disease is usually caused by type A, B and E, rarely by types C, G and F. The toxin is absorbed from the intestine into blood. Symptoms appear 12 to 36 hours after consumption of contaminated food. Symptoms are – vomiting, thirst, constipation, difficulty in speaking and breathing. Diarrhoea is not symptom. Mostly prognosis is poor with 25-70% fatality and death ensues due to respiratory failure.

Source of botulism

Home preserved vegetables, meat, fish (raw or tinned fish) may cause food borne botulism.

Mode of action of toxin

After absorption of toxin into blood (toxaemia), the toxin acts by blocking the release of acetylcholine at synapses and neuro-muscular junction which leads to neurological signs and symptoms (oculomotor and pharyngeal paralysis, vomiting and constipation).

(b) Infant botulism

Though this condition is rare, usually 6 months old infants are affected with the start of mixed feeding. This condition is not due to ingestion of preformed toxin but due to consumption of food contaminated with **Cl. botulinum.** Honey has been reported as source of infection. The spores after germination produce botulinum toxin, which causes toxaemia. The disease is manifested by constipation, weakness, lethargy and cranial palsies. It may be very mild or fatal depending on the absorption of toxin into blood. Infected infants are managed by supportive care and assisted feeding.

(c) Wound botulism

It is extremely rare. During wound infection toxin is produced at the site of wound infection and absorbed into blood. This toxaemia may be responsible for neurological manifestations similar to those of blood-borne botulism.

Pathogenesis and clinical features : Botulism is not an infection, but is an intoxication resulting from the ingestion of food in which Cl. botulinum has grown and produced toxin (preformed toxin).

The toxin acts by blocking release of acetylcholine at neuromuscular junctions. Flaccid paralysis results.

Symptoms begin 18-24 hours after ingestion of toxic food with visual disturbances (incordination of eye muscles, double vision), inability to swallow and speech difficulty); signs of bulbar paralysis; death is due to respiratory paralysis and cardiac arrest. Gastrointestinal symptoms are not always prominent, there is no fever, the patient remains fully conscious until shortly before death; the mortality rate is high.

Laboratory Diagnosis

Toxin can be demonstrated in the patient's serum and in contaminated food, can be neutralised by specific antitoxin in mice and also can be detected by passive haemagglutination and radioimmunoassay.

Presence of toxin in suspected residual food, patient's serum and intestinal content can be demonstrated by injecting the filtrate—obtained by macerating specimen of food, stool, vomitus in sterile isotonic saline—into mice. The test animal (unprotected) develops dyspnoea, flaccid paralysis and dies within 24 hours.

2. Demonstration of organisms

Gram-positive spore forming bacilli can be demonstrated in smears made from suspected food, and intestinal content. Specimens should be heated first at 65°C to 80°C for 10 minutes (to destroy non-sporing bacilli) and then inoculated on blood agar (incubated anerobically) and Rebertson's Cooked Meat (RCM) medium. Toxigenicity test in mice should be performed to detect toxin culture filtrate. In absence of toxin, mere demonstration of bacilli in food and stool is of no significance.

Treatment and prophylaxis : Potent antitoxin to 3 types should be given intramuscularly. Tin containing contaminated food may "swell" due to gas production by **Cl. botulinum. Food** from such can should not be consumed.

Since botulism is due to consumption of contaminated canned or preserved food, home processing of meat and vegetables (peas, beans, carrots) for preservation is not advisable. Since a low pH inhibits the growth of **Cl. botulinum,** acid fruits may be preserved in bottle at home. Once the toxin has entered into the nervous tissue and gets fixed in the synapses, the symptoms develop. This toxin can no longer be inactivated by antitoxin. Only supportive care may bring down the mortality rate from 85% to 20%. When an outbreak occurs, antitoxin can be given intramuscularly to those who consumed the suspected food.

46

Clostridium Difficile

It has been so named because of the difficulties encountered in its isolation. The bacterium with its toxin is found in the stool of patients suffering from **acute pseudomembranous colitis.**

Morphology and staining

Cl. difficile is a large Gram-positive bacillus with oval subterminal spore. In old culture, it may become Gram-negative.

Toxins

C. difficile produces two toxins :

(1) **enterotoxin** (type A) responsible for intestinal symptoms; (2) **cytotoxin** that produces cytotoxic effect in cell culture.

Symptoms of colitis are from mild diarrhoea to a fatal disease of the colon with fulminant diarrhoea. Diarrhoea may be profuse with about 20 motions per day with abdominal cramps and fever.

Pathogenesis

In antibiotics associated colitis, the pathogenic role of **Cl. difficile** was well-understood. Many antibiotics (ampicillin, tetracycline, chloramphenicol, lincomycin, clindamycin) alter the balance of the normal flora of the intestine **Cl. difficile** colonies and multiply with the production of toxin in the colon. If this condition is not quickly diagnosed, it may terminate fatally.

Laboratory Diagnosis

1. **Culture :** Isolation of **Cl. difficile** from stool can be done by inoculating into selective media.
2. **Direct demonstration of toxin** in the faeces of the patients can be done by inoculation of cell culture (Vero or human embryo and lung cells) with the stool. The toxin in the faeces may cause cytotoxic effect on the cell culture. **Cl. difficile** toxin can be neutralised by **Cl. sordelli** antitoxin which can also be shown in cell cultures. **C. sordelli** is serologically identical species. All strains of **Cl. difficile** are not toxigenic.

Treatment and prevention

Only oral metronidazole and vancomycin is effective against **Cl. difficile.** Current antibiotic therapy should be avoided as early as possible.

Demonstration

1. A Gram-positive stained smear of **B. anthracis,** arranged in long chain with central spores, from culture.
2. Appearance of **B. anthracis** smear from blood or tissue showing distinct capsule stained by polychrome methylene blue—Methylene blue reaction of McFaydean.
3. "Inverted fir tree" growth appearance of **B. anthracis** in gelatin stroke.
4. Gram stained smear from culture of **B. subtilis chains** are smaller.
5. Hanging drop preparation showing motility of **B. subtilis.**
6. Medusa head appearance colonies of **B. anthracis.**
7. A smear of **Cl. tetani** showing bacilli with spherical terminal spore - drum-stick appearance (Fig. 43.1).
8. Anaerobic jar (McIntosh jar) used for anaerobic culture of **Cl. tetani, Cl. welchii.**
9. A smear showing **Cl. welchii** showing oval and subterminal spore.
10. Culture of **Cl. welchii** in litmus milk medium showing production of acid (pink colour), clotting of milk and gas which disrupted and pushed up the clot—"Stormy clot" appearance reaction.
11. Antitetanus serum (ATS) poly anti-gas gangrene serum (AGGS) used for passive immunisation of tetanus and gas gangrene, respectively.
12. Tetanus toxoid available as triple vaccine used for active immunisation of tetanus.

Practical work

Stain the given smear by Gram stain.

Questions

1. When is methylene blue reaction of McFaydean useful?
2. What is zoonotic disease, malignant pustule, Wool sorter disease?
3. Describe in brief the most common methods of anaerobiasis.
4. What are the principle and use of Ascoli's test?
5. For what are ATS and AGGS used?
6. Which organism produces medusa head appearance colony.
7. How will you differentiate between **B. anthracis** and **B. subtilis**?
8. Which organism shows drum stick appearance?
9. What is trismus, lockjaw. How it occurs?
10. Why cultures of **Cl. tetani** have an unpleasant slightly pungent odour? Why meat particles are blackened in RCM?
11. What is the difference between the toxin and toxoid?
12. Which are the ions present in the wound which favour the toxin production by **Cl. tetani** and **Cl. welchii**?
13. In which medium can **Cl. welchii** be identified biochemically?
14. What is lecithinase, Nagler reaction?
15. What is the minimum lethal dose of **Cl. tetani** and **Cl. botulinum** toxin to a mouse? What is the most potent toxin amongst them?

47
Non-Sporing Anaerobes

Non-sporing anaerobes have been recognised as important causes of human and animal infection during recent years. Many of these organisms have been isolated from necrotic lesions though they are commensal flora of mouth, oropharynx, gastrointestinal and genital tract of men and animals. In the gut they outnumber the aerobes (Esch. coli). by a ratio of 1,000 : 1 when the body resistance is lowered, they act as opportunistic pathogens by setting up the infection in the damaged and necrotic tissue.

Due to difficulties for their isolation in pure culture and diverse properties, there is no generally accepted classification for these organisms.

However, a widely accepted recent classification is :

Classification
(Non-sporing anaerobes)

(A) **Cocci**

(I) Gram-positive	1. Peptococcus
	2. Peptostreptococcus
	3. Sarcina
(II) Gram-negative	1. Veillonella
	2. Acidoaminococcus

(B) **Bacilli**

(I) Gram-positive	1. Lactobacillus
	2. Bifido bacterium
	3. Propioni bacterium
	4. Actinomyces
(II) Gram-negative	1. Bacteroides
	2. Fusobacterium
	3. Leptotrichia

Besides these medically important anaerobic non-sporing bacteria, there are some anaerobes present in soil and water e.g. **Butyri vibrios** and **Methanobacteria.** Treponeme and **Borrelia** are non-sporing anaerobic **spirochaetes.**

Table 47.1 Normal anaerobic flora of human body

Organism	Mouth, naso-pharynx	Gut colon	Vagina, skin
Actinomyces	+	++	
Bifidobacterium	+	++	+
Propionibacterium			++
Bacteroides fragilis		++	
Bacteroides Melaninogenicus	++	+	++
Fusobacteria	++	+	
Gram-positive cocci	++	++	++
Gram-negative cocci	++	++	++
Spirochaetes	+		

Anaerobic cocci

These anaerobic cocci are usually found as normal flora on the skin, mouth, intestine and vagina. In the Bergey's Manual (8th edition) they are classified into four groups—**Peptococcus, Peptostreptococcus, Sarcina** and **Veillonella** on the basis of Gram reaction and cellular arrangement (Table 47.2).

Table 47.2. Species of Gram-positive anaerobic cocci

Peptococcus
Peptostreptococcus anaerobius
Peptostrep. heliotriniedoucens
Peptostrep. indolicius
Peptostrep, magnus
Peptostrep. productus
Peptostrep. tetradius
Peptostrep. micros
Peptostrep. prevoti

1. Peptococcus : They are Gram-positive cocci (0.5 to 1 μm in size) arranged in pairs or clumps. They cause pyogenic infection of wound puerperal sepsis, urinary tract infection.

2. Peptostreptococcus : These are Gram-positive cocci (0.3 to 1 μm) arranged in chains and produce a foetid odour in culture. At first these organisms were isolated from puerperal fever and were named **Peptostreptococcus anaerobicus** (or **putridus**). They are the commonest anaerobic cocci recovered from human infection (pleuropneumonia, brain abscess and puerperal infection).

3. Sarcina : They are large spherical Gram-positive cocci (2-3 μm in size) and are arranged in packets of eight or more. They grow on ordinary media, form heat resistant spores. They are non-pathogenic and found in soil and faeces of vegetarians.

4. Veillonella : They are small (0.3-2.5 μm), Gram-negative cocci, arranged in short chains, clusters, pairs. Though they are non-pathogenic, they occasionally invade blood stream after operation on mouth.

Anaerobic Gram-negative Bacilli (Bacteridaceae)

(A) Bacteroides (bacilli with rounded ends)

1.	Fragilis group	**B. fragilis, B. vulgatus, B. distasonis, B. ovitus, B. thetaiotaomicron**
2.	Melaninogenicum group	**B. melaninogenicus, B. ovalis**
3.	Asaccharolytic group	**B. asaccharolyticus B. gingivalis, B. ureolyticus**

(B) Fuso-bacterium (bacilli with pointed ends) species : **F. necrophorum, F. nucleatum** and **F. necrogenes**

(C) Leptotrichia (large bacilli)

Species : **L. buccalis** (Tables 47.3, 47.4)

I. Habitat

(a) **Mouth** : Bacteroides (anaerobic Gram-negative bacilli) are normal commensals of mouth. Seventy percent strains belong to melaninogenicus group (mainly **B. oralis**) and the remaining to **Fusobacterium** and **L. bacilli** (Table 47.1).

(b) **Respiratory tract** : **B. fragilis** is sometimes encountered in respiratory tract.

(c) **Gut** : Bacteroides are normal flora of the intestine and 80% belong to **B. fragilis.**

(d) **Female genital tract** : 80% Bacteroides (normal flora of cervix and vagina) belong to Melaninogenicus group and 15% to Asaccharolytic group.

II. Morphology and staining. They are Gram-negative non-motile bacilli (a. Bacteroides – small, oval or coccobacillary; b. Fusobacteria and **L. buccalis** are long 5-10 μm and spindle shaped, (Table 47.3).

III. Culture : They are strict anaerobes and grow in enriched media with blood or haemin for growth and also in Robertson's Cooked Meat (RCM) medium.

Anaerobic Gram-positive Bacilli

1. Lactobacillus : They are Gram-positive bacilli showing bipolar staining due to metachromatic granules, non-motile, large, thick (1.5 × 1 μm), occurring in chains, pairs filaments.

Habitat

They are distributed as saprophytes and ferment animal products (milk, cheese), though they are common flora of man and animals in the mouth, gut, and vagina.

Classification

Lactobacilli are separated into 6 species on the basis of precipitation test : **L. bulgaricus, L. casei, L. casei-helveticus, L. fermentus, L. lactis-brevis, L. plantorum.** Each species is again separated by agglutination tests.

Lactobacilli may be (a) Homofermenters, or (b) Heterofermenters; Homofermenters convert glucose into 95% of lactic acid and little CO_2; heterofermenters produce 50% lactic acid and other organic acids. The intestinal lactobacilli are homofermentative. **L. acidophilus, L. fermentus** and **L. salivarius** are commensals of the lower intestine. **L. acidophilus** is commensal of vagina. **L. casei, L. adontolyticus** and **L. salivarius** are commensals of mouth.

Culture

Lactobacilli are microaerophilic and grow at 5% CO_2 (at pH 3-6). Enriched media with glucose or blood will support of Lactobacilli. On nutrient agar medium their colonies are small. Selective acid media are Hadley's tomato juice agar and glucose yeast extract acetic acid agar of Rogosa *et al.*

Their role in health and disease

1. In the intestine, they synthesise biotin. Vitamin B_{12}, vitamin K.

2. Though Lactobacilli are commensal flora of vagina, they ferment glycogen deposited on vaginal epithelium and form lactic acid; vaginal acidic pH is maintained by Lactobacilli. Similar lactobacilli—described by Doderlein (1892) in the vaginal secretion—are called **Doderlein's bacilli.** Some Lactobacilli are non pathogenic.

2. Bifidobacteria : This name is derived because of its bifid Y-shaped appearance. They are commensals of mouth, urino-genital tract and intestine and are related to **Lacto-bacillus** and **corynebacterium.** They are rarely pathogenic.

3. Propionibacterium : As they are related to **Corynebacterium,** they are called non-pathogenic diphtheroid. Though they are commensal of the skin **(P. acne),** they are often found in acne pustules of the skin, in abscess. Its pathogenicity is not yet understood.

Anaerobic Infection

The non-sporing anaerobes are now recognised as "opportunistic pathogens" and they may produce the disease when the body resistance is lowered by trauma, tissue necrosis, impaired circulation, cytotoxic agents or by antibiotics, corticosteroid therapy. Predisposing factors (diabetes, malnutrition or malignancy) can help the bacterium to initiate the infection. The anaerobic infection is usually polymicrobial, mostly remain localised and bacteriaemia may be due to dissemination of these organisms. In anaerobic infection, the resultant pus is usually putrid and cell units are most common.

1. Bacteroides : B. fragilis is the most common isolate from clinical specimens. It is also found in association with other organisms (notably coliform bacteria). They play an important role in gynaecological and abdominal sepsis.

2. Fusobacteria and L. buccalis : Dental sepsis and Vincent's angina associated inelanino genicus/oralis strains and **Borellia** are caused by this **Fusobacterium.** The combined infection most probably potentiates the ability of each bacterium to cause infection i.e. pathogenic synergy.

3. Anaerobic cocci : They cause local sepsis in mixed infections in association with other aerobes (coliform) or anaerobes (bacteroides, fusobacteria).

4. Lactobacillus : They are associated with dental caries.

Laboratory Diagnosis

Specimen

Specimens should be collected very carefully to avoid normal flora. Maximum care should be taken as these bacteria cannot survive in presence of oxygen. Specimens should fill the bottles completely without any air space and kept in airtight containers. Swabs, if collected, should be preserved in Stuart's transport medium.

1. Direct Smear Examination : Gram staining of pus shows a variety of organisms and pus cells.

2. Culture : A suitable culture medium is blood agar medium with neomycin, yeast extract, haemin and vitamin K; inoculated medium can be incubated at 37°C for 2-3 days anaerobically. Gas Pak system can maintain anaerobiasis.

Treatment

These anaerobes (except **B. fragilis**) are sensitive to penicillin, chloramphenicol, fucidin, trimethoprim and tetracyclines. **Bacteroidaceae** are sensitive to metronidazole and it is used now-a-days as prophylaxis in large bowel surgery.

Table 47.3. Characteristic features of Gram-negative non-sporing bacilli

Properties	Bacteroides	Fusobacteria	Leptotrichia
Morphology	Bacilli; Cocco-bacilli, pleomorphic, occurs singly, in pairs, short chains, rounded ends, capsule in some strain (**B. fragilis**)	4.6 × 0.5-1 μm with pointed ends L-forms, spheroplasts common (spherophorus)	5-15 × 1 μm with pointed ends, slightly curved rods. In culture separate filaments (200 μm). Tangled mass
Cultivation Bile salt	Resistant, **B. fragilis** grow in 20% bile salt	Inhibitory	Inhibitory
Fermentation			
Glucose, Maltose	A, G	A, G	Negative
Indole, H_2S	Negative	Positive	Negative
Metabolic end products	Acetic, succinic acid	Butyric acid (sufficient), acetic, propionic acids (scanty)	L. buccalis produces mainly lactic acid
Antibiotic sensitivity (Penicillin)	R (Some Melanino) (genicus sensitive)	S	S
Neomycin (1,000 μgm)	V	S	V
Metronidazode	S	S	S
Cefoxitin	S	V	V
Chloramphenicol	V	S	S

S = Sensitive, R = Resistant; V = Variable

Table 47.4. Taxonomy of clinically-important species of Bacteriodaceae (Gram-negative non sporoing anaerobes)

Group	Number of species	Genus	Species (important)
Fragilis group (Saccharolytic group)	12	**Bacteroides**	**B. fragilis, B. caccae, B. distasonis, B. eg gerhii, B. merdae, B. evatus, B. ster coris, B. thetaiotao-micron, B. inhiformis B. vulgaus**
Melaninogenicus group (moderately) Saccharolytic gorup)	17	**Prevotella**	**B. melaninogenicus, B. bucalis, B. tenicola, B. bivius, B. buccae, B. disiens, B. intermedius, B. oris, B. ruminicola, B. veroralis, B. zoogleo fermans.**
Asaccharolytic group	10	Porphyromonas	**B. asaccharolyticus B. gingivalis, B. endo dontalis**
Other (uncertain taxonomic group)	10		**B. achraceus, B. levil, B. ureolyticus, B. gracilis**

Table 47.5. Anaerobic infections and their causative anaerobes

Site & Nature of infection	Causative anaerobes	Associated facultative aerobes	
1. Central Nervous System	Brain abscess	**B. fragilis, pepto-streptococcus**	**Staphylococcus**
2. Ear-nose-throat	Otitis media, mastoiditis, orbital cellulitis, Chronic sinusitis.	**Fusobacterium**	**Staphylococcus Pseudomonas, Proteus, Enterobacter**
3. Mouth, Jaw	Ulcerative gingivitis (Vincent's angina) dental abscess, cellulitis abscess, sinus of jaw	**Fusobacterium Spirochaetes Actinomyces Mouth anaerobes**	**Staphylococcus Pseudomonas, Klebsiella**
4. Respiratory	Aspiration pneumonia, Lung abscess, bronchi-ectasis, chronic sinusitis	**Fusobacterium B. melaninoge-nicus, Pepto streptococcus peptococcus B. fragilis Propioni bacterium Spirochaetes**	**Klebsiella Staphylococcus Streptococcus Pseudomonas**
5. Abdominal	Subphrenic abscess hepatic abscess, appendi-citis, peritonitis, ischio-rectal abscess, wound infection after colorectal surgery	**B. fragilis Peptococcus Clostridia**	**Esch. coli, Proteus Enterococcus Klebsiella Pseudomonas Staphylococcus**
6. Female genitalia	Wound infection following genital surgery, puerpe-ral epsis, tubo-ovarian abscess, Bartholin's abscess, septic abortion	**B. fragilis, B. melaninogeni-cus, Fusobacterium, Peptostreptococcus, genital anaerobes Cl. welchii**	do
7. Skin, tissue	Infected sebaceous cyst, breast abscess, axillary abscess, cellulitis, diabetic ulcer, gangrene	**Peptococcus Peptostrepto-coccus, an-aerobic cocci B. melanino genicus B. fragilis**	**Staphylococcus Pseudomonas**

SECTION IV
VIRUSES, RICKETTSIAE AND SPIROCHAETES

48
Viruses, Rickettsiae and Spirochaetes

Virus

General Introduction to Virology

History : Many common contagious diseases of animals and man were clinically known since ancient time for which no bacterial aetiology has been assigned. From pre-Christian times Small pox was considered as a deadly infection and Hippocrates (C. 430 BC) described swollen neck in mumps. In 1884, Pasteur believed that Rabies of dogs is caused by a "microorganism infinitesimally small" as he could not detect bacteria in the infective material of rabid dogs. In 1892, Iwanowsky showed that the mosaic disease of tobacco plants was caused by a minute agent which was so small that it was ultramicroscopic and could pass through pores of bacteria stopping filters. In 1898, Loeffler and Frosch have shown that foot and mouth disease of cattle was caused by a filterable infectious agent. In 1901, Walter Reed et al proved that yellow fever was caused by a mosquito borne virus.

Viruses were originally described as ultramicroscopic and filter passing. Later, it was shown in animals such as foot and mouth disease and rinderpest in cattle, distemper and rabies in dogs and fowl pest in poultry. Rous in 1911 demonstrated that certain sacromata of fowls could be transmitted with cell free filtrates of the tumours. Since that time, it was established that virus can cause tumour in animal and they are called **"Oncogenic viruses"**. Fibromas, papillomas, and related tumours in rabbit and other mammals; mammary carcinomata, leukemias and parotid tumours (polyoma virus in mice and leucosis in poultry were caused by **oncogenic viruses**).

Insects are vectors of viruses which attack man, animals and plants. Nematodes, parasitic to pigs, spread swine influenza virus as in case of plant nematodes.

Twort in 1915 and d'Herelle in 1917 observed independently that viruses can infect and cause lysis of bacteria (clear zone of lysis-plaque), these viruses are called as Bacteriophage—a name now abbreviated as "phage." This phenomenon of lysis was first noted in **Shigella shigae**—causative agent of bacillary dysentery. Because of this, knowledge of mechanism of phage infection and reproduction is much advanced than knowledge of the corresponding mechanism of animal viruses.

Denfinition of Virus : Virus (*Vira,* poison) were earlier defined as an ultramicroscopic agent which can be seen only under electron microscope, and can pass through the bacteria stopping fillers, reproduce by replication, can grow only in living cells, resist the action of antibiotics and contain Ribonucleic acid (RNA) or Deoxyribonucleic acid (DNA) covered by a protein coat.

Luria, in 1967, produced a composite definition incorporating all the accepted essential features of viruses.

A virus is one of a group of minute infections agents characterised by a lack of independent metabolism and by the ability to replicate only within living host cells.

They range from 15-300 nm in size and are morphologically, heterogeneous (Dorland's Medical Dictionary).

"Viruses are entities whose genome is an element of nucleic acid, either DNA or RNA, which reproduces machinery to direct the synthesis of specialised particles, the virions, which contain the viral genome and transfer it to other cells."

Following are two cardinal features of viruses :

1. They possess the genetic material which, when it is within the host cell, behaves as a part of the cell;
2. They also exist in an intracellular form, which is the product of the host cell under the control of the virus itself. The extracellular form—the virion—serves as a vehicle to carry the viral genome to other cells.

Viruses can reproduce only when they are within their host cells and are of necessity intracellular parasites. They have no ribosomes, no enzymes to generate high energy bonds, no mitochondria. They lack a rigid cell wall. Thus, there is no muramic acid in their outer coatings, hence they are unaffected by antimicrobial agents. Indeed, viruses have no real cell structures and it is difficult to regard them as microorganisms. True microorganisms multiply by binary fission.

Table 48.1. Differentiating features of prokaryotes and viruses

Properties	Bacteria	Mycoplasma	Rickettsia	Chlamydia	Virus
Cell wall	+	+	+	+	–
Muramic acid in cell wall	+	+	+	+	–
Ribosome cellular enzyme	+	+	+	+	–
DNA, RNA	Both	Both	Both	Both	only one type
Division by binary fission	Yes	Yes	Yes	Yes	No
Growth in inanimate ongelium	+	+	+	–	–
Sensitivity to antibodies	+	+	+	+	–
Sensitivity to infection	–	–	–	+	+

Structure : A complete infective virus particle is called virion and the genome is in the core and consists of **either** deoxyribonucleic acid (DNA) or ribonucleic acid (RNA) but not both; the outer shell of protein covering the nucleic acid is known as **capsid.** The protein and nucleic acids are closely integrated to form a nucleoprotein of distinct symmetry. When a virion enters the host cell, its protein capsid is stripped off and its nucleic acid is liberated within the host cell. At this stage, it ceases to exist as a particle although its nucleic acid is still present and intact. Component parts are still detectable. This

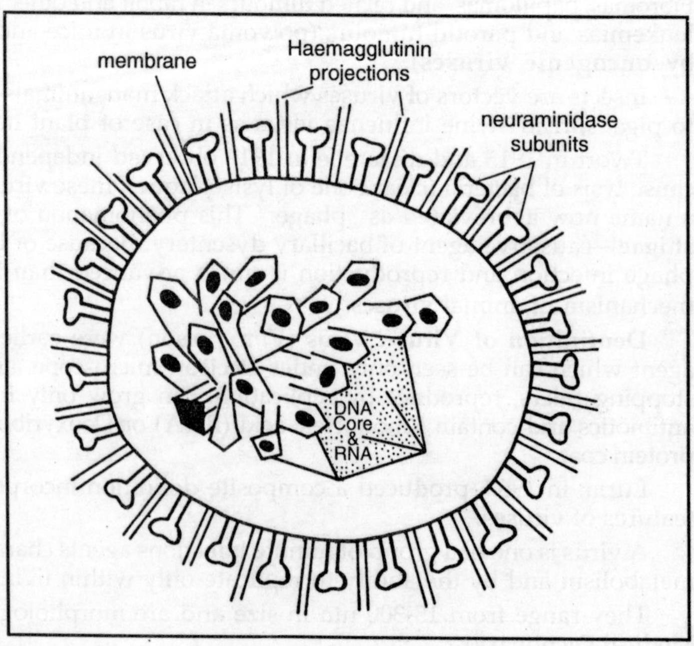

Fig. 48.1: Structure of virus

stage in viral multiplication is known as the eclipse phase. All true viruses have an eclipse phase in their reproductive cycle (Fig. 48.1).

Classification of Viruses

Animal viruses may be arranged into groups—the names of these groups and in the suffix—Virus, e.g. adeno virus, herpes virus and pox virus. Members of these groups share similar features and constitute families ending with the suffix—idae, i.e. the family **Hepres viridae** would have as its type genus Herpes virus which is a group that contains the **Herpes simplex,** varicella zooster.

Following are the important distinguishing features of animal viruses : 1. Type of nucleic acid; 2. Chemical composition; 3. Susceptible to chemical and physical agents; 4. Size and measurement; 5. Design and construction of virus; 6. Antigenic characters.

Deoxyribo viruses at present are placed in five groups (Pox virus, Herpes virus, Adeno virus, Papova virus, Parvo virus) and ribo viruses in nine groups (Orthomyxo virus, Paramyxo virus, Rhabdovirus, Togavirus, Arenavirus, Reovirus, Picornavirus, Leukovirus, Coronavirus).

There are many viruses that do not fit neatly into these groups. They are known as Arbo viruses, because they are transmitted by the bite of arthropods.

Types of nucleic acid

DNA or RNA carries in their nucleic acids the genome and infectivity of viruses.

Most deoxyribo viruses have linear double stranded DNA; whereas, in the parvo viruses, the molecule is single stranded RNA.

When the protective capsids of the viruses are removed, some fragile viral nucleic acid retains their infectivity for some time, they can be seen and measured under electron microscope. Most of them are linear but some are circular.

Chemical Composition

Proteins are the main components of all viruses. The most important function of these proteins is to provide the shield for the underlying delicate nucleic acid molecules. The surface proteins of the virion have special affinities for specific receptor sites on the host cell and provide a means of attachment of the particle to a position where it can enter the host cell and initiate the process of infection.

Viral strength, which are protein in nature, stimulate the host immune response during infection. They are responsible for the distinctive serological characteristics of the viruses.

The capsomeres of most pathogenic viruses contain several different polypeptides. These polypeptides make up the surface configuration. They constitute the haemagglutinin prickles of ortho and paramyxo viruses and form a part of the mushroom shaped projections of neuraminidase subunits.

Viral enzymes : There are many enzymes coded in the nucleic acids.

Lipids : When some mature viruses are liberated from nuclear and cytoplasmic membrane, they acquire a surface layer of lipoprotein derived in part from the host cell. The lipids may cement the proteins in the envelopes of the viruses. These viruses are inactivated by lipid solvents (ether, chloroform, bile salt).

Carbohydrates : Some viruses contain minimal amounts of carbohydrates.

Effect of Physical and Chemical Agents

Heat and Cold : The viruses causing the diseases in man and animals are readily inactivated by moderate heat (56°C to 60°C for 30 minutes) except serum hepatitis and poliomyelitis viruses. Viruses are resistant to extremes of cold; freezing at – 35°C or – 70°C is satisfactory common method for their preservation in the laboratory. The majority of viruses can be well preserved by freezing drying method, pH variation. Viruses remain viable within a range of pH 5 to 9, but they are destroyed by extreme acidity or alkalinity.

Tricidal agents : The most efficient disinfectants for use against viruses are oxidising agents (hydrogen peroxide, potassium permanganate and organic iodine derivatives). Chromaldehyde (a reducing agent) is slower in action but is valuable in defined concentration in the preparation of inactivated poliomyelitis vaccines. Glutaraldehyde has an important role in the disinfection of apparatus used in renal dialysis units. Phenol and certain cresol disinfectants (i.e. lysol) are active against only a few viruses and are not to be recommended for material contaminated with the poliomyelitis or small pox viruses. Acyclovir, amantadine, idoxuridine, trifluridine, vidarabine, ribavirin and azidothymidine are currently licensed antiviral agents. However, ideal antiviral agents remain to be developed.

Table 48.2. Action of antiviral agents

Replicative stage	Potential target	Licensed antiviral agent
Attachment	Block virus attachment	Ab to viral binding site
	Down-regulation to cell receptor	Ab to cell receptor
Penetration/ Uncoating	Stabilise viral capsid in endo-somal membranes	Amantadine, Rimantadine
Viral macro-nuclear synthesis	RNA & DNA polymerase inhibitors	Nucleoside analogue: vidarabine, acyclovir ganciclovir, ribavirin zidovudine
	Termination of nucleic acid chain by incorporation	Foscarnet
	Translation inhibitors caping inhibitors	Interferon
	Antisense oligonucleotides for inhibitors inhibitors of active enzyme formation	
Assembly	Prevention of virus specific cleavage polypeptides inhibitors of glycosylation and myrisylation	

Ether : Viruses containing lipids in their envelopes are sensitive to ether. Naked viruses (Polio, echo, coxsackie, adeno, papova and parvo viruses and some pox viruses) are resistant to ether, whereas herpes, orthomyxo and paramyxo, rhabdo, corona and leuko viruses are inactivated by ether.

Vital dyes : Acridine dyes, neutral red and toluidine blue permeate the nucleic acid and render virions vulnerable to ultraviolet rays. **Herpes simplex** and vaccinia viruses are more severely damaged then polio viruses. Double stranded DNA viruses stained with acridine dyes fluoresce with a yellow colour when seen under electron microscope while single stranded DNA viruses fluoresce red.

Antibiotics and chemotherapeutic agents have no effect on viruses, but the agents of psittacosis lymphogranuloma group are susceptible to these drugs.

The unit measurement of whole virus particle is the nanometre (nm) or millimicron (mμ) or one thousandth part of a micron (μ) or micrometre (μm) or 0.000001 mm or it is 10^{-9} metre; whereas the component parts or the internal structure (capsomere) of the virus is expressed as Angstrom (A°) which is one tenth of a millimicron (0.000001 mm). The Angstrom is the unit used to measure the wave length of light in microscope.

Virions vary in diameter from 300 to 18 nm. The largest ones are nearly half the size of small bacteria and can just be seen under an optical microscope. Most viruses can be seen only under electron microscope. Largest virus is vaccinia virus (330 × 100 nm), smallest one is picorna virus and parvo virus (40-20 nm).

It is customary to include in a suspension of purified viruses some latex particles of known size (e.g. 88 nm) in electron microscope, so in electron micrographs, the size and shape can be determined accurately; vaccinia virus is brick shaped; influenza virus is round or filamentous; bacteriophage is sperm-like with head and tail.

Formerly, the size of viruses was measured by their capacity to pass through the filters or by their rate of sedimentation in a suspended fluid.

Design and Construction of Virus

A virion (the old term which is still in use) in its simplest form is a single molecule of nucleic acid enclosed within a protein capsid. It was known as "elementary body". The shape taken by the capsid is that of rigid spherical cage or of a tube; mainly the capsid protects the nucleic acid.

Viral capsids are made up of large number of "morphological units" or capsomeres" that are attached to each other by their bonds.

Cubical capsids : Viruses with cubical symmetry take the form of an icosahedron. An icosahedron has 20 facets, each an equilateral triangle and 12 vertices or corners.

Virus haemagglutinin : Many different viruses agglutinate red blood cells when viruses and erythrocytes are in a suspension, they collide and adhere to each other, the cells become speckled with attached virions and they are bound to each other by viral bridges.

Inclusion bodies : During the course of multiplication, the viruses are associated with the appearance of large distinctive structures known as "inclusion bodies". They may be situated either in the cytoplasm (intracytoplasmic inclusion bodies) or in the nucleus (intranuclear inclusion bodies)—as in the case of measles—in both. The inclusion bodies are usually acidophilic and appear as pink masses in smears stained with Giemsa stain or Mann's eosin methylene blue stain; basophilic inclusion bodies are characteristic of psittacosis-lymphogranuloma group. They vary in size from 1-30 μ in diameter.

The presence of large intracytoplasmic acidophilic inclusion bodies in the nerve cells of hippocampus of the brain is the presumptive diagnosis of Rabies.

Acidophilic intranuclear inclusion bodies are of two types : Cowdry Type A is granular in appearance and of variable size (herpes simplex, zoster varicella, yellow fever). Type B is more round and multiple (Poliomyelitis, adenovirus).

Virus tropism : Viruses are classified according to their particular tissue predilection as dermotropic, neurotropic, pneumotropic, enterotropic and viscerotropic.

Viral pathogenicity : When the virus multiplies in the cell, it may spread from cell to cell producing a small focal lesion (Wart or molluscum contagiosum). When the viruses are deposited on the mucosa membrane of respiratory tract, they infect, multiply inside the mucosa and spread over a large area producing common cold; when trachea and bronchi are infected, influenza ensues.

Pathogenesis of viral infections depends upon the viral interactions and host factors :

1. Entry of virus into host cell
2. Multiplication of virus and spread
3. Effect of virus on cell functions
4. Host immune response
5. Viral establishment and infection
6. Viral shedding.

Viral entry

Viruses enter the host through skin, respiratory, gastrointestinal, urogenital route or conjunctiva. Mostly they enter through respiratory mucosa (e.g. **chicken pox**) or gastrointestinal mucosa (e.g. **Polio virus**).

Virus may be introduced into the blood stream by needles **(Hepatitis B; HIV)** or by insect bite **(Arbo virus)** Congenital infection of **Rubella** and **Cytomegalo virus** may lead to maldevelopment or severe neonatal disease. Mammary tumour viruses of mouse are transmitted through breast milk.

Milk viruses (small pox, chicken pox, entero virus) produce lesions in organs distant from the site of entry. After **primary multiplication** at the site of entry these viruses pass along the lymphatics to local lymph nodes. After further multiplication in lymph nodes, they enter the blood stream causing **primary viraemia** (short-lasting), then they spread along blood to **"central foci"** (liver, spleen). They reenter blood stream after extensive multiplication in **central foci**, thus resulting into **secondary viraemia** with onset of clinical signs. The viruses are spread into **target organs** during secondary viraemia. The distinctive lesions are produced in these organs after their further multiplication in these target organs. These changes are variable from one species of virus to another. **The incubation period** is the time taken by the viruses to enter the body and to reach the target organs. Rabies virus spread by **neural route.**

Target organs

Main target organs are skin and central nervous system; other organs are also involved. Generalised viral infections with skin rash.

Table 48.3. Skin rashes due to generalised viral infection

Type of rash	Viral infection
Maculopapular	Measles, Rubella, Echo virus, Coxsackie A
Vesicular	Herpes simplex, Varicella Zoster, Vaccinia, Coxsackie
Haemorrhagic	Small pox, Measles, Arbo viruses

Effect of virus on cell

Viruses have cell and organ specificity. They act on target cell surface receptors (cell tropism). As a result of virus and host cell interaction, there may be (a) **cytotoxic or cytolytic growth;** (b) **non-cytocidal productive growth**; (c) **abortive infection** and (d) **cell transformation.**

(a) In **cytotoxic** or **cytolytic growth,** viruses replicate inside host cells, release progeny viruses which ultimately infect new cells, produce the disease after destroying target cells by their cytopathic effect (CPE) in the form of inclusion bodies they produce and cell necrosis. This is referred to as **cytolytic cycle** and the susceptible host cells are termed **permissive** cells.

(b) In **non-cytocidal productive growth,** the viruses infect the host cells and do not destroy or kill the cells during replication without affecting the host cell metabolism. The infection is productive but non-cytolytic (e.g. this type of co-existence of virus and host cells can be demonstrated by **Influenza virus** growth in monkey kidney cell culture). This co-existence may result in persistent infection which may be **latent, inapparent,** subclinical or may progress to chronic infection.

(c) In **abortive infection,** the viruses infect cells but do not replicate and there is no loss of cell function.

(d) **Transformation** virus infects the cell and its nucleic acid gets integrated in the host cell DNA leading to cell **transformation.** The virus is not generally released from the infected cell.

Table 48.4, Virus groups and their target organs in man

Classification by target organ	Specific virus	Portal of entry	Other affected organs
Respiratory	[Influenza A, B, C	Respiratory tract	
	Para influenza	Respiratory tract	
Viruses	Respiratory syncitial	Respiratory tract	
	Measles	Respiratory tract	Brain, lung, skin
	Mumps	Respiratory tract	CNS, testes, ovaries
	Adeno virus	Respiratory tract	
	Rhino virus	Respiratory tract	
	Coxsackie virus	Respiratory tract	CNS*
	Echo virus	Respiratory tract	CNS* skin
	Reo virus	Respiratory tract	?
	Lymphocytic meningitis	Respiratory tract	CNS
	Corona virus	Respiratory tract	
Enteric virus	Polio viruses	Gastrointestinal tract	Muscles, CNS*
	Coxsackie virus	Gastrointestinal tract	CNS*, skin
	Echo virus	Gastrointestinal tract	CNS*, skin
	Rota virus	Gastrointestinal tract	
	Hepatitis A	Gastrointestinal tract	
	Hepatitis B	Blood	Liver
Neurotropic virus	Polio virus	Gastrointestinal tract	Upper respiratory tract
	Coxsackie virus	Gastrointestinal tract	Upper respiratory tract
	Echo virus	Gastrointestinal tract	Upper respiratory tract
	Rabies	Skin, blood	CNS
	Mumps	Respiratory tract	Testes, ovaries, pancreas
	Measles	Respiratory tract	Skin, lung
	Arbo virus	Blood	
	Herpes simplex	Respiratory tract, genitalia	Skin
	Varicella zoster	Respiratory tract	Skin, cornea
	Lymphocytic meningitis	Respiratory tract	Respiratory tract
	Kuru	Gastrointestinal tract	
	Creutzfeldt Jakob	Unknown	
	BK and JC	Unknown	

Contd.

Classification by target organ	Specific virus	Portal of entry	Other affected
Dermotropic virus	Poxvirus	Respiratory tract	Resp. tract, viscera
	Measles	Respiratory tract	Lung, brain
	Varicella zoster	Respiratory tract	CNS, cornea
	Coxsackie virus	Gastrointestinal tract	Upper respiratory tract
	Echo virus	Gastrointestinal tract	CNS, gastrointestinal tract
	Herpes simplex	Skin	Peripheral ganglia
			Cornea, genitalia
	Rubella		
	Human wart	Skin	
	Molluscum contagiosum	Skin	
Human T-cell Tropic viruses	HTLV-I, HTLV-II	Blood	Spleen, lymph node
	Human immuno-deficiency virus (HIV)	Blood	Organs containing lymphocytes, macrophages

* Major involvement in clinical disease; CNS—central nervous system

Host Resistance to viral infection (viral immunity)

The host can resist the viral infection by (a) **Immunological**, or (b) **non-immunological response** (non-specific) response.

(A) Immunological response

After primary infection or immediately, an immune response develops in immunised host against viral infection. It may be antibody and cell mediated immune response. Antibody plays an important role as the principal immunodefence for some diseases (entero and arbo virus infections), while in others (HSV, CMV), cell mediated immunity (CMI) plays a more important role.

(I) Circulating antibody

In an immunised individual, IgA may limit viral attack on mucosal surface and serum Ig G may act on lower respiratory tract. Ig M and Ig G cannot dislodge the virus from the site of primary entry in an immunised host. Both prevent the spread of some virus (polio virus) to target organ and also help in recovery from viral disease.

The degree of protection is related to the level of neutralising antibody in the blood. Ig M and Ig G antibodies may act **in vivo** in the following ways :

(a) **Neutralisation** of virus may prevent attachment, penetration and subsequent events.

(b) **Immune opsonisation** of virus for phagocytosis and destruction of virus by macrophages and neutrophils.

(c) After **interaction** with virus on cell membranes, the antibodies render the infected cells susceptible to complement dependent destruction by killer lymphocytes (K cells) or by phagocytosis.

(II) Cell mediated immunity

This immunity plays an important role at a later stage of infection. It prevents infection of target organs and promotes recovery from the disease. Infected cell surface contains virus-specific antigens. Activated T-cells release **lymphokines.** Recruited activated macrophages destroy some viruses better than macrophages of infected persons. Cytotoxic T-cells also destroy infected target cells.

(B) Non-specific defence against virus

This non-specific defence also plays an important role in adults than in young animals, which involve three factors : **humoral, cellular,** and **environmental factors** which may be present before infection or induced by the virus:

(a) **Humoral factors** may be (i) humoral inhibitors, or (ii) Interferon.

(i) **Humoral inhibitors** contain non-specific inhibitors (lipid and non-lipid) that inhibit attachment of virus to cell receptors. When viruses attach to cells, cell nuclease may remain free in the cytoplasm which may destroy the viral nucleic acid.

(ii) **Interferon** virus phagocyte **interaction** leads to production of **interferon** and **endogenous pyrogen** which mediates fever and sometimes affects replication of virus.

Three human interferons are recognised : α produced by leucocytes; β-by fibroblasts; and γ by T-cells. α and β interferons are potent antiviral **agents** γ is an immunomodulator. If IFN α and β induce several biochemical reactions with the help of three enzymes (synthetase, RNase, protein kinase), each of them inhibit synthesis of viral protein, but do not affect host protein synthesis.

(b) **Cellular factors**

(i) **Polymorphonuclear leucocytes (PMN).** Migrate to the site of viral infection, adsorb to the virus and ingest some viruses. They help the body defence by inhibiting viral growth or by destroying them, though viruses inhibit **chemotaxis.**

(ii) **Mononuclear phagocytes** (MN). Both blood and tissue macrophages ingest and destroy some viruses; some may resist ingestion. Sometimes ingested viruses may resist killing and replicate intracellularly.

(iii) **Environmental factors.** Certain viruses inactivated non-specifically by lymphocytes and certain virus infected cells are killed by natural killer (NK) lymphocytes without the help of antibody. Thus they act non-specifically.

Transmission of virus infection : Inclusion conjunctivitis is transmitted by the direct contact between persons during intercourse from one person to another. Later it reaches the eyes of the newborn at it passes through the infected birth canal. Polio viruses and other entero viruses may be transmitted after the ingestion of food or drink.

Interferon : Among animal viruses, interference of one virus with the reproduction of another may be mediated by a protein called **"interferon"** which is produced by the cell after infection with the first virus.

Interferon is a protein with a molecular weight of 30,000 daltons. Because of its size, the interferon is released from cells and can diffuse in the body throughout the extracellular fluids.

Types of interferon

There are three antigenically and chemically distinct types of interferon :

(1) **α-interferon** (IFN-α)—produced by monocytes and B lymphocytes.

(2) **β-interferon** (IFN-β)—produced by fibroblasts and epithelial cells.

(3) **γ-interferon** (IFN-γ)—a lymphokine produced by T-cells.

IFN-α and IFN-β are produced only by cells in response to presence of viruses and certain intracellular bacteria; but IFN-γ is produced from antigen activated T-lymphocytes.

Mechanism of action

Interferons inhibit viral replication and are also able to modify immune response. They also act as anti-tumour agents.

Interferon binds to specific cell surface receptors. Both IFN-α and IFN-β share a common receptor; while IFN-γ binds to its own specific receptor.

Properties

1. **Species specific :** Interferon produced by one species can protect only cells of the same species against viral infection.

2. **Non-specificity :** Interferon activity is not virus specific. Interferon induced by non-virus renders cell resistant to infection by the same broad spectrum of viruses.

3. **Virus susceptibility :** Though all viruses are inhibited by interferon, they vary in their susceptibility to interferon e.g. RNA viruses are more susceptible to interferon than DNA viruses.

Cultivation of Virus : Viruses can be grown in (1) The animal; (2) Chick embryo (Fig. 48.2), (3) Tissue culture.

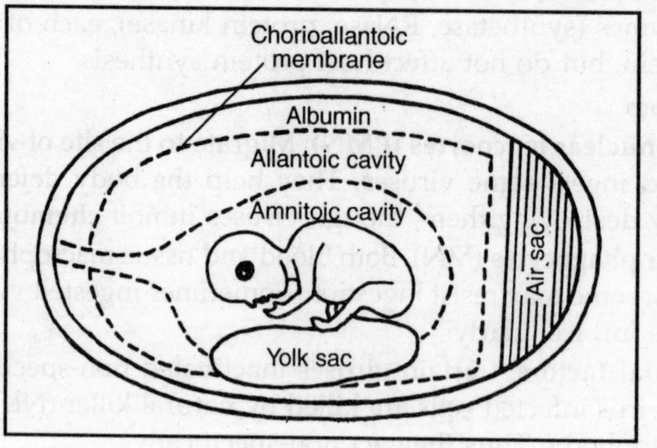

Fig. 48.2: Chick embryo

Cultivation

1. **Animal :** Many animals and man are susceptible to rabies. Certain species (skunks, opossums, fowls) are resistant. Mice are the animals of choice for the experiment at Rabies infection.

Animal can be inoculated by any route; intracerebral intoculation may cause encephalitis and the animal dies in 5-30 days.

Viruses freshly isolated from natural infection, which have not undergone any modification in the laboratory, is known as **"Street"** virus. They cause fatal encephalitis in the laboratory animals (with an incubation period of 21-60 days in dogs). They also produce intracytoplasmic inclusion bodies **(Negri bodies)** in brain.

After several serial intracerebral passage in rabbits some strains of rabies virus are adapted to laboratory animals. They are called **"fixed virus"**. These fixed viruses can cause fatal encephalitis if inoculated intracerebrally with a short incubation period of 4-6 days. As they are **neutro**-neurotropic, they are less effective by other routes and do not produce Negri bodies in most of the cases.

1. Animal inoculation

White mice (infant mice) are animal of choice for cultivation of virus. Toga and coxsackie viruses grow only in suckling infant mice after inoculation by intracerebral or intranasal routes. Animal inoculation is still carried out for (a) **primary isolation** of certain viruses and for studies of (b) the **pathogenesis of viral diseases** and of (c) **viral oncogenesis.**

Other animals : Monkeys can be used for selective viruses, e.g. viral hepatitis. Animals can be inoculated by intraperitoneal, subcutaneous intracerebral or intranasal routes. After signs of disease or death, the animals should be sacrificed and their tissue are tested for the presence of virus by microscopic examination of stained smear for **inclusion bodies** and by **neutralisation** and **haemagglutination inhibition** (NI) tests.

2. Chick embryo (embryonated egg)

After incubation in the incubator, the hen's egg embryoes of 7 to 12 days are used for cultivation of viruses. They can be inoculated by (a) **Chorioallantoic membrane** (CAM); (b) **Allantoic cavity,** (c) **Amniotic cavity** route, incubated and examined daily for virus growth.

(a) **Chorio-allantoic membrane** (CAM) : Pox viruses can grow on CAM, produce visible lesions **(pocks)** which indicate replication of single virus. The morphology of pocks is variable according to different viruses.

(b) **Allantoic cavity :** Influenza virus, yellow fever (17 D strain) and rabies (flury strain) vaccines were produced by inoculating allantoic cavity. Duck's egg yields more viruses than hen's egg.

(c) **Amniotic sac :** Primary isolation of influenza virus is done in this amniotic sac.

(d) **Yolk sac :** Some viruses, some bacteria (chlamydiae and rickettsiae) are inoculated in yolk sac.

2. Tissue culture

Small pieces of organs **(organ culture),** fragments of minced tissue **(explant culture)** from man and animal are inoculated into tissue culture growth medium. This medium is balanced salt solution and contains 13 essential amino acids, glucose, salts, buffering system, protein supplement (lactalbumin hydrolysate), calf serum (5%), antibiotics (penicillin, streptomycin) and phenol red (indicator).

Cell culture

Tissue is trypsinised and the dissociated cells are washed, counted and suspended in a growth medium. These cells undergo a very slow cell division and are distributed in tubes, bottles, Petri dishes. Fibroblastic cells adhere and grow on glass surface of test-tubes, bottles. They grow on incubation and spread out on the glass surface to form a **confluent monolayer sheet** of cells in a week period.

Types of cell culture

On the basis of their origin, chromosomal characters and the number of generations through which they can be maintained, cell cultures are classified into three types :

(a) **Primary cell culture :** Normal fresh cells are cultured and get attached to the glass surface and form a confluent **monolayer of cells** by their mitotic division. These primary cell cultures are commonly used for **primary isolation** of viruses and in **preparation of vaccine.** They are **monkey kidney cell** and **human amnion cell culture.**

(b) **Semi-continuous cell (diploid cell strain) culture.** These **fibroblasts,** having same number of chromosomes as in parent cells, are **diploid,** grow rapidly and can be subcultured for a limited time, they undergo **"senescence"**—hence they are lost. These fibroblasts are derived from **embryo tissue** (human embryo lung cell), are susceptible to large number of human viruses, and are also used for **primary isolation** of some viruses and **production of viral vaccine.**

(c) **Continuous cell culture :** These cells of single type are able to grow infinitely **in vitro,** are derived from cancer cells, grow faster and their chromosomes are **haploid.** They can be cultivated indefinitely, they are called **"continuous cell lines".** They are derived from cancer cells e.g. HeLa cells. These cells are from cervical cancer of a lady, HeLa; hence the name HeLa. Other cells are Hep 2; KB cells. These continuous cells can be stored in deep freeze at – 70°C or subcultured and used for **primary viral isolation** but **not** for preparation of viral vaccines because they are considered unsafe for human use as they are cancer cells. Rhesus monkey kidney cell culture are very commonly used as they support the growth of many viruses.

Table 48.5. Common Cell Cultures

Type	Cells derived from
Primary cell culture	Rhesus monkey kidney cell culture, Human amnion cell culture, Chick embryo fibroblast cell culture
Semi-continuous cell lines (diploid cell culture)	Human embryonic lung strain, Rhesus embryo cell strain
Continuous cell lines	HeLa (Human carcinoma of cervix cell line); Hep-2 (Human epithelioma of larynx cell line); KB (Human carcinoma of nasopharynx cell line); Vervet monkey (kidney cell line), BHK-21 (Baby hamster kidney cell culture)

Recognition of virus growth in cell culture

Viral growth can be detected by :

(1) Cytopathic effect (CPE)

Microscopical examination of culture will reveal cell degeneration or death caused by viruses. This CPE can help to identify the viral isolates:

(a) **Syncytium formation :** This syncytium (multi-nucleated giant cells) due to fusion of monolayer cells can be noticed in measles virus.

(b) **Cell necrosis and lysis :** It can be caused by entero viruses.

(c) **Cellular clumping :** This resembles clusters of grapes (but no fusion) which is produced by adeno viruses.

(d) **Inclusion bodies :** These are virus-specific intracellular globular masses produced during viral replication. They are visible under light microscope after staining as acidophilic or basophilic inclusion.

(e) **Discrete focal degeneration :** It is characteristic of herpes virus infection.

(f) **Transformation :** Tumour or oncogenic virus can transform cells into "microtumours".

(2) Haemadsorption

When guinea pig erythrocytes are added to tissue culture infected by haemagglutinating viruses (orthomyxo, paramyxo and toga viruses), these erythrocytes will adhere to the infected cells. This haemadsorption can be blocked by the addition of specific antiserum against these haemagglutinating viruses.

(3) Immuno-fluorescence (direct or indirect)

It can detect viruses in infected cells by antiviral serum labelled with a fluorescent dye.

(4) Interference

Rubella virus multiplies within the host cells and it produces direct cytopathic changes. These host cells are not susceptible to superinfection with CPE producing virus due to viral interference.

(5) Neutralisation test

Known antiviral serum is allowed to react with unknown virus patients. Specific antiserum neutralises virus activity and the consequent mixture fails to produce CPE. This test can be used to type the haemadsorption viruses.

Microscopical examination of culture will reveal cell degeneration or death caused by viruses. This CPE can help to identify the viral isolates.

Bacteriophage : (Fig. 48.3) The structure of bacteriophage is complex and sophisticated than that of virus. The basic design is sperm shaped with a polyhedral head and a cylindrical tail.

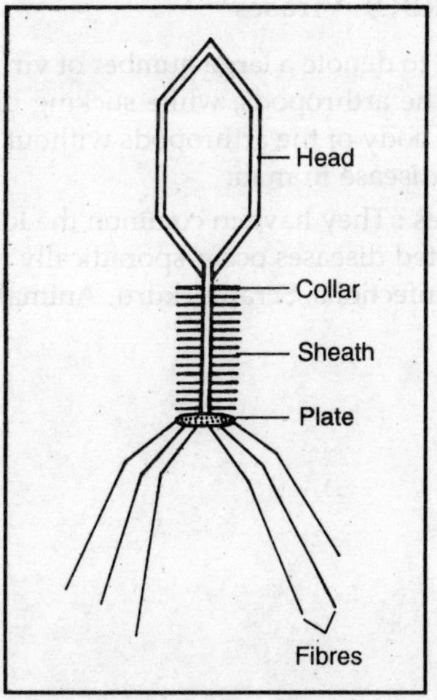

Fig. 48.3: Bacteriophage

The head of T_2 phage of **E. coli** is bipyramidal hexagonal prism and consists of an outer shell of about 1,000 subunits of a protein with a molecular weight of 30,000 and an inner central mass of DNA. The tail is about 100 mμ long and 25 mμ wide and is composed of contractile sheath surrounding a central hollow core. At the distal extremity of the tail, there is a hexagonal plate to which six fibres are attached. The sheath of the tail contracts less than half of the original length. The central core extrudes through the bacterial wall to enable the transference of DNA to the host cells. The epidemiology of the disease can be studied by bacteriophage typing. The choleraphage typing method has obvious epidemiological uses in tracing the epidemic spread of cholera.

The genome of most bacteriophages contain double stranded DNA (T-even phages of **E. coli,** T_2, T_4, T_6, T_3, T_5, T_{17}) and lambda phages of **E. coli;** P_{22} of **Salmonella**). Some contain single stranded DNA (S_{13}, M_{13} phages of **E. coli**); some others contain only single stranded RNA (mu, M_{52} of **E. coli**).

Temperate and virulent phages

There are two types of bacterial phages—**virulent** or **temperate** phage.

Infection of a bacterium with a **virulent** phage results in replication of virus and subsequent release of virus particles causing death and lysis of the host cell.

On the contrary, **temperate** phage persists indefinitely in a quiescent state (**prophage** state) without phage production. When in the latent state, the phage genome is called **prophage.** Since phage DNA is integrated in the host cell chromosome, the prophage multiplies synchronously with bacterial DNA as an inheritable entity. The prophage acts as an additional element of chromosome and expresses new characters. The state of indefinite persistence of phage DNA in host cell without phage production is called **lysogeny** and bacteria carrying prophage are called **lysogenic**; only double stranded DNA phage can be integrated in host cell chromosome as prophage.

Arthropod Borne Virus (ARBO) Viruses

The term arbo virus is used to denote a large number of viruses transmitted by arthropod. These viruses are taken in by the arthropods, while sucking blood of man or animal. These viruses, multiplying within the body of the arthropods without causing damage to the tissues of the arthropod, produce the disease in man.

Slow and oncogenic viruses : They have in common the long continued association with the host. In general, the associated diseases occur sporadically and they exceptionally assume epidemic features (slow virus infections, Scrapie, kuru, Animal virus tumours).

49
Rabies (Hydrophobia)

Rabies is primarily a disease of animals caused by neurotrophic virus. It is a dreaded viral zoonotic disease known to mankind since antiquity before 2,300 BC. It has been reported that over 3 million persons are bitten annually by dogs in India. Over 30,000 Indians die of Rabies every year. It is incurable but preventable by immunoprophylaxis.

Morphology

(1) Under electron microscope, Rabies (*Latin rabidus to rave*) viruses (Fig. 49.1) are large rod or bullet-shaped (*rhabdos,* meaning rods) measuring 76 × 175 nm.

(2) Nucleo capsid shows helical symmetry and contains a single stranded unsegmented RNA genome and viral transcriptase.

(3) Outer lipoprotein envelope contains producing haemagglutinating peplomer spikes, 10 nm long.

Rabies virus is bullet shaped. It forms eosinophilic intracytoplasmic inclusion bodies in the nerve cells of the hippocampus—known as "Negri bodies" which are specific in rabies infection and enable a diagnosis of rabies. Rabies virus is more resistant to disinfectants : 0.5 per cent formaldehyde fails to kill in two months at 4°C; but 1 per cent formaldehyde, 3 per cent cresol and 0.1 per cent mercuric chloride inactivate in 15 minutes; also it is inactivated at 60°C in 10-15 minutes. It is destroyed by a 5 per cent phenol solution and other disinfectants.

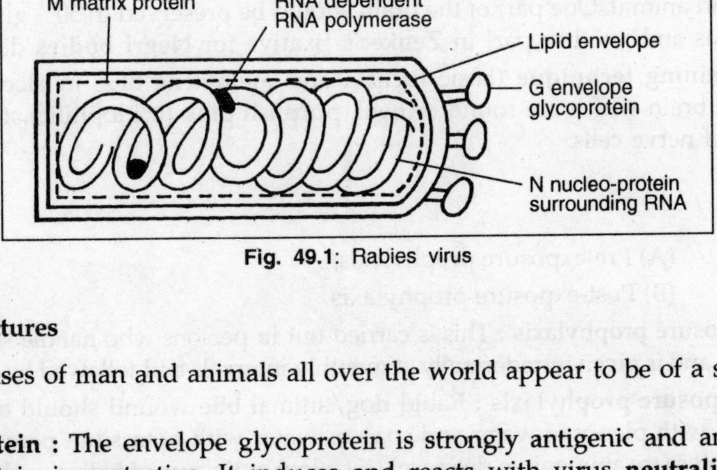

Fig. 49.1: Rabies virus

Antigenic structures

Rabies viruses of man and animals all over the world appear to be of a single antigenic type:

(a) **G. protein** : The envelope glycoprotein is strongly antigenic and antibody against G. protein is protective. It induces and reacts with virus **neutralising antibody.**

G. protein also stimulates T-lymphocytes expressing helper, suppressor or cytotoxic activity. Antibody to G protein lyses infected cells in presence of complement.

(b) **M. protein** (internal membrane protein) and **N. protein** (nucleoprotein) have no virus neutralising activity.

(c) **Haemagglutin** (NA) has haemagglutinating activity with goose erythrocytes.

Pathogenesis and disease in man : The portal of entry is the bite and the rabies virus in the infected saliva is introduced into the wound or scratch or abrasion contaminated by saliva. The virus multiplies locally in the tissues, invades the damaged nerve fibres and spreads centrally to reach the brain and spinal cord.

The incubation period is ten days to two years after the bite of rabid animals, its duration depends on the distance between the point of entry and the brain : bite on the legs, 60 days; on the arm, 40 days; on the head, 30 days. It is short in children than in adults.

The first symptoms of the disease are headache, fever, a profound sense of apprehension and a feeling of irritation at the site of the bite. The patients complain of dry throat, but they will not drink. High fever, difficulty in swallowing and a fear of water (hydrophobia) become dominant symptoms and the patient passes into delirium with generalised convulsion. The outcome is invariably death.

Laboratory diagnosis

First diagnosis should be made in rabid animals.

(I) Then **diagnosis in man** should be carried out on the basis of clinical findings.

Rapid immunofluorescence test can detect viral antigen in skin biopsy or in corneal impression smear. Virus can be isolated from saliva and CSF. Antibodies to virus appear very slowly.

Postmortem diagnosis can be done by

(a) demonstration of **Negri bodies** in hippocampus major of brain (80% positive) of animals or men died of rabies.

(b) isolation of virus by mouse inoculation with infected brain, CSF, saliva and urine.

(c) Immunofluorescence test can detect viral antigen in impression smear.

(II) **Diagnosis in animal** : First one must wear hand glove and remove very carefully the brain of rabid animal. One part of the brain should be preserved in 50% glycerol saline for isolation of virus and another part in Zenker's fixative for **Negri bodies** demonstration.

Steller's staining technique (basic fuchsin and methylene blue in alcohol) can reveal Negri bodies in brain which are round or oval, purplish pink (acidophilic) structures within the cytoplasm of nerve cells.

Prophylaxis

It may be (A) Pre-exposure prophylaxis;
(B) Post-exposure prophylaxis.

(A) **Pre-exposure prophylaxis :** This is carried out in persons who handle severely infected animals and is given intradermally at monthly intervals and followed by yearly boosters.

(B) **Post-exposure prophylaxis :** Rabid dog/animal bite wound should be **immediately** washed with plenty of water and soap or water with potassium permanganate, then with quaternary ammonium detergent (cetavlon) or tincture of iodine or alcohol. Damaged tissue debris should be removed and wound should not be sutured. The suspected animal should be under strict isolation/observation for 10 days under veterinarian through public health office. If the animal remains alive without any symptom for more than 10 days, rabies can be excluded. If rabies is suspected, post-exposure prophylaxis should be adopted by (i) hyperimmune serum, and (ii) vaccine.

Table 49.1. Post-exposure prophylaxis in Rabies

Biting animal	Physical state of animal	Prophylactic measure
(A) Domestic	(i) Healthy, alive for 10 days	None, unless rabies develop
	(ii) Rabid or suspected rabbit	HRIG and HDCV
	(iii) Unknown (escaped)	consult public health dept. if needed, HRIG, HDCV
(B) Wild bat, fox, skunk, other carnivores	To regard as rabid unless proved negative by laboratory tests	HRIG and HDCV
(C) Live-stock rodents, hares, guinea pig, squirrels	Cases to be considered individually	To seek advice from public health officer

1. HRIG – Human Rabies Immune Globulin
2. HDCV – Human Diploid Cell Rabies Vaccine

Table 49.2. Different antirabic vaccines

Nature	Name	Use
1. Neural Inactivated fixed virus grown in sheep brain inactivated by chemical and physical method	**(a) Semple vaccine** vaccine developed by Semple (1911) at Central Research Institute, Kasauli 5% suspension of infected brain inactivated by 5% phenol at 37°C	Widely used anti-rabic vaccine
	(b) Betapropiolactone (BPL) Vaccine Modified Semple vaccine with BPL—an inactivating agent—instead of phenol, believed to be more antigenic than Semple vaccine	Major Indian Laboratories manufacture
	(c) Infant brain vaccine Vaccine prepared in brain of suckling mice inactivated by ultraviolet radiation, BPL or phenol (Fuenzalida type vaccine)	Used widely in South America, similar type rat brain vaccine in use in CIS, rabbit brain vaccine used in Netherlands
2. Non-neural (i) Inactivated	**(a) Duck egg vaccine**	Discontinued
	(b) Tissue culture vaccine (HDCV). Fixed virus grown in WI-38 or MRC 5 human normal fibroblast cell line inactivated by BPL	Highly antigenic, free from side-effects but costly

Contd.

(ii) Live attenuated	Chick embryo vaccine, 2 types—low egg passage of 40-50 (LEP) and high egg passage of 180 (HEP)	LEP for only dogs above 3 months old; HEP for cattle, cats
3. Subunit vaccine	Surface glycoprotein protective antigen cloned and recombinant vaccine produced	Experimental stage

Table 49.3. Schedule of Semple and BPL vaccine

Groups	Semple vaccine	BPL vaccine
1. Person with slight risk	2 ml × 7 days	2 ml × 7 days
2. Person with moderate risk	5 ml × 14 days	3 ml × 10 days
3. Person with great risk	10 ml × 14 days	5 ml × 10 days

Table 49.4. Presently available antirabic vaccine

Vaccine	Substrate	Type
Semple	Brain, sheep, goat	Phenol-inactivated BPL-inactivated
HDCV+	Human diploid cell	BPL-inactivated
PCECV++	Chick embryo cell	BPL-inactivated
PVRV+++	Vero cells	BPL-inactivated
PDED++++	Duck embryo	BPL-inactivated

+, Human diploid cell vaccine; ++, purified chick embryo cell vaccine; +++, purified vero cell rabies vaccine; ++++, purified duck embryo vaccine

Dose schedule of vaccine

(a) **In Europe** HDCV vaccine 1 ml is given intramuscularly on days 0, 3, 7, 14, 30 and 90. HDCV is only licenced vaccine in U.K. and USA.

(b) **In India** HDCV is recommended rabies vaccine available in market and is costly. So people prefer less costly Semple or BPL vaccine.

Vaccine for animal : Cell culture vaccine containing BPL is adsorbed on aluminium hydroxide before vaccination. A simple dose of 0.1 ml is given intramuscularly, followed by booster at 1-3 years' interval.

Prevention and control

Vaccination of domestic dogs by a Flury (Live) canine vaccine, and destruction of stray dogs are most effective control measures. In bats, the virus may remain as latent infection for long time. Man may get the infection by inhaling, contaminated dust in caves housing infected bats. Man should wear mask while frequenting old abandoned house or cave.

Vaccine

Passive immunisation : In case of severe bites, anti-rabies serum or hyperimmune horse serum is injected for passive protection around the bite wounds.

Active immunisation : Various vaccines are used to confer active immunity.

(1) **Semple vaccine :** which contains a 4 per cent suspension of the brain of sheep infected with the "fixed virus" inactivated by 0.5 per cent phenol. This vaccine has a

drawback that it may contain nervous tissue which may sensitise a small proportion (1 : 4,000 to 1 : 10,000) of person who may develop an allergic type of encephalitis.

(2) **Avianised vaccine** contains no nerve tissue, it avoids the neuroparalytic accidents. The inactivated duck embryo vaccine was first introduced in United States of America and is mainly used in Britain; it is less effective than brain tissue or tissue culture vaccine.

A similar vaccine prepared from Rabies virus grown in primary chick embryo cell culture and purified to remove cell proteins and nucleic acids has been made available in India through Hoechst India Ltd., Mumbai. It is given intramuscularly one dose (1 ml) in the deltoid muscle of alternate arms on days of 0, 3, 7, 14, 30 and 90 days. O indicates the day of the first dose.

(3) Human diploid cell vaccine (HDCV) is recently used for immunoprophylaxis without side-effects. This vaccine is prepared from rabies virus grown in human diploid cells.

50
Poliomyelitis

Picorna Virus

Picorna (***pico*, small, rna,** RNA) virus contains single stranded RNA.

Classification

Picorna viruses of medical importance comprise two genera : enteroviruses of enteric tract and rhinoviruses of upper respiratory tract.

Table 50.1. Classification of human Picorna viruses

Genus	Species	Antigenic types	No. of types
1. Enterovirus	Polio virus	Types 1-3	3
	Coxsackie virus		
	Coxsackie A	Types 1-22, 24*	23
	Coxsackie B	Type 1-6	6
	Echo virus	Type 1-9, 11-27, 29-34+	32
Enterovirus		Types 68-72xx	5
2. Rhinovirus	Rhino virus	Types 1-113	113

* Coxsackie A-type 23 now classified as Echo-9
+ Echo10 reclassified as Reovirus-1 and Echo-28 as Rhino-1
xx Entero 72 now designated as hepatitis A virus

Table 50.2. Properties of Picorna viruses

Property	Enterovirus	Rhinovirus
Size (nm)	22-30	30
Capsid form	Icosahedral	Icosahedral
Polypeptide	VP1, VP2, VP3, VP4	VP1, VP2, VP3, VP4
RNA type	Single stranded	Single stranded
Acid	stable (pH 3-9)	Labile (pH 3-5)
Optimal growth temperature	37°C	33-44
Density of calcium chloride (g/ul)	1.34	1.39-1.42

Though poliomyelitis is known as one of the most ancient contagious diseases, its infectious nature was ascertained only in 1905 by Wickman; later, in 1908-09, it was proved to be of viral aetiology.

Polio virus ranges from 8-27 nanometre (nm) (1 nm = 10^{-9} metre) or equal to millimicron (mµ) and forms intranuclear inclusions. It is cultivated **in vitro** in tissue culture of monkey kidney or HeLa cells.

There are three types of viruses which do not possess common immunogenic properties:

Type I viruses include Brunhilde strains which are pathogenic to man and monkey;

Type II viruses include the Lansing strains which are responsible for disease in man, monkey and rodents (rats, mice, hamsters etc.);

Type III viruses (the Leon strain) are pathogenic only to man and monkeys and differ immunologically from the first two types.

Resistance : The poliomyelitis virus survives in sterile water at room temperature for more than 100 days; in milk for 90 days; in faeces in cold for more than 6 months and in sewage for several months. It withstands exposure to 0.5-1 per cent phenol solution and remains viable for several weeks at pH 3.8-8.5. It is very sensitive to calcium chloride, formalin, potassium permanganate and hydrogen peroxide. It is rapidly killed on boiling.

Pathogenesis and disease in man : The virus is extremely neurotropic. It causes the degenerative inflammatory process in the anterior horns of spinal cord and in the grey substance of the brain. However, the virus circulates in the blood. It may be discharged in the faeces of patients and convalescents for 2-7 weeks and is discharged through the nasopharyngeal mucous membrane secretion and sometimes up to 4 months and during the incubation period. Healthy carriers also excrete the virus with the faeces. This virus may be found in the nasopharyngeal mucus and tonsils approximately 3 days before the temperature rises and for 3 days after the onset of the disease. According to the clinical symptoms, three forms of poliomyelitis are distinguished—abortive, non-paralytic, and paralytic.

(a) **Abortive** or **Inapparent infection without symptom**

It is the most common form (90%) of the disease **(abortive poliomyelitis).** Patient recovers in a few days.

(b) **Non-paralytic poliomyelitis (aseptic meningitis)**

In this category, the patient shows clinical symptoms of stiffness, pain in back and neck for 2-10 days. There is rapid and complete recovery.

(c) **Paralytic poliomyelitis**

Due to damage of lower nerve motor neurons, flaccid paralysis develops and it is classified into **spinal, bulbar,** and **bulbospinal** on the basis of nerve involvement. Muscle involvement is most frequent. Within six months, the recovery is maximum, but the residual paralysis may last longer.

Laboratory diagnosis

1. **Isolation of virus :** Virus can be recovered from the pharyngeal aspiration during first 1-5 days and from the faeces up to 5 weeks and it cannot be usually recovered from CSF. It is cultivated in human or similar cell culture and its cytopathic effect is observed in 2-3 days. Its identification is performed by neutralisation test with standard era of 3 types.
2. **Direct demonstration of virus** in stool is done by dried electron microscopy and by immune electron microscopy.

3. **Serology** : Paired serum samples can be tested for neutralising complement fixing antibodies.

Immunity : There are three immunologically distinct types of polio viruses : I, II and III. Immunity to one does not confer immunity to another. A very stable immunity is produced following the disease. No case of reinfection has been described. Immunity is associated with the presence of virus neutralising antibodies in the blood.

Antigenic structure of Polio virus

Each type of polio virus contains 2 types of specific antigens—C and D. C antigen of all types are cross-reactive but D antigen is not. One attack of poliomyelitis gives permanent immunity only against the type causing the infection.

Both live and killed vaccines are available and offer excellent protection. Killed vaccine induces only humoral antibodies (Ig M and Ig G) but does not produce intestinal immunity. Live vaccine induces humoral antibodies (Ig M and Ig G) and local secretory and circulating Ig A antibodies and makes intestine resistant to reinfection. This **live oral attenuated polio vaccine** (OPV-**Sabin vaccine)** is administrated orally and is indicated for active immunisation of all infants of 2 months of age simultaneously with the first DPT injection. The second and third doses are administrated at 2 month intervals. The fourth dose is administrated at 1½ years of age.

Epidemiology

Poliomyelitis caused by three types of polio virus is distributed worldwide mainly affecting children in tropical countries with poor sanitation. The most important source of dissemination of polio virus in the community is usually due to sewage contamination of drinking water with faeces of poliomyelitis patient, sometimes pharyngeal (tract) secretions may spread the virus in the early stage of disease; about 90% of children of tropical countries with poor hygiene have antibodies to all three types of polio virus by the age of 5 years and hence epidemics do not occur; 80% paralysis occurs before the age of 3 years in developing countries. Immunisation has brought down the incidence to 20-40/100,000 population. Vaccination of whole population may eradicate the disease.

Coxsackie viruses

These viruses was first isolated in 1949 in Coxsackie of New York State. They resemble polio viruses in properties and epidemiology. They are divided into two groups : A (23 types) and B (6 types). They can be isolated from throat secretions or faeces in suckling mouse brains. Coxsackie B and A9 grow in monkey kidney tissue culture. Due to existence of several types in each group, sero diagnosis is difficult. Similarly, vaccination is not susceptible to physical, chemical agents; is similar to those of entero viruses.

Clinical findings

Incubation period is 2-9 days. Infection is transmitted by faecal-oral routes. Clinical manifestations of coxsackie virus infection are :

1. **Herpangina (Vesicular pharyngitis)**

   The syndrome caused by certain group A viruses (2, 4, 5, 6, 10) is characterised by abrupt onset of fever, pharyngitis, headache and pain in abdomen. Pharynx becomes hyperaemic with discrete vesicles. It is a self-limiting disease.

2. **Aseptic meningitis**

   Both group A and B viruses are responsible for this condition. Sometimes clinical picture may resemble paralytic meningitis.

3. **Pleurodynia (epidemic myalgia, Bornholm disease)**

   This disease is caused by group B virus and is characterised by fever and substernal chest pain intensified by movement. Its duration is 2 to 15 days.

4. **Myocarditis**

   In children and adults, coxsackie B virus may result in myocarditis.

5. **Transplacental passage**

   Transplacental passage of Coxsackie B virus may result in disseminated lesions (hepatitis, myocarditis, meningoencephalitis and adrenal-cortical disease).

6. **Juvenile diabetes**

   Coxsackie is associated with this condition.

Table 50.3. Clinical manifestations of Coxsackie virus infections

Group	Types	Clinical manifestations
A	1-22, 2n	Aseptic meningitis, paralytic disease Herpangina, Hand, foot and mouth disease
B	1-6	Neonatal disease, Bornholm disease Myocarditis, hepatitis, meningitis

Echo Virus

Echo viruses (enteric cytopathic human orphan viruses) infect human enteric tract. Only man is infected. They were called "Orphan viruses" as they are not related to any particular clinical disease. There are 34 serotypes which cause asymptomatic infection; only few are responsible for overt disease (outbreak of fever and aseptic meningitis (echo 4, 6, 9, 16), infantile diarrhoea (echo 18, 20), and mild respiratory disease (echo 28).

Echo viruses resemble other picorna viruses in their properties. Diagnosis is by isolation of virus from throat secretion, stool, CSF in monkey kidney CPF, and neutralisation test. Serology is difficult due to existence of many types of echo viruses. When echo viruses were first identified they were not pathogenic to laboratory animals.

Table 50.4. Clinical manifestation associated with Echo viruses

Manifestations	Common epidemic types	Uncommon types
Aseptic meningitis	4, 6, 9, 16, 30	3, 7, 11, 16, 18
Paralysis	–	4, 6, 30
Rash fever	4, 9	16, 18
Respiratory disease	–	19, 28
Pericarditis, myocarditis	–	1, 6, 9, 19
Neonatal infection	–	4, 9, 17-20

Entero Virus (Types 68-72)

Out of five types of viruses of this group, four (68, 70, 71, 72) are associated with human diseases and type 72 is now designated as hepatitis A virus.

Table 50.5. New entero viruses and their diseases in man

Serotype	Disease
68	Pneumonia, bronchitis
69	–
70	Acute haemorrhagic conjunctivitis
71	Meningitis
72	Hepaitis A (HAV)

Pathogenesis

Coxsackie virus A24 and entero virus 70 caused two massive epidemics of acute haemorrhagic conjunctivitis. Its incubation period is about 24 hours.

Rhino virus

Rhino virus cause common cold and are isolated usually from nose and throat and rarely from faeces. Because of their adaptation to grow in the nose ***(rhine*, nose)**, they are called Rhino virus.

Properties

These viruses resemble other picorna viruses except that they are destroyed at pH 3-5 and are more heat stable. There are about 113 serotypes of Rhino virus.

Host range and cultivation

Only man harbours rhino viruses, chimpanzees can be infected experimentally. Based on growth in human or monkey kidney cell cultures with cytopathic effect, rhino viruses are divided into three groups : M (Monkey) strains and H (Human) strains. H strains can grow in both human and monkey cells. O (Organ) strains grow in organ cultures of nasal or tracheal ciliated epithelium.

Pathogenesis

Human rhino viruses cause common cold which is an acute respiratory tract infection. Its transmission is mainly in droplet inhalation and the incubation period is 2-3 days. During this period the virus is present in the nasopharyngeal secretions.

Laboratory diagnosis

Isolation of virus is performed by inoculation of nasopharyngeal secretion in human or monkey kidney cell cultures and incubated at 33°C. Due to multiplicity of serotypes, it is not possible to isolate serologically.

Epidemiology

Rhino virus infection is widespread and is transmitted by inhalation. Rhino virus 13 inactivated vaccine gave in volunteers protection against some strains for a very short period depending on Ig A antibodies. It is difficult to prepare an effective vaccine due to multiplicity of antigenic types.

Polio vaccine : In 1949, Enders, Weller and Robbins (Nobel Prize winners) were able to cultivate poliomyelitis virus in tissue cultures, made from human, monkey kidneys, human intestinal tissues, human embryonic tissues and human cancer (HeLa cells). This virus multiplies and kills the tissue cells.

The **Salk vaccine** was prepared by Jones Salk by cultivating polio virus Types I, II, III in live monkey kidney tissue cells and, after an incubation, the dead tissue cells and other debris are removed and the remaining fluid containing polio virus is collected and formaldehyde (1 : 4,000) is added to kill the virus and allowed to act for one week, and excess of formaldehyde is removed. Safety tests were then carried out to determine whether the virus is really killed and the fluid is not contaminated with bacteria. If satisfactory, the preservative is added and the vaccine is ampouled and used.

Use and effectiveness of Salk vaccine

Three doses are recommended : first two doses at an interval of about four to six weeks apart and the third at an interval of 1-3 years or more.

This vaccine does not prevent poliomyelitis, but the incidence is reduced to a very low level, when it is used consistently, because of the antibodies in the blood and the tissues of vaccinated persons which interpose a barrier between the gastrointestinal source of virus and the central nervous system. Thus, the most important effect of the vaccine is to prevent severe **paralytic polio** (e.g. crippling and deadly "spinal paralysis"). This vaccine is 90 per cent effective in preventing the **paralytic polio.**

Vaccination in Pregnancy : Immunisation of the mother with the vaccine probably gives some passive protection to the infants for a few months.

The Sabin or Oral Polio vaccine : On cultivation, the polio virus would probably lose its virulence for man and become available as living, attenuated virus vaccine. Sabin and World Health Organisation conducted a large scale experiment with this living attenuated virus vaccine and the vaccine was found to be excellent and approved in 1962 for general use. The vaccine is given routinely by oral route to millions of people by incorporating it in candy, food, beverage.

Following the oral administration of the Sabin vaccine, the virus multiplies in the alimentary canal and the virus is discharged in the faeces. No symptoms are observed. In addition to the excellent antibody response, the intestinal infection apparently results in an immunisation of the intestinal tract as well, thus preventing subsequent reinfection.

51
Viral Hepatitis

Viral hepatitis is a systemic disease with primary inflammation in the liver. Most of the viral hepatitis resemble each other in clinical symptoms; whereas Hepatitis B viral infection is mostly severe and fatal. Many cases of hepato-cellular carcinoma are due to Hepatitis B and C viruses.

Pathology

The lesions in liver produced by all types of hepatitis viruses are similar and consist of infiltration of mononuclear cells (mainly lymphocytes), necrosis of hepatic cells, hyperplasia of Kupffer cells and variable degree of cholestasis. Parenchymal cell damage is due to hepatic cell degeneration and necrosis, ballooning of single cells and acidophilic degeneration of hepatocytes as they die.

In healthy carrier and chronic hepatitis due to Hepatitis B virus (HBV), large hepatocytes with a ground glass appearance of the cytoplasm may be seen; these cells contain Hepatitis B surface Antigen (HB_sAg). In chronic hepatitis, there is piece meal necrosis at first and later on fibrosis occurs which ultimately leads to cirrhosis, hepatocellular carcinoma.

Pathogenesis

Though Hepatitis viruses differ antigenically, their clinical features are almost similar. These viruses cause acute inflammation of the liver with a clinical picture characterised by fever, anorexia and malaise followed by nausea, vomiting and liver tenderness **(pre-icteric phase)**. This phase may last for a few days and sometimes it may continue longer (3 weeks or more). As this phase subsides, the **icteric phase** appears with jaundice with dark urine, pale stools, obstructive jaundice with a slow recovery period of 4-6 weeks and longer severe cases.

Symptomless or minor infection is also common in HAV and HEV types.

Hepatitis vaccine

Potato vaccine offered hope against Hepatitis A virus vaccine grown in genetically engineered potatoes—seemed to protect more people who ate them, reported by Times of India in February 2005.

About 60% of the volunteers who ate these potatoes showed an immune response that should protect against infection with hepatitis B virus that is shown to stimulate the immune system response.

Antibodies raised in most of 60% volunteers who ate more than three pieces of the genetically engineered potatoes and more than those who ate two pieces.

Hepatitis B virus vaccine shot should be kept refrigerated and expensive—meaning that it cannot be used in many poor countries. People prefer edible vaccine than to get a shot.

Scientists are working to grow the vaccine in banana, tomato or tobacco.

In 1996, 115 million people were infected with HBV even though vaccine isolated from yeast became available in 1986.

Global mortality due to HBV was to be one million cases per year. Hepatitis B vaccine **booster** was not required as published in Lancet, 2005—reported in Times of India (Oct. 2005) because of immunising effect of Hepatitis B vaccine lasts for ten years. Infants and adolescent immune system recalls the response to Hepatitis B virus for more than 10 years after immunisation.

There are six major types of primary hepatotrophic, acute hepatitis viruses. Besides, other viruses are also responsible for acute viral hepatitis.

Table 51.1 Classification

Hepatitis type	Previous description
Hepatrotrophic viruses	
1. Hepatitis A (HAV)	Infectious hepatitis
2. Hepatitis B (HBV)	Serum hepatitis (a) Wide type (b) African HB_SAg—anti HBc + mild disease course (c) Mediterranean HB_c Ag – HBV-DNA + aggressive liver disease
3. Hepatitis C (HCV)	Parenteral non-A non-B hepatitis
4. Hepatitis D (HDV)	Delta hepatitis (agent)
5. Hepatitis E (HEV)	Enteric non-A non-B hepatitis
6. Hepatitis F (HFV)	
Others :	
Cytomegalovirus (CMV) Epstein-Barr Virus (EBV) Herpes simplex virus Coxsackie B virus Echovirus, Yellow fever virus	All these viruses cause acute hepatitis in which involvement of other organs is more common and more prominent than evidence of liver involvement

52
Hepatitis A Virus (HAV)

In 1973, HAV (Fig. 52.1) was discovered in faeces of infected patients by immune microscopy. World Health Organisation (WHO) considered that this infection is prevalent worldwide, in countries where overcrowding; poor hygiene and sanitation are common. HAV was classified as picorna virus. It is a 27 to 32 mm spherical with cubic symmetry. However, there is now more evidence to support that HAV is different from other well defined four genera. The pathogenic mechanism of liver cell damage in acute HAV infection is not yet understood. HAV is destroyed by boiling in water for 5 minutes. Usually it causes a minor or unnoticed illness in children and young adults and high mortality in patients over 60 years of age.

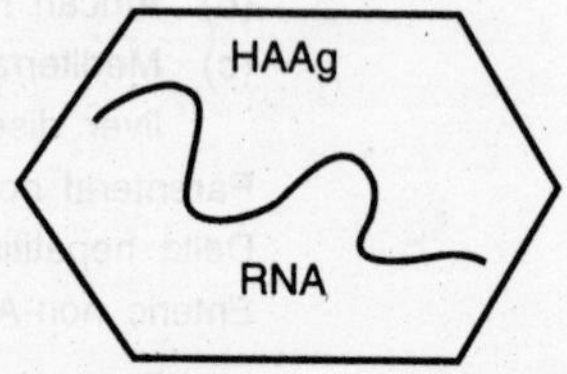

Fig. 52.1: Hepatitis A Virus (Morphology)

More sensitive serological assays, the microtiter solid phase immunoradiometric assay and immune adherence could detect HAV in stools, liver homogenates and bile and to measure specific antibody in serum.

High titre serum immunoglobulin preparations have value in the prophylaxis of HAV infection. Killed HAV vaccine is under clinical trials.

Resistance

(a) HAV is stable to treatment with 20% ether; pH 2.4 and at a temperature of 60°C for one hour.

(b) It can be destroyed by autoclaving, boiling for 5 minutes, dry heat, ultraviolet radiation (UV) and by formalin (1 : 4,000 for 3 days at 37°C).

Laboratory Diagnosis

Laboratory diagnosis can be done by demonstration of virus and its antibody alongwith biochemical tests:

(A) **HAV antigen tests :** Only one type of Hepatitis A virus (HAV) is known—HAV viraemia—occurs only transiently in the incubation period and the excretion of the virus occurs only for 7-10 days after onset of clinical illness.

(1) **Isolation :** It is not possible to grow routinely from faeces of patients, though HAV was grown in human and simian cell culture.

(2) **Immuno-fluorescence :** It can detect HAV in faeces during their excretion in faeces.

(B) **Hepatitis A virus antibodies :** Since it is difficult to isolate HAV from faeces, it is possible to demonstrate specific Ig M antibody to HAV which is found in the blood during early stage of clinical illness and at the time of jaundice appearance. Though Ig M antibody can be detected in serum for 2-6 months after onset of clinical symptoms. After 3 months the titre falls to a low level. Ig G anti-HAV appears during convalescence and persists for many years. It indicates immunity and past infection.

(C) **Biochemical tests :** The pathological and clinical diagnosis is supported by biochemical tests (Liver function tests like ALT and bilirubin).

(1) **Alanine amino-transferase (ALT) :** Alanine amino-transferase (ALT, previously called as SGPT), a cytoplasmic enzyme and asparagine amino-transferase (AST formerly known as SGOT) are present in cytoplasm and mitochondria. Normal serum contains low activities of these two enzymes. The source of which is not known. ALT and AST are not specific to the liver, but ALT occurs in much higher concentration in hepatic cells than elsewhere; thus a rise in serum ALT activity reflects more specifically liver damage.

Serum concentration of ALT

(a) During recovery phase of **Acute Hepatitis A,** titre of 500-2,000 units **decrease** progressively.

(b) In HAV infection, there is a **sharp rise of ALT** with short duration (4-20 days).

(c) In HBV infection, there is **gradual rise** over a longer period (35-200 days).

(d) In non-A-non-B hepatitis, there is **fluctuation** in serum ALT levels.

(2) **Bilirubin and protein :** With the appearance of jaundice, serum bilirubin level usually reaches 5 to 20 mg/dl. Serum globulin is increased with fall in albumin level.

Epidemiology

The spread of the infection is usually from case to case, through contaminated food (raw oysters, shell fish milk) and water.

Prophylaxis

The prevention can be by (a) improving the sanitation; (b) by avoiding the faecal contamination of food and water; (c) by administrating immune human globulin (Ig G) before or within 1-2 weeks after exposure to HAV infection; (d) by disinfecting water by sodium hypochlorite (0.5%) for half an hour inactivates virus; one attack can give life-long protection.

53
Hepatitis B Virus (HBV)

Blumberg et al (1965) described an antigenic substance (protein) in serum of an Australian aborigine that gave a positive precipitation reaction with sera of two multiple transfused haemophiliacs. This antigen was designated as **Australia antigen.** Later it was confirmed that this antigen was the surface component of Hepatitis B virus and named Hepatitis B surface Antigen (HB_s Ag).

Hepatitis B virus is 42 nm in diameter with one molecule of double-stranded DNA and DNA dependent DNA polymerase core of 27 nm diameter, with 2 nm thick shell and an envelope of 7 nm thickness. The core has an icosahedral symmetry. Replication of HBV occurs in primary duck hepatocyte culture system. Only 10% of the duck hepatocytes become infected in tissue culture.

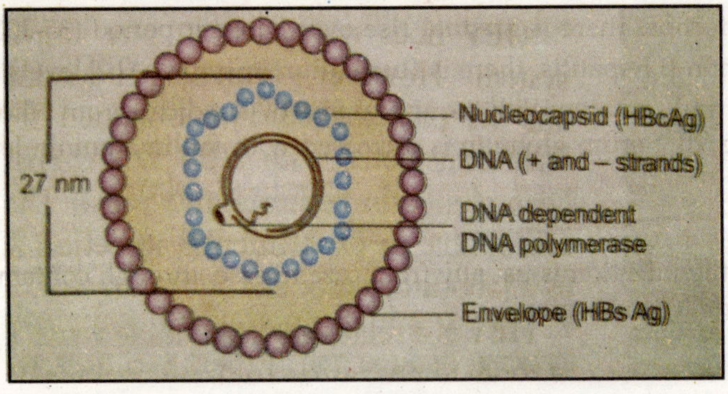

Fig. 53.1: Structure of Hepatitis B virus

Antigenic structure

1. HB_s Ag : surface antigen (envelope protein).
2. HB_c Ag : 27 nm core (nucleocapsid) of the virus with group specific protein which is not detected in patient's blood.
3. HB_e Ag : Hidden antigenic component of core which may be a conversion product of HB_e Ag. It is soluble and appears in serum with HB_s Ag. Later it disappears within a few weeks.

The particles of HB_s Ag are complex and are of four **antigenic types : adw, adr, agw**, and ayr. These types are useful in the study of epidemiology spread through Iran, Pakistan to India.

Additional surface antigens of HBV (q, x, f, t, j, n, g) are yet to be characterised.

Table 53.1. Subtypes of HB_s Ag

Types	Subtype	Distribution
adw	adw 2	Worldwide
	adw 4	Worldwide
adr	adr	Asia
ayw	ayw 11	Africa, India, Russia
	ayw 2	Africa, India, Russia
	ayw 3	Africa, India, Russia
	ayw 4	Africa, India, Russia
ayr	ayr 1	Africa, India, Russia
others	adyw	
	adywr	

Hepatitis B carriers

There are two types of Hepatitis B carriers :

(a) Simple carriers; (b) Super carriers.

(a) **Simple carriers** are persons who do not have HB_e Ag but low titre of HB_s Ag in blood. They contain anti-HB_e in blood and the infection is transmitted only with large volume of blood.

(b) **Super carriers** are persons with HB_e Ag in blood. They are highly infectious as very little (0.0001 ml) quantity of infected plasma can transmit the disease. Their blood contains high titre of HB_s Ag and DNA polymerase. HBV can be demonstrated in blood.

Persistence of HBV infection is indicated by :

(1) The presence of HB_s Ag for more than 6 months.

(2) The infection in 5-10% adults, 30% children, and 90% newborn.

(3) The susceptibility of immuno-compromised hosts to persistent infection.

Transmission

It is mainly due to artificial inoculation of infected blood and blood products. Therapeutic, prophylactic and diagnostic procedures by percutaneous route may also transmit the infection.

Immune Response

(I) Antibody to HBV

(a) **Anti-HB_c** : Following the HBV infection, anti-core antibody rises rapidly. It is not protective; during viral replication in liver and in carrier state, it is persistent in serum in high titre.

(b) **Anti-HBe** : Its presence in serum is an indication of past infection and recent immunity. It rises between 3 and 26 weeks. Later it persists in blood for indefinite period. Both B and T cells response is induced by core and surface antigens. By both antibody-dependent and cytotoxic action of T-cell, the hepatocyte can be damaged.

(II) Cell mediated Immunity (CMI)

With development of chronic liver damage, T-cell function becomes defective. However, in self-limited courses of hepatitis B, T-cell function is within normal limits.

Laboratory Diagnosis

Since there is limitation in the isolation of HBV in tissue culture, enzyme linked immunosorbent assay, radioimmunoassay, latex agglutination and haemagglutination tests, which are sensitive and specific laboratory tests, can be used for the diagnosis.

(I) HBV antigens

(a) **HB_s Ag :** It can be detected in blood a month after exposure to infection. It reaches its peak during pre-icteric phase, it disappears mostly with recovery from clinical disease and persists only in small number of cases. After disappearance of HB_s Ag in serum, anti-HB_s Ag antibody appears and persists for decades.

(b) **HB_c Ag :** It can be detected in liver cells, **by immunofluorescence** not in patient's serum, by immunofluorescence **Anti-HB_c antibody** is detected in the early stage of illness and persists in blood for longer period.

(c) **HB_e Ag :** HB_e Ag and HB_s Ag appear in patient's blood at the same time. HB_e Ag disappears in a few weeks and its persistence in blood is indicative of adverse prognosis, sera of such patient is highly infectious.

(d) **Viral polymerase :** During pre-icteric phase, it appears transiently in serum.

Prevention of HBV can be carried out by **Active immunisation :**

(i) **HB_s Ag vaccine** is prepared by purifying small 22 nm particles of HB_s Ag from plasma of healthy carriers and by inactivating with formalin, urea or heat. These particles are separated by ultra centrifugation, protection is offered by antibody to the "a" antigen (group specific). The product is safe and immunogenic. It is successfully used.

(ii) **Hepatitis B vaccine** is produced by a recombinant DNA technique in yeast cells or in continuous mammalian cell lines in which a plasmid containing the gene of HB_s Ag has been incorporated. The product is particulate and 15-30 nm in diameter with morphological characteristics of free HB_s Ag (surface antigens) in plasma. This vaccine is claimed to be as immunogenic as that derived from plasma of carriers.

Both vaccines are safe and local swelling and reddening may occur in some 20% cases accompanied by slight fever. Three doses at 0, 1 and 6 months are administrated (with alum as adjuvant) intramuscularly into deltoid muscle.

Hepatocellular carcinoma

Chronic infection with HBV is an important aetiological factor in hepato-cellular carcinoma (HCC). In areas where HBV infection is highly endemic, HCC is more frequently observed. It occurs at a very early stage. An interval of 30-40 years is needed between infection and development of tumour. Precise mechanism of oncogenesis is not yet clear. DNA of hepatitis B virus most probably gets integrated with the nucleus of liver cells. Tumour cells collected from Hepatitis B carriers show integrated viral DNA with the tumour cell.

Table 53.2. Hepatitis B infection-outcome

EXPOSURE
↓
INFECTION
↓

- **Death** 0.5-2% Fulminant hepatitis (~1%)
- **Recovery** 90-95% Immune
- **Persistent infection**. Asymptomatic carrier chronic persistent hepatitis
  ↓
  - Clearance Immune
  - Chronic active hepatitis Cirrhosis Hepatocellular Carcinoma

Table 53.3. Differential characteristics of Hepatitis A and B viruses

Properties	Hepatitis A	Hepatitis B
1. Virology		
Diameter	27 nm	42 nm
Symmetry	Icosahedral	Icosahedral
Nucleic acid Inactivation	RNA (enterovirus 72)	DNA (circular)
60°C × 1 hour	Survives	Survives
100°C × 1 min	Inactivated	Inactivated
Envelope	Non-enveloped	Enveloped
2. Transmission		
Primary route	Faecal-oral	Parenteral
Secondary route	Rarely parenteral	Faeces, saliva
3. Clinical	15-40 days	40-200 days
Onset	Acute	Insidious
Fever over 38°C	Common	Uncommon
Chronicity	Rare	Common
HB_s Ag	–	Positive (68-81 days)
Mortality	0.1%	1-10%
4. Carrier state		
Blood	8 months	up to 5 years
Faeces	1-3 months	Negative

HBV, (Table 53.3) the cause of serum hepatitis is a hepadna virus. Hepatitis B surface Antigen (HB_s Ag) is associated with hepatitis B infection. Electron microscopy of HB_s Ag reactive serum revealed 3 morphological forms: (1) the most numerous are small spherical particles of 22 mm in diameter made up of HB_sAg; (2) tubular or filamentous forms; (3) large, 42 nm spherical particles (HBV) called Dane particles—are less frequently observed. These particles are more complex. Their envelope contains HB_cAg. A form of HB_cAg designated as HB_eAg may be present in the serum during HBV infection. HB_cAg and HB_eAg are serologically distinct.

HBV (but not HB_sAg) is sensitive to high temperature. HBV infectivity is lost at pH2, but HB_sAg is stable. HB_sAg is not destroyed by ultraviolet irradiation of plasma and blood product. Transmission can be during **dental surgery.**

Immunofluorescence studies indicate that during HBV infection HB_cAg is found primarily in the nucleus, whereas HB_sAg is localised in the cytoplasm. HB_sAg and HB_cAg are rarely found in the same cell.

In man, HBV is not cytopathogenic because there is existence of HBV carrier state for many years without evidence of parenchymal liver damage.

54
Hepatitis C Virus (HCV)

Hepatitis C virus infection is curable if the treatment is undertaken at the right time, if untreated it can prove fatal in the long run.

The infection involves an initial (acute) phase which is often asymptomatic and can last up to six months. In 65 to 85 percent cases the immune system is not able to eradicate the virus and these people develop a long term (chronic) infection. Chronic infection, after many years can lead to cirrhosis, liver failure, liver cancer and death.

The virus can be transmitted to other members of the family via blood or blood transfusion or blood products from the infected person.

Since Hepatitis C virus infection is blood borne it is compulsory to check blood before transfusion to the patient. Articles (razors, syringes, tampons) used by the patients are to be completely destroyed as they can become a potential source for viral spread. HBV and HCV can be transmitted during **dental surgery.**

This infection can be confirmed by a special test called HCV RNA. Pegylated interferon in combination with an oral drug (Ribavirin) is available. It can cure the infection up to 80 per cent cases. No vaccine is available.

Hepatitis C virus (HCV) or Non-A Non-B (ANB) Virus in **dental operation.**

Cases of clinically viral hepatitis without defined aetiology, after isolation of HBV in 1960s and HAV in 1970s, occurred after **blood transfusion** and led to chronic hepatitis. Thus the term non-A non-B (NANB) hepatitis was used. NANB virus is 30-60 nm in diameter and has been recently identified by molecular cloning technique and termed as HCV which can spread during **dental surgery.**

Hepatitis D virus (HDV)

A new viral antigen was found in the nuclei of hepatocytes of patients infected with HBV and found to be related to a new virus—now named as HDV. HDV (Fig. 54.1) is an incomplete single stranded circular RNA virus. HDV requires HB_sAg for its hepatotropism and propagation, but does not depend on HBV for replication. Replication of HDV is associated with liver damage suggesting that HDV may be directly hepatotoxic.

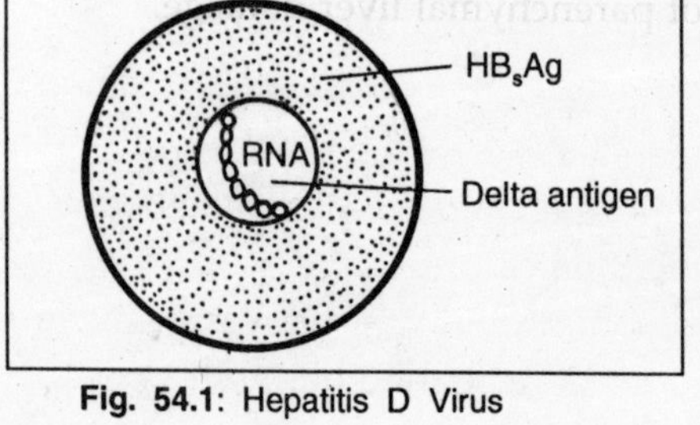

Fig. 54.1: Hepatitis D Virus

Delta Hepatitis (Delta Agent)

A new antigen-antibody system, termed antigen (delta antigen) and antibody (anti-delta) is detected in some HBV infection. The antigen is found in certain HB_sAg particles and is distinct from antigenic determinants of HB_sAg. It has a particle size of 35-37 nm. The delta antigen is believed to be a defective virus that replicates in HBV infected cells and acquires an HB_sAg coat.

Hepatitis E virus (HEV) or Enteric Non-A Non-B Hepatitis

In 1983, Virus—like particle (VL P_s) measuring 27-32 nm were demonstrated by immune electron microscopy in the stools of the cases of HEV infection in CIS.

The first and massive outbreak of enteric non-A non-B epidemic was reported in 1955 in New Delhi (India) when drinking water was contaminated by overflow of an open sewer. Out of 29,000 affected, 10% women were in their third trimester of pregnancy and died of fulminant hepatic failure. It is confirmed as faecal orally transmitted type non-A non-B hepatitis. The treatment is purely supportive.

Clinical features : Clinical distinction among hepatitis A, hepatitis B and non-A, non-B hepatitis is not possible. In viral hepatitis, onset of jaundice is often preceded by gastrointestinal symptoms—nausea, vomiting, severe anorexia and fever that may mimic influenza, jaundice may appear within few days, but anicteric hepatitis is clinically mild. Extrahepatic manifestations of viral hepatitis include (1) a transient serum sickness-like prodrome (urticaria, rash, polyarthralgia or arthritis; (2) glomerulonephritis.

Laboratory Diagnosis : HAV antigen has been detected in the liver, stool, bile and blood by Radioimmunoassay (RIA).

The most specific and sensitive methods to detect HB_sAg or anti-HB_s are RIA and ELISA. These assays and the red cell agglutination (RCA) technique or Reverse Passive Haemagglutination (RPHA, Fig. 8.8) which employs anti-HB_s-coated cells in a microtiter system has replaced counter immuno-electrophoresis as the method of choice for detecting HB_sAg.

A Recombinant Immunoblot Assay (RIBA) is more sensitive and specific to diagnose HCV infection. Polymerase Chain Reaction (PCR) and molecular hybridisation could detect successfully serum HCV RNA. The diagnosis of different forms of HDV infection relies in detection of HD Ag in liver biospies and Hd Ag, HDRNA, IgM and IgG in serum.

Control and Prevention

(1) Clothes of jaundice patients should be washed separately in boiling water;
(2) Jaundice patients should be kept in isolation wards;
(3) All syringes, needles and equipments should be autoclaved to prevent the entry of hepatitis B virus in the body;
(4) Australia antigen test should be conducted by the most sensitive method to detect HB Ag in :
    (a) Jaundice patients
    (b) Blood donors
    (c) Persons to be operated;
(5) Cleanliness and hygiene should be maintained at all public places;
(6) Drinking water should be chlorinated;
(7) Laboratory investigators should wear gloves, while testing sera of patients;
(8) Used materials and glass wares should be discarded in formalin (1 : 4,000).
(9) Laboratory and hospital ward should be fumigated.

55
Human Immunodeficiency Virus (HIV)

Retro virus

Retrovirus (***retro,*** L. backward) belong to the **lenti virus** subgroup of **Retro viridiae** family. They are RNA viruses. It was believed that RNA was the only source of genetic information during multiplication of host cells; later it was found that they reverse the process. Retro viruses contain **reverse transcriptase** (RNA dependant DNA polymerase) which prepares a DNA copy of the RNA genome in host cell. The DNA copy is integrated with the chromosome of host cell.

Table 55.1. Classification of Human Retrovirus

Sub-families	Human pathogens
1. Onconvirinae (Exogenous)	Human T-cell Leukaemia virus I, II, (HTLV-I and II)
2. Lentiviridiae (Exogenous)	Human Immunodeficiency virus 1, 2 (HIV- 1 and HIV-2, formerly known as HTLV-III and HTLV-IV, respectively)
3. Spuma viridiae (Endogenous)	Human foamy virus (HFV)

Onco viruses include both strains of that cause tumour and that do not produce tumours though in man tumour producing strains are found in normal human placenta and tetracarcinoma cell lines, they are not associated with the disease. So they, most probably, are endogenous human virus.

Lentiviruses are so named because they give rise to slowly developing disease in man. HIV-1 and HIV-2 infections are exogenous in origin.

Human T-cells Leukaemia viruses

Human T-cell leukemia/lymphoma virus (HTLV) first reported in Japan, has been isolated in 1980.

Pathogenesis

Human T-cell leukaemia is an acute T-cell malignancy. This virus affects CD4+ T cells of adults—hence it is called as adult T cell leukaemia/lymphoma virus. Both HTLV-I and HTLV-II transform CD4+ T-cells **in vitro.** HTLV-I is also responsible for a neurological disease, spastic para paresis or slowly progressive encephalopathy with spastic or ataxic features. There is a long latent period of many years. The T-cell proliferation may be due to protein coded by **tart** gene of virus. T-cell leukaemia in man is reported in Japan, tropical America and West Africa.

Laboratory Diagnosis

(a) **Serology :** Antibody to HTLV is detected by immunofluorescence, ELISA and confirmed by Western Blot test.

(b) **Antigen :** HTLV antigen is rarely detected in CSF.

(c) **PCR :** Gene amplification by polymerase chain reaction can be applied to lymphocytes of sero-positive patients.

Human Foamy virus

Human foamy virus (HFV) produces a characteristic foamy or vacuolated appearance of infected cell in human live cell culture, hence its name, HFV. Its pathogenic role in human disease is not yet established.

In 1981, Virus was believed hypothetically to be responsible for Acquired Immunodeficiency Syndrome (AIDS). AIDS was first detected in homosexuals at USA. All victims suffered a depletion of a specific subset of T-cells (T_4 cells)—as a result they were susceptible to pathogens that will be controlled by a healthy immune system.

In 1983, it was observed that Human T-Lymphotropic virus (HTLV) had affinity for T_4 lymphocytes **in vitro** and **in vivo.**

In USA, Gallo (Chief of the Laboratory of Tumour cell Biology at the National Cancer Institute, USA) hypothetised that AIDS is caused by HTLV virus or related virus. The two agents known in human pathology at that time (HTLV-I and II) induced leukaemic lymphoid proliferation, while, in case of AIDS, lymphocytes depletion was observed.

Montagnier (Professor of Virology, Pasteur Institute, Paris) discovered a new **retro virus** known by him as Lymphadenopathy associated virus (LAV) from a patient affected with chronic lymphadenopathy. Later, LAV was found similar to HTLV-III. Gallo (1984) isolated HTLV-III similar to be morphologically and immunologically identical to LAV after molecular cloning.

In 1986, HIV (Fig. 55.1) was well-established as aetiological agent of AIDS. Montagnier has also isolated a new virus, HIV-II. The source for a new focus of AIDS in West Africa was HIV-II. In 1987, it was realised that HIV may be a mutant, dating to 20-40 years, of a human virus

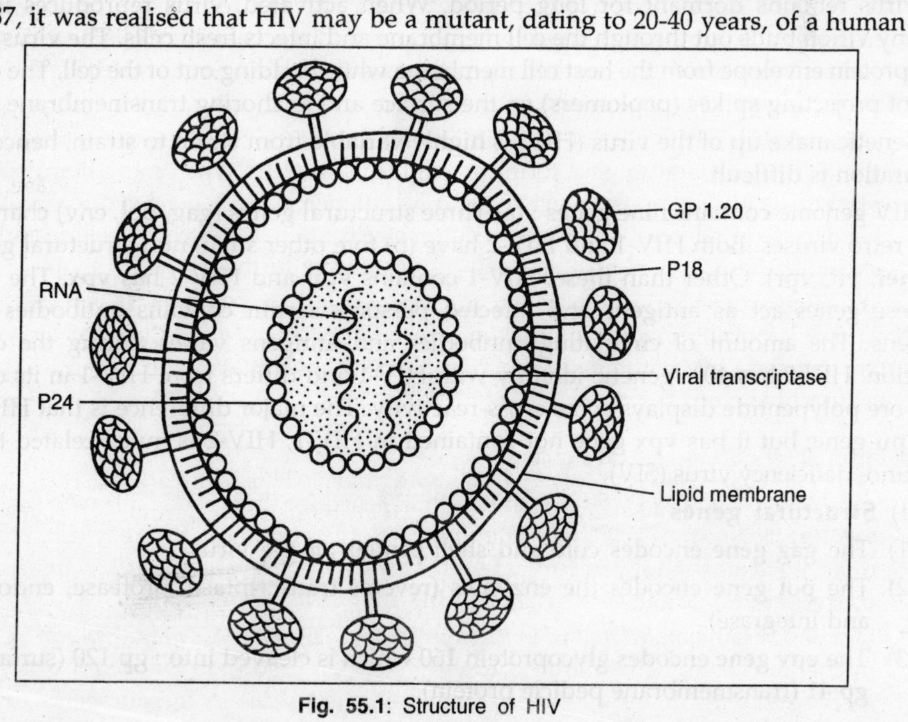

Fig. 55.1: Structure of HIV

not much pathogenic or of a simian virus. Existence of vector of this disease was also demonstrated. HIV and HTLV-III are the same. To eliminate the confusion, an international commission had changed its name to HIV. It is isolated from blood, semen, cerebrospinal fluid, urine, saliva, tears, vaginal secretions, milk, cerebral nervous tissue and spinal marrow. It has tropism for cells; (1) Tropism for T_4 lymphocytes; (2) for macrophages—hence it is isolated in CNS.

HIV is 110-120 nm particles. Its envelope is external part. It has small core (nucleotide) which contains viral RNA. HIV is a RNA retrovirus. It has 9,200 nucleotides in length.

Its genome contains 3 genes of retrovirus respectively coding for :

(a) internal protein in core

(b) inverse transcriptase necessary for replication

(c) glycoprotein on the envelope (Fig. 55.1).

HIV genome also contains :

(1) gene coding for small protein, known as "tat" (for transactivation)

(2) gene coding for small protein 'art' which has same role as 'tat';

(3) gene coding for 2 proteins Q and F whose role is unknown.

New virus—lymphadenopathy associated virus (LAV)—grew in T_4 cells, not in related T_8 cells. Later, LAV were identified as HTLV-III and were found to be the best cause of AIDS. LAV, HTLV-III, HIV are the same.

HIV is the cause of AIDS and is now firmly established. It could affect T_4 cells and macrophages. HIV binds with marker for T_4 cells, infects and kills T_4 cells.

In the host blood cell (CD4 cells), HIV releases RNA which is transcribed by one of its enzymes, **reverse transcriptase,** first into single stranded DNA and then into double stranded DNA **(pro virus)** which becomes integrated into the cell's chromosome by another enzyme. The virus remains dormant for long period. When activated, virus reproduces itself and progeny virion buds out through the cell membrane and infects fresh cells. The virus acquires a lipoprotein envelope from the host cell membrane while budding out of the cell. The envelope has got projecting spikes (peplomers) on the surface and anchoring transmembrane pedicles.

Genetic make up of the virus (HIV) is highly variable from strain to strain, hence vaccine preparation is difficult.

HIV genome contains nine genes : (a) Three structural genes (gag, pol, env) characteristic of all retro viruses. Both HIV-1 and HIV-2 have (b) five other small non-structural genes (**tat, rev, nef,** vif, vpr). Other than these, HIV-1 contains **vpu** and HIV-2 has **vpx.** The products of these genes act as antigens and infected person's serum contains antibodies to these antigens. The amount of circulating antibodies and antigens varies during the course of infection. HIV-2 has 40% genetic identity with HIV-1 and differs from HIV-1 in its envelope. The core polypeptide displays some cross-reactivity. The major difference is that HIV-2 lacks the **vpu** gene; but it has **vpx** gene not contained in HIV-1, HIV-2 is much related to Simian Immuno- deficiency virus (SIV).

(I) **Structural genes**

(1) The **gag gene** encodes core and shell protein of the virus.

(2) The **pol gene** encodes the enzymes (reverse transcriptase, protease, endonuclease, and integrase).

(3) The **env gene** encodes glycoprotein 160 which is cleaved into : gp 120 (surface spike); gp 41 (transmembrane pedicle protein).

Table 55.2. Genetic products of HIV

Gene	Coding for HIV antigens	Indicated by Mass in Kilo daltons
1. **gag**	(a) Core antigen	Principal core Ag-P24/25
		Other core Ag. P15, P55
	(b) Shell antigen	Nucleocapsid protein-P17/18
2. **pol**	Polymerase antigen	P31, P51, P64
3. **env**	Envelope antigen	Spike Ag-gp 120 (Principal envelope Ag)
		Transmembrane Ag-gp 41

(II) **Non-structural, regulatory genes**

1. **tat** (transactivation) **gene.** In collaboration with a cellular protein, it enhances expressions of all viral genes to increase the production of active messengers.
2. **rev** (regulatory of virus) **gene** is required for expression of the **gag, pol** and **env** genes, but not for **tat** and **rev.**
3. **nef** (negative factor) **gene** may be responsible for the regulation of latent state of virus.
4. **vif** (viral infectivity factor) **gene** confers infectivity of the virus.
5. **vpv gene.**
6. vpu (in HIV-1) and **vpx** (in HIV-2). They code for small viral proteins of unknown function.

Antigenic variation

Most HIVs are considered to be variants of HIV-1 which was original isolate (LAV/HTLV-III). Pandemics of AIDS is due to HIV-1. HIV-2 is less virulent. Antigenic variation occurs within both HIV-1 and HIV-2. Strains of HIV differ from each other due to **mutations, deletions** and **insertions.** HIV-1 does not cause disease in animals whereas HIV-2 infects Rhesus monkey.

Animal lenti virus

Simian AIDS virus (SN) is more closely related to HIV-2 than HIV-1, causes natural asymptomatic infection in the primates. Non-primates AIDS viruses are **Feline T Lymphotropic** virus (FTLV) causing AIDS–like syndrome in cats and **bovine lenti virus** (BTLV) causes degenerative wasting disease with defects in CNS in cattle.

Tropism

The spikes (gp 120) of the viral envelope selectively binds to the 58 kd CD4 protein of T helper lymphocytes. Antibodies to CD4 protein block the viral binding site. Mere attachment of virus to CD4 will not suffice for virus infection, but a second human receptor component is of great necessity for viral entry, mediated by gp 41.

Any human cell with CD4 protein on its surface is susceptible to HIV infection. However, the principal target cells are CD4+/lymphocytes.

Two cleavage products of envelope glyco-protein (gp 160) i.e. gp 120 and gp 41 play a great role in the replication of virus. At first gp 120 binds to CD4 protein of host cell, then gp 41 terminus is exposed, thus helping the host cell membrane to fuse with the viral membrane. Hence, the viral core directly enters the cytoplasm of host cell. The infected CD4 cells express a high level of gp 120 protein on their surface which ultimately fuses to CD4 protein of uninfected neighbouring cells, with formation of **multi-nucleated syncitial cells.** These fused cells die finally, thereby causing a depletion of large number of un-infected cells in the circulation.

Evolution usually virus remains hidden (latent) in host cell for a short period.

Window period is the interval period between HIV infection and appearance of antibodies and lasts for 2 to 3 weeks; sometimes it may last for more than six months. During this window period the seronegative person may transmit the virus.

After about 2 weeks of infection, free p 24 Ag and RT **(reverse transcriptase)** Ag circulate in the blood (antigenaemia), which is difficult to identify—particularly in sexually contracted infection.

But it is easier in infection acquired by blood transfusion as the blood contains free virus and large number of infected cells.

With the onset of **acute infection** or seroconversion (about one month after infection), antibody titres becomes detectable and the level of antigens in the blood declines, disappears from the blood and remains absent throughout the asymptomatic phase.

With the formation of antibody, there is disappearance of the virus antigens in the blood. It indicates the immunological suppression of virus multiplication. Mostly **serum p 24 antigen** and viral replication remain suppressed during the first few years of infection. The antigen appears again in the blood when the immune system is damaged. Hence p 24 antigenaemia corresponds to the loss of anti p 24 antibody in patients with **chronic HIV infection.** Virus is easily cultured from a full-blown AIDS than from the asymptomatic person.

Resistance

1. **Temperature :** HIV is inactivated at 56°C in half an hour; at 100°C in less than a second. It withstands **lyophilisation,** hence, the virus in lyophilised blood products can be inactivated by heating at 68°C for 72 hrs.
2. **Disinfectants :** 50% ethanol, 35% isopropyl alcohol, 0.5% formalin, 3% hydrogen peroxide, 0.5% lysol, 0.5% iodine can inactivate HIV in 10 minutes.

Transmission

1. Sexual contact : Sexual transmission occurs among homosexual and heterosexual individuals. There is exchange of body fluid during intercourse. HIV has been isolated from semen, vaginal secretion and breast milk. Genital ulcers may enhance transmission. HIV can also be transmitted by large quantity of saliva.

2. Transmission in blood : Infected blood transfusion, blood products, sharing needles as in drug abusers or accidental inoculation can transmit HIV.

3. Perinatal transmission : HIV can be transmitted from an infected mother to her foetus through placenta. At birth, an infant may be infected when infected placental blood or fluid cut animates abrasions of infant. Post-natal infection is acquired from breast milk.

Pathogenesis

After entry into blood stream, HIV attaches itself to CD_4 lymphocytes. Once in the host cell, the virus releases RNA which is transcribed by reverse transcriptase into DNA (provirus) which gets integrated into host cell chromosome causing **latent infection.**

HIV grows slowly in CD_4 lymphocytes and monocytes. There will be depletion of T4 cells and macrophages. It results into **impaired responses** of T4 cells leading to recurrent life-threatening opportunistic infections characteristic of AIDS.

Table 55.3. Classification of HIV infection

Group illness	Manifestation
I. Acute infection	Characterised by fever, sore throat, lymphadenopathy
II. Asymptomatic infection	Usually well, but HIV antibody positive
III. Persistent generalised lymphadenopathy (PGL)	PGL for 3 months without any other explanation for lymphadenopathy
IV. AIDS and AIDs related complex (ARC)	CD4+ T cells count decrease Other diseases A. Constitutional illness B. Neurological disease C_1. Secondary infections diagnostic of AIDS C_2 Other specific secondary infections D. Secondary cancers E. Other HIV related diseases

Group **I** : Acute HIV infection : The acute illness is characterised by malaise, fever, sore throat, rash and lymphadenopathy. Peripheral blood shows lymphocytosis. Acute HIV illness is mistaken for infectious mononucleosis. Some cases are accompanied by transient signs of meningitis, encephalitis or neuropathy. Infection of CNS occurs early due to initial viraemia.

Group **II** : Asymptomatic HIV infection in this group, all infected persons are well but HIV antibody positive.

Group **III** : Persistent generalised lymphadenopathy.

In this group, lymph node is enlarged (more than 1 cm) at two or more extra-genital sites for three months.

Group **IV** : AIDS or AIDS related conditions (ARC).

The immune system is overwhelmed by viruses. During this stage, the patients suffer from fever, night sweat, diarrhoea, muscle pain and weight loss. The T_4 lymphocytes count decreased. In case of full blown AIDS, the ratio of CD4 (helper) to CD8 (suppressor) cell reversed from 2 : 1 to 1 : 1 or 0.5 : 1. The total T cell count is less than 200/cu mm.

Clinical types

Incubation period varies from 1-14 years, average of 6 years.

(1) **AIDS in adults** : anal and genital intercourse, intravenous drug abuse, haemophiliacs treated with blood or blood products, and blood transfusion are risk factors for transmission of AIDS in adults.

(2) **AIDS in paediatrics** : Infected mother can transmit HIV to babies. Children may be infected after transfusion of HIV infected blood or blood products. Symptoms develop within 2 years in paediatric AIDS. In human immunodeficiency in children, there is opportunistic infections (interstitial pneumonitis, candidiasis and recurrent bacterial sepsis) and death due to Kaposi's sarcoma.

Complications

A. **Infections**

1. Protozoal : **Pneumocystis carinii**, pneumonia, toxoplasmosis, cryptosporidosis.

2. **Fungal :** Candidiasis, cryptococcosis, aspergillosis, histoplasmosis.
3. **Bacterial : M. tuberculosis,** M. avium, salmonellosis, nocardiasis.
4. **Viral :** Cytomegalovirus (CMV); **Herpes simplex.**

B. **Malignancies**

They are common in about 40% homosexuals with AIDS.

1. Kaposi's sarcoma 90%
2. Lymphoma 10%

(Hodgkin's and non-Hodgkin's type)

Almost 90% of HIV infected individuals die due to supervening infections.

Immuno-pathology

1. Humoral response : Repeated infections result in massive antigenic stimulation of B cells. Depletion of regulatory T4 cells may result into the formation of polyclonal immunoglobulins. Inspite of adequate circulating Igs, an AIDS patient shows deficient immune response to new antigen.

2. Cellular response : In asymptomatic HIV infection, immune response does not recognise the latent provirus, Cell Mediated Immunity (CMI) is undisturbed and cytotoxic T-cells are capable of lysing cells that are producing HIV particles. As the disease progresses, there is destruction of T4 (helper) cells; as a result of which there is a decline in cell mediated response to all antigens.

Laboratory Diagnosis

A. Specific tests for HIV infection
   1. Isolation of virus
   2. Detection of HIV antigens : p 24 antigenaemia, polymerase chain reaction
   3. Detection of HIV specific antibodies

ELISA (Screening test)

Western Blot (confirmatory test)

B. Non-specific tests
   1. Total and differential white cell count
   2. Assay of T-lymphocyte subsets
   3. Platelet count
   4. Estimation of Ig G and Ig A levels
   5. Skin test for CMI

C. Tests for opportunistic infections and tumors.

1. Isolation of virus

It can be done during window period and acute infection from CD4 lymphocytes of peripheral blood, bone marrow, serum or plasma.

2. HIV antigen detection

Shortly after HIV infection (after about 2 weeks) free p 24 Ag and Reverse Transcriptase (RT) can be detected in sera. The serum level of p 24 Ag is an useful guide to monitor the virus suppression, when the patient is under Azidothymidine (AZT) therapy.

Polymerase chain reaction (PCR) : In HIV infection, PCR can detect viral gene (provirus) during window period.

3. Antibody detection

During "window period", HIV infected person is seronegative; in most laboratories, the diagnosis of HIV infection is made by detection of serum antibodies to viral protein both core (p 24) or envelope (gp 120, gp 41). There are two types of serological tests (screening and confirmatory). The screening test is easy to perform and are highly sensitive for a broad spectrum of antibodies. Sera positive in screening (ELISA) test can be confirmed by confirmatory (Western Blot) test for HIV infection.

ELISA kit contains both HIV-1 and HIV-2 and thus either detected in routine screening.

Western blot test

There are three types of electro-blotting tests : **Southern blot,** in human of Edward Southern who invented the process of analysing fragments of DNA and **Northern blot** (named factiously) employed to analyse transferred RNA. These two tests can detect antigen by known antibody. The third electro-blot test is commonly termed Western blot to maintain the geographical contour and is used to detect unknown antibodies by known antigen. It is also known as "Immuno blot test."

In Western blot test, HIV is broken down (speared) into protein fragments in a polyacrylamide gel. The separated proteins are blotted electrophoretically from the gel into a strip of nitro-cellulose sheet. These strips are incubated with test sera. Antibodies to HIV protein, present in test serum, combine with all or any fragment of HIV. The strips are washed and treated with enzyme conjugated anti-human gamma globulin and allowed to react. Then a suitable substrate is added that produces colour bands. The position of colour bands on the strips indicates the fragment of antigen to which serum antibodies combined. In a typical case of HIV infection, usually bands with multiple proteins are formed.

B. Non-specific tests

The following parameters can detect immuno deficiency and monitor therapeutic response:

1. **Blood count :** In a full blown AIDS, there is leucopenia with a lymphocyte count of less than 400 per cu mm and thrown leucocytopenia.
2. **T-cell subset :** In AIDS, the count of CD4 lymphocytes fall below 200/cu mm. The count of CD4 lymphocytes rises with effective therapy.
3. **Hyper-gamma globulinaemia :** Ig G and Ig A levels are raised in blood.
4. **CMI** is diminished as evident from tuberculin skin test.

Other investigations

1. **Opportunistic infections** are diagnosed by direct microscopy cultural or serological tests.
2. **Malignancy** is frequently associated with AIDS in homosexuals (4%); Kaposi's sarcoma (38%) is a malignant vascular tumour which appears pink on the skin and mucous membrane.

Epidemiology

It is well-established that HIV is mainly a sexually transmitted disease, though it was originally observed in homosexuals. It may be transmitted through blood, semen, vaginal fluid, via breast milk, from infected mother to her child through placenta. Because of the educational programme, homosexual contacts have fallen. Through routine screening test, HIV infection through blood transfusion is virtually eliminated. An infected person may transmit the virus unknowingly during latent period and asymptomatic phase.

Though AIDS has spread in 1970s or 1980s in America, Western Europe, East and central Africa, about 8 to 12 million individuals are infected with HIV and about 1.5 million AIDS cases may have occurred in adults worldwide (WHO, 1993). By August 1994, about 650 cases of AIDS have been reported from India; incidence is higher in males than females (2 : 1).

On World AIDS Day—2000 it was reported on December 1, 2000 that about 3.5 lakh persons are already infected and most of them are in the prime of youth. 89% of the reported cases, are inactive and economically productive age group of 18-40 years, over 50% of new infection taking place among youth below 25 years. HIV infection has reached over 1% among women attending antenatal clinic. 80% of all new infection, are through sexual transmission, 6% by injecting drugs, 4% through blood transfusion in India (National AIDS Control Organisation, NACO, New Delhi, India).

Further it was reported that there are mainly two types of HIV : HIV type 1 and type 2. Within HIV-1 there are various subtypes.

In India, the most common type of HIV is HIV subtype 1 and subtype C which are more virulent. Subtype C spreads faster and—if not controlled—kills faster.

In much developed countries, HIV-1 and subtype B are more common (Northern America and Europe). Subtype O is also reported in India. However, HIV type 2 is generally less common and as well as less dangerous as it does not spread as fast as other subtypes. HIV type 1 is more common and consists of innumerable subtypes M N O.

As per NACO figures, in India about 80% cases are due to HIV type 1; 1.8% due to HIV type 2; 1.5% have HIV type 1 and 2 combined. HIV type C is more dangerous, spreads faster and kills faster.

Prevention

Following preventive measures should be adopted through health education:

1. **Sexual contact :** Safer sex should be followed by avoiding exchange of body fluids (semen, vaginal discharge). The use of condoms should be encouraged to prevent the transmission of the virus.
2. **Sharing needles :** During drug abuse, needle and syringe should not be shared.
3. **Blood** and blood products should be screened before transfusion. The same procedure should also be practised for donation of semen, cornea, bone marrow, kidney, since HIV can spread through any tissue.
4. **Control of infection** can be done by screening the individuals from risk group.
5. **Isolation of AIDS patients** is of great necessity to check the spread of infection. Then treatment against virus and other opportunistic infections is also essential.
6. **Risk factors** are female sex workers, intravenous drug abuse, men and women with multiple sex partners.

Prophylaxis

No effective vaccine is available till date. Vaccine maker Yax Gen Ine President Dr. Donald Francis reported in February 24, 2003 that his first attempt to develop a vaccine to prevent AIDS has failed.

Treatment

Azidothymidine (Zidovudine, AZI) is still a drug of choice. Alternative drugs (dideoxynosine, dideoxycytidine) are under evaluation.

Table 55.4. Laboratory diagnosis of HIV infection

Markers	Window period	Acute infection phase	Asym-ptomatic ARC	AIDS and
1. Virus infection	++	+	–	+
2. Antigen : p 24 RT	–	+	–	+
3. Antibody				
Anti p 24	–	+	+	+
Anti p 120, p 41	–	+	+	+
ELISA test (Screening test)	–	+	+	+
Western blot test (Confirmatory test)	– (Partial p 24) gp 120	+ (Full pattern)	+ (Absence) of p 24 AB	+

Table 55.5. World-wide cases of AIDS by 'UNAIDS' – Nov. 2010

Country	Cases
Sub-Saharan Africa	22.5 million
North Africa and Middle East	460,000
Asia	4.9 million
Oceania	57,000
Central and South America	1.4 million
Europe	2 million
North America	1.5 million
Total (Adult and Children living with HIV/AIDS)	33.3 million

Table 55.6. Epidemiological pattern of HIV infection – Nov. 2010

Areas	Transmission
Pattern I	
• Typical of industrialised countries – large no. of cases were reported • eg, North America, Western Europe, Austrialia, New Zealand, Latin America etc.	• Mainly homosexual or bisexual men, • Intravenous drug abusers, • Small no. of heterosexual cases

Contd.

Areas	Transmission
Pattern II • Sub-Saharan Africa • North Africa • Caribbean Countries	• Mainly heterosexual • Perinatal infections were also significant in no. • Low numbers of IV drug abusers or homosexuals
Pattern III • Eastern Europe • Middle East • Asia • Most of the Pacific	• Mainly homo and heterosexual contacts

Table 55.7. Seroprevalence rates in risk groups in India

Risk groups	Size	Seroprevalence
High Risk Group		
Intravenous drug abusers	15,000-50,000	30-50%
Female sex workers	0.5-1 million	2-30%
Intermediate Risk Group		
Men and women with multiple sex partners	1.5 million	5/1000
Low Risk Group		
Men, women and children	800 million	1/10,000-1/1000

Table 55.8. Opportunistic infections in AIDS and diagnosis

Organism	Habitat	Human lesion	Laboratory diagnosis
Pneumocystis carinii	Widespread (man, animals) dormant in lung, aerial transmission	Pneumonia	Trophozoites, cysts in human alveoli
Toxoplasma gondii	Intestine of cat and other animals; faecal transmission	Toxoplasmosis of brain and CNS	Demonstration of intracellular protozoa in CNS and brain after Giemsa staining; detection of Ag more useful than antibody; culture of exudate in mice
Cytomegalo virus (CMV)	Man	Hepatitis, Pneumonia	1. Demonstration of cytomegalic inclusion in urine, saliva and body fluids 2. Cultivation in fibroblasts
Herpes simplex	–	Mucocutaneous ulcerations	Inclusion bodies in smear prepared from lesions after Giemsa stain
Candida albicans	Normal inhabitant of skin and mucosa	Oropharyngeal candidasis extending to trachea	1. Budding Gram-positive cells can be seen in smears prepared from lesions 2. Grow in Sabouraud's agar medium
Coccidioides immitis	Soil and rodents	Coccidiomycosis (influenza like) causing severe damage to CNS granuloma	Dimorphic fungus occurs as yeast in tissue and as mycelium in culture Tissue form as a sphericle (15-17 μm) filled with endospores; cultured in Sabouraud's medium
Cryptococcus neoformans	Soil, saprophytes	Cryptococcosis in pigeon faeces	Capsulated budding yeast cells in CSF (cryptococcal meningitis) lesions; cultured in Sabouraud's medium
Mycobacterium tuberculosis	Man	Pulmonary tuberculosis	Sputum shows AFB; Growth in L.J. medium
Myco. avium	Birds	Pulmonary tuberculosis	1. AFB in sputum smear 2. Growth in L.J. medium 3. Aryl sulphatase, animal inoculation test

HIV is diagnosed by IgG to viral protein not to virus of antigen.

(A) **ELISA** is an immunoenzymatic technique, rapid, sensitive, reproducible, less specific, less costly. This test can detect antibody against viral protein.

(B) **Western Blot** or Immuno Blot. Denatured viral protein is the basis for this test. This technique can detect antibody against denatured viral protein or antibody against fragments of gp 120 (glycoprotein of the envelope).

(C) **RIPA test** (Radio immunoprecipitation test) can detect antibody against glycoprotein and also native viral protein by radioisotopic technique. This test is more specific, less sensitive, more costlier than ELISA test.

Seropositivity is observed between 1 to 4 months after contamination. Possible HIV transmission is through **dental** surgery.

Arthropod Borne Rickettisal Infections

Rickettsiae occupy a biological position which is intermediate between the smallest bacteria and the largest virus. Rickettsiae are small prokaryotic cells that have an obligate intracellular existence. They resemble bacteria as they are visible under light microscope and are known to divide by binary fission. They have cell wall containing the amino sugar (muramic acid) and are susceptible to the action of antibiotics.

Like viruses, they are obligate intracellular parasites except **Rickettsia quintana** which grows extracellularly in the louse gut and has been cultivated on modified blood agar medium. Under natural conditions, they are present in the alimentary canal of blood sucking arthropods (lice, ficks, flea, mite) but when they are transmitted to man they cause the disease "Typhus" characterised by fever and rash.

Diseases arranged according to the arthropod vectors :

1. **Louse borne typhus**	
(a) Epidemic typhus	**Rickettsia prowazekii**
(b) Trench fever	**R. quintana**
2. **Flea borne typhus**	
Murine endemic typhus	**R. Mooseri**
3. **Tick borne typhus**	
Rocky mountain spotted fever	**R. rickettsii**
4. **Mite borne typhus**	
(a) Scrub typhus	**R. tsutsugamushi**

Rickettsiae are coccobacilli. Though they are Gram negative, they can be stained with Castaneda or Giemsa stain. In general, they are easily destroyed by heat, drying and chemical disinfectants.

Rocky mountain spotted fever, first recognised by Ricketts in America, is caused by R. rickettsii and is transmitted by a tick **(Dermacentor andersoni).** Fresh tick faeces are infectious.

Louse borne typhus fever (epidemic typhus fever) is caused by **R. prowazekii** and is spread by the human body louse **(Pediculus corporis).** Though it is worldwide in distribution, it is confined to Middle East, Asia, Africa, Mexico. Lice become infected while biting infected patients or carriers, when the infected blood reaches the intestine of the louse, rickettsiae invade the epithelial cells until the host cells distend and rupture. As a result, the faeces of louse become heavily laden with the organisms and when they are discharged on the skin, they enter the blood stream through the abrasions or fresh bite wounds, causing rickettsiaemia.

Typhus is characterised by an onset about two days during which there are nausea, headache, dizziness and high fever, then appears a rash which may cover the whole body. The patient is lethargic and delirious. The blood of the patient is infectious to the louse. The organism cannot be demonstrated microscopically in the blood, but it can be cultivated in yolk sac. However complement fixation test (CFT) is most accurate and specific as the antigen is derived from the rickettisae cultivated in yolk sac.

56
Oncogenic Virus

In 1908 Ellerman and Bang first discovered virus causing leukaemia in chicken. Later Rous (1911) proved that the virus can cause chicken sarcoma. Now it is well estimated that about 20% of human tumours are caused by virus.

Classification

Oncogenic viruses are those viruses that produce tumours in their natural hosts, experimental animals, or in cell cultures. They are classified according to their nucleic acid content in their genome. Many classes of RNA viruses are responsible for tumour production in animals but only one family of RNA viruses **(Retro viridae)** can produce the tumour.

Mechanism of viral oncogenesis

In cell transformation by tumour viruses, the initial stage of adsorption, penetration and uncoating are exactly the same as for productive infection, but in subsequent two stages, they differ

1. **In case of oncogenic DNA viruses,** the DNA is integrated in the host cell genome as prophage. The integrated viral genome is rearranged. As the integrated viral DNA is either defective or incompletely, no infectious virus is produced, instead the host cell undergoes neoplastic transformation under its influence.
2. **Retroviruses** replicate by a unique manner by an enzyme, reverse transcriptase (RT) carried by the viruses. RT constructs a DNA copy of the RNA genome of the virus and the **DNA copy (prophage)** becomes integrated with DNA of the host cell, where it may remain latent for variable periods. Only when activated, the integrated **provirus** acts as template for translation of progeny viral RNA and cell transformation.

Oncogenes

Genes that are responsible for the induction of tumours are known as **oncogenes** which were first discovered in **retro virus, Rous sarcoma virus** (RSV) that can transform cells. Besides their important role in new plastic transformation, they are also responsible for normal cell growth, division, and differentiation. The process of transformation and neoplasia is due to **in correct or illegimate expression** of these genes. Martin and Vogt first identified viral gene **(v-sre)** in Rous sarcoma virus and later a similar **src gene** was identified in genome of normal chicken cells which is called **cellular src (C-src) gene.** More than 30 oncogenes have been identified.

A new class of human cancer genes called "tumour suppressor genes", growth suppressor genes or anti-oncogenes have been identified.

Oncogenic retroviruses

They are responsible for tumours of reticulo-endothelial and haemotopoietic system (leukaemia, lymphoma) or of connective tissue (sarcoma). They are also called as **"acutely transforming viruses"** (ATVS), because they produce tumours within a short period of six months after injection into a suitable host.

1. Avian Sarcoma leukosis viral (ALV) Complex : They are caused by antigenically related viruses which caused lymphoma, leukaemia and sarcoma.

2. Murine leukosis virus : There are several strains of murine leukaemia and sarcoma viruses which are derived from Mo-Mu Lv during passages in mice and rats.

3. Mouse mammary tumour viruses (MMTV). They may be endogenous or exogenous viruses. The endogenous ones have no oncogenic role, whereas the exogenous ones are oncogenic. Mammary cancers develop only in susceptible females after a latent period of 6-12 months.

4. Sarcoma leukaemia viruses of **animals :** Leukaemia, lymphosarcoma in cat is induced by **Feline leukaemia virus** (Felv); Lymphosarcoma in cattle is due to **bone leukaemia virus.**

5. Human T-cell leukaemia virus (HTLV) : Adult T-cell leukaemia is induced by HTLV-1 but having cell leukaemia of T-cell type is due to HTLV-II.

Oncogenic DNA viruses

1. **Papova viruses :** They induce benign warts and papilloma in natural hosts. **Human papilloma virus** (HPV) type 6 and 11 are incriminate in pre malignant lesions of the female and male genital tract.

   SV 40 **polyoma viruses** produce tumours in mice when injected.
2. **Herpes virus :** Herpes simplex type 1 and 2 and **Cytomegalovirus** transform cultured cells at a very low frequency. They transformed hamster cells, when injected into another hamster, form tumours. In woman, **Herpes simplex** type 2 is responsible for cervical carcinoma. No transforming gene is involved **Epstein-Barr** (EB) **virus** is associated with Burkitt's lymphoma in Africa and nasopharyngeal carcinoma in Chinese male population. It is believed that EB virus transforms normal lymphocytes into lymphoblast in immuno-compromised child.
3. **Hepatitis B virus** is implicated in hepato-cellular carcinoma. It does not carry any oncogene and is integrated in tumour cells as Hepatitis B virus DNA.
4. **Pox virus : Yaba virus** produces histiocytoma (benign tumour) in natural host (monkey) while **shope fibroma virus** induces fibroma in rabbit. **Molluscum contagiosum** virus produces benign growths in humans.

57

Pox Viruses

Pox viruses are most complex and largest so they can be seen under light microscopes. They replicate in the cytoplasm unlike other DNA viruses. Elementary bodies (Paschen bodies) are found in smears from the lesion.

Morphology

Pox virus are brick shaped. They measure 300 × 240 × 100 nm; they are largest and are complex as they do not show any discernible symmetry. This virus consists of double stranded DNA surrounded by double layered membrane and it contains more than 100 different polypeptides and enzymes which include **transcriptase.** It affects man, monkeys, calves, sheep and rabbit.

Cultivation : They can grow in chorio-allantoic membrane (CAM) of chick embryo and tissue culture (Fig. 57.1).

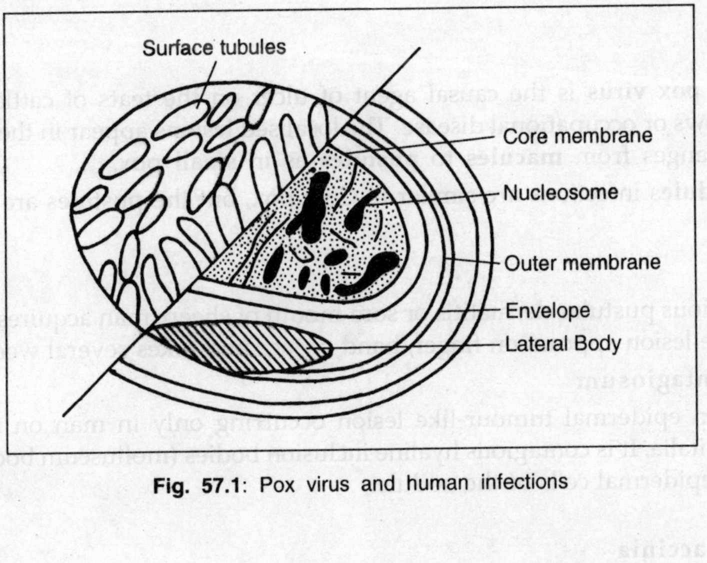

Fig. 57.1: Pox virus and human infections

Classification

Orthopox virus, Parapox virus and some unclassified species cause human infections. They share a common nucleo-protein antigen in their inner core.

Table 57.1. Pox virus and human infections

Genus	Virus	Primary host	Diseases
Orthopox virus	**Variola**	Man	Small pox (eradicated)
	Vaccinia	Man	Small pox vaccine preparation (used)
	Monkey pox	Monkeys	Human infections (rare)
	Cow pox	Cows	Human infections (rare) localised ulcerating lesion
Parapox virus	**Orf**	Sheep	Human infection (rare)
	Milker's node	Cows	localised lesion
Unclassified	**Molluscum contagiosum**	Man	Benign skin lesion
	Tana pox	Monkeys	Human infection (rare) localised
	Yaba pox	Monkeys	Human infection (very rare localised)

Small pox

Pathogenesis

In all pox virus infections, pathogenesis is almost similar. First pox virus enters the respiratory tract by inhalation, settles in the respiratory mucosa, multiplies in the draining lymph nodes and thereby resulting into **primary viraemia** which favours the dissemination of the virus throughout the body **secondary viraemia.** During this stage, the virus settles in the skin and mucosa, produces skin rashes after an incubation period of about 12 days. The rash appears on the buccal mucosa (**exanthem**), then develops into **macules, papules, vesicles** and finally **pustules** which dry up in 10-12 days after the first rash.

Cow Pox

Mainly **cow pox virus** is the causal agent of ulcer on the teats of cattle. In man, it is acquired from cows or occupational disease. The localised lesions appear in the fingers of man and undergo changes from **macules** to **pustules** as in small pox.

Milker's nodules infections are similar to Cow pox, but the pustules are rare.

Orf

It is a contagious pustular dermatitis or sore-mouth of sheep; man acquires. This infection by contact; single lesion appears on finger, hand or face and takes several weeks for healing.

Molluscum contagiosum

It is a benign epidermal tumour-like lesion occurring only in man on the arms, legs, buttocks and genitalia. It is contagious hyaline inclusion bodies (molluscum bodies) are within the proliferated epidermal cells of the nodule.

Variola and Vaccinia

Variola virus causes small pox only in human and monkeys. In the past, small pox epidemics appeared in two forms : (1) florid and fatal disease occurred in India; (2) mild, non-fatal disease (**alastrim**) in Latin America. The virus causing classical small pox was named variola major; the other one causing **alastrim** is variola minor. These two viruses are antigenically identical, but differ in certain biological properties only.

Vaccinia virus causes vaccinia which is a localised skin infection and infects mice, rabbit. It is from Jenner's original cow pox vaccine and is used for small pox vaccination. Now, it is distinct from **Orthopox virus** and is maintained by arm to arm passage in man. During this passage, it underwent some permanent changes differing from the freshly isolated cow pox. Virus may, be a product of recombination of cow pox and a hybrid of variola.

Prophylaxis

Vaccination with vaccinia produces protection against small pox for about 5 years. A natural infection of small pox gives a complete protection against reinfection.

58
Herpes Virus

Herpes viruses (100 nm in diameter) contain icosahedral capsid made of 162 capsomeres, DNA genome and are surrounded by a lipid envelope. Electron microscope cannot distinguish different members of Herpes virus. Because of their multiplication in the nucleus of cell, they produce Cowdry type A inclusion body (Fig. 58.1).

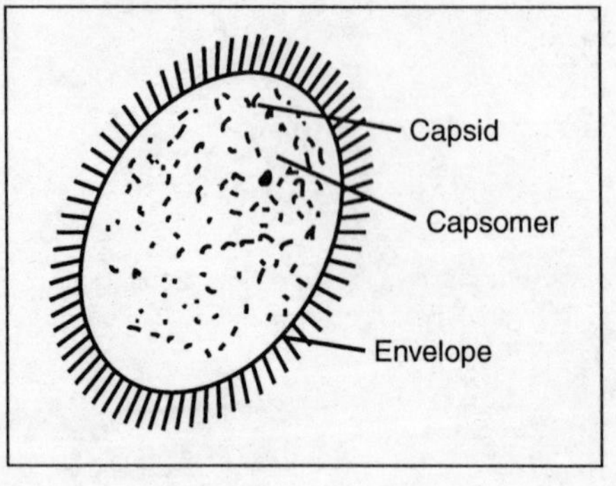

Fig. 58.1: Herpes virus

Classification

Herpes viruses are divided into 3 subfamilies on the basis of their biological properties. Both man and animals are affected. Antigenically, they differ from each other except Herpes simplex types 1 and 2—which share common antigens. Human B-lymphotrophic virus, a new virus designated as human herpes virus type 6, has been recovered from lymphoproliferative disordered patients. Herpes viruses frequently cause recurrent infection.

Herpes Simplex virus

It infects only humans. **Herpes virus type 1** causes oral and ocular lesions, whereas Herpes virus type 2 causes genital infection; congenital malformation may occur due to transplacental passage of both types of Herpes virus.

Pathogenesis

The primary mode of entry is through the skin, oral mucosa, or eyes. It may result into a vesicle formation under the layer of keratinised squamous epithelial cells. The vesicle fluid contains multinucleated giant cells and eosinophilic intranuclear inclusion with inflammatory cells and cellular debris. The virus infects draining lymph nodes causing lymphadenitis which may heal with little soon.

After primary infection the virus travels by retrograde intra-axonal flow to sensory root ganglia which innervate the area of infection. They settle with the neurones (trigeminal, sacral). The Herpes virus DNA gets integrated in the host cell genome.

(1) **Initial (primary) infection** due to type 1 is mostly acquired at 6 months to 3 years of age through eye or oral mucosa; it is often **asymptomatic;** only 10-15% of infected children show **acute gingivo stomatitis.** About 75% of adults harbour antibodies against these viruses. Saliva, skin lesions, or oropharyngeal lesions of patients or carriers. **Recurrent infections** are common (e.g. recurrent **herpes labialis**) and may lead to **dendritic keratitis, corneal ulcers, acute keratoconjunctivitis** vesicles on eyelids. The transmission of type 1 virus is by direct contact or droplet spreads. Type 1 virus may also produce **eczema herpeticum** (crops of vesicles on the body) and encephalitis.

2. Sexual transmission is common in **genital infection** due to types 1 and 2 virus. Neonate may be infected from mother's birth canal. Lesions are common in the penis and urethra of male; cervix, vulva, vagina and perineum of the female.
3. The causal relation of type 2 virus in cervical and valvular carcinoma is yet to be evaluated. Patients with these malignancies show high titre HSV-2 type antibody.

Table 58.1. Classification of human herpes viruses

Sub family	Growth cycle	Cytopathology	Latent infections	Official name	Common name
Alpha herpes virus	Short	Cytolytic	Neurons	Human herpes virus 1	Herpes simplex virus type 1
				Human herpes virus 2	Herpes simplex virus type 2
				Human herpes virus 3	Varicella zoster Virus
Beta herpes virus	Long	Cytomegalic	Glands Kidneys	Human herpes virus 5	Cytomegalo virus
		Lymphotrophic	Lymph node	Human herpes virus 6	Human B cell Lymphotropic virus
				Human herpes virus 7	RK virus
Gamma herpes virus	Variable	Lympho-proliferative	Lymphoid tissue	Human herpes virus 4	Epstein Barr (EB) virus
				Human herpes virus 8	Kaposis's sarcoma associated herpes virus

Immunity

Type 1 antibodies appear in early childhood. Type 2 antibodies during adolescence.

Table 58.2. Herpes simplex virus disease

Virus	Diseases
HSV-1	Gingivostomatitis Herpes labialis Kerato-conjunctivitis Dendritic keratitis Eczema herpeticum Encephalitis, Genital ulcer
HSV-2	Genital lesions (penis, urethra, cervix, vulva, vagina, perineum) Neonatal herpes Cervical and valvular carcinoma

Clinical diagnosis is important.

1. Smear from the base of the vesicle is stained by toluidine blue. **Mutinucleated giant cells** and cowdry type A intranuclear inclusion bodies can be seen.
2. Herpes virus can be grown in human embryonic tissue, HeLa cells or in chorio-allantoic membrane (CAM) of chick embryo.
3. Serological tests (CFT, neutralisation test) are positive.

Varicella Zoster

It is a single virus which is known as **varicella zoster** (V-Z) virus. It causes both varicella (**chicken pox**) and herpes zoster (shingles). Chicken pox may be transmitted by **primary contact** of a non-immune host with this virus, whereas zoster is a **reactivation** of the **latest virus** in individuals with ineffective immunity.

Varicella (Chicken pox)

Varicella zoster virus enters the respiratory tract, multiplies locally, enter the blood circulation (viraemia) and localise in the skin, mucous membranes and other organs (Table 58.1). Incubation period is 10-21 days. The disease is highly infectious in childhood and is characterised by vesicular rash on the trunk. This rash transforms into macule, papule, vesicle, pustule and scab. Pneumonia is a common complication, Post-viral encephalitis and haemorrhagic (fulminating) varicella.

Herpes Zoster

It is a disease of old age occurring several years after chicken pox. The V-Z virus remains latent in the cranial nerve ganglia (sensory). There is inflammatory reaction in these nerve ganglia which results into eruption of crops of painful vesicles in areas of skin supplied by the affected sensory nerves. The vesicles are similar to those of varicella. The eruption is often unilateral. When the thoracic nerves are involved, there is sudden pain and rash around the trunk. When the ophthalmic branch of trigeminal nerve is affected. There is **ophthalmic zoster.** Within 2-3 days the rashes clear. When a patient is under radiotherapy or on immunosuppressive drugs, the disease may disseminate further.

Immunity

One attack of varicella confers lifelong immunity, though both the clinical entities are caused by a single virus.

Laboratory diagnosis is similar to that of Herpes simplex virus.

Prophylaxis

1. Convalescent pooled serum contains V-Z virus immunoglobulin and gives passive protection and is ineffective in treatment.
2. Alive attenuated varicella vaccine has been developed by serial passage in tissue culture in Japan which gives lasting protection for several years.

Cytomegalovirus

Cytomegalo virus infections are always apparent with antibody prevalence of 80% in adults. The exact mechanism of transmission of this virus is still unknown except in congenital infection and those spread by organ transplantation and blood transfusion. This virus is shed in urine, saliva, tears, semen, cervical secretion and breast milk. This virus has been recovered in cervix of 10% of healthy women.

Pathogenesis

Cytomegalo virus is transmitted from a mother with a latent infection to the foetus. **In utero,** this congenital infection may cause the death of foetus, congenital cytomegalic inclusion disease or may remain apparent (**asymptomatic**) at birth.

Cytomegalic inclusion disease is characterised by hepatosplenomegaly, jaundice, thrombocytopenic purpura, pneumonitis, CNS damage (microcephaly). Clinically the disease in adults resembles infectious mononucleosis. Post-natal infections are usually asymptomatic, but sometimes they show hepatitis.

Diagnosis

1. Enlarged cells with large intra-nuclear "owl's eye" appearance inclusions (cytomegalic cells) are often seen in involved organs (salivary glands, kidney, liver, spleen).
2. This virus can be grown in embryonic tissue (fibroblast) culture.

Epstein-barr Virus (EBV)

Epstein and Barr isolated EBV from Burkitt's lymphoma. Hence its name. EBV affects mostly lymphoid tissue and EBV infections are clinically inapparent, though 80-90% children are seropositive. The primary B lymphocytes have receptors for EBV and these infected cells are transformed in such a way that they multiply continuously. The transformed cells contain EBV genome and expresses EBV DNA. EBV is the aetiological agent of infectious **mononucleosis** and is associated with **Burkitt's lymphoma** and nasopharyngeal sarcoma.

Burkitt's lymphoma is a malignant neoplasm of B lymphocytes (tumour of jaw) which occurs mainly in children and young adults in Africa and New Guinea. This disease occurs in endemic or sporadic form, but endemic form is more common. All cells of Burkitt's lymphoma and nasopharyngeal carcinoma carry multiple copies of EBV genome and express the antigen EBV NA. The aetiological role of the virus is strongly suggestive in the two malignancies.

Infectious mononucleosis (Glandular fever)

EBV causes infectious mononucleosis which is a self-limiting disease in children and young adults; it is characterised by fever, an increased number of monocytes, and large lymphocytes in the blood, enlarged lymph nodes and spleen. Its incubation period is 4 to 7 weeks. The transmission may occur by kissing (kissing disease) and by respiratory tract. The virus can be recovered from saliva and throat washings. An associated subclinical hepatitis is detected in mononucleosis.

EBV activates B lymphocytes to produce immunoglobulin. The virus is a potent polyclonal activation of antibody production by B cells. Ig M producing B lymphocytes predominate. However, other immunoglobulins (Ig G 3, Ig A, Ig D) are also produced.

Diagnosis

Blood count. Total leucocyte count ranges from 10,000 to 90,000 cu mm, with a predominance of abnormal lymphocytes—B cells.

Serological tests

(a) **Paul-Bunnell test.** The heterophilic antibody agglutinating sheep erythrocytes can be removed by absorption with OX erythrocytes. Paul-Bunnel test makes use of this differential absorption and haemagglutination test with sheep erythrocytes.

(b) **Virus specific serological test.** Indirect immuno-fluorescence test can detect the specific serum antibody.

Table 58.3. CMV infection

Group	Mode of infection	Manifestation
Congenital	Transplacental	Hepato-splenomegaly, jaundice, haemolytic anaemia, mirocephaly mental abnormalities
Children	Post-Immuno suppression	Insidious hepatitis, pneumonitis
Reactivation	Post-Immuno suppression	Hepatitis, intestinal pneumonia
Post-perfusion syndrome	Repeated transfusion	Fever, Infectious mono-nucleosis-like blood picture

59
Adeno Viruses

These viruses were first detected by Rowe et al (1953) in human adenoid tissue (**adeno,** from adenoid) and are non-enveloped DNA viruses of medium size.

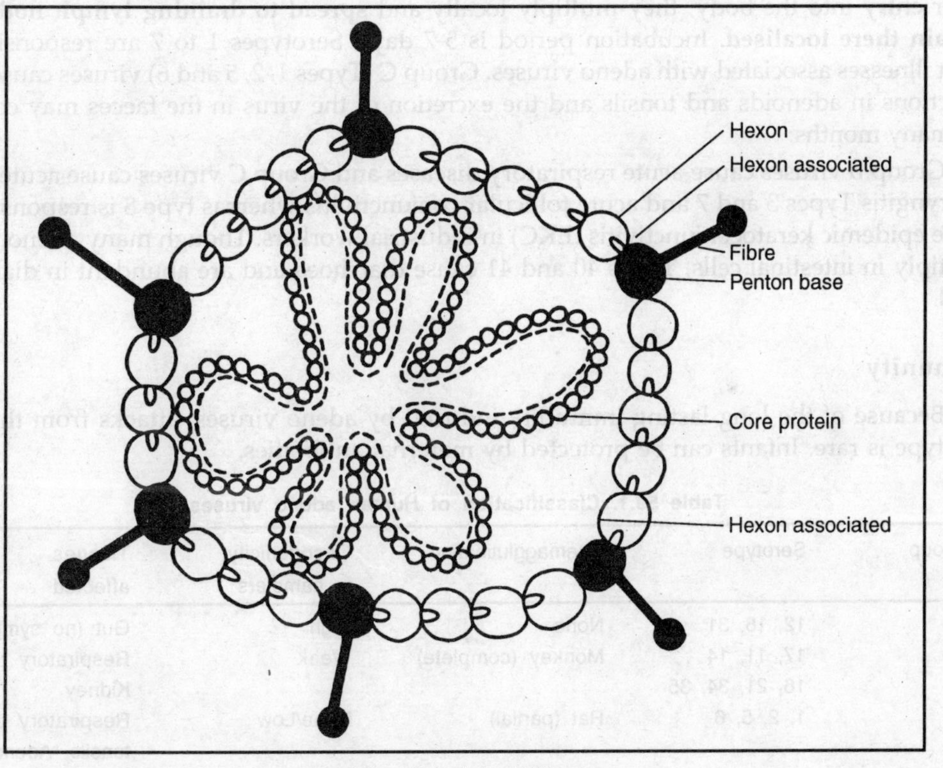

Fig. 59.1: Adeno Virus

Virology

Adeno viruses are 70-90 nm in diameter with an icosahedral capsid which encloses a double stranded DNA in association with polypeptides. The capsid is made of 252 capsomeres arranged as an icosahedron with 20 triangular facets and 12 vertices. The capsid consists of 240 **hexons** and 12 **pentons** and a thread-like structure projects from each of the 12 vertices for red cell.

Each of the 12 capsomers at the vertices is surrounded by 5 others and are called **pentons,** whereas the **hexons** are surrounded by 6 neighbours (capsomer).

Classification

Adeno viruses are grouped into two genera : (1) **Aviadeno viruses** (adeno viruses of birds) and **Mastadeno viruses** (adeno viruses of mammals).

Human adeno viruses are divided into 6 subgenera – A to F, on the basis of haemagglutination and oncogenic potential. There are about 47 known human adeno virus serotypes. They share a common complement fixing antigen.

Pathogenesis

Adeno viruses cause infection of the respiratory, gastrointestinal, urinary tract and eyes. After entry into the body, they multiply locally and **spread to draining lymph nodes and remain there localised.** Incubation period is 5-7 days. Serotypes 1 to 7 are responsible for most illnesses associated with adeno viruses. Group C (Types 1, 2, 5 and 6) viruses cause latent infections in adenoids and tonsils and the excretion of the virus in the faeces may continue for many months.

Group B viruses cause acute respiratory diseases and Group C viruses cause acute febrile pharyngitis Types 3 and 7 and acute follicular conjunctivitis whereas type 8 is responsible for acute epidemic keratoconjunctivitis (EKC) in industrial workers. Though many adeno viruses multiply in intestinal cells, Types 40 and 41 cause diarrhoea and are abundant in diarrhoeal stool.

Immunity

Because of the long lasting immunity induced by adeno viruses, attacks from the same serotype is rare. Infants can be protected by maternal antibodies.

Table 59.1. Classification of Human adeno viruses

Group	Serotype	Haemagglutination	Oncogenicity in hamsters	Tissues affected
A	12, 18, 31	None	High	Gut (no symptom)
B	17, 11, 14 16, 21, 34, 35	Monkey (complete)	Weak	Respiratory tract Kidney
C	1, 2, 5, 6	Rat (partial)	None/Low	Respiratory tract tonsils, Adenoids
D	8, 9, 10, 13 15, 17, 19 20, 22, 30 33, 36, 39 42, 47	Rat (complete)	None transform cells	Conjunctivitis Respiratory tract Gut
E	4	Rat (partial)	None/Low Respiratory tract	Conjunctiva
F	40, 41	None	None	Gut

Table 59.2. Association of Adeno viruses in diseases

Serotypes	Diseases	Individuals at risk
1, 2, 3, 4, 5, 6, 7	Acute febrile Pharyngitis	Infants, young children
3, 7	Pharyngoconjunctival fever	Older children
4, 7, 14, 21	Acute respiratory disease	Adults
1, 2, 3, 7	Pneumonia	Infants
3, 4, 11	Follicular conjunctivitis	Any age
8, 19, 37	Epidemic keratoconjunctivitis	Adults
11, 21	Haemorrhagic cystitis	Infants, young children
40, 41	Diarrhoea, vomiting	Infants, young children
1, 2, 5	Intussusception	Infants
5, 34, 35 43, 47	Disseminated infection	AIDS, renal, heart, lung, bone marrow, transplant recipients

Laboratory diagnosis

(1) **Isolation of virus.** By tissue culture in human epithelial cell lines i.e. HeLa, Hep 2 or KB, adeno virus can be isolated from throat, conjunctiva or stool. The cytopathic effects (CPE) are rounding, and grape-like clusters of swollen cells after 10-28 days of incubation. Fluorescence antibody CF and haemagglutination tests can identify the virus.

(2) **Serological tests.** Rising titre of CF antibodies can be seen in paired sera. Neutralisation (N+), Haemagglutination (HI) tests can be carried out for specific identification.

Epidemiology

Transmission of adeno virus infection from man to man is via respiratory and alimentary route, whereas eye infection is by hand to eye transfer. Adeno virus can be transmitted to the recipient from donor by bone marrow transplantation.

60
Orthomyxo Viruses

Orthomyxo Viruses (*Ortho*, free; *Myxo* mucus) are so called because they have affinity for mucins. They are spherical or filamentous with single stranded segmented RNA genome.

A single genus, **Influenza virus,** with three immunological types, designated A, B and C. These viruses have a unique antigenic variation occurring continuously within type A; in type B it is lesser, but in type C it is stable. They cause influenza, an acute respiratory illness. Animals (pigs, horses, birds) are also infected by Influenza virus type A strains.

The term myxo virus was at first proposed for a large group of enveloped RNA viruses which get attached to cell surface receptors of RBC and have affinity to mucin. They are now separated into two distinct families—**Orthomyxovirus** and **Paramyxovirus**—because of their difference in replication pattern, structures and other properties.

Influenza virus

Smith et al (1933) first isolated **influenza** type A from throat washing of a patient and in 1940 Type B virus was isolated along with type A in cell culture; **Influenza virus** type C, the third serotype, was isolated by Taylor (1949).

Morphology

Types A and B are morphologically identical but Type C differs from them in some aspects. They are pleomorphic :

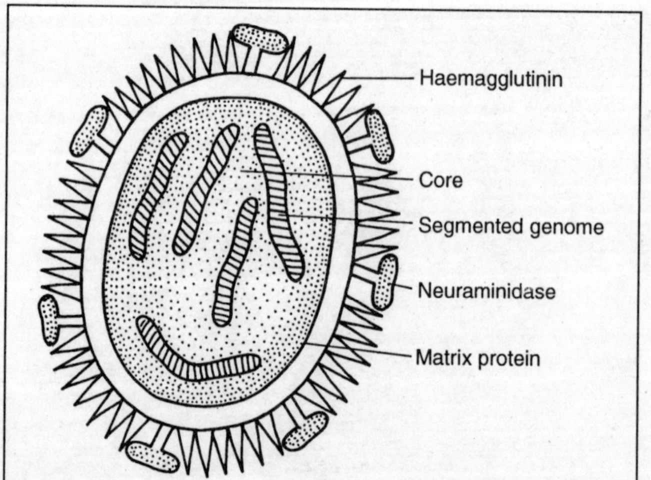

Fig. 60.1: Influenza virus

1. **Spherical particle :** diameter 80-100 nm.
2. **A lipid envelope** derived from the host cell membrane separates the spikes from the inner core.
3. Attached to lipid layer of the envelope are densely arranged radial projections of two types of peplomers-haemagglutinin (HA) spikes and neuraminidase (NA)-mushroom shaped. Distal tip of HA contains sites for binding to host cell.
4. Single stranded RNA genome is segmented.

Table 60.1. Classification of Orthomyxo, Paramyxo Viruses

Family	Genus (Types)	Species (sub types)
Orthomyxo virus	Influenza virus A	H_1, N_1 (A, human, H_s W N_1) H_2 N_2 (A_2) H_3 N_2 (A_3, A Hongkong)
	Influenza virus B	B (human)
	Influenza virus C	C (human)
Paramyxo virus	Paramyxo virus	Para influenza 1-4 Mumps, Newcastle disease (NDV), Simian (SV_5), para influenza
	Morbilli virus	Measles, Rinderpest, Canine Distemper
	Pneumo virus	Respiratory syncytial

Table 60.2. Differential characteristics of Orthomyxo and Paramyxo Viruses

Property	Orthomyxo virus	Paramyxo virus
Size	80-120 nm	100-300 nm
Shape	Spherical filamentous	Pleomorphic
Genome	Single stranded RNA in 8 species	Single stranded RNA in single species
Inner RNA (protein helix)	9 nm diam.	18 nm diam.
Site of ribonucleo-protein synthesis	Nucleus	Cytoplasm
Genetic reassort-ment (recombination)	Common	Absent
DNA dependent RNA synthesis	Necessary for multiplication	Not required
Rate of antigenic change	High	Low
Haemolysin	Absent	Present

Antigenic Classification

Influenza virus possesses four antigens (structural proteins) : (1) the internal or nucleo-capsid (nucleo-protein-NP) is closely associated with ss-RNA protein core); (2) matrix protein of the viral envelope (M); and (3) two surface glycoproteins (HA, haemagglutinin; NA, neuroaminidase). Three polymerase polypeptides, PA, PB and PB_2 are also present.

Influenza viruses are divided into three types—A, B, C—on the basis of antigenic structure differences of NP and M proteins.

Again, the types are divided into subtypes on the basis of antigenic variation of HA and NA. Till now, 15 types of HA (H1-H13) and 9 types of NA (N1-N9) in different combination have been isolated from influenza viruses of birds, animals or humans. Human viruses have 3 HA (H_1, H_2, H_3) and 2 NA (N_1, N_2) types. Type A human virus has 2 main subtypes; A_1 (H_1 N_1) and A_2 (H_2 N_2).

Non-human influenza viruses belong to type A whereas human influenza viruses belong to type A, B and C.

Non-human viruses do not infect man but play an important role in the emergence of pandemic influenza by genetic reassortment with human viruses.

Nomenclature system of influenza virus : type/host origin/strain number/year of isolation and subtypes of HA and NA in parenthesis e.g. A/Hong Kong / 03/68 (H_3 N_2).

1. Haemagglutinins

These are glycoprotein spikes on the surface of each influenza virus particle. Each virus contains 500 haemagglutinin spikes. When influenza virus is mixed with a suspension of fowl erythrocytes, the virus is adsorbed on to the **mucoprotein receptor** on the surface of red cells by its haemagglutinin spikes and also with adjacent red cells causing haemagglutination—an important property of influenza virus.

2. Neuraminidase

The enzyme neuraminidase, a glycoprotein, is present on viral surface. Neuraminidase of influenza A and B viruses hydrolyses specific glycoprotein on the cell receptor and splits off N-**acetyl muramic acid** from the receptor and causes **Haemagglutination and elution.** Due to enzymatic action of neuraminidase, (Receptor Destroying Enzyme, RDE) the virus is eluted from RBCs and remain free in the solution.

Haemagglutination action can be inhibited (HIT) by specific homologous anti-serum.

Antigenic variation

Influenza viruses show remarkable ability to undergo variation due to frequent changes in the antigenicity of HA and NA. The variation is highest in Type A and less in Type B but none in Type C. This antigenic variation is of great importance in the epidemiology of the disease.

Two antigenic variation forms are :

(1) **Antigenic rift**; and (2) **Antigenic shift**.

(1) Antigenic rift refers to **minor** antigenic changes in haemagglutinin and neuraminidase, or both, and results from mutation in the HA and NA genome.

(2) **Antigenic shift** is **major** antigenic changes in NA and HA and results in emergence of new subtype.

Pathogenesis

The portal of entry of influenza virus is respiratory tract. Ciliated cells of respiratory tract are mainly susceptible, because its mucous membrane contains the specific mucoprotein receptors, for influenza virus. After entry they encounter respiratory secretions with mucoprotein. Viral neuraminidase lowers viscosity of the mucus. Then a large number of cells are infected and killed.

Clinical features

Usually the incubation period is 1 to 4 days; subclinical infection are common. Influenza is an acute respiratory illness and clinical manifestations vary from a mild coryza to fulminating pneumonia.

During acute illness, due to necrosis of virally infected cells, there is extensive desquamation of respiratory epithelium.

Influenza is characterised by fever, chills, headache, dry cough, and generalised myalgia. Fever lasts for about 3 days and respiratory symptoms last for 3 to 4 days. An uncomplicated case usually resolves within 7 days. It is self-limiting disease secondary bacterial pneumonia due to staphylococcus aureus and Haemophilus **influenzae** is usually observed in 10% cases.

Laboratory Diagnosis

Very frequently Influenza is diagnosed clinically:

1. **Isolation of virus :** Nasal and throat washings or secretion (within 3 days of illness) are inoculated into amniotic sac of 11-13 days old chick embryo or on monolayers of monkey kidney tissue culture.
2. **Immuno-fluorescence** can detect the viral antigen. ELISA and RIA have also been developed to detect viral antigen.
3. **Serology : Haemagglutination inhibition test** (HI) is a convenient and widely used technique for identification of the strain of the virus. CFT is sensitive.
4. **Antigens :** Immuno-fluorescence, ELISA, RIA have been developed to detect influenza antigens in the clinical material.

Immunity

An attack of influenza produces active immunity against the strain. Local secretion of Ig A plays the dominant role. The short duration of immunity is due to antigenic variation of influenza virus.

Epidemiology

Its patterns are variable in three types of influenza virus. Type A causes severe and wide spread epidemics; B causes sporadic and sometimes epidemics, but C does not cause epidemics, but does cause inapparent infections.

Epidemics and pandemics of influenza is associated with **antigenic shift** which is exhibited by only Type A virus. Periodical epidemics can be caused by antigenic drift also, which is exhibited by all three types. Type B, and C are confined to humans, while Type A viruses circulate in ecosystem (birds, swine, horses). These animal viruses infect man.

Since antiquity epidemics occurred at regular intervals. Influenza epidemic starts abruptly, spreads rapidly and often distributed worldwide.

Prophylaxis

Artificial immunisation is the primary means of prevention of influenza. Its efficiency is about 80%. Vaccine is prepared by incorporating the circulating latest strains of Type A and B virus specified by WHO.

Composition of vaccine

Types A and B viruses, grown in allantoic cavity of chick embryos, are inactivated by formalin or betapropiolactone. This vaccine administrated is in a single dose but requires to be repeated each winter.

Indication

Vaccine is administrated in cold countries to protect elderly people with pre-existing cardiovascular or renal disease. Side effects are few and mild, but few cases of polyneuritis are reported.

Chemo-prophylaxis with antiviral **amantadine and rimantadine** inhibits absorption of all influenza A viruses, but it is without any effect on B viruses.

Table 60.3. Prevalence of antigenic subtypes of influenza virus type A in Man, 1918-1990

Antigenic structure	Period of prevalence	Type of antigenic variation	Possible mechanism of origin
H1 N1	1918	Shift	Not known
	1918-57	Progressive antigenic drift	
	1957	Shift	Genetic recombination between human H1 N1 and A virus of unknown source (H2 N2)
H2 N2	1957-68	Progressive antigenic drift	
H3 N2	1965	Shift	Genetic recombination between H2 N2 and influenza virus A of unknown origin (H2 N2)
H2 N2	1957-68	Progressive antigenic drift	
H3 N2	1965	Shift	Genetic recombination between H2 N2 and influenza virus A of unknown origin (H3N2)
	1968-90	Progressive antigenic drift	
H1 N1	1976	Reappearance of swine H1 N1	Swine virus 1918 pandemic strain
H1 N1	1977	Reappearance of 1950 H1 N1 virus	1950 H1 N1 virus maintained by unknown mechanism
	1977-78	Progressive antigenic drift	
	1989	Reappearance of H1N1 virus	Swine virus related to 1950 pandemic
	2009-2010 (Pandemic H1N1/09)	Antigenic shift	Quadraple genetic reassortment of two swine strains, one avian strain of influenza

Avian Influenza (Bird Flu)-H5 N1 Virus

Avian Influenza is normally known as bird flu affecting human with influenza striking the lungs.

Malik Peiris, a top microbiologist in Hong Kong, battled the bird flu virus since 1997 when it made its first known jump to humans in Hong Kong and killed six people.

After interaction of bird flu from wild birds to poultry it was not a major risk, but it becomes endemic—that is a big problem.

Once the virus multiple in poultry, there is a golden opportunity for continued interaction with human population. WHO reported 20 cases contracted bird flu virus, directed from poultry, which caused 50% mortality in humans. The virulent strain H5N1 of bird flu has been isolated from migratory bird in Canada. It was also reported from Iraq, China, Turkey. Gujarat (India) got the first suspected case of bird flu who later died (human death) in February 16,

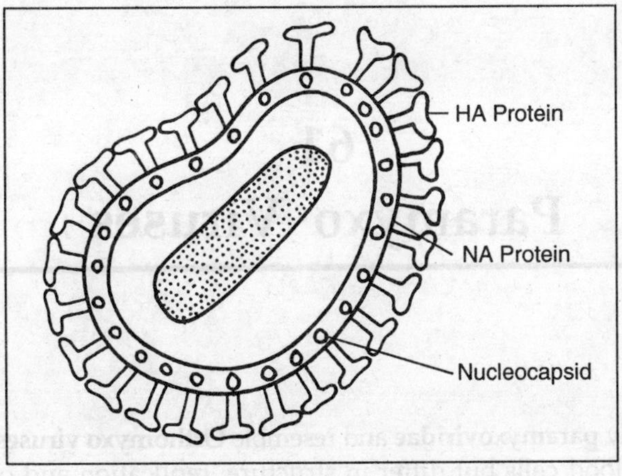

Fig. 60.2: Avian Influenza Virus (H5N1)

2006, when 27 year old poultry farmer from Navapur of neighbouring Maharashtra State died in Surat Hospital (Gujarat). It was confirmed that it was due to Avian Flu virus.

India has become the first country in South Asia to report H5N1 virus, a deadly bird flu virus strains—after 36,000 birds died in Maharashtra (India). It was also reported by high security Laboratory, Bhopal (Madhya Pradesh) India, where samples (blood, stool) were tested and confirmed eight birds and diagnosed the H5N1 virus on February 18, 2006.

Prophylaxis : A prophylactic dose of Tamiflu was given to those who are undertaking the culling of birds. This drug has side effects.

Swine Flu (H1N1 rivus)

This novel Influenza 2009A/H1N1 virus contains a combination of 2 swine, one avian and one human influenza virus genes.

Initially recognised in Mexico, swine flu or H1N1 influenza was declared as a pandemic by WHO on June 11, 2009. The virus had killed more than 19,633 people worldwide, whereas 1,632,258 laboratory confirmed cases were reported. The global infection rate was 11-21% and case fatality ratio was 0.03%. Number of cases steeply declined since May 2010 and on 10th August, 2010 WHO announced the end of H1N1 pandemic.

India had reported a widespread, low intensity epidemic with 29,599 confirmed cases and 2024 deaths. Cases occurred mainly in Maharashtra, Kerala, Karnataka, Andhra Pradesh and Delhi.

61
Paramyxo Viruses

They belong to the family **paramyxoviridae** and resemble **Orthomyxo viruses** in morphology and haemagglutinate red blood cells but differ in structure, replication and other properties.

Properties

They are spherical enveloped particles (100-300 nm diameter, giant form 800 nm diameter). They contain single stranded RNA genome and haemagglutinin in envelope and are sensitive to lipid solvent.

Classification

The family **Paramyxoviridae** consists of three genera and infects man and animals:

1. **Paramyxo virus** : Para influenza, Mumps, Newcastle disease (NCD) virus, Simian virus 5 (SV5) contain both haemagglutinin and neuraminadase.
2. **Morbilli virus : Measles virus, Canine distemper virus, Rinderpest virus,** possess haemagglutinin and no neuraminadase.
3. **Pneumovirus** : Respiratory syncytial **virus** (RSV), **Pneumonia virus of mice** (PVM) and **Turkey rhinotracheitis** virus have neither haemagglutinin nor neuraminadase.

Differentiation of the genera : The nucleocapsid of all paramyxo viruses is 18 nm in diameter except **pneumo virus** (14 nm in diam.). The spikes (peplomers) of **Pneumo virus** are longer than those of other paramyxo viruses.

Table 61.1. Properties of human paramyxo viruses

Properties	Para influenza	Mumps	Measles	RSV
Serotypes	4	1	1	1
Haemagglutinin*	+	+	+	–
Haemadsorption	+	+	+	–
Haemolysin	+	+	+	–
Neuraminadase	+	+	+	–
Inclusion	C	C	n, C	C

* Chicken and guinea pig red cells; C = cytoplasm; n = nucleus

Paromyxo Viruses

The envelope surface of paramyxo viruses is of lipoprotein membrane and is covered by projections of 12-14 nm × 2-4 nm. These projections are of two types : HN (haemagglutinin and neuraminidase) and F (fusion of protein) and glycoproteins. Here HN projection of paramyxoviruses have both haemagglutinin and neuraminidase functions, but in myxo viruses separate projections carry each function.

Cultivation : Primary isolation is done in human and monkey kidney cell and in amniotic cavity of chick embryo. Cytopathic effects (CPE) are formation of large syncytia containing eosinophilic cytoplasmic inclusion bodies; viruses are identified by haemadsorption of fowl or guinea pig red cells.

Replication

Paramyxo viruses attach via the haemagglutinin glycoprotein (HN or H protein) to the sialic acid containing receptors on the host cells. The virus penetrates the cell by means of fusion of viral and cell membrane which is mediated by **Fo glycoprotein. Fo glycoprotein** becomes activated when it is cleaved into two subunits F_1 and F_2. If Fo protein fails to cleave, the virus will attach but will not fuse with the host cell membrane and the viral genome cannot penetrate the cell.

The viral RNA polymerase transcribes m RNA in the cell cytoplasm; then viral components are synthesised in the cytoplasm. The surface HN and F proteins are incorporated in the membrane forming envelope. The enveloped virus buds out of the cell into the exterior.

Activated fusion protein (Fo) causes fusion of adjacent cell membrane of host cells producing syncytium (multinucleated giant cells).

Para Influenza virus

These viruses have four antigenitically distinct serotypes—types 1, 2, 3 and 4—of which only the first three are associated with severe respiratory disease.

Pathogenesis and clinical features

Incubation period of is 2-6 days. These viruses are widespread, cause common cold with sore throat in all ages, severe respiratory tract disease in infant and children (laryngo tracheo bronchitis—especially by types 1 and 2) and group (6-9%). The group is characterised by a harsh brassy cough in children due to respiratory obstruction as a result of swelling of larynx and related structures. The infection may further spread down causing pneumonia and bronchiolitis if it is due to type 3.

The transmission is by droplet aerosols or by direct person-to-person contact. Infection may produce both antibody and cell mediated immunity which may cause termination of illness with complete recovery in 10-14 days.

Immunity

Reinfection may occur in children; clinical picture of common cold may be modified by preexisting antibodies.

Laboratory Diagnosis

1. **Isolation :** Throat swabs and mouth washings can be inoculated in monkey kidney tissue culture, CPF is minimal in tissue culture. Virus in infected tissue culture cells is identified by haemadsorption with guinea pig's red cells. Typing is done by inhibition of haemadsorption by type specific antisera before adding the guinea pig red cells.

2. **Direct demonstration :** Viral antigen can be demonstrated in exfoliated respiratory cells with mixture of monoclonal antiviral antibodies of 4 types of virus by immuno-fluorescence or ELISA.
3. **Serology :** Rising antibody titre can be detected by ELISA or CFT.

Mumps virus

The term mumps is derived from the mumbling speech of patients incubalio.

Pathogenesis and clinical features

Mumps (epidemic parotitis) of childhood is transmitted from direct contact with infected saliva or aerosols from infected patients. The incubation period is 16-18 days. First the virus multiplies in epithelial cells of nasal or upper respiratory tract and spreads by viraemia to the salivary glands, testes, ovaries, pancreas, kidney and brain. In about 95% cases, non-suppurative inflammation of the parotid glands (salivary adenitis) is a characteristic feature.

Six days before the onset of clinical parotitis, the virus is shed in saliva. Children of 5-10 years of age are commonly affected. The infection is more severe in adults. Salivary-adenitis is often associated with low grade fever and subsides in one week with complete recovery.

Complications

1. **Meningitis** and **meningoencephalitis** occur in mumps which resolve without sequelae.
2. **Orchitis** in males and **oophoritis** in females, **polyarthritis, pancreatitis, nephritis** are other complications. Orchitis and oophoritis usually develop with the resolution of parotitis.

Laboratory Diagnosis

1. **Direct demonstration of virus** by immuno-fluorescence in throat secretion and saliva.
2. **Isolation** of virus can be done by inoculating secretion in monkey kidney or HEp-2 cell cultures. Growth of virus is identified by haemadsorption.
3. **Serological tests** indicate rise in antibody titre by CFT using soluble (S) and viral (V) antigens.

Immunity is permanent after a single infection.

Epidemiology. It is a contagious disease but less than measles and chicken pox. Mumps is an endemic disease with worldwide distribution affecting only man.

Control

An attenuated mumps virus vaccine prepared after growing in chick embryo cell culture is available and gives protection. This vaccine contains Jeryl Lynn or Urabe strains and is available in monovalent form (mumps only) or in combination with measles and rubella (MMR) live virus vaccine.

Respiratory Syncytial virus

Respiratory Syncytial virus (RSV) has no haemagglutinin and neuraminidase, but it contains a G glycoprotein (receptor for cell component) and a F (fusion) protein that induces fusion of neighbouring cells into large mononucleated **syncytia,** from which the virus gets its name.

Pathogenesis and Clinical features

The RSV is shed for 1-3 weeks. It is transmitted by large droplets or by contact with contaminated hands and surfaces and so nosocomial infection does take place in nurseries and paediatric wards. The virus multiplies in epithelial cells of nasopharynx, then spreads down into lower respiratory tract via secretions:

1. RSV causes **bronchiolitis** (60%), pneumonitis (30%) in infants of 1-6 months of age when the maternal antibody levels are decreasing.
2. It causes **asymptomatic** or **febrile rhinitis** or common cold in older children or adults.

Immunity

Secretory Ig A in nasal secretion protects against reinfection, whereas CMI is responsible for recovery from infection. RSV has antigenically only one type; monoclonal antibodies studies show 2 subtypes—A and B. Subtype A is more virulent than B.

Laboratory Diagnosis

1. **Isolation** : RSV is fragile, hence specimens should not be frozen. In acute phase of illness virus can be isolated by inoculating nasal and pharygngeal specimens/secretions in human (HeLa, Hep-2) or monkey kidney cell culture which will yield the growth of giant cells and syncytia.
2. **Direct demonstration** of virus can be done by immuno-fluorescence test in less than an hour.
3. **Serology** : Since there is no detectable antibody titre in serum, serology is not of much use. However, CFT and NT may detect rising antibody titre.

Epidemiology and control

RSV is ubiquitous and causes a winter epidemic in infants and children of one year of age. Formalin **inactivated** crude whole virus vaccine and **live** vaccine (cold adapted, temperature sensitive) have not been found satisfactory. Preparation of vaccine with purified F and G surface glycoprotein is in progress.

Measles (Rubeola) Virus

Measles is the most common cause of childhood fevers and is highly infectious in nature.

Description

Measles virus is antigenically related to canine distemper virus (CDV) in dog and rinderpest virus in cattle. Spikes on envelope contain only haemagglutinin but not neuraminidase. Besides, Matrix M protein is located below the envelope lipid bilayer and F protein is also a projection (spike).

Pathogenesis

Inhalation is the mode of entry. The incubation period is 9-12 days. The virus multiplies in lymphoid tissues of respiratory tract and invades the blood circulation (**primary viraemia**) and localises in the reticulo-endothelial system. Secondary viraemia is characterised by flu-like high fever, cough, conjunctivitis. **Koplik's spots** (red spots with a bluish white centre on the buccal mucosa) appear in the prodromal phase. After secondary viraemia the virus settles in epithelial surfaces of skin, respiratory tract and conjunctiva. As the acute symptoms decline in 1-2 days maculopapular rash appears on skin, mucous membrane and conjunctiva. Rash is due to interaction of immune T cells with virus infected cells in small blood vessels. The rash fades out in a week. Immuno-competent patients recover in 10-14 days.

Complication

1. **Giant cell pneumonia, otitis media, post-measles encephalitis** may occur in smaller number.
2. Mortality is high in malnourished and immuno-compromised children.
3. Sub-acute sclerosing panencephalitis (SSPE) is a complication of measles and is considered to be a slow form of measles virus encephalitis due to a defective form of measles virus in infected cell. Patient's condition deteriotrates over several years and finally develop CNS symptoms.

Immunity

There is only one serotype of measles virus and an infection confers lifelong immunity.

Laboratory Diagnosis

1. Direct smear stained by Giemsa's stain show giant cells and inclusion bodies (Cowdry type A). Immuno-fluorescence test can detect virus particles in exfoliated respiratory cells.
2. **Isolation :** Specimens collected during febrile period can be used to cultivate in human fibroblasts, monkey or human kidney cells. Growth is slow with CPE.

Serology : H1, CF and NI tests can detect measles-specific Ig M antibody.

Epidemiology

The disease is endemic throughout the world and epidemics occur in **late** winter and early spring. Man is the only natural host of measles and monkeys acquire the infection from man. Transmission is through respiratory route, conjunctivitis may be the source.

Control

1. **Active immunisation :** Live vaccine in use is 90% effective. It is administrated in one dose subcutaneously.
2. **Passive immunisation :** Pooled sera containing antibody against measles virus confer passive immunity to infants.

Rubella (German Measles)

Rubella or German measles virus is a sole member of the Rubi virus genus under **To gaviridae** family. It is discussed with **Paramyxo virus** as it forms **rash** of German measles similar to measly rash. Rubella is a mild childhood fever characterised by transient macular rash and posterior circular and suboccipital lymphadenopathy. Exposure of the foetus in early (first trimester) pregnancy to rubella infection may result into congenital malformation. Rubella may be acquired congenitally or post-natally.

Virology

1. Rubella virus is pleomorphic, 50-70 nm, enveloped, RNA virus.
2. It agglutinates goose, pigeon, day-old chick & human RBC at 4°C.
3. It grows in rabbit kidney cell line-RK 13 and in embryonated duck egg.

Pathogenesis and clinical features

A. **Post-natal rubella :** Infection is acquired through mucosa of upper respiratory tract. The virus replicates locally, followed by multiplication in the cervical lymph nodes, after an incubation period of 2 to 3 weeks.

Viraemia occurs with fever. These viruses are disseminated in the target organs with the formation of rash suggesting an immunological reaction.

Macular rash appears on the face, then trunk and legs and lasts for less than 3 days. Infection in children is asymptomatic and common in children than in adults. Transient arthralgia and arthritis occur in about 60% women but uncommon in children.

Post-infectious encephalomyelitis, thrombocytopenic purpura are rare complications.

B. **Congenital rubella :** During viraemia, rubella virus crosses the placental barrier and replicates in the differentiating cells of the embryo and infects a limited number of cells in affected organs. The foetal cells are not destroyed by the virus. In the first trimester of pregnancy, the risk is common (50-70%), followed by second trimester (20%), and only 4% in 7th month of pregnancy.

Abnormalities of eyes (cataract); **ears** and **heart** are the classical rubella syndrome.

Diagnosis : A. Post-natal rubella

1. **Isolation :** Virus in blood or throat swabs can be grown in various tissue culture cell lines of monkey or rabbit kidney. CPE is not inconspicious.
2. **Serology :** ELISA is the method of choice to detect rubella specific Ig G or Ig M.

B. **Congenital rubella**

1. **Isolation of virus** can be done from the pharyngeal secretion or urine for first 4 months of life.
2. **Serology :** Demonstration of rubella-specific Ig M is diagnostic of intra-uterine infection.

Epidemiology

Rubella is worldwide in distribution and is endemic in all countries when the vaccination is not successful. Epidemics occur every 5-6 years in spring and are transmitted by respiratory route. Inapparent maternal infection can cause foetal anomalies. Congenitally infected infants can transmit the infection to others.

Immunity

One attack of rubella confers life-long immunity; immune mother can transmit antibodies to breast fed infants for 4-6 months.

Control

Since 1989, a combined measles-mumps-rubella (MMR) vaccine has been advocated. This vaccine is given in two doses. Pregnant women are not vaccinated.

62
Arbo Viruses

The arthropod viruses or **Arbo viruses** are a group of RNA viruses of diverse physical and chemical properties, that are transmitted by blood sucking arthropod from one vertebrate host to another. The viruses multiply in arthropods without producing disease vectors acquire life-long infection.

The Rodent-borne (robo) viruses are maintained in nature by direct transmission from rodent to rodent by contact of body fluids or excretions of infected rodents. It is not transmitted by Arthropods.

Robo viruses consist of the arena viruses of the family **Arena viridae** (Zoonotic in rodents).

Classification

Arbo viruses were designated according to the disease with which they are associated e.g. Yellow fever, Rift valley fever, Chikungunya and Kyasanur Forest disease. Sometimes they were named after the geographic area e.g. St. Louis encephalitis and West Nile fever. They contain about 450 viruses and infect man, mammal, bird, snake. They include five families : **Togaviridae, Flaviviridae, Bunyaviridae, Reoviridae, Rhabdoviridae. Togaviruses** of medical importance are **Alpha virus** and **Rubi virus.**

General properties

1. Arbo viruses cause fatal encephalitis within 1 to 10 days after the intra-cerebral inoculation in 48 hour old suckling mice.
2. They have haemagglutinin for erythrocyte of newly hatched chicks and geese.
3. They multiply in continuous polypoid tissue culture at 37°C, but dengue and Ross River viruses multiply in continuous tissue cultures of **Aedes albopictus** mosquito cells.
4. Mosquito borne arbo viruses multiply in **Aedes** and **Culex** mosquitoes after blood sucking infected individuals.
5. Tick borne arbo viruses multiply in Ioxodid ticks.

Replication

The replication of arbo viruses differ from each other significantly. This feature is considered for their classification.

Alpha viruses

They attach to the receptors of host cells by means of E_1 and E_2 glycoproteins of envelope and by endocytosis they enter into host cells. The single stranded RNA genome may act as messenger molecule release of virus occurs by budding from cell membrane.

Flavi viruses

They are similar to alpha viruses in many respects, but they differ by the composition of envelope glycoprotein and RNA.

Buniya viruses

They are larger than alpha and flavi viruses and their nucleic acid genome contains three molecules (M, S and L strands) of circular single stranded RNA. The virus contains an RNA polymerase to initiate the transcription.

Table 62.1. Properties of Arbo Viruses

Properties	Alpha virus	Flavi virus	Buniya virus	RNA code virus	Reo virus
Symmetry	Cubic	Cubic	Helical	Bullet shaped	Cubic
Size (diam. in nm)	60-65	40-50	90-100	179×100	60-80
Nucleic acid	+ ss RNA	+ ss RNA	– ss RNA	– ss RNA	ds RNA
MW ($\times 10^6$)	4.2-4.4	4.2-4.4	0.45.0	3.5-4.6	0.2-0.3
No molecules	1	1	3	1	10-12
No serotypes	29	69	251	50	74
Inactivated by diethyl ether Sodium deoxy-cholate	+	+	+	+	–

Toga viridae

The name **Toga viridae** is derived from Latin ***toga,*** cloak, a reference to the envelope contained by the virus, and this family contains mainly alpha viruses.

Virology

Toga viruses are spherical, enveloped and contain single stranded RNA in a core having cubic symmetry. **Alpha viruses** and **pesti-viruses** (60-70 nm diam.) are larger than Flavi viruses (30-50 nm diam.).

Pathogenesis

Virus enters the body through the skin when infected insect vectors suck the blood. It multiplies in local lymph node and invades the blood into **target organs** (CNS in encephalitis, capillary endothelium in haemorrhagic fever, and liver in yellow fever).

Clinical features

Incubation period is 4-21 days. The infection is characterised by sudden onset with headache, nausea, vomiting, bodyache, sometimes arthralgia. Subclinical infections are common; they may be severe. Table 62.3 shows the common arbo virus diseases in India.

Table 62.2. Important Arbo viruses

Family Genus	Disease Category Encephalitis	Febrile illness	Haemorrhage fever
(I) **Togaviridae**			
(a) Alpha virus	1. Western equine encephalitis	4. Chikungunya fever	Chikungunya fever
(Mosquito borne)	2. Eastern equine encephalitis	5. Ross river fever 6. Senliki fever	
	3. Venezuela encephalitis	7. Sindbis Rubella	
(b) Rubi virus (not known arthropod vector)			
(II) **Flaviviridae** **Flavi virus**			
(i) Mosquito borne	1. St. Louis encephalitis 2. Japanese B encephalitis 3. Murrary valley encephalitis	4. Dengue 5. West Nile fever	Dengue 6. Yellow fever
(ii) (Tick borne)	1. Tick borne encephalitis		2. Kyasanur Forest Disease
(III) **Bunya viridae**			
(a) Bunya virus (mosquito borne)	California encephalitis	1. Sand fly fever	
(b) Phlebo virus (Phlebo tomus or mosquito bite		2. Rift valley fever	
(Tick borne)			Nairobi sheep disease
(d) Uniku virus (Zoonotic)			Korean haemorrhagic fever
(IV) Reoviridae oris virus (Tick borne)		Colorado tick fever	
(V) Rhabdo viridae vesiculo virus (Mosquito borne, sand fly-borne)		1. Vesicular stomatitis 2. Chandipura virus	

Table 62.3. Incidence of Arbo viruses in India

Virus	Reservoir	Vector	Disease	Location
Toga virus	Not known	Mosquito	Chikungunya fever	India, Asia, Africa
Chikungunya	Monkeys			
Sindbis	–	Mosquito	Sindbis fever	Philippines, Australia, India
Flavi virus				
Dengue	Monkeys, Man	Mosquito **(Aedes aegypti)**	Dengue, haemorrhagic fever	India, Far East, Carribean Islands
Japanese B. Encephalitis	Wild birds Pigs	Mosquito (Culex tritaeniorhynchus)	Encephalitis	Japan, India, S.E. Asia
Kyasanur Forest disease	Forest birds animals	Tick **(Ixodes ricinus, Ixodes Persulcatus**	Haemorrhagic fever	India, (Karnataka)

Laboratory Diagnosis

1. Isolation of virus : The specimen of blood, CSF from acute disease is inoculated intracerebrally into suckling mice which later develop fatal encephalitis. These arbo viruses can be grown in tissue culture or in egg embryo and can be identified by **haemagglutination inhibition** test up to group. **Neutralisation test** can establish the species.

2. Serology : Rising titre of haemagglutinating and neutralising antibodies can be demonstrated in the blood after a few days of onset of illness.

Alpha viruses

Twenty five serotypes of alpha viruses are mosquito-borne:

(A) Encephalitis viruses : Western, Eastern and **Venezuelan encephalitis viruses** are three important strains producing encephalitis in horses and men. Wild birds are reservoirs of viruses that are transmitted by **Culex** and **Anopheles mosquitoes.**

(B) Viruses causing febrile illness

1. Chikungunya virus : The name is derived from the which language native word for "double up" which occurs in the disease due to severe joint pain. The term was first coined by the people of Makonde Tribe in Tanzania, Africa in their native language.

This virus produces only a viraemia phase characterised by fever, creeping joint pain and rash and is transmitted by **Aedes aegypti.**

Epidemics of chikungunya virus infection have been reported from Africa, Thailand (1958) and India (1963, Kolkata and Chennai) along East coast of India and Maharashtra, the disease was endemic till 1975.

2. Semiliki Forest virus : In 1942 this virus was first isolated in Semiliki forest of Uganda from **Aedes** mosquitoes and it is pathogenic for mice, not for man, although **neutralising** antibodies to this virus are detected in serum of African people.

3. Sindbis virus : In 1952, this virus was first recovered from **Culex** mosquitoes in Sindbis district of Egypt. Febrile illness in man was caused by this virus in Philippines, Australia and India.

Flavi viruses

Out of 60 serotypes some are **mosquito-borne,** others are tick-borne:

(A) **Mosquito-borne flavi viruses**

1. Encephalitis viruses : In this group, there are five viruses which cause encephalitis and are named after the geographical zones. **St. Louis encephalitis virus** (North and Central America); **Ilheus virus** (South and Central America); **West Nile virus** (West Nile province of Uganda), **Murray valley encephalitis virus** (Australia and New Guinea) and **Japanese B encephalitis virus.** These viruses are transmitted by **Culex** mosquitoes.

Japanese B encephalitis (JBE) Viruses

This (JBE) virus was so named to distinguish it from **Japanese A encephalitis virus** which was prevalent at that time. It was first reported in Japan in 1935; later, in South East Asia, Korea, Malaysia and India, it caused most serious illness.

Pathogenesis

This JBE virus spreads from bird to bird through **Culex tritaeniorhynchus.** Human infection occurs from **herons** (reservoir) by several species of **Culicine mosquitoes.** The disease was first recognised in Tamil Nadu in 1955 during an outbreak of encephalitis. In Tamil Nadu (India) the JBE occurs during June to October. Several outbreaks of JBE have been reported in different parts of India—Bankura and Burdwan of West Bengal, Dibrugarh in Assam, Uttar Pradesh, Goa, Karnataka.

Clinical features

JBE has a sudden onset, with fever and vomiting. After an incubation period of 1-6 days, shows signs of encephalitis—neck rigidity, convulsions, drowsiness, deepening coma, neurological signs (paralysis, tremor). All parts of CNS (basal structures of brain, cerebral cortex-spinal cord) are involved. Perivascular cuffing and mononuclear cell infiltration of meninges are common.

Acute phase lasts for about two weeks. Mortality rate is 50% in some epidemics. Convalescence may last for many weeks; paralysis (residual) persists in about 50% survivors.

Prevention

The spread of this disease can be prevented by the control of mosquitoes and taking away piggeries from the residential areas. A formalin in activated vaccine is useful for the pigs during epidemics.

2. **Yellow fever :** It is an acute febrile illness transmitted by mosquito. Rapid and extensive destruction of liver can be seen in severe cases.

Incubation period is 3-6 days and this illness occurs in two forms : **"Urban cycle"**—where man is the reservoir and **Aedes aegypti** is the vector; **Forest** or **Sylvatic cycle**—where wild monkeys act as reservoirs, forest mosquitoes as vectors.

In many countries, yellow fever is still endemic. In India, it does not exist due to strict vigilance on vaccination and quarantine of travellers from other countries (endemic areas).

Attenuated live vaccine of 17 D strain is protective against yellow fever.

3. **Dengue :** This infection is also transmitted by **Aedes** mosquito and is characterised by the sudden onset of fever, headache, pain in bone joints and muscles. Hence it is called **"break-bone fever".** Lymphadenopathy and maculopapular rash. Though endemic, is often epidemic in tropical and subtropical countries (India, South East Asia, Pacific Islands). In East Coast of India, dengue is common.

There are four serological subtypes of Dengue virus (1-4). Though Dengue and Yellow fever are antigenically related, there is no cross-immunity.

Clinical features

Clinically, the disease is manifested in two forms :

(a) **Classical dengue fever** has relatively benign course with fever, headache, pain in muscle and bones. Incubation period is 5-8 days. Rash may appear on 3rd or 4th day. Febrile illness lasts for about a week and terminates by crisis. It is rarely fatal.

(b) **Dengue haemorrhagic fever** appear to be a hyperimmune response and is seen in patients previously infected with dengue fever virus. On reinfection with a different strain of virus within a period of 2 years of first infection, antibodies formed against the first virus reacts with the second subtype forming immune complex **(virus-antibody complex).**

Initial symptoms are associated with haemorrhagic rash, thrombocytopenia and shock. The mortality rate is 5-10%.

Type 2 dengue virus is often responsible for the haemorrhagic fever. The disease is epidemic in Thailand, South East Asia and India, where dengue serotypes are present. The disease can be controlled by anti-mosquito measures. No effective vaccine is available.

(B) Tick-borne flavi viruses

1. Tick-borne encephalitis virus

Russian spring summer encephalitis (RSSE) has been reported in Central, Eastern Europe, CIS countries. The ticks are the vectors and the bats are reservoirs. Infected goats excrete the virus in the milk. Clinically, patient develops ascending paralysis and hemiparalysis with 30% mortality.

Control can be conducted

(1) by avoiding tick-bite

(2) by formalin inactivated RSSE.

Vaccine

In North USA, Canada, Powssan virus can cause **Powssan encephalitis.**

2. Tick-borne haemorrhagic fever

(a) **Kyasanur Forest Disease** (KFD) is an Indian haemorrhagic disease appeared, in 1957, in Kyasanur forest of Karnataka (India) and is caused by a virus which is antigenically related to RSSE and isolated in National Institute of Virology, Pune (India). This KFD virus affects **haemopoietic system**. Birds and small mammals are reservoirs of the virus which is transmitted by the bite of tick **(Haemaphysalis spinigera).**

Clinical features

Incubation period is 3-7 days. KFD is characterised by sudden onset of fever with headache, vomiting, myalgia, severe prostration. Massive haemorrhage in alimentary canal, chest cavity and epistaxis may occur in some cases. The fatality is about 10%.

Epidemiology

KFD virus is responsible for the natural infection in langur and bonnet monkeys; then in man in South and Western India (Shimoga district of Karnataka, Kutch and Saurashtra). A killed vaccine is found to be satisfactory in field trial.

(b) **Omsk haemorrhagic fever** has been reported in CIS countries, Rumania. The virus is related to KFD and causes clinical symptoms similar to KFD.

Bunya viridae

The name of this virus family **(Bunya-viridae)** is derived from a place Bunyamvera in Uganda of Africa from where this virus was first isolated.

Virology

They are spherical (901-00 nm) particles, replicate in cytoplasm and enveloped. They contain single stranded RNA genome which is trisegmented.

Classification

Bunya viridae	Contains four genera :
1. **Bunya virus** (Mosquito borne)	California encephalitis group virus
2. **Phlebo virus** (Phlebotomous) or mosquito borne	Sand fly fever and Rift Valley fever
3. **Nairo virus** (Tick borne)	Nairobi sheep disease
4. **Unku virus** fever	Korean haemorrhagic

California Group

1. **California encephalitis virus** was first isolated from mosquitoes in 1942 in California.
2. **la Crossie virus** was isolated in Wisconsin (USA).
3. **Chitor virus** was isolated in Chitor (India).

All three viruses are antigenically related and similar in clinical features except that **Chitoor virus** causes mild fever. Clinically, there is fever, headache and mild or severe central nervous system involvement. All infections are mosquito-borne and are more common among children. Recovery is usually complete with rare fatality.

Phlebo virus group

1. Sand fly fever (Phlebotomous fever)

It is transmitted by female sand fly **(Phlebotomous papatasi).** After an incubation period of 3-5 days, patient develops fever, malaise, headache, and nausea which lasts for 3-4 days. This infection has been reported in India, Pakistan, Central Asia and Mediterranean countries.

Sand flies breed in sand, dust and soil. **Phlebotomous virus** has two serological types: Sicily and Naples strains.

Chandipura virus

This Chandipura belongs to same family as Rabies virus. This rare virus was first found at Chandipura in Northern Maharashtra (India) in 1965—called as killer virus claiming 108 children—though it had spread in epidemic form in Andhra Pradesh killing 165 children in 2003.

The killer virus with a very high fatality rate of 60 per cent had made its appearance in Gujarat for the first time claiming lives of 16 children and affecting at least 26 others in Chota Udaipur and Kwant talukas in the year 2004. Chandipura is the name of first patient.

In view of similar symptoms found in Andhra Pradesh, National Institute of Virology (NIV), Pune (India), suggested that this causative organism could be "Chandipura virus' and its mode of transmission was through sand flies which are vectors carrying virus. This deadly virus earlier, it was suspected, as virus causing Japanese encephalitis—a disease endemic to Asia. Studies on the vector population and symptoms ruled out the possibility of viral encephalitis.

Most children developed dramatic symptoms as the disease progressed much faster than normal—from chills, fever, vomiting and convulsions to coma and death.

Treatment

Since there is no definite cure, the patients were given supportive treatment.

Prevention and control

Luckily 11 sand flies (vectors) are susceptible to pesticides, they can be eradicated by spraying the insecticides.

2. Rift Valley fever

It is mainly a disease in sheep and other domestic animals in Rift Valley (Kenya) and Middle East. Human beings are secondarily infected during **epizootics** in domestic animals. The clinical features resemble influenza-like illness and dengue fever.

Nairo (or Nairobi) sheep disease virus

In Equatorial Africa this virus causes economic loss in sheep. **Ganjam** virus caused a disease in India in sheep. It is related to Nairo virus.

Haemaphysalis tick is the vector. The Nairo virus sometimes infects man causing haemorrhagic fever.

Orbi virus

Three genera—**Reo virus, Orbi virus** and **Rota virus** belong to the family **Reoviridae.** Arthro borne infection is caused by **Orbi virus** only. In the genus, **Orbi virus,** only **Colorado tick borne virus** is recognised pathogen which is maintained in wild rodent population; it is spread by wood tick, **Dermacenter Anderson.** This illness is characterised by a mild fever and it is self limited in Western USA.

Vesiculo virus

In 1967, **Chandipura virus** was isolated in Nagpur (India) from blood of patients during dengue-chikungunya fever. The pathogenic role is not yet well-understood. Sand-flies and **Aedes aegypti** are the vectors in which **Chandipura** virus multiplies.

Rodent-Borne Haemorrhagic fevers

Arena viridae

Arena (*aeronosus,* Latin for sandy) viruses are of grainy appearance of virions under electron microscope. They are spherical, 85-120 nm diameter and contain single stranded segmented RNA genome. They are maintained in nature in rodent without the help of arthropod vectors. Man gets the infection by contact with excreta (urine and faeces) of infected rodents.

Clinical features are fever, petechiae, or purpura, gastrointestinal, nasal and uterine bleeding, leucopenia, thrombocytopenic and shock. Central nervous system involvement may often terminate into death.

Table 62.4. Arena Virus diseases

	Virus	Reservoir	Human disease	Distribution
1.	Lymphocytic Chorio meningitis (LCM)	House mouse	Meningitis, pneumonia	Wide-spread North & South America, Europe
2.	Lassa fever	Multi man-mate, mouse	Haemorrhagic fever	West Africa
3.	Junin	Field mouse rodents	Haemorrhagic fever	Argentina
4.	Machupo	Field mouse	Haemorrhage fever	Bolivia

Filo virus

This virus does not belong to Arbo virus group, but they are described under Arbo virus group as they have similar clinical features.

Marburg virus and **Ebola virus** are two members of **Filoviridae** and are enveloped, tubular (800-1500 × 80 nm) and contain single stranded RNA genome. They possess 7 nm surface spikes. The incubation period is 3-10 days. These viruses cause acute febrile haemorrhagic fever.

(1) The **Marbug virus** was first isolated in Marburg, Germany, and Yugoslavia. Fatality rate was about 35%. This virus was epidemiologically linked to monkeys imported from the same area and was isolated from blood and tissue of these monkeys. Infection may be due to accidental needle sticks or abrasions. This virus was demonstrated in the semen of one patient and is grown in vero cell.

(2) **Ebola virus** was first described in 1977 following an outbreak of haemorrhagic fever in Southern Sudan and Northern Zaire between July and November 1976 in rodents. Serological tests show serum antibodies in rodents and are suggestive of suspected reservoirs. **Ebola virus** has been isolated from Asian Macaques (natural reservoirs of infection). They grow in cell cultures and guinea pigs.

63
Miscellaneous Viruses

Papova viruses

Papova (from ***pa,*** papilloma, ***po,*** polyoma, ***va,*** vacuolaling agent) **Viridae** family comprises of papilloma virus of man and rabbits, polyoma virus of mice and simian virus 40 (SV 40)—the vacuolating agent (virus) of rhesus monkeys.

Table 63.1. Papova viruses infecting man

Genus	Types
Papilloma virus	1 to 57
Polyoma virus	JC virus, BK virus
Vacuolating virus	Simian virus 40 (SV 40)

Virology

These viruses are small 42-55 nm diam., icosahedral, enveloped, contain double stranded circular DNA and replicate in cell nucleus. They can produce tumours.

Human papilloma virus

It causes infectious warts in hand, face, feet, larynx or genitalia. These warts are transmitted by direct or indirect contact (sexual). Incubation period is 2-8 months. The virus multiplies in the connective tissue of dermis followed by proliferation and hyperkeratinisation of the epidermis. Regression of most lesions is spontaneous. As long as the virus multiplies in warts, antibody (Ig M) is present in serum of patient. More than 50 types of human papilloma virus (HOV) are known to produce lesions associated with human papilloma. Papilloma virus can remain latent in normal epithelium. Viral DNA may be detected in about 80% cytologically normal cervices of women.

Pathogenesis

1. **Cutaneous warts :** They are common in children and disappear spontaneously within 2 years of onset. Recurrence is due to persistence of the virus in the skin surrounding the original wart.
2. **Genital warts** are commonest in sexually active women. Lesions are on vulva, within vagina, and on cervix. In men, the lesions are on shaft of penis, perianal skin, and anal canal. Subclinical infection may be present in both men and women.

3. **Recurrent respiratory papillomatosis** : Benign squamous papilloma appears on larynx. Children below 5 years of age may acquire the lesions during passage through an infected birth canal. Adults are infected by orogenital contact.
4. **Oral papillomatosis** : It occurs during oral genital contact with infected sexual partner. Buccal mucosa with multiple papillomatous lesions are called **"Oral florid papillomatosis"** which may progress to malignancy in which HPV DNA has been demonstrated.

Relation of HPV with Cancer

Cervical intraepithelial neoplasia (CIN) precedes cervical cancer and progresses from grade 1 to grade 3. HPV DNA has been detected in all grades of premalignant lesions of the female and male genital tract (HPV types 6, 11). HPV types 16, 18 and 31 have been detected in 60-100% of cervical cancers. Papilloma virus **(Shope papilloma)** causes a benign wart in rabbit which often progresses to cancer after several months.

64
Polyoma Virus

It causes latent infection in rabbit and produces a variety of malignant tumours in newborn mice, hamsters and guinea pigs; hence the name polyoma (***poly***—many, ***oma***—tumour). Till date there is no report on association of polyoma virus with naturally occurring tumour in man. Important members are polyoma virus and two viruses in man—JC virus and BK virus. JC and BK viruses were recovered from brain of a child with Hodgkin's disease, and urine of a renal transplant recipient, respectively.

The names JC and BK are derived from the initials of the persons from whom these viruses were isolated. The child with JC virus developed progressive multifocal leucoencephalopathy.

Vacuolating agent

This agent and SV_{40} (Simian virus 40) was isolated from rhesus monkey's kidney tissue cultures. This virus is morphologically similar to polyoma virus. It causes cytopathic effects (CPE) of monkey kidney cell culture (Vero, BSe 1 and CV 1 cell lines) and sarcoma in newborn hamsters.

Polyoma virus and SV_{40} vacuolating agent are not immunologically related.

Laboratory Diagnosis

Warts are clinically diagnosed. Subclincal infection in female genital tract is common. Diagnosis can be done by histological and cytological methods. Culture of virus can be done in organ culture of human skin epithelium; viral antigens can be demonstrated by electron microscopy or by **DNA hybridisation.**

Epidemiology

The infection from genital tract wart is transmitted by sexual contact, but that of common wart (verruca vulgaris) is by direct contact.

65
Parvo Virus

It is a small (20 nm) and simplest DNA virus that replicates autonomously in rapidly dividing cells. They are distributed in nature and cause disease in animals. Some Feline Parvo virus (FPV) and Canine Parvo virus (CPV) are most important animal pathogens. In developed countries, immunisation is done routinely against these diseases.

Table 65.1. Animal Parvo Viruses

Virus	Host	Lesion
H1	Rat	Subclinical
Minute virus of mice (MVM)	Mice	Subclinical
Feline Parvo virus (FPV)	Cat	Enteritis, Leucopenia, Cerebellar ataxia
Canine Parvo virus	Dog	Enteritis, Myocarditis
Porcine Parvo virus (PPV)	Pig	Reproductive failure
Mink enteritis virus (MEV)	Mink	Enteritis
Aleutian disease virus (ADV)	Mink	Pneumonitis, Hypergammaglobulinaemia Renal failure
Human Parvo virus		
B19	Man	Respiratory tract disease Aplastic crisis, Erythema infection Hydrops fetalis

Parvo virus B19 infects only man. It was first isolated in 1983 in blood of symptomless blood donors. About 60% blood donors are seropositive. This virus causes aplastic crisis in sickle cell and other haemolytic anaemia, erythema infectiosum. It is common in children of early school age and is transmitted by respiratory tract. This virus grows in developing red cell serum containing virus. By counter immuno-electrophoresis (CIE), antibody can be detected in serum at the late stage of disease. Viraemia can occur one week after infection of B19 into the volunteers. The virus can cross the placental barrier and infect the foetus if viraemia occurs during pregnancy.

Table 65.2. Diseases caused by Parvo virus B19

Disease	Host
Asymptomatic rash illness Respiratory tract illness, Arthralgia	Normal
	Chronic haemolytic anaemia
Severe anaemia	Immuno-suppressed
	Intra-uterine infection

66
Corona Viruses

Corona viruses (*Corona,* meaning crown) are spherical (100-150 nm in diam.), pleomorphic, enveloped RNA viruses containing petal- or club-shaped peplomers (spikes) on the surface.

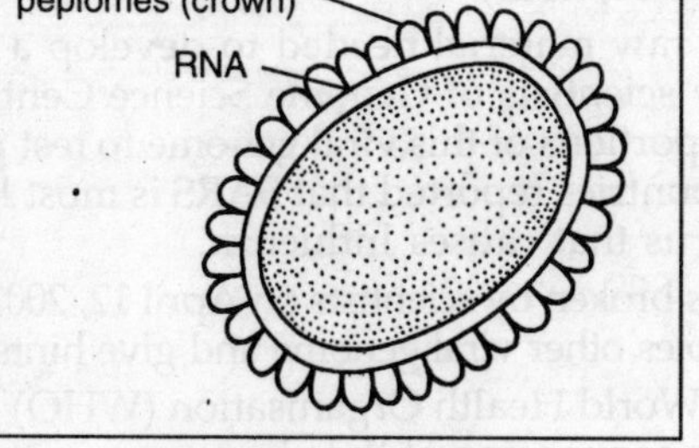

Fig. 66.1: Corona virus

Pathogenesis

They are widespread in nature and infect a wide range of hosts. They have a variable tissue tropism in man. They cause Severe Acute Respiratory Syndrome (SARS).

Table 66.1 Corona Virus groups

Group	Virus	Host
1.	Avian infectious bronchitis virus (IBV)	Bird
2.	Turkey corona virus (TCV)	Turkey
3.	Human corona virus (HCV) 229 E	Man
	Porcine transmissible gastrointestinal virus (PTGEV)	Pig
	Canine corona virus (CCV)	Dog
4.	Feline infectious peritonitis virus (FIPV)	Cat
	Human corona virus (HCV) OC 43	Man
	Rat corona virus (RCV)	Rat
	Rat sialodacro-adenitis virus (RSDV)	Rat
	Bovine haemagglutinating encephalomyelitis virus (HEV)	Pig
5.	Porcine epidemic diarrhoea (FEDV)	Pig

Corona virus family contains 11 recognised species which are divided into five groups on the basis of antigenic structure of N and M peplomer protein. Corona viruses have tropism for respiratory and gastrointestinal tract epithelial cells.

Human Corona virus 2(HCV)

In man, they cause upper respiratory tract diseases like common cold, severe acute respiratory syndrome (SARS). This HCV is responsible for 10% cases of common cold. It causes more coryza and discharge than rhino virus. Acquired immunity is not absolute. Reinfection with the same type of HCV is common in children of 4-10 years of age group.

SARS was reported first in China, then Hong Kong, Singapore. In India, the first SARS case has come from the place of sea and sand (Goa); Prasheet Warclhe (32 year old Goa), engineer who had sailed to Hong Kong and Singapore on March 30, 2003. He remained at the port for four hours before returning to Mumbai (India) on April 1, 2003. His blood, sputum was found positive for SARS by National Institute of Communicable Disease (NICD) New Delhi (India), admitted at Goa Medical College Hospital, treated in isolation ward, a second round of test confirmed that he was SARS positive based on sample drawn on April 18, 2003. Later, he was discharged after few days' treatment.

This disease, which is fatal in more than five per cent of cases and has no known cure has now killed 203 people and infected 3,900 around the world after first surfacing in southern China (Times of India, April 31, 2003).

The genetic code is the raw material needed to develop a diagnostic test for SARS. The genetic code was broken by scientists of Genome Science Centre, Canada, on April 12, 2003. One could use these broken portions of this viral genome to test patients for infection by corona virus. Scientists in several countries reported that SARS is most likely caused by a virulent new corona virus the type of virus that causes Influenza.

The genetic sequence was broken by scientists on April 12, 2003. This new information will tell if SARS virus genome resembles other viral genome and give hints about the biology of this virus.

A team of experts from World Health Organisation (WHO) has introduced in China a safe testing method based on the sequencing of the virus genome to test the virus within an hour.

This new method uses the specially modified protein of the virus to detect the presence of a type of antibody which the body produces as a response to infection with the virus. This is **"quick new test for virus, corona virus"** (Times of India, April 22, 2003).

Suspected SARS cases were reported from different parts of India (New Delhi, Nasik, Jaipur, Kerala, Kolkata, Pune, Mumbai). (Times of India, April 25, 2003).

The total number of SARS cases in India had now gone up to seven confirmed. (Times of India, April 27, 2003).

Nine more SARS cases, mostly of health workers had been confirmed from Pune taking a total number of those WHO have tested positive to 19. In Amritsar (Punjab) a 85 year old man, who did not travel to any of the SARS affected countries, was tested positive for SARS in the initial tests (Time of India, May 1, 2003).

The global toll from SARS climbed above 500 dead, 7,000 infected on Thursday (May 8, 2003 as the World Health Organisation (WHO) declared that the disease is far more deadly than it was previously thought (Times of India, May 9, 2003).

Heinz Felfmann, head of WHO investigating team, confirmed SARS virus spreads by droplets and is not borne (Times of India May 17, 2003).

By July 3, when the pandemic was controlled, it had affected over 30 countries, with many thousand cases & over 800 deaths. India escaped the epidemic. No further outbreak has occured after that till 2011.

Laboratory Diagnosis

1. **Isolation** of human corona virus in cell culture is difficult. Some strains have been grown in organ cultures of human embryonic trachea in research centre.
2. **Direct demonstration** of virus respiratory secretions can be made by ELISA test with high titre anti-serum.
3. **Serological test :** CFT, ELISA and haemagglutination test become positive.

67
Reoviridae

The name Reo is derived from "Respiratory Enteric Orphan" virus because of their frequent occurrence in respiratory tract and enteric tract. Since its pathogenicity was not known, it was called Orphan. **Reo viruses** show wide range of hosts (man, birds, plant and insects). The RNA genome is double stranded and divided into two segments.

Classification

The family **Reoviridae** contains three genera:

1. **Orthoreo virus :** There are three serotypes (1, 2, 3) of mammalian reo viruses found mostly in animals and sometimes in man. Although reo viruses are found in fever, respiratory tract illness and diarrhoea in children, it has not been well established that it produces human disease. Amongst the reo viruses, rota virus is recognised as important cause of gastroenteritis throughout the world.
2. **Orbi virus :** It is an arbo virus and is already described.
3. **Rota virus** causes gastroenteritis in mammals and birds.

Rota virus (*rota,* Latin wheel) virus is similar to Reo virus with a double walled icosahedral capsid resembling a wheel. Its genome consists of double stranded segmented RNA. Electron microscopy shows two types of rota viruses, complete (65-70 nm in diam.) and incomplete particles.

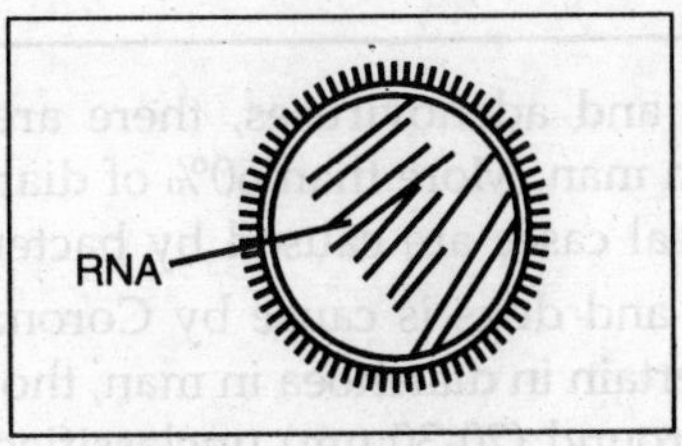

Fig. 67.1: Rota virus

Pathogenesis

There are 4 serotypes of rota viruses. They are now recognised as common cause of infantile diarrhoea and also diarrhoea in calf and infant mice. The virus multiplies in cytoplasm of epithelial cells of small intestine and are excreted in the stool during the first few days of diarrhoea.

Laboratory diagnosis

1. **Virus** in the stool can be demonstrated by immune electron microscopy—ELISA Immuno diffusion test.
2. **Antibody** titre can be measured by ELISA and CFT.

Epidemiology

Infection occurs by faecal-oral route; nosocomial infection is common. Rota virus diarrhoea is common in children of 6 months to 2 years. Antibodies appear in serum of 60-90% children of 6 years of age.

Table 67.1. Characteristics of Reoviridae

Genus	Size	Capsid	No. of RNA segments	M.W. genome	Host range
Ortho reo viruses	80	Double layered	10	10×10^6	Man, vertebrate
Orbi virus	60-80	"	10 or 12	12×10^6	Man, vertebrate, arthropod
Rota virus	70-75	"	'	$12\text{-}13 \times 10^6$	Man, other vertebrates

Virus Causing Gastroenteritis

Table 67.2. Viruses of gastroenteritis in children

	Virus	Disease	Diagnosis
1.	Rota virus	Infantile diarrhoea (in infants, children)	Electron microscopy of stool, ELISA for viral antigen in stool
2.	Adeno virus	Diarrhoea in children	do
3.	Astro virus		
4.	Norwalk		do
5.	Calci virus		do

In addition to rota viruses and adenoviruses, there are other viruses which are also associated with gastroenteritis in man. More than 60% of diarrhoeal diseases are due to viral infection, whereas 30% diarrhoeal cases are caused by bacterial and parasitic agents.

Diarrhoea in calves, piglets and dogs is cause by Corona viruses which are recognised pathogens. Their role is still uncertain in diarrhoea in man, though they are detected in human diarrhoeic stools. Several small round (20-30 nm) unclassified viruses have been detected in stools of acute diarrhoea of children.

Slow virus disease

Certain number of viruses cause slow, progressive infections in animals and man characterised by a very long incubation period, slow course, fatal termination after involvement of central nervous system, absence of immune response. Sigudsson (1951) a veterinary pathologist, first observed slowly progressive disease in sheep (scrapic, visna and maedi) and proposed the term **"Slow infection agent"** for the causative agents. Slow virus disease may be described under two groups:

A. Animal infection

1. Visna

It is caused by viruses which are classified under the family lentiviridae (See AIDS) as retro viruses and also cause a demyelinating disease in sheep with incubation period of 2 years. Pathological changes are observed in brain, lungs, and reticulo-endothelial system. The disease has an insidious onset with paresis, total paralysis and death. The virus can be isolated from CSF, saliva or blood of infected sheep and by tissue culture of choroid plexus. CNS manifestation appears to be an **antigen-antibody** reaction on the surface of infected glial cells.

2. Maedi

Maedi virus is closely related to visna and belongs to subfamily lentiviridae. Incubation period is about 2-3 years. Maedi is a slowly progressive haemorrhagic pneumonia of sheep with fatal termination.

3. Scrapie

It is a slow virus encephalopathy of sheep. Different breeds of animals are susceptible to scrapie. Incubation period is 2 years. The infection remain confined to nervous system and exhibits reactive astrocytosis. The animal becomes irritable and later dies of paralysis. The virus has been maintained in brain tissue explant cultures by serial passages.

4. Mink

Mink encephalopathy is similar to scrapie in all aspects except that it occurs in minks. The causative agent may be a strain of scrapie virus.

B. Human infection

1. Kuru

It is a unique disease affecting only the members of cannabalistic fore tribe of Eastern highlands of New Guinea. It is a slow viral infection with an incubation period of 5-10 years and is transmitted by the tribal practice of eating infected brains of relatives after a **"non-sterilising"** ritual cooking. Grey matter of CNS is degenerated, most marked in cerebellum. This degeneration causes progressive ataxia and tremors. The disease ends fatally in 3-6 months.

2. Creutzfeldt-Jacob disease (CJD)

It is a subacute encephalopathy which develops gradually and is characterised by progressive dementia, epilepsy, myoclonus and extrapyramidal motor neuron signs. It may be accidently transmitted to man from corneal transplant from infected inadequately sterilised neurological instruments and implanted ECG electrodes.

3. Subacute sclerosing panencephalitis (SSPE)

It is a rare disease of children and young adults and develops as a very late complication of measles many years after the initial infection. The disease is characterised by slowly progressive demyelination in the CNS with gradual loss of mental and motor function and as a result there is death in 1-3 years.

Electron microscopy and serological test of brain cells of SSPE patients show measles virus infection. A defective virus closely resembling measles virus has been isolated from lymph node and brain material by co-cultivation with He La cells.

Long after administration of live measles virus vaccine, SSPE may also develop. Similar illness may rarely occur in parents with congenital rubella. SSPE may represent a tolerant infection of latent measles virus due to defective CMI.

4. Progressive multi-focal leuco-encephalopathy (PML)

In old patients whose immune system is impaired as a result of malignancy (chronic leukaemia, Hodgkin's disease lymphoma) or immunosuppression, PML is a progressive demyelinating disease (multifocal encephalopathy) resulting from infection of oligodendrocytes by **papova virus**. PML is a rare complication of CNS and is characterised by progressive loss of motor function, speech and vision — death occurs in 3-4 months.

Table 67.2. Slow and atypical agents

Disease	Host	Organ involved	Virus
Visna	Sheep	Brain	Retro virus
Maedi	Sheep	Lung	Retro virus
Scrapie	Sheep	Brain	Unknown/vivioid/Prim
Mink encephalopathy	Mink	Brain	Unknown/vivioid
Kuru	Man	Brain	Unknown
CJD	Man	Brain	Unknown
SSPE	Man	Brain	Measles, rubella
PML	Man	Brain	Papova (SV40, BK, JC)

68
Bacteriophage

Bacteriophage (Greek *phagein*—to eat; **bacteriophage,** bacteria-cater) are viruses that infect and parasitise bacteria. They cause lysis of bacteria. They are abbreviated as **phages.**

Twart (1915) and d'Herelle (1917) observed an invisible minute parasite of bacteria that caused lysis of the culture of dysentery bacilli **(Sh. shiga)** and named it bacteriophage.

Phages occur widely in association with bacteria in the environment (faeces, sewages).

Bacteriophages are highly host specific and, on the basis of phage, typing of bacteria is done.

Morphology

Coliphages, called T-even phages (T_2, T_4, T_6... series) which attack **E. coli** are extensively studied. T-even phage is a prototype of bacterial viruses.

The phages are tadpole-shaped and have a head and tail:

1. **Head.** It is hexagonal and contains a tightly packed core of nuclei acid (double-stranded DNA) covered by a protein coat (capsid). The head of phage T_4 has a diameter of 65 nm and is 100 nm long.
2. **Tail.** The tail is cylindrical and is composed of a central hollow core or tube (7 nm thick) surrounded by a contractile sheath (protein) and a terminal base plate with tail fibres (usually six in number). Each corner of base plate contains a short pin or spike and a 130 nm long tail fibre. The tail of phage T_4 is 100 nm in length and 25 nm in diameter.

Life cycle

There are two categories of bacteriophages based on their life cycle (a) **Virulent,** (b) **Temperate.**

(a) **Virulent** or **lytic phage** produces lysis of infected cell releasing large number of progeny viruses.

(b) Temperate or lysogenic phage becomes integrated with bacterial chromosome and remains in a dormant state **(prophage). The prophage** is replicated synchronously with the bacterial chromosome and segregated to the daughter cell during bacterial division without harming the host cell.

Phages are usually specific for a few bacterial strains, because of the presence of phage specific receptors.

A. Lytic cycle

The replication cycle of virulent phage is divided into five sequential phases : **Adsorption, Penetration, Synthesis of phage components, Maturation and assembly, and Release of progeny viruses:**

1. **Adsorption.** The phage particles come into contact by random collision and a phage attaches to a specific receptor site on the host cell membrane by means of tail fibres. Adsorption occurs within minutes of contact.
2. **Penetration.** After adsorption of phage to bacteria, the tail sheath of phage contracts and the base plate and tail fibres are held firmly against the bacterial cell. As a result the hollow core is pushed downwards through the already weakened part of cell-wall caused by a phage muramidase present on the base plate. The viral nucleic acid passes down the hollow tube similar to injection through a syringe. The tube does not penetrate the cell wall and the empty head (capsid) and tail remain outside as shell or ghost.
3. **Synthesis of phage components.** After the release of nucleic acid into the bacterial cell, the viral genome directs the biosynthetic machinery of host cell to shut down the normal cellular metabolism and to produce components of new virus particles. This is effected by synthesis of specific enzymes (called **early proteins**) necessary for synthesis of phage components. Subsequently, **late protein,** subunits of phage head and tail appear. Some of the components appear in the nucleus and others in the cytoplasm of host cell.
4. **Maturation and assembly.** During maturation there is spontaneous assembly of phage DNA head protein and tail protein of phage. Each component of phage nucleic acid acquires a protein coat and finally the tail structures are added forming a virion (infective virus particle).
5. **Release.** The progeny phages are rapidly released by the lysis of the infected bacterium. Phage enzyme (probably muramidase) weakens the cell wall during replication of phage. As a result the infected bacterium assumes a spherical shape. Muramidase concentration rises in the late stage of growth cycle, which acts on the already damaged cell-wall causing lysis of cell with release of progeny phage.

Eclipse phase

The time interval between the entry of phage nucleic acid into the bacterial cell to the appearance of first infectious intra-cellular phage particle is called **"eclipse phase",** because viruses cannot be detected within the host cell during this period.

The time interval between infection of host cell and sudden increase in extracellular virus is called **"latent period"**. The duration of eclipse phase is about 15-30 minutes in phages.

B. Lysogenic cycle

In lysogenic cycle, the lytic (vegetative) phage becomes integrated with the host cell chromosomes and is converted into **prophage** without lysis of bacterial cell. The prophage may be converted into a virulent vegetative (lytic) phase spontaneously or by physical and chemical agents (UV rays, H_2O_2, nitrogen mustard).

"Prophage" is a latent bacteriophage retaining its DNA. Host bacteria carrying prophage without being lysed by it is called **"lysogenic bacteria"**. Bacteriophage that parasitises a host bacterium without lysing it is called **"temperate phage"**. Prophage may be lost during multiplication of lysogenic bacteria by means of excision. The excised prophage can infect other bacterial cells making the lysogenic.

Significance of Phages

1. Phage typing

On the basis of the susceptibility of different strains of bacteria to different bacteriophages, the typing of bacteria can be done for identification and epidemiological studies. Epidemics of **V. cholerae, S. typhi,** S. paratyphi and **Staph. aureus** can be detected by phage typing. Phage typing is most useful in intra-species typing of bacteria e.g. to distinguish **V. cholerae** (classical) from **El tor biotype V. cholerae.**

For testing bacteriolysis phage preparations are standardised by titration. Serial dilutions of phage preparations is applied on a lawn culture of a susceptible bacterial strain. The plate is incubated and lysis of bacteria is observed. The **"routine test dose"** (RTD) of phage is defined as the highest dilution of phage preparation required to produce just confluent lysis.

2. Phage assay

When phages are applied on a lawn culture of susceptible strain, clear zones appear after incubation. These clear zones are known as **plaques.** A single phage produces only one plaque. Phage assay is an useful method in titrating the number of viable phages.

B. Temperate phage

Prophage genes may change the properties of host bacterium e.g. toxins of **C. diphtheriae** and **clostridium** are determined by genes carried in prophage DNA. Bacteriophage infection in **S. typhi** confers a new antigenic surface structure on the host. Such acquisition of new properties by bacteria following phage infection is called **"phage conversion". In transduction,** phages act as carriers of genes from one bacterium to another.

69
Rickettsiae

Cultivation

All rickettsiae cannot be grown on cell free media, except **R. quintana** which will grow on blood agar medium.

They can be cultivated in yolk sac of chick embryo, grow on mouse fibroblast, HeLa, Hep2 and on continuous cell lines. Pure preparations of rickettsiae can be obtained by differential centrifugation of yolk sac suspension. For primary isolation, tissue cultures are not satisfactory. Rickettsiae of Typhus group grow in cell cytoplasm, whereas those of spotted fever in nucleus and coxiellae in cytoplasmic vacuoles.

Animal inoculation

Isolation of Rickettsiae from clinical materials can be done by inoculating into mice and guinea pigs.

Q fever is an acute systemic infection usually characterised by an interstitial pneumonia clinically resembling influenza; unlike other rickettsial infections, it has no rash. There is only high fever. The name of the disease is derived from the letter "Q" in Query as its aetiology was uncertain, though it was recognised in Queensland (Australia). The causal agent, named **Coxiella burnetii,** was first recognised by Cox and Burnett. Q fever is quite widespread in Europe and Egypt. It is an obligate intracellular parasite. It can be cultivated in animals and chick embryo. It remains viable for several days in water or milk or butter. Pasteurisation at temperature 145°F or 62.7°C kills **C. burnetti.**

C. burnetti differs from other members of rickettsiae by the following properties : it is filterable, highly resistant to heat and disinfectants, does not produce rash in infected patients and does not elicit the agglutination to the non-motile Proteus strains which is characteristic to typhus fever (Weil Felix test is negative for C. burnetti); hence it is not considered as the true member of rickettsiae and has been designated as a new member Coxiella.

Q fever is spread throughout the world mostly in animals. Infected animals may excrete coxiella in the milk and also during parturition; hence plenty of the organisms are present in the placenta and birth canal. Man may be infected by drinking, contaminated milk or by inhalation of infected dust from the straw or dried placenta. **C. burnetti** is conveyed from animal to animal by the bite of tick. Ticks rarely transmit the infection to man. The risk of person to person transmission is small; so strict isolation procedures are not needed.

Laboratory Diagnosis

Isolation of causative agent is done in animals or chick embryo. Laboratory workers may easily get infected, so they should be careful.

Resistance

Rickettsiae are destroyed at 56°C and at room temperature when they are free from host components.

Serology : Some non-motile strain of proteus and rickettsiae are antigenically similar. Proteus organisms can be grown artificially in plenty. Therefore antigens from Proteus OX2, OXK, OX19 are used in Weil-Felix test which is positive for Typhus fever, except Q fever. This test is useful but not reliable as it is strongly positive in patients with Proteus infection than Typhus fever. CFT is accurate and specific.

Treatment : Tetracyclines, Chloramphenicol and paraaminobenzoic acid exhibit a rickettsiostat effect; but, in Q fever, chloramphenicol and tetracycline are effective therapeutically.

70
Chlamydial Infection

The genus chlamydia includes organisms previously called as Psittacosis-Lymphogranuloma venereum, Trachoma group (PL T) organism. The generic name Bedsonia has also been used in recognition of Bedson; but by the rules of nomenclature chlamydiae has priority. It is now clear that the chlamydiae are small prokaryotic that have evolved to a highly parasitic existence in the cytoplasm of cells. These organisms are small, non-motile, Gram-negative obligate intracellular parasites. They occur in two forms :

Table 70.1. Properties of species of Chlamydia

Properties	C. trachomatis	C. psittaci	C. pneumoniae
Elementary body (EB)			
Size (diam)	300-350 nm	300-350 nm	310 × 400 nm
periplasmic space	very little	very little	Large
Reticular body (RB)			
Size (diam)	800-1000 nm	800-1000 nm	800-1000 nm
Shape	Circular	Circular	Circular
Nucleic acid			
Weight	660×106	660 × 106	660 × 106
Plasmid DNA	+	+	–
(Most strains)	(Most strains)		
Antigenicity			
Outer membrane			
proteins (h) major one	Species specific	Species specific	Species specific

Lipopolysaccharide (LPS) Genus specific genus specific genus specific

(a) There is a small, 300 nm diameter form, which has a compact electron-dense nucleoid which is highly infectious, stable, extracellular form or elementary body.

(b) There is a large form, 800-1200 nm in diameter without a dense nucleoid, the 'initial body' which is intracellular, replicating form. The organisms grow in the cytoplasm of their host cells forming characteristic microcolonies or inclusion bodies which are made up of a mixture of the larger and smaller cells. Both forms stain well with Castaneda or Giemsa stain.

Chlamydiae have 2 subgroups—A, B

Subgroup A has compact inclusions with a glycogen matrix. Subgroup B has no glycogen matrix. These two groups also differ in their susceptibility to sulphadiazine.

Chlamydial infection of man takes two main clinical forms :

(a) organism of psittacosis ornithosis causes respiratory illness with fever; and

(b) trachoma-inclusion conjuctivitis (TRIC)—Lympho-granuloma venereum (LGV) organism of sub group A causes the clinically quite dissimilar ocular, **genital infection.** TRIC-LGV subgroup A chlamydia contains a group of infections transmitted by contact—mainly sexual—in developed countries but also eye to eye in underdeveloped countries where trachoma is endemic.

LGV is more invasive; it starts as a small painless papula or ulcer (Lymphogranuloma chancre) on the external genitalia, or internally some 5 to 10 days after exposure. The infection spreads to the regional lymph nodes (inguinal, perirectal) with suppuration in many cases and sometimes a generalised infection with fever and rash, arthritis, conjunctivitis and meningo-encephalitis. In late stage of the disease chronic inflammation around lymphatics in the genital and rectal area leads to fibrosis with elephantiasis of the genitalia. Rectal structures are common in women and male homosexuals. The treatment of genital infections is by 21 days' course of tetracycline, 250 mg, 4 times a day.

Pathogenicity

Chlamydial infection in man occur in three forms : (a) febrile respiratory disease caused by **C. pneumoniae** and **C. psittaci**, (b) ocular, and (c) genital lesions caused by C. trachomatis.

Antigenic structure : Chlamydiae have two types of antigens:

1. **Heat-stable complement fixing antigen** is a lipo-polysaccharide protein complex similar to cell wall of Gram-negative bacteria. It can be extracted by deoxycholate, ethanol, chloroform.
2. **Heat-labile antigen** is a type-specific antigen left on cell wall after extraction of cell with trypsin or deoxycholate.

Genital tract infection

Recently more interest was focused on chlamydia because of its involvement in genital tract infection, this infection was known since the first decade of this 20th century. Most of the ophthalmologists who worked on patient with ocular disease, traced the infection chain from the genital tract. In 1959, Chlamydiae were isolated from cervix and by 1964 they were recovered from men with urethritis and women with cervicitis.

Table 70.2. Incidence of C. trachomatis infection in the genital tract

Heterosexual males		Females	
Primary diagnosis	Range (%)	Primary diagnosis	Range (%)
Non-specific urethritis	30-50	Contact of chlamydia positive males	45-60
Gonorrhoea	26-30	Contact of chlamydia negative males	4-20
Asymptomatic	3-7	Gonorrhoea	27-60
Attending genitourinary clinic	12-30		
Attend other clinics	1-20		
Requesting termination of pregnancy	10-20		

Table 70.3. Human Chlamydial infections

Site of infection	Lesions	Chlamydia (serovar)
Eye	Trachoma	**C. trachomatis** (A, B, Ba, C)
	Inclusion conjunctivitis	**C. trachomatis** (D-K)
	Ophthalmia neonatorum	**C. trachomatis** (D-K)

Contd.

Site of infection	Lesions	Chlamydia (serovar)
Genital tract		
Male	Urethritis, epididymitis, proctitis	**C. trachomatis** (D-K)
Female	Urethritis, cervicitis, proctitis	**C. trachomatis** (D-K)
	Salpingitis, perihepatitis	
	Peri-appendicitis, infertility	
	Abortion, stillbirth	**C. psittaci** (ovinestoinus)
Male and female	Lympho-granuloma venereum	**C. trachomatis** (L-1-L-3)
Respiratory tract	Pneumonitis of infants	**C. trachomatis** (D-K)
	Pharyngitis, pneumonia	**C. pneumoniae**
	Psittacosis	**C. psittaci** (ovire strain)
	Pneumonia	**C. psittaci** (ovire strains)

LGV : Usually, the inguinal lymph nodes of males are involved in LGV. Fistula or anogenital disease may occur in travellers (having sexual exposure) returning from South East Africa or Central America or South America.

Diagnosis is not easy by physical examination but the serological test (CFT or micro-immuno-fluorescence test) may be useful.

Cultivation. C. psittaci is the first to be propagated in mice by intraperitoneal inoculation and in chick embryo and tissue cultures.

Resistance. Chlamydiae are heat labile and are inactivated at 56°C within few minutes. They are susceptible to dilute solution of formalin and phenol N-acetyl-muramic acid is lacking in cell membrane.

Frei test—a delayed hypersensitivity skin test—is not useful as it was once, and is no longer available in United States.

Therapy : Tetracycline or sulphonamides are not very much effective.

Erythromycin with full systemic doses is very useful in patients allergic to tetracyclines.

71
Mycoplasma

Mycoplasma are small prokaryotic cells—probably the smallest organism to grow in cell-free culture medium. The first member of this group, **Mycoplasma mycoides**, was isolated in 1898 from bovine pleuro-pneumonia. The most popular group is Pleuropneumonia. Like Organism (PPLO) this term PPLO is replaced by Mycoplasma. The human Mycoplasma consists of 8 or 9 species. **M. pneumoniae** is the only unequivocal pathogen, although **M. hominis** may act as a low grade pathogen. T strain Mycoplasma (T for tiny colony) splits urea, requires cholesterol, low pH optimum for growth than classical Mycoplasma.

Table 71.1. Characteristics of Human Mycoplasmas

Mycoplasma	Frequency of isolation from: Respiratory tract	Urogenital tract	Metabolism of	pH of medium	Aerobic reduction of Tetrazolium	Phosphatase phas acti vity	Haem adsorp tion	Susc-petibi-lity to Thal-lium
M. genitalium	Rare	Rare	Glucose	7.5	W	–	+	+
M. hominis	Rare	Common	Arginine	7.0	–	–	–	+
Ac. laidlawii	Rare	Not reported	Glucose	7.5	W	–	–	–
M. baecale	Rare	Not reported	Arginine	7.0	–	+	–	–
M. faucium	Rare	Not reported	Arginine	7.0	–	–	+	–
M. fermentans	Not reported	Rare	Glucose and Arginine	7,5	–	+	–	–
M. lipophilum	Rare	Not reported	Arginine	7.0	–	+	–	–
M. ovale	Common	Not reported	Arginine	7.0	–	–	+	–
M. pneumoniae	Rare	Very rare	Glucose	7.5	+	–	+	–
M. primatum	Not reported	Rare	Arginine	7.0	–	+	–	–
M. salivarium	Common	Rare	Arginine	7.0	–	–	–	–
M. spermato-philum	Not reported	Rare	Arginine	7.0	–	W	–	–
U. urealyticum	Rare Common	Urea	≤ 6.0	–	+	+	+	

W, weak; b, serotype 3 only; a, rare except in disease outbreaks

M. hominis and T. strain Mycoplasma cause genito-urinary tract infection. Vaginitis, cervicitis, urethritis, ovarian abscess, salpingitis, pueperal sepsis, haemorrhagic cystitis are caused by **M. hominis.**

Laboratory diagnosis

Swabs should be collected and sent to the laboratory by transport medium. It should be inoculated into diphasic medium. The best known character of Mycoplasma in the "fried egg" colony is solid medium. Mycoplasma grows best at 35°C-36°C. Most species are aerobes or facultative anaerobes.

Isolates are identified by glucose fermentation, β-haemolysis, haemadsorption and growth inhibition by specific antiserum.

Serum is collected as soon as after onset of illness as possible again after 3 weeks. Sera are tested by CFT.

Treatment : Tetracycline is the drug of choice, less sensitive to erythromycin, chloramphenicol, streptomycin.

72

Spirochaetes

The pathogenic and commensal spirochaetes are slender flexuous spirals 4-16 μ in length and 0.6-0.8 μ thick. They are composed of regular, tight coils or of loose irregular spirals of varying amplitude. They are more highly organised than other bacteria. In addition to cell wall and cytoplasm they contain from one to twelve long filaments applied to their bodies and it is due to these structures that they have their shape, their elasticity, and characteristic movements (angulation). Some cells are visible by dark field microscopy, many may be cultivated except **Treponema pallidum** Nichol's strain.

The family Treponemataceae included three genus : Treponema, Borrelia and Leptospira.

Syphilis : The causal agent of Syphilis **Treponema pallidum** was first discovered in 1905 by a German scientist Schaudinn in the primary sores **(Chancres,** pronounced shankers) of a syphilitic patient.

In electron micrograph, **T. pallidum** is seen to be covered by an outer periplast which covers the whole organism when the periplast is removed by digestion with trypsin or pepsin, the fine filaments are seen twisted around the organism. It seems likely that they are contractile and maintains the characteristic shape of motility of the organism. **Tr. pallidum** shows rotary corkscrew like highly characteristic motility (Angulation) which can be easily seen under dark field microscope.

Staining : Tr. pallidum can be stained by Giemsa stain in 1 : 10 dilution over a long period, it appears pink in colour in contrast to the purplish colour of non-pathogenic spirochaete. The organism can be demonstrated by India Ink or by Fontana's silver impregnation method using the exudate from the chancre. In tissues, spirochaetes can be stained by Levaditi's silver impregnation method in which silver salts are allowed to penetrate the inside of the cells. Metallic silver is then precipitated inside the spirochaetes by means of a reducing solution. The organism appears black against a yellowish black background.

Cultivation : Tr. pallidum cannot be cultivated artificially, but the pathogenic strain (Nichol's strain) can be grown in the testicles of experimentally inoculated rabbit. Certain other non-pathogenic strains (e.g. Reiter strain) can be cultivated under strict anaerobic condition in Smith Noguchi medium.

Viability : Outside the body, **Tr. pallidum** cannot live. It is a strict parasite; it dies rapidly in water and is very sensitive to drying. Soap and other detergents quickly destroy it. It is readily killed by heat at 41.5°C in an hour. Secretions containing Tr. pallidum are possible source of infection to nurses, doctors and technicians who handle the syphilitic patient. The infections are virtually acquired by direct contact with an infected patient.

Pathogenesis : There are three stages in the untreated cases of syphilis :

(a) **Primary syphilis : Tr. pallidum** gains entrance into the body through the skin and mucous membrane. During sexual intercourse, it generally infects genitalia, occasionally the lip during kissing; and it is not homosexually acquired. After an incubation period of 4-6 weeks, the initial sore of primary syphilis appears on the genitalia. This lesion is at first small red purple (chancre), it gradually enlarges, becomes indurated and necrosis in the centre of an ulcer; then a generalised lymphadenopathy of the inguinal gland develops. Spirochaetes are present in large numbers in the exudate of the primary chancre. As the sore heals, the organism becomes less numerous and may not be demonstrated in the exudate, but, at this stage, it may be possible to find them in fluid aspiration by lymph gland puncture.

(b) **Secondary syphilis :** After 6 to 12 weeks of the appearance of primary chancre, the secondary syphilis develops with the invasion of blood stream and widely distributed throughout the body. The clinical manifestations in this stage are fever, a generalised roseolar skin rash, mucous patches in the mouth and condylomata of the anus and vulva. The severity of the lesion is extremely variable. Sometimes the lesions heal up and disappear completely.

(c) **Tertiary syphilis :** In the tertiary syphilis, the spirochaetes become localised producing low grade inflammatory lesions in the cardiovascular and central nervous systems and in chronic granulomata (gummata) in the skin, bone and internal organs. This is also called **chronic stage.** Thus tabes dorsalis and meningo, encardiovascular syphilis may be detected 5-15 years after the appearance of primary chancre.

The late symptoms of syphilis depend on the organ that is attacked by the spirochaetes. The most frequent, serious and disabling results of syphilitic infection are disease of heart, arteries, causing sac-like dilatation called **aneurysm.** These may burst and the patient may die of the haemorrhage. Syphilis is one of the principle causes of diseases of the **aortic valves,** but not responsible for **arteriosclerosis**; and cerebral haemorrhage may occur in young person.

In untreated cases, **Tr. pallidum** lodges in the central nervous system (brain and spinal cord) where they cause a chronic inflammation and destroy the nerve tissue. Various forms of insanity result. These lesions result in paresis (general paralysis) and locomotor ataxia or tabes. In paresis, spirochaetes are present in the tissue of the brain; in tabes, in the spinal cord.

Congenital syphilis : Tr. pallidum can cross the placental barrier and a syphilitic mother especially in secondary syphilitis—may transmit the infection to her foetus. The lesions of congenital syphilis are similar to those already described when the infection is massive, the child may be stillborn or survive for a short time. The most important defects of late congenital syphilis are mental deficiency, chronic meningitis, blindness and deafness.

Table 72.1. Spirochaetal diseases of man

Organism Species	Disease	Primary mode of transmission
Tr. pallidum	Syphilis	Sexual, congenital
Tr. pertenue	Yaws	Skin to skin contact
Tr. carateum	Pinta	Skin to skin contact
Tr. endemicum	Bejel	Mouth to mouth via utensils
B. recurrentis	Relapsing fever	Biting insects (lice)
B. vincenti	Vincent's angina	Biting insects (ticks)
B. burgdorferi	Lyme disease	Biting insects (ticks)
L. interrogarns	Leptosporosis	Rodent, domestic animals
L. biflexa	Saprophytes	Free-living in pools, stream
L. icterohaemorrhagiae	Weil's disease	Infected rats, dogs,
	Leptospiral jaundice	Cattle, pigs

Table 72.2. Diagnostic tests in syphilis

A. Direct demonstration of syphilis	1. Dark field microscopy
	2. Direct immuno-fluorescence (DFTA-TP) test
	3. Fontana's stain (Ag impregnation)
	4. Demonstration in tissue Levaditi's stain (Ag-impregnation) or immuno-fluorescence
B. Serological tests	
1. Non-treponemal (reagin) tests	VDRL, RPR (KT and WR are no more in use)
2. Treponemal tests	
(a) Immuno-flourescence	FTA, FTA-ABS
(b) Immobilisation	TPI test
(c) Haemagglutination	MHA TP, TP HA

Table 72.3. Reactivity of sero-diagnostic tests in untreated syphilis

	STAGE OF DISEASE		% POSITIVE		
Test	Primary	Secondary	Latent	Tertiary	Congenital
VDRL	59-87	100	73-91	37-94	100
FTA-ABS	86-100	99-100	96-99	96-100	100
TPHA	64-87	96-100	96-100	95-100	
MHA-TP	74-87	96-100	94-100	95-108	

Laboratory Diagnosis

Syphilitis exudate : In primary and secondary lesions, it is possible to find and identify Tr. pallidum by dark field microscope.

Serology

A specimen of 5-10 ml clotted blood is needed. It should be collected in a sterile dry container without any preservative. If **Tr. pallidum** immobilisation test is required, information must be provided about recent antibiotic treatment, because traces of penicillin or other antibiotics in the blood interfere with this test. Specimens from the newborn babies should be taken by heel stab, cord blood from the newborn is not satisfactory.

Tests for lipoidophil antibody

Standard Test for Syphilis (STS). These tests, made with cardiolipin antigen, are usually the first investigations arc carried out to confirm the diagnosis of syphilis. A rapid slide flocculation test, such as VDRL test, is often used for screening, although some prefer the Kahn test. A second test, i.e. Wassermann test, is carried out quantitatively, so that besides confirming previous tests, it also provides a baseline in assessing the effect of treatment.

In primary syphilis, Wassermann antibody is usually detectable about one week after the appearance of the primary chancre. In the secondary stage, virtually all cases give positive findings with high titre.

There are many microbial infections and pathological lesions that may liberate lipid antigen in the tissues with the consequent formation of lipoidophil antibody and the occurrence of biological false positive reaction.

Persons who were vaccinated against small pox or were suffering from various infections (e.g. leprosy, typhus) give weakly positive reaction.

Tests for Treponemal antibodies

When complement fixation test (CFT) is employed to diagnose syphilis, it is called Wassermann test. CFT may be Reiter Protein complement fixation test (RPCFT) when the antigen of Reiter strain of treponemes is used.

Absorbed fluorescent Treponemal antibody test (FTAABS) or Treponema pallidum immobilisation (TPI) is more specific and can be used to verify STS positive reaction.

An indirect haemagglutination test for the serodiagnosis of syphilis has been developed by using the antigen of the Nichol's strain of **Tr. pallidum.** The specific test is claimed to be similar to that of TPI test and its sensitivity is comparable to that of FTA test.

Tr. pallidum antibody : Of all serological tests, the more reliable, highly specific antitreponemal test is Treponema pallidum immobilization (TPI) test in which the patient's serum is incubated with living virulent **Tr. pallidum** (Nichol's strain) in the presence of complement. TPI is not useful in the diagnosis of early syphilis. It is able to distinguish between true and false positive STS. TPI is technically difficult and costly—so it is not frequently used.

If the brain or spinal cord is affected by syphilis, a positive serological test is usually given by CSF. The reactions are practically always positive and frequent in locomotor ataxia.

Of the classes of Immunoglobulins that take part in the TPI and FTA ABS, the most important is IgG though IgM is detectable in early syphilis.

Chemotherapy : Penicillin is lethal to Treponema pallidum in a concentration of 0.003 unit/ml and is the drug of choice.

Oral spirochaetes : (Vincent's angina)

Borrelia vincenti is commonly present in the normal mouth in small numbers. It is anaerobic and is very difficult to grow in the laboratory. It is implicated in a painful, ulcerative disease of the gums, cheeks and throat called "Trench Mouth," because it was common amongst military troops in the trenches during World War I (1914-1918). It is also known as "Vincent's angina." It is believed to be infectious disease causing a superficial gangrenous ulceration or stomatitis often with an offensive odour (oral fetor). It may be that certain vitamin deficiencies are the basic cause of the lesions in **Vincent's angina** and the spirochaetes then multiply in the lesions as secondary invaders or opportunists. They are always found in large number in the ulcers, associated with fusiform bacilli **(Fusobacterium fusiformis).** They can be seen under microscope as Gram-negative spirochaetes and fusiform bacilli.

The disease can be transmitted by sneezing, speaking, by improperly disinfected drinking glass, eating utensils, kissing and articles that pass undisinfected from an infected mouth to another. Vigorous mouth washing with disinfectant may cure the infection. In some cases, **Treponema pallidum** may occur in mouth of primary syphilis.

Genus Leptospira

Leptospirae are small, delicate, slender, flexuous organisms. They are composed of tight coils and curved into a hook at both ends like hockey stick. There are many pathogenic leptospirae. They are highly organised than other bacteria. In addition to cell wall and cytoplasm, they contain from one to twelve filaments which are responsible for corkscrew-like motility. They may be seen readily under darkfield illumination method in the infected urine or tissue—wriggling and twisting. They grow at 22 to 37°C in liquid media containing animal serum.

Resistance : Leptospira withstands low temperature and survives in water over a period of many months. They are very sensitive to desiccation and acids. Exposure to 56°C kills the organism in 30 minutes. They are lysed in bile.

Pathogenesis and disease in man : Infected rats, dogs, cattle, pigs are the main source of leptospira. They discharge them into their surrounding environment (water, soil, foodstuffs) with the urine. Contaminated water and foodstuffs are transmission factors. Human beings acquire the disease after swimming in contaminated water, drinking contaminated water or milk from infected cows. Leptospiral jaundice is an occupational disease for people in constant contact with water contaminated by rats. The same hazards occur during work in rice fields (Japan, Indonesia).

The pathogenic leptospirae are responsible for the Zoonotic diseases which are subdivided into icteric and anicteric leptospirosis. Icteric leptospirosis (leptospiral jaundice, Weil's disease) is caused by l. icterohaemorrhagiae.

This organism enters the host body by the gastrointestinal tract and by injured skin and mucous membrane. The disease is characterised by a sudden onset of high pyrexia, headache and pain in the muscles. The disease involves the central nervous system. Jaundice develops and the liver becomes enlarged and painful. Haemorrhagic eruptions, nose bleeding, gastric and intestinal haemorrhages may occur and the spleen becomes enlarged. Nephritis and anuria are also observed.

Leptospiraemia developed in the first seven days of the disease plays an important role in the pathogenesis of leptospirosis. At the end of the first week, the organism accumulates in the liver, spleen, lymph node and bone marrow. Then they penetrate the kidneys and are discharged in the urine for 4 to 6 weeks.

Anicteric leptospirosis (Water fever) is characterised by a sudden onset, fever, severe headache and pain in the bones and muscles. The patient looses his appetite. Nausea and lassitude are observed. The spleen and liver are enlarged. A typhoid condition, mental depression; delirium, dulled consciousness and insomnia occur.

Laboratory diagnosis can be done : 1. by direct dark field microscopy of blood smear, by blood or urine culture; 2. by agglutination and lysis reactions with convalescent sera (dilution not less than 1 : 400) which are of diagnostic value and by complement fixation test or indirect haemagglutination test.

Prophylaxis can be done by destruction of rats; by general sanitation; by prohibition of infected swimming pool; Prophylactic vaccination with vaccine prepared from a suspension of more common types of Leptospira.

Treatment : Penicillin, chlortetracycline, oxytetracycline are drugs of choice.

SECTION V
CLINICAL MICROBIOLOGY

73
Diarrhoeal Diseases

Gastroenteritis is inflammation of the mucus membrane of the stomach and intestine resulting in frequent loose motions with or without blood, with or without mucus, abdominal pain, with or without rise in temperature. Acute gastroenteritis with or without vomiting is a common complaint in diarrhoeal diseases.

Dysentery, literally, means presence of blood and mucus in stool.

Acute infectious diarrhoeal disease can be divided into *non-infective* and *infective* types:

(I) Non-invasive bacterial pathogens–The organisms, which are toxin-mediated (toxic type), cause gastroenteritis or food poisoning:

1. Enterotoxigenic E.coli (ETEC)
2. Enteropathogenic E. coli (EPEC) — Non-toxic, non-invasive pathogen.
3. 01 *V. cholerae* and non 01 *V. cholerae*
4. Cl. *perfringens* type A
5. *Staph. aureus*
6. *Bacillus cereus*
7. Cl. *difficile*
8. *Sh. dysenteriae*–1.

(II) Invasive bacterial pathogens–These organisms, which are *non-toxic* produce gastroenteritis or food poisoning by their tissue invasive properties:

1. Salmonella species
2. Campylobacter species
3. Shigella species
4. Enteroinvasive *E.coli* (EIEC)
5. Enterohaemorrhagic *E.coli* (EHEC)
6. *V. parahaemolyticus*
7. *Yersinia enterocolitica*
8. *Yersinia pseudotuberculosis.*

(I) Non-invasive bacterial pathogens

1. Enterotoxigenic *Escherichia coli* (ETEC) *Pathogens.*

   ETEC produce two types of toxins :

   (a) heat stable enterotoxin (ST)

   (b) heat labile enterotoxin (LT); or both.

In addition to these toxins, they also have plasma mediated colonisation factor which favour *E. coli* to adhere to the mucosa of small intestine. LT is related to enterotoxin of *V. cholerae* and is a protein complex consisting of one A and five B sub-units. Sub-unit A is activated to give two fragments—A_1 and A_2. Sub-unit B are responsible for binding of the toxin to the epithelial cells. A_1 catalyses activation of adenylate cyclase to cause an increase in the concentration of cyclic adenosine 5′ monophosphate (cAMP) which inhibits the absorption of sodium by epithelial cells and increases sodium secretion. It causes loss of chloride and water which results into a profuse watery diarrhoea.

Whereas, the other enterotoxin, ST, exerts its effect through stimulation of guanylase cyclase (cGMP) in the intestinal mucosa. Its action is more rapid than that of LT. Some important ETEC serogroups are O6, O8, O15, O25, O115, O148 and O167.

ETEC strains cause diarrhoea in children under 5 years of age (*infantile diarrhoea*). They also cause *Traveller's diarrhoea* in persons of developed countries who visit unhygienic under-developed countries.

The incubation period is 24–72 hours. In severe cases, its symptoms last for 24–72 hours like Cholera. Patients respond well to intravenous (IV) electrolytic repletion therapy, and Oral Rehydration therapy (ORT) recommended by WHO.

(b) Enteropathogenic E. coli (EPEC)

Though these pathogens are *non-toxic* and *non-invasive*, they cause infantile gastroenteritis in tropical countries, by their plasmid-encoded adherence to the mucosa of small intestine which is associated with dissolution of glycocalyx and loss of brush border microvilli. However, the exact mechanism is yet to be known. They respond to IV fluid therapy. Important EPEC strains are O26, O25, O86, O111, O126, O128, O142.

Laboratory diagnosis of ETEC and *EPEC diarrhoea*: *Faeces* from diarrhoeal patients can be inoculated in MacConkey's agar medium. The isolates were used for *Biochemical test, Agglutination test*. The organism is first tested by polyvalent antisera for the EPEC serogroups, and then by individual O antisera.

(3) Vibrio cholerae

On the basis of their polysaccharide O antigen, these organism are classified into two groups: (a) O1 *Vibrio cholera* ; (b) non–O1 *Vibrio cholerae* (non-agglutinating vibrios).

Within the group *V. cholerae* O1, the strains are categorised into one of the two biotypes *classical* or *el' tor*. Both biotypes are separated into Inaba and Ogawa and Hikojima serotypes.

V. cholerae cause cholera (acute diarrhoeal disease) which may result into severe and rapidly progressive dehydration causing death within hours unless quickly treated with IV electrolyte and ORT.

Some non-O1 *V. cholerae* (non-agglutinating vibrio) cause diarrhoea only, it is rarely severe.

Other vibrios, *V. parahaemolyticus, V. fluvialis* cause human diarrhoea. *V. parahaemolyticus, V. mimicus, V. vulnificus* cause invasive diarrhoea.

Pathogenesis

Incubation period is 8–24 hours. V. cholerae adhere to the mucosa of small intestine by mean of their adhesions. Once adhered, they produce Cholera toxin (CT) similar to LT enterotoxin of ETEC, which is plasmid-coded CT and has two sub–units, a single sub-unit A and 5 sub-units

B. These 5 sub-units B mediate binding of the toxin to receptors of jejunal mucosa. Then a single sub-unit A is transported into the cells which is responsible for the increase in the level of intracellular cyclic AMP (cAMP) causing an increase in the flow of water and electrolyte into the lumen. This fluid contains high concentration of bicarbonate and potassium. The loss of large volumes of isotonic body fluid is the cause of Cholera.

Klebsiella and *Enterobacter* and other enterotoxigenic *Enterobacteriaceae* can sometimes cause acute diarrhoea in developing countries.

Laboratory diagnosis of *V. cholerae* is similar to that of *E.coli.*

V. cholerae is grown on selective media (TCBS).

4. Clostridium perfringens type A

This organism is distributed in soil and in faeces of man and animal. Its heat-resistant spore can survive cooking, spores germinate into vegetative forms during slow cooking and unrefrigerated storage of food.

Consumption of such contaminated food with *Cl. perfringens type A* can cause food poisoning and gastroenteritis in man.

Pathogenesis

The disease (food poisoning), caused by *Cl. perfringens type A* , is characterised by diarrhoea, abdominal pain following ingesting of food (meat, poultry product) contaminated with this organism. Incubation period is 6 to 12 hours, and its duration is 10–24 hours, and the illness is self-limited. The heat-labile enterotoxin produced by this organism acts mainly on the membrane permeability of the small intestine.

Besides, *Cl. perfringens* types C and D strains have been reported to produce enterotoxin which is responsible for food poisoning. Antibiotic therapy has no value. Presumptive diagnosis is done by isolation of the same serotype from a large numbers of the victims of an outbreak of food poisoning.

Laboratory diagnosis

Faeces from large numbers of victims and food samples should be inoculated in aminoglycoside blood agar and incubated anaerobically colonies may be β-haemolytic or non–haemolytic. Gram-staining shows Gram-positive rod with subterminal spore. Identification of the organism can be done by Nagler reaction and serotyping by agglutination test.

4. Staphylococcus aureus

Strains of staph. aureus belonging to phage group III (type 6/47) and group IV (421) produce enterotoxin. There are five serologically distinct enterotoxins (A to E). Of these, enterotoxin A is most often incriminated in outbreaks of staphyococcal food poisoning; this enterotoxin A is toxic protein and is heat-stable.

Preformed enterotoxin (toxic-dose = 1µgm of toxin) in contaminated food can cause acute staphylococcal food poisoning after its ingestion. During acute illness the causative organisms are absent in the stool. The illness is characterised by acute onset of nausea and vomiting within few hours after ingestion of contaminated food followed by diarrhoea. It is self-limiting illness and rarely severe. Acute staphylococcal food poisoning differs from other non-invasive bacterial diarrhoea by its prominence of vomiting. Treatment is by intravenous electrolytic repletion therapy. Antibiotic therapy is of no value.

Pathogenesis

Preformed toxin acts locally on the intestinal mucosa. Vomiting is apparently mediated by a direct effect of the toxin on the central nervous system. The outbreaks depend on the food habits of the country. *Staph. aureus* can multiply in a variable temperature, 4°-46°C. If contaminated food is left at room temperature after cooking, the organisms multiply on potato, salad, cream, sauces. A staphylococcal lesion on the fingers of the cook or food handlers may contaminate the food.

Laboratory diagnosis

Suspected food, vomit, or faeces specimens are inoculated on selective media, Mannitol-salt agar. Selective media are preferred for stool culture because of mixed flora. The isolate is identified by Coagulase test and epidemiology is traced by phage typing.

Demonstration of enterotoxin

Enterotoxin of food, vomit, or culture filtrate of isolate can be detected by ELISA and Reverse Passive Latex Agglutination (RPLA) kits which are commercially available.

5. Bacillus cereus

The infection occurs after ingestion of food contaminated by non-pathogenic organism, *B. cereus,* which is capable of producing two distinct enterotoxins—one resembling LT of E. coli and other that of staphylococcal enterotoxin.

They cause two distinct clinical syndromes:

1. Short incubation period (1-2 hours) types : Symptoms are nausea, vomiting, often followed by diarrhoea, similar to these of staphylococcal food poisoning. This type is associated with bulk prepared rice. This is also called as "emetic form of *B. cereus* food poisoning".

2. Long incubation period (6-16 hours) type : This type of gastroenteritis is characterised by sudden onset of diarrhoea and abdominal pain and is similar to those caused by enterotoxin producing *E. coli* (ETEC). Soups and sauces contaminated with *B. cereus* can cause this type of illness.

Epidemiology

B. cereus are distributed in soil and cereals. Their spores resist cooking. When food is stored at a warm temperature, the spores germinate into vegetative forms which produce enterotoxin.

The short incubation period of *B. cereus* food poisoning is associated with contaminated fried rice served in mass feast or in restaurants. Brief rewarming of the contaminated food does not destroy heat stable toxin.

Laboratory diagnosis

Suspected food, vomit, faeces can be inoculated on nutrient agar, blood agar. Overnight incubation shows "curled hair" colonies typical of *B. cereus. They* are Gram-positive spore-bearing bacilli seen in smear.

6. Clostridium difficile

Cl. difficile is associate with about 20-30% cases of antibiotic associated diarrhoea and pseudomembranous colitis.

The most common antibiotics (lincomycin, clindamycin, ampicillin and cephalosporins) are associated with pseudomembranous colitis.

Pathogenesis

When the antimicrobial therapy has suppressed the growth of competing gutflora there is overgrowth of antibiotic resistant *Cl. difficile*—which is quite common in the faeces of neonates.

Cl. diffcle produces two toxins: enterotoxin (toxin A); cytotoxin (toxin B). Toxins A and B act synergistically. Toxin A causes tissue damage and accumulation of fluid in the lumen of experimental animal. Thus Toxin A has both histotoxic and enterotoxic effects. Cytotoxin causes cytopathic effect (CPE) in cell culture which is a diagnostic marker for *Cl. difficile*. In antibiotic associated diarrhoea, the colonic mucosa shows a mild erythema with oedema. Sometimes the colitis is more severe and is characterised by an exudate membrane (*pseudomembrane*). The mucosa may be haemorrhagic. Withdrawal of antimicrobial therapy may lead to early resolution of symptoms.

Laboratory diagnosis

1. *Demonstration of toxin* may be done by the cytopathic effect of faecal filtrate on vero or human embryo fibroblast and by neutralisation of toxic effect by specific antiserum.
2. *Culture* is done by inoculating faeces on selective media and subsequent toxigenicity test.

B. Non-invasive bacterial pathogens

1. Salmonella gastroenteritis

The common food poisoning serotypes of *salmonella* are *S. enteritidis* (poultry egg), *S. typhimurium* (rat, mice), *S. dublin* (cattle), *S. hador* (turkey), *S. choleraesuis, S. helderberg,* and *S. thompson*.

Incubation period of salmonella food poisoning is 12-36 hours. This illness is characterised by self-limited fever and diarrhoea, vomiting and abdominal pain.

Common sources of salmonellae are food derived from domestic animals and poultry (meat, egg, sausages). Sometimes, human cases and carriers (food handlers) may transmit this infection.

Pathogenesis

Ingestion of contaminated food may cause salmonella food poisoning. Salmonellae multiply in the food and later in the intestine of victim—only large doses of salmonellae are required for human infection. Sometimes septicaemia may develop due to infection with *S. enteritidis.*

Sporadic cases of salmonella gastroenteritis may go unnoticed; but large outbreaks—often called "food poisoning"—are investigated and diagnosed.

Laboratory diagnosis

Faecal sample or food can be cultured on selective media (MacConkey's agar, deoxycholate citrate agar, Wilson and Blair medium) Pale non–lactose fermenting colonies appear on MacConkey's agar and DCA; black shiny colony on Wilson and Blair medium.

Identification can be done by biochemical tests, later by agglutination test with polyvalent group sera (O and H). Epidemiology is confirmed by phage typing.

Treatment consists of fluid repletion therapy. Antibiotics are not advised as they may contribute to reemergence of antibiotic-resistant strain.

2. Shigella

Sh. dysenteriae, Sh. flexneri, Sh. boydii, Sh. sonnei cause bacillary dysentery as they are invasive pathogens; but *Sh. dysenteriae* type I (*Sh. shigae*) also produce a powerful enterotoxin (neurotoxin) and cytotoxin.

Pathogenesis

Infection is spread via *food, flies, fomites*. Ingestion of contaminated food may cause bacillary dysentery. The organisms invade the colonic mucosa. Then cell-to-cell spread of infection occurs. Infected cells are killed, DNA inflammation develops in the submucosa and lamina propria resulting into necrosis and ulceration of epithelium of intestine. They do not invade deeper layer and blood (no bacteriaemia). Stool contain blood mucus.

Laboratory diagnosis

Stool and rectal swabs can be inoculated on MacConkey's agar and DCA; after 26 hours incubation non-lactose fermentating pale colonies are formed; except *Sh. sonnei* which is late lactose fermenter.

Identification : (1) Biochemical test; (2) Agglutination test by group specific polyvalent antisera to shigella.

3. Enteroinvasive E. coli (EIEC)

They cause bacillary dysentery quite similar to that of shigellosis, but *without vomiting*. They invade the mucosa of large intestine and multiply intracellularly. The incidence of diarrhoea caused by EIEC is about 5% of all diarrhoea. The illness is short lived and antibiotic therapy is of no use.

Diagnosis can be done in the laboratory by culturing the stool on MacConkey's agar and by serotyping of isolate. Serogroup O124 is most common, others are O128 and O112.

Verocytotoxigenic E. coli (VTEC)

VTEC was previously called enterohaemorrhagic *E. coli* (EHEC). It is associated with two clinical conditions–haemorrhagic colitis (HC) and haemolytic uraemic syndrome (HUS).

In *haemorrhagic colitis* there is blood stained diarrhoea preceded by abdominal pain and watery diarrhoea, sometime pyrexia. All age group are affected. *E. coli* sero group O157 is vero cytotoxigenic strain. VTEC is non-invasive and produces verocytotoxin similar to Shiga toxin and, hence, it is called "Shiga Like Toxin" (SLT)—food is the source of VTEC infection.

Laboratory diagnosis

Faeces can be *cultured* on MacConkey agar, lactose fermenting pink colonies appear on this medium after overnight incubation.

Identification

1. About 95% *E. coli* are sorbitol fermenters, whereas O157 VTEC is sorbitol non-fermenter.
2. Production of Vero cytotoxin (VT) is determined by its cytotoxic effects of isolated strain on vero cells.
3. *Agglutination test* is done by serotyping of the strain. Rising titres of VT neutralising antibodies may be detected in patient's serum.

4. Campylobacter jejuni

C. jejuni is major cause of diarrhoea. It occurs in the intestine of wild and domestic animals (poultry). Milk and water are common sources of outbreak of diarrhoea due to *C. jejuni.* Its incubation period is 3-10 days. The illness is characterised by diarrhoea with blood mucus in the stool with abdominal pain. It is self-limiting; septicaemia is common in severe cases.

Duration : Usually 3-4 days rarely it may persist for 3–4 weeks

Laboratory diagnosis

Specimen Faeces

Culture selective media containing vancomycin, polymyxin are used. Optimum temperature for growth is 43°C. Faeces is inoculated in Thayer Martin medium and incubated at 5-10% CO_2 at 42-43°C. *C. jejuni* and *E. coli* selectively grow against other faecal bacteria.

Identification : These organisms are Gram-negative, curved, slender bacilli; showing darting motility. They are oxidase positive.

Treatment. Campylobacter enteritis is self-limiting and does not require treatment. Severe cases respond to erythromycin therapy which also reduces the duration of excretion of the organism.

5. Vibrio parahaemolyticus

It is a Gram-negative, curved, non-motile aerobic bacillus present in coastal waters throughout the temperate zones.

It is a common cause of diarrhoea (food poisoning) in Japan and Singapore. Man gets infected after ingestion of raw sea food (fish and shell fish). Other symptoms are abdominal pain and vomiting; stool may contain blood.

Kanagawa positive strains of V. parahaemolytics produce a cytotoxin which causes diarrhoea in volunteers. These strains also adhere to human intestinal cells. They produce a heat labile enterotoxin like that of E. coli.

Laboratory diagnosis

Specimen Faeces

Culture MacConkey' agar, TCBS and alkaline peptone water containing 1% NaCl are used as they are halophilic vibrios. After overnight incubation, pale colonies develop.

Identification: Isolates are identified by biochemical tests and agglutination test.

Other halophilic vibrios

Vibrio mimicus and *V. vulnificus* cause sporadic cases of diarrhoeal diseases in men who ingest raw or under-cooked sea fish occurring along the Gulf Coast. *V. mimicus* diarrhoea follows after taking oysters while *V. vulnificus* occurs after ingestion of shellfish. They do not produce cholera enterotoxin. The illness is self-limited. *V. vulnificus* causes septicaemia. They grow in alkaline peptone water with 1% NaCl and on thiosulphate bile salt sucrose agar.

6. *Yersinia enterocolitica*

It is common in Canada and Northern Europe (Belgium and Scandinavian countries), and is distributed worldwide. Sources of infection are birds, wild and domestic animals. The infection spreads via faecal-oral route from animals by contaminated drinking water or directly from person to person.

Symptoms vary with age. Predominant symptom in young children is acute watery diarrhoea, lasting for 3-14 days; about 5% children have blood in stool. In older children and young adults there is pain in right upper quadrant of abdomen, fever, and moderate leucocytosis which mimics appendicitis. In debilitated patients, the infection may progress to septicaemia.

This organism can be isolated from stool or from blood culture. It is non-lactose fermenting gram-negative aerobic bacilli. It is susceptible to chloramphenicol, aminoglycosides, tetracycline, and cotrimoxazole.

Table 73.1. Microbial agents and their diarrhoeal diseases

Causative agents	Usual source	Mode of transmission
Salmonella sp.	Animal gut	Poultry, meat, milk
Campylobacter sp.	Animal gut	Poultry, meat, milk
Shigella sp.	Human gut	Faecal-oral route
E. coli (ETEC, EHEC, EIEC, EPEC)	Human gut	Faecal-oral route
V. cholerae	Human gut	Water, food
V. parahaemolyticus	Human gut	Water, food
Yersinia pseudotuberculosis	Animal gut	Faecal-oral route
Staph. aureus	Septic lesions on food-handlers	Cooked meat, dairy products
Cl. perfringens	Animal gut	Meat pies, stews
Bacillus cereus	Environment (soil)	Rice
Cl. difficile	Human gut	Faecal-oral route

74

Monsoon Diseases in India

The monsoon-diseases in India are :

1. Gastrointestinal diseases
2. Enteric fever (Typhoid)
3. Hepatitis A virus infection (Jaundice)
4. Hepatitis E virus infection
5. Dengue fever (less common)
6. Malaria (common).

During the rainy season, rain water contaminated with micro-organism (bacteria, virus, fungus) may gain entrance into city drinking water supply system through leaking waterpipe, causing gastroenteritis, viral hepatitis (Jaundice), and enteric fever.

Enteric fever (Typhoid) will show an alarming rise during monsoon. It is contracted by consuming contaminated food or drinking water. Hepatitis A virus and Hepatitis E virus can enter the alimentary canal after drinking water contaminated via leaking city waterpipe line, or consuming contaminated food.

Malaria

In rainy season, there is water logging which may be a congenial habitat for breeding of mosquito which transmits malaria which may become rampant. Only night-time biting female Anopheles mosquito can transmit malaria.

Dengue fever, less common viral infection in India, is transmitted by day-time biting Aedes mosquito which breeds in clean water.

The human body is adjusted to certain level of temperature (37°C) and climate. If there is sudden change in temperature and in the level of humidity, there is disturbance in the body's defence mechanism with the rise in humidity, the replication of virus is highest. This may lower the body's resistance. Thus the susceptibility to viral infection will become quite imminent.

Cold, cough, runny nose and bodyache are some common symptoms of viral fever.

Prevention and control

The viral infection can be prevented by avoiding pollution congested atmosphere and contact with person suffering from a viral infection. Hygiene should be maintained by drinking boiled water and keeping away from roadside food as adopted in gastroenteritis and enteric fever.

In Dengue fever, the water tank used to store clean water should be covered with a tight lid so that the mosquito cannot enter; if they enter they may die of suffocation.

Spray of insecticides with kerosene may kill mosquitoes which have not developed resistance to insecticide.

Life cycle of mosquito from egg to adult is completed in twelve days. Therefore, weekly once (particularly during holidays–Sunday), water in the container should be replaced. In this way, the life cycle is intercepted and there will be no mosquito to transmit Dengue fever.

Malaria can be treated by anti-malarial drugs.

Leptospirosis in India (Gujarat)

Leptospirosis mainly affects farmers working in fields with stagnated rain water contaminated with Leptospira infected rat urine.

Leptospirosis—which strike South Gujarat following fresh floods in 2004—among 540 suspected cases, 71 persons reportedly died in 4 districts namely, Surat, Valsad, Navsari and Bharuch.

75
Bacterial Food Poisoning

The term "Bacterial food poisoning" is referred to acute gastroenteritis that results from the presence of bacteria, usually in large numbers, or the products (toxin) in food. Contamination of food occurs either at source or during preparation of food.

It may be divided into three types :

1. *Infection type* in which multiplication of the organism occurs *in vivo*, e.g Salmonella;
2. *Toxin type* in which the disease follows ingestion of food with *preformed toxin*, e.g. staphylococcal entero-toxin, and
3. *Intermediate type* in which bacteria release the toxin in the bowel, e.g. *Cl. perfringens.*

Causes of food poisoning

A. Infection Type

1. Salmonella sp. (*S. typhimurium, S. enteritidis, S. thompson*)
2. *Campylobacter jejuni*
3. *Vibrio parahaemolyticus*
4. *Vibrio mimicus.*

B. Toxin type

1. *Staphylococcus aureus*
2. Bacillus cereus.

C. Intermediate type

1. Cl. perfringens type A
2. E. coli verocytotoxigenic (neurocytotoxin producing)
3. Clostridium botulinum.

Food borne botulism

It is a severe, often fatal, form of food poisoning which is due to the ingestion of *preformed toxin* in food contaminated with *Cl. botulinum*. It is characterised by pronounced neurotoxic effects. Incubation period ranges from 1-2 days. There may be initial nausea, vomiting and abdominal pain but no *diarrhoea*.

Source of infection

Cl. botulinum is widespread in nature and its spores can withstand boiling in water (100°C) for several hours. This illness has been associated with home canned food ingestion.

Pathogenesis

Antigenically there are seven types of Cl. botulinum (A–G) which produce antigenically distinct toxins with pharmacologically identical actions. Toxin types A, B, E are mostly associated with human disease and, rarely, F is responsible. Botulinum toxin (neurotoxin), whether ingested or produced in the intestine, is absorbed from the intestinal tract and enters the vascular system and is transported to peripheral cholinergic nerve terminals and blocks the release of acetylcholine.

Clinical features

Cranial nerve involvement is an indication of the onset of symptoms and affects the oculomotor muscles leading to diplopia and drooping eyelids with a squint. There may be vertigo, blurred vision and dry mouth. There is progressive symmetric descending flaccid paralysis that may lead to respiratory failure and death.

Diagnosis

Specimens : Food, vomitus, faeces, and blood.

Toxin in the specimen may be detected by toxin–anti-toxin neutralisation test in mice.

Non-bacterial Infective Diarrhoea

In addition to bacterial diarrhoea, viral, fungal, and protozoal diarrhoeas are also encountered in human beings.

Table 75.1 Non-bacterial infective diarrhoea

Causative agent	Usual source	Transmission
Viruses		
Rota virus		
Astro virus		
Calci virus	Faeces	Faecal-oral
Adeno virus		
Protozoa		
Entamoeba histolytica	Faeces	Faecal-oral
Giardia lamblia	Faeces	Faecal-oral
Cryptosporidium	Faeces	Faecal-oral
Balantidium coli	Faeces	Faecal-oral

Laboratory diagnosis

Specimen : Faeces

A. Microscopy

(a) Saline preparation

1. Amoebic dysentery–cyst and motile trophozoites of *E.histolytica* .
2. Giardiasis. *G. lamblia* cysts in formed stool or trophozoites in fresh stools, duodenal, secretions or jejunal biopsies.

(b) Iodine mount

1. Amoebiasis and giardiasis–cysts take up iodine and appear distinct.
2. *Balantidium coli*–cysts in formed or trophozoites in fresh stool.

3. *Cryptosporidium*–Oocyst excretion maximum during first 3-5 days of illness, 5 μm diam oocysts fail to take up iodine stain.

(c) Acid fast staining

It shows acid fast oocyst of *Cryptosporidium* in stained faecal smear.

(d) Electron microscopy of faeces

Morphology of virus particles can be demosntrated.

B. Serological tests

1. Amoebiasis—Significant antibody titre persists for months after cure. Indirect haemagglutination and ELISA are most sensitive.
2. Viruses in stool can be detected by fluorescent antibody and ELISA test.

76
Respiratory Tract Infections

Upper respiratory tract is frequently the site of localised or general infections. Infections of the respiratory tract may be divided into four groups :

1. Infections of the throat and pharynx.
2. Infections of middle ear and sinuses.
3. Infections of trachea and bronchi.
4. Infections of lungs.

Infections of Throat and Pharynx

I. Sore throat

It is an acute pharyngitis and/or tonsillitis; causes—

1. Prodromal stages of infectious diseases
2. Sore throat syndrome
3. Diphtheria
4. Vincent's angina.

Viruses are most common causes of sore throat (about two-thirds of all cases are of viral origin). Besides, there are non-infective causes and infection due to *Candida sp*.

Sore throat syndrome (STS)

Streptococci and viruses cause similar signs and symptoms of sore throat, i.e., pain on swallowing, congested tonsils, pharynx, enlarged tonsillar lymph nodes and pyrexia. *Aetiology*: Bacteria, virus and mycoplasma.

Bacteria Group A–haemolytic streptococcal, *Str. pyogenes* (most common). Group C and G are rarely involved, sometime *Staph. aureus, H-influenzae*.

Streptococcal sore throat

Source of infection : Carrier or case: Children of 5-8 years of age are commonly affected with this disease. In mild cases, there is redness of tonsils and pharynx. The actual illness is characterised by infection and oedema involving the fauces and soft palate with exudate–acute follicular tonsillitis. Incubation period is 3-5 days.

If untreated, streptococcal tonsillitis may give rise to septic complications (peritonsillar abscess, sinusitis, otitis media or to immune complex diseases (glomerulonephritis, rheumatic fever). When the infecting strain of str. pyrogenes is erythrogenic toxin producing (lysogenic), the throat infection is accompanied by erythematous rash (scarlet fever).

Laboratory diagnosis (sore throat)

Specimen : throat swab from fauces inoculated in blood agar incubated aerobically and anaerobically.

Identification

(a) Colonies are small, dry, beta haemolytic.

(b) Lancefield grouping

Rheumatic fever (RF)

Latent period, 2-3 or up to 6 weeks after throat infection. Rheumatogenic serotypes M types 5, 18, 24 are mostly responsible.

Serology : ASO titre 200 (significant) or more.

Treatment : Rheumatic fever is due to repeated attacks. Therefore long term basis penicillin therapy is necessary to eliminate streptococci.

Acute glomerulonephritis (AGN)

It is an immune complex hypersensitivity reaction:

1. *Latent period* : 1-3 weeks after streptococcal sore throat or skin infection (impetigo).
2. *Nephritogenic serotypes* : Acute glomerulo-nephritis is liable to follow infection with certain serotypes—mostly M type 12, 1, 25, 4, 3 in throat infection, M types 49, 52–55, 57–61 in skin infection.

Serology : Serum ASO titre is usually not elevated Anti-DNAse B is raised and C3 reduced.

Treatment : AGN does not recover. Antibodies are of no use in established AGN.If skin infection is treated with penicillin or erythromycin, AGN may be prevented.

Diphtheria

Corynebacterium diphtheriae gravis intermedius, mitis causes diphtheria, mitis type is common in India.

Type : Faucial diphtheria is common, fauces covered with patches, serocellular exudate forming a greyish-white pseudomembrane. Nasal diphtheria (mild), laryngeal diphtheria is serious because of laryngeal obstruction.

Incubation period : 2-5 days.

Source : Throat and nose of carriers.

Pathogenesis : Bacilli remain localised, multiply, produce powerful exotoxin. This exotoxin diffuses through the body, affects myocardium, adrenal glands, and nerve endings.

Treatment : (a) Large dose of antitoxin should be injected without delay.

(b) Antibiotics (penicillin, erythromycin) can eliminate C. *diphtheriae* from throat without any effect on toxin already produced. (c) In case of obstructive respiration, tracheostomy is necessary.

Candidiasis

Oral candidiasis (oral thrush) in neonates is caused by *candida albicans* and is characterised by loosely adherent white patches superimposed on red, raw mucous membrane of tongue, cheek and gums.

Source : Neonates contact the infection from mother's genital tract or by cross-infection in nurseries.

Though *C. albicans* is commensal of mucous membrane of mouth and may become an opportunist pathogen of respiratory tract.
Treatment : Local application of Nystatin or Amphotericin.

Vincent's angina

Acute ulceromembranous *gingivitis* (AUMG) is synergic infection with fusobacterium and spirochaete.

1. **Bacterial aetiology**
   (a) *Spirochaete–Borrelia vincenti.*
   (b) Anaerobic bacilli–*Fusobacterium fusiform* (now called Leptotrichia buccalis, the present name of vincent's bacillus).
   (c) Oral *Bacteroides sp* (B. intermedius) are now believed to be responsible for infection.

Source : Endogenous, the organisms are present in the normal mouth.

Pathogenesis : AUMG usually develops in patients with poor oral hygiene or dental caries; malnutrition and debility resulting in overgrowth of the offending organisms.

Treatment : Penicillin and Metronidazole.

Infectious mononucleosis

Presenting feature–Exudative tonsillitis.

Cause : Epstein-Barr virus (EBV).

Source : Oropharyngeal secretions (the kissing disease of young adults).

Diagnosis : 1. Atypical lymphocytosis; 2. Presence of heterophilic antibodies in serum (Paul–Bunnel test); 3. *Isolation* of EBV from oropharyngeal washing or blood is laborious.

Treatment : No specific treatment.

Laboratory diagnosis of throat and pharyngeal infections

Specimen : Throat swabs should be rubbed over the affected area and quickly sent to the laboratory. If delay in transit is anticipated, swabs should be preserved in the refrigerator.

Microscopy

(a) Gram stain : *C.albicans* are Gram-positive oval yeast cells with germ tube. *Vincent's* infection shows Gram-negative spirochaete (*B. Vincenti*) and Gram-negative fusiform bacilli (*Fusobacterium sp.*).
(b) Albert staining of smear shows V and L shaped bacilli with metachromatic granules (barred appearance). This is useful for presumptive diagnosis of *C. diphtheriae*. For confirmatory diagnosis, smear of diphtheriae must be isolated on culture and it should be subjected to toxigenicity test.

Culture

1. Blood agar
2. Crystal violet blood agar — selective for *Str. pyogenes* when incubated anaerobically.
3. Sabouraud's dextrose agar — selective for *C.albicans*.
4. Loeffler's serum, Potassium tellurite agar for isolation of *C. diphtheriae*.

Other test

(a) Lancefield grouping *Str. pyogenes.*

(b) Toxigenecity test for *C. diphtheriae.*

(i) Elek's test

(ii) Guinea pig inoculation for *C. diphtheriae*

Infection of middle ear and sinuses

Aetiology

The direct spread of pathogen from throat via Eustachian tube may cause the infection of middle ear and sinuses, viruses, mycoplasma, bacteria may be responsible for this infection. The infection may be acute or chronic.

H. influenzae and *Str. pneumoniae* are bacterial pathogens in *acute infection* whereas *Ps. aeruginosa and Staph. aureus (aerobic pathogens), Peptococcus, Pepto-streptococcus, Bacteroides* (*B. fragilis, B. melanino-genicus*—anaerobic pathogens) cause *chronic infection* of middle ear and sinuses in pathogenesis, the obstruction is an important features.

Table 76.1. Bacterial pathogens of sinusitis and Otitis media

Syndrome	Bacterial pathogens
Acute otitis media and sinusitis	*H. Influenzae, Staph. aureus, Str. pneumoniae, anaerobic*
Chronic suppurative Otitis media and sinusitis	Aerobes
	Staph. aureus, Ps. aeruginosa, Proteus sp (Pr. mirabilis, Pr. vulgaris)
	Anerobes
	Bacteroides, (B. fragilis) B. melaninogenicus, *Fusobacterium,* Anaerobic cocci

Laboratory diagnosis

Specimen : Swabs or pus, antral washings (collected carefully for anaerobic culture by disposable sterile syringe, needle which is bent at right angle immediately after collection).

A. *Microscopy*. Gram stained film is not helpful.

B. *Culture*, Blood agar, nutrient agar, RCM incubation–aerobically and anaerobically.

C. *Other tests* : Coagulase test–staph. *aureus*, oxidase test–Ps. *aeruginosa* urease test–*Proteus sp*. Biochemical tests help to distinguish different species.

Treatment

A. *Acute infection* : Ampicillin, amoxycilin or erythromycin.

B. *Chronic infection* : Drug resistant organisms are often encountered.

(1) Treatment should be guided by antibiotic sensitivity test.

(2) Anaerobes are sensitive to metronidazole, many are sensitive to lincomycin, Chloramphenicol, and Cefoxitin.

(3) Topical applications of neomycin, polymyxin, bacitracin is useful. *Staph. aureus* shows multidrug resistance, particularly in the hospital.

Many strains of *Staph. aureus* and *Bacteroides* produce a penicillin destroying enzyme (B-lactamase) that hydrolyses the beta lactam ring in the penicillin nucleus.

Infection of trachea and bronchus. Many infections of trachea (tracheitis), larynx((laryngitis) and bronchus (bronchitis) are caused by viruses.

Table 76.2. Causative agents of laryngitis, tracheitis

Syndrome	Infective agents
Acute epiglottitis	*H. influenzae* type 6, Para-influenza virus 1, 2, 3
Acute laryngitis, tracheobronchitis (Croup)	
Bronchilts	*H. influenzae*, *Str. pneumoniae*, Br. catarrhalis, *Mycoplasma pneumoniae*, viruses, influenza, Rhino and Adenovirus.
Whooping cough	Bord. pertussis, *Bord. parapertussis*

A. Acute laryngo-tracheo-bronchitis (Croup)

1. *Cause* : Bacteria, H. influenzae type 6, virus, parainfluenza virus 1, 2, 3
2. *Incidence* : Infants and young children (2-7 years)
3. *Symptoms* : Croaking cough
4. Blood culture is positive in septicaemia, pharyngeal swab culture is positive for *H. influenzae*.

Treatment : Ampicillin or Chloramphenicol.

B. Chronic bronchitis

1. *Clinical features* : At the beginning cough is dry and painful, later it becomes productive with expectoration of yellowish green sputum, most marked in early morning samples.
2. *Pathogenesis* : It is a relapsing condition. Predisposing factors are smoking, previous lung damage, atmospheric pollution, cold damp weather.
3. *Pathological changes*
   (a) Mucous secreting cells in bronchi are increased in number resulting in hypersecretion of mucus.
   (b) Inflammation, fibrosis, collapse, dilatation, cyst formation occur in bronchi and alveoli leading to irreversible damage.
4. *Laboratory diagnosis*
   Sputum culture.

C. Whooping cough

It is an acute tracheobronchitis of childhood. Incubation period is 10 days. Patients with catarrhal stages can be the source of infection. Transmission is by airborne or droplet infection.

Clinical features

Initial catarrhal stage with cold lasts for 2 weeks. It is followed by a stage of 2 weeks' paroxysmal coughing. Then a persisting residual cough for another month.

Fatality is low; morbidity high; 50 times higher in children under one year than 4 year olds. Whooping cough appears in epidemic preparation.

Immunity : Immunity by infection or by vaccination is long lasting.

Laboratory diagnosis

Specimen : Perinasal swab passed by gently along the floor of the nose and nasopharyngeal secretions is collected.

(a) *Culture* : Specimen is inoculated in Bordet Gengou medium agar or charcoal medium. Alternatively, medium is held in front of mouth of patient during a paroxysm of coughing, plate is incubated for 3-5 days at 35–36°C; colonies are moist "mercury drop" like.

(b) *Agglutination* : Organisms are identified by slide agglutination with specific anti- serum.

(c) *Serology* : Rising antibody titres may be found in serum in children over one year.

Infections of lungs

Pneumonia may be defined as inflammation and consolidation of the lung substance. It may be caused by (a) microorganisms, (b) physical, and (c) chemical agents.

Table 76.3. Bacterial causes of lung infection

Disease	Causative organism
Pneumonia	Str. pneumoniae
Lobar pneumonia	Str. pneumoniae
Bronchopneumonia	Str. pneumoniae, H. influenzae (rarely, Staph. aureus, Kl. pneumoniae)
Atypical pneumonia	M. pneumoniae, C. psittaci, C. pneumoniae, Coxiella burnetti
Legionnaire disease	Legionella pneumophila
Lung abscess	Str. pneumoniae, Staph. aureus
Aspiration pneumonia	
	Anaerobes – Bacteroides, Prevotella.
	Fusobacteria sp. P. melaninogenicus, peptococcus, peptostreptococcus
Empyema	Str. pneumoniae, Staph. aureus, H. influenzae.

Types of Pneumonia

Infective pneumonia are to three types :

1. *Lobar pneumonia* is an acute inflammation characterised by homogeneous consolidation of one or more lobes or segments of lung.
2. *Bronchopneumonia* is a secondary pneumonia preceded by bronchial infection. It is an acute inflammation of bronchi, especially the terminal bronchioles which are filled with pus, the consolidation is scattered and distributed bilaterally in small patches.
3. *Atypical pneumonia.* There is patchy consolidation of lungs. "Mycoplasma pneumoniae" causes atypical pneumonia in which upper respiratory tract infection progresses to pneumonia.
4. *Nosocomial pneumonia.* Patient admitted in hospital for more than 48 hours may develop pneumonia–hospital acquired infection. The most common causes are : *Str. pneumoniae, Staph. aureus, M. pneumoniae, Legionella pneumophila, E. coli.*

Pneumonia in the immuno-compromised patients. Pulmonary infection is common in patients receiving immuno-suppressive drugs or in congenital or acquired immune deficiencies (AIDS). The common causes are *Pneumocystis carinii, Ps. aeruginosa, Staph. aureus, Aspergillus fumigatus,* Candida albicans, viral infections (CMV), Herpes and *Mycotuberculosis.*

Viruses. Respiratory syncytial virus causes most severe infection in young children as bronchiolitis and broncho-pneumonia. Influenza and para-influenza viruses in a previously healthy adult is rare.

Laboratory diagnosis of Lung disease

Specimen : Early morning sputum sample is most purulent. Sample taken properly with minimal salivary contamination should be despatched immediately to the laboratory. In the diagnosis of lobar pneumonia, blood culture should be helpful.

Microscopy

1. *Gram stained smear*. Adequate number of pus cells and presence of organisms is due to the probable pathogen.
2. *Ziehl-Neelsen or Auramine stained smear*. Presence of Acid Fast Bacilli (AFB) is an indication of tuberculosis.

Culture : Purulent sputum is best for culture.

Blood agar. After inoculation, the medium is incubated aerobically at 37°C. Isolate later confirmed.

Chocolate agar is a selective medium for *H. influenzae*. It is incubated at 37°C in 5-10% CO_2.

Culture for mycobacteria

Lowenstein-Jensen medium is inoculated with three samples of sputum collected on three successive days, then incubated aerobically at 37°C for 6-8 weeks (long incubation period) LJ medium is screw capped to avoid evaporation of medium during long incubation period.

Detection of bacterial antigens

A rapid diagnosis of Pneumocystis carinii and Legionella pneumophila can be done by fluorescent antibody staining of bronchial lavage and respiratory secretions, respectively.

Serological tests

When the causative organisms are difficult to isolate, serological tests should be undertaken:

Table 76.4. Serological tests in atypical pneumonia

Causative bacteria	Serological test	Diagnostic titre
Mycoplasma pneumoniae	Complement fixation	256
Coxiella burnetti	Complement fixation	256
Legionella Pneumophilia	Indirect immuno-fluorescence	256
Chlamydia pneumoniae	Complement fixation, ELISA	256
Chlamydia psittaci	Complement fixation; ELISA	256

77
Urinary Tract Infections

After respiratory tract infection, the next common site for infection is the urinary tract. Infection of urinary tract (UTI–Urinary tract infection) is defined as bacteriuria, i.e. the multiplication of the organisms in urinary tract and the presence of more than a hundred thousand (10^5) organisms per ml in the midstream sample of urine (MSU).

Pyuria means the presence of pus cells in urine and it occurs after the urinary tract infection. Normally, urinary tract (renal tissue, ureters, bladder and proximal urethra) is sterile, in distal urethra, many species of bacteria are encountered as transient flora, they are derived from the faecal flora (E. coli, Klebsiella sp., etc).

Types of UTI

UTI is divided into two categories :

A. **Lower tract infection** : (1) Urethritis; (2) Cystitis; (3) Prostatitis.

B. **Upper tract infection** : (1) Acute pyelitis–infection of pelvis of kidney; (2) Acute pyelonephritis–infection of parenchyma of kidney.

Factors limiting multiplication of organism

Certain factor normally play an important role in limiting the bacteria multiplication as the urine is a good culture medium :

1. A high rate of urine flow.
2. Regular complete bladder emptying.
3. Constant dilution of residual urine in the bladder by inflow from kidney.
4. Mucosal defences act by rapid clearing of bacteria from the mucosa.
5. Local antibody, complement and lysozyme may also give protection.
6. Secretions of prostate and periurethral glands possess antibacterial activity.

Factors favouring multiplication of organism

The ability of urine to support the growth of bacteria depends on pH, osmolality and chemical constituents:

1. pH 6.0–7.0 favours bacterial growth.
2. *Osmolality.* Lowered osmolality of urine encourages bacteriurial multiplication and decreases with the return of increasing concentrating ability.

3. *Glucose* provides source of energy for bacterial growth.
4. *Obstruction*–to urine flow.

Clinical features

1. **Asymptomatic :** Symptomless urinary tract infection or "Covert bacteriuria" is common. Adult women (5%), girls (1–3%), and boys (0.3%) have covert bacteriuria that can be detected only by urine culture.
2. **Symptomatic :** Symptoms are dysuria, frequency, suprapubic pain along with loin pain and tenderness. There may be fever and rigors. Fever is associated with pyelonephritis.

UTI is more frequent in women than men. Almost 50% women suffer from UTI during their adult lives. In males, incidence is much less and, in persons over 60, UTI due to enlarged prostate is common.

Predisposing factors

1. *Gender and sexual activity.* Females are more frequently affected by UTI (particularly cystitis) due to following reasons :
   (a) *Female urethra* is prone to colonisation of Gram-negative bacilli because it is close to anus.
   (b) *Short length of urethra* favours the introduction of bacteria into the bladder.
2. *Pregnancy.* Pregnancy predisposes the upper urinary tract due to :
   (a) Dilatation of ureters and renal pelvis.
   (b) Stasis in ureter up to the brim of pelvis. Dilatation and stasis are partially caused by pressure of the enlarged pregnant uterus on the ureter of the brim of pelvis.
   (c) Temporary *incompetence* of vesico-urethral valves.
3. *Other factors* :
   (a) *Obstruction* to flow the urine (tumour, stone, stricture, prostatic hypertrophy)
   (b) *Neurogenic bladder dysfunction* (spinal cord, injury, multiple sclerosis).
   (c) *Vesico-ureteral reflux* (reflux of urine from bladder into ureters and sometimes in the renal pelvis).
   (d) *Bacterial virulence.*
   (e) *Genetic factors* (genetically determined receptors on uroepithelial cells).

Causal organisms

A. Gram-negative bacilli

They are the most infecting agents :

1. *Escherichia coli* is the commonest cause of UTI in acute infection (60–90%) in general population without urologic abnormalities or calculi and 50% of hospital acquired infection.

Sero groups (02, 04, 06, 07, 08, 075) of *E. coli* are well adapted to enter the urinary tract and form majority of isolates of UTI.

Factors associated with *virulence* of *E. coli* are :

(a) *K. antigens* that inhibit phagocytosis and bactericidal effects of complement.
(b) Bacterial *adhesion* to receptors on urò-epithelium by specialised fimbriae .

2. Klebsiella sp.
3. Proteus sp. specially P. mirabilis.
4. Enterobactor, Ps. aeruginosa, serratia.

Though *Klebsiella, Proteus, Pseudomonas, Enterobacter*, and *Serratia* are responsible for a small number of uncomplicated infections. They gain importance in hospital acquired infection and infections associated with urologic manipulation, calculi or obstruction. Proteus sp. due to production of urease and *Klebsiella sp.* through the production of extracellular lime and polysaccharide predispose to formation of stone and are more frequently associated with UTI with Calculi.

B. Gram-positive cocci

They are not much associated with UTI :

1. *Enterococci* are normal flora of the intestine. They are common in urine as contaminants. Sometime they cause urinary tract infection after invasive procedure.

2. *Staph. saprophyticus* is a true primary pathogen of urinary tract and causes urethritis and cystitis (2–3%) in sexually active or healthy young females. *Staph. epidermidis* and micrococci are common contaminants of urine.

Staph. aureus and *Enterococci* cause urinary infection in individuals with renal calculi or after instrumentation. Isolation of *Staph. aureus* in urine is suggestive of localised lesions of the kidney or is secondary to prostatectomy or catheterisation.

Acute uncomplicated urinary infection is caused by one predominant organism (*E.coli*).

Chronic complicated infection is often associated with more than one type of organisms (*E.coli*–commonest; *Klebsiella, Enterobacter, Proteus, Citrobacter*)

Table 77.1 : Bacteria in Urinary tract infection

Organism	Domiciliary—Uncomplicated	Hospital—Complicated
Escherichia coli	80	50
P.mirabilis; other Proteus	8	12–15
Klebsiella sp.	8	12–20
Staph. saprophyticus	0.1	1–2
Staph. epidermidis	0–1	1–2
Enterococci	0–1	4–5
Enterobacter Citrobacter sp Acinetobacter sp	<1	<1
Ps. aeruginosa	0–1	5–12
Staph. aureus	0	<1

Pathogenesis and source of infection

1. *Ascending route.* In most of the cases, urinary infection is ascending from the perineum; aided in females by short distance between urethra and anus, interposition of the vaginal introitus and the shortness of urethra.

The distal urethra and vaginal introitus are normally colonised by lactobacilli, streptococci, diphtheria and staphylococci but not by enteric bacilli that are normally responsible for urinary tract infection.

Factors predisposing to periurethral colonisation by enteric bacilli :

(a) alteration of the normal perineal flora by antibiotics or by contraceptives, especially diaphragm and spermicide.

(b) faecal incontinence in infants.

(c) entrance of periurethral bacteria inside bladder during intercourse.

(d) poor hygienic habits in adults.

2. Haematogenous route

In the aetiology of UTI, haematogenous spread is rare. It may play an important role in renal infection of the newborn. In many infections, bacteriaemia occurs. Bacteriaemia may lead to abscess formation in renal parenchyma or mere excretion of the organism in the urine.

Laboratory diagnosis

Before treatment, culture of urine is of great necessity for identification of the organism, antimicrobial susceptibility test and assessment of the result of treatment.

Specimen

Specimen of urine should be in sufficient quantity, and it should be free from urethra and genital tract contamination.

1. **Mid-stream specimen of urine** (MSSU/MSU). Before collecting a sample of urine, the women should be instructed to swab the vulva and men to retract the foreskin and clean the glans penis. The patient begins to pass urine in toilet or bedpan. The first portion is allowed to pass, then without interruption of the urine flow, midstream of the urine is collected in sterile wide-mouthed container or test tube and the terminal portion of urine stream is passed into the toilet or bed pan.

   The first portion of urine flushes out the normal flora. MSU is most ideal for culture for diagnosing bacterial cystitis and quantitative examination for presence of significant bacteria.

2. **Catheter specimen (CSU).** In catheterised patients, urine should be collected directly from the catheter which should not touch the container.

3. **Urine specimen from infants.** A clean catch specimen obtained carefully produces excellent result, the catheterisation should not be advocated because of the risk of introducing infection.

Transport

It there will be delay in transporting within 2 hours to the laboratory, the specimen should be preserved as :

(a) Refrigeration at 4°C.

(b) Dip slide coated on both sides, with culture medium is inoculated by dipping into freshly passed urine and keeping in a sterile container for transport and growth can be observed after incubating.

Laboratory methods

After sending a portion of urine sample to the laboratory for cultural test the rest is examined immediately under microscope.

I. **Microscopy**

(a) Direct examination of deposit bacteria, pus cells, epithelial cells can be detected by microscopic examination of centrifuged deposit of urine.

Pyuria is associated with most of the clinical infections but may be absent in symptomless bacteriuria. Pus cells with RBCs are usually found in haemorrhagic cystitis. Pyuria without bacteriuria may indicate renal tuberculosis.

Microscopical examination of deposit also reveals urinary casts, red cells, tubular epithelial cells or atypical cells that will indicate non-infective renal lesion such as glomerulonephritis or tumour.

(b) *Gram stained smear* of deposit may show white cells and bacteria that may have come from genital or urinary tract.

B. Culture

I. *Media* : (1) Blood agar; (2) MacConkey's agar

II. *Semiquantative culture* . Most laboratories use this technique by *standard loop*. Dip slide technique is useful while examining large quantity of urine specimens.

Standard loop technique

A standard calibrated loop is used for transferring a fixed volume of undiluted urine to culture medium and incubated overnight. Next day the number of colonies obtained is counted.

Say, the fixed volume loop used can hold 0.04 ml. The total viable bacterial count per ml sample = Number of colonies × 250. When number of colonies formed in plate, say 400 — i.e. 100, 000 or 10^5 organisms per ml. of unspun urine sample.

Dip Slide

Commercially available plastic slides coated with Cysteine lactose electrolyte deficient (CLED) agar on one side and MacConkey's agar on the other side is dipped into the freshly voided urine and replaced in a sterile container and incubated. Viable count is obtained by comparing the growth on the media with the manufacturer's charts. Though this technique is costly, it avoids the problems of transport of specimen to the laboratory and is useful in screening for significant bacteriuria in busy out-patient department (e.g. antenatal clinic).

Interpretation of results

(a) More than 100,000 (10^5) viable bacteria of a single species per ml : *Significant growth*, sensitive test is to be done.

(b) Between 10,000 to 100,000 bacteria per ml : of *doubtful significance*, further specimens are to be cultured.

(c) Less than 10,000 bacteria per ml : no *significant growth* regarded as contaminants.

III. *Identification of the organism* is performed by biochemical and/or serological tests.

Bacteriuria of pregnancy

The prevalence of significant bacteriuria in pregnancy is 5% in first trimester rising to 10% at term. About 25% of these women with symptomless bacteriuria eventually develop clinical episodes during pregnancy. These women require antimicrobial treatment. If these infections persist and become chronic, they may progress to cause hypertension and ultimate renal failure.

If the bacteriuria responds to treatment during pregnancy, the risk of pyelonephritis is prevented; but if the patients have not received treatment or did not respond to treatment, acute pyelonephritis develops in 30% bacteriuric women with pregnancy.

Hospital urinary infection

About 75% hospital acquired urinary tract infections occur after urethral catheterization or instrumentation.

Source of infection

1. *Endogenous* : Contamination of individual's urethra and perineum by his own intestinal flora.
2. *Exogenous* : Cross-infection with bacteria from urinary tract of another patient through instrument (Cystoscope, Catheter) or hands of nurses and doctors.

Tuberculosis of kidney and urinary tract

Tuberculosis of kidney is a blood-borne infection. Early lesions occur in blood vessel surrounding the glomeruli. Then these microscopic foci expand and erode into pelvis and spread downwards to bladder. In many cases, epididymis and seminal vesicles are infected.

The patients present with increased frequency and painless hematuria and urine shows numerous pus cells and RBCs but routine culture does not show any urinary pathogen. Tuberculosis can be considered in cases of pyuria without bacteriuria.

Specimen

Tubercle bacilli are excreted from kidney intermittently, so MSU is not useful. Early morning urine should be collected in sterile container on three consecutive days which are to be preserved in the refrigerator till examined.

Laboratory methods

Preparation of concentrate (Petroff's method)

Urine is decontaminated by treatment with 4% sodium hydroxide for 15–30 minutes. After centrifugation the deposit is neutralised with N/10 or 8% hydrochloric acid in presence of an indicator (e.g. phenol red) :

1. *Ziehl–Neelsen film* : Smear made from decontaminated deposit may reveal acid-alcohol fast bacilli which have to be excluded from saprophytic mycobacteria (e.g. *M. smegmatis)* that may be present in normal urine.
2. *Culture* : Lowenstein-Jensen medium is inoculated with the uncontaminated urine deposit and incubated for 6-8 weeks.

78

Meningitis

Leptomeningitis is an inflammation of the membranes surrounding the brain and spinal cord (paraarachnoid). It may be caused by viruses, bacteria, fungi and protozoa.

Infection may occur either through the blood (blood borne) or by direct spread along sinuses and veins from other parts of the body.

Acute pyogenic meningitis may be caused by pyogenic organisms and tuberculous meningitis by *M. tuberculosis*.

Acute pyogenic meningitis

Diagnosis of acute pyogenic meningitis is done by the direct examination of cerebrospinal fluid (CSF).

A clear indication of the causal organisms of meningitis can be obtained by chemical and cytological examination of CSF (Table). The CSF usually contains more than 1,000 leukocytes per cu. mm, 90–95% of which are polymorphonuclear leukocytes. The protein content is elevated, often more than 100 mg % and the glucose level is markedly diminished or even absent.

Table 78.1 : Cerebrospinal fluid in meningitis

Features	Normal CSF	Pyogenic meningitis	Tubercular meningitis	Viral meningitis
Pressure	Normal	Highly increased	Moderately increased	Slightly increased
Chemical				
(Total protein)	30–45% mg	Highly increased 100–600mg %	Slightly increased (100–120 mg %)	Slightly increased (60–80 mg %)
Sugar	40–80 mg %	Diminished (10–20 mg % or absent)	Diminished (30–50 mg %)	Normal
Cell count				
Total cell per cu. mm.	1–3	1000–20000	50–500	4–10
Type of cell	Lymphocytes	Neutrophils (3–98%) Lymphocytes 10%	Lymphocytes 90%	Lymphocytes 2%
Bacteriological				
Gram film	Nil	Gram negative/positive cocci/bacilli found		
Acid fast film	Nil	Acid fast bacilli found		

A. Causative organism

1. *N. meningitidis*
2. *Str. pneumoniae*
3. *H. influenzae*
4. *Staph. aureus*
5. *Listeria monocytogenes*
6. *Gram positive/negative organisms*
7. *E.coli, Proteus, Klebsiella, Citrobacter, Enterobacter, Serratia.*

B. In neonates

1. *E.coli*
2. *Str. agalactiae group B*
3. *L. monocytogenes*
4. *Klebsiella*

The incidence of various types of meningitis varies greatly with the age of the patient. *E.coli,* Str. haemolyticus group B and Staph. aureus are important causes in infants of first few months. Meningitis due to H. influenzae is common between 3 months to 5 years of age. Meningococcal and pneumococcal meningitis can occur at any age.

Infection due to *L.monocytogenes* is found in neonates and immuno-compromised host.

Certain fungi (*Cryptococcus neoformans, Histoplasma capsulatum, Coccidioides immitis, Candida albicans and* Aspergillus) may occasionally cause meningitis. They are found in immuno-compromised patients (e.g. those with leukemia, lymphoma, AIDS or on immuno-suppressive drug).

Laboratory diagnosis

CSF is obtained by lumbar puncture. The fluid should be examined immediately after collection. The fluid is collected in 3 separate sterile vials — one for cell count; one for chemical examination and one for culture The type of meningitis can be indicated by routine chemical examination and cell count.

A. *Microscopy*

Microscopy examination of smear made from centrifuged deposit will show plenty of pus cells and few Gram-negative or Gram-positive bacteria.

B. *Culture*

1. CSF Blood agar, Chocolate agar, and cooked meat medium are inoculated with the centrifuged deposit and incubated for 24 hours in 5–10% CO_2.

   The isolates were identified by biochemical and serological test.
2. *Blood.* Blood culture is useful and may be positive in about 50% of cases of meningitis due to N. meningitidis, *H. influenzae* and *Str. pneumoniae.*

C. *Demonstration of bacterial products.*

1. *Bacterial antigens* can be detected by immunological test (latex agglutination) counter current immunoelectrophoresis. (CIEP) and ELISA using specific antisera to common sero group A, C of N. meningitidis, H. influenzae and Str. pneumoniae.
2. *Bacterial endotoxins.* The limulus lysate test is specific and sensitive for the detection of bacterial endotoxin.

Tubercular meningitis

In this infection CSF shows moderate rise in :

(a) Cell count (50–500 per cu.mm) — most of them are lymphocytes.

(b) Protein (80–120 mg %).

(c) Sugar is diminished (30–50 mg %).

Ziehl-Neelsen stained smear of centrifuged deposit reveals few lymphocytes with few *M. tuberculosis*.

Culture : After inoculation of centrifuged deposit of urine on L-J medium and incubation for 6-8 weeks, M. tuberculosis colony is formed.

79
Common Nosocomial Infections

1. *Urinary tract infection*–About 40% of hospital acquired infections occur in the urinary tract and are usually associated with catheterisation and instrumentation of urethra, bladder or kidneys. Initial infection is caused by *Esh. coli*, *Staph. epidermidis* and *Enterococcus*, but later on invaded by *Klebsiella*, *Proteus*, *Serratia*, *Pseudomonas* and Providencia sp.
2. *Infection of the lower respiratory tract*–Some (15–20%) of all hospital acquired infections are of the lower respiratory tract which are the leading causes of mortality. The important pathogens are Gram-negative bacilli, *Staph. aureus*. The most frequently recovered Gram-negative bacilli are *Klebsiella*, *Enterobacter*, *Serratia*, *Proteus*, *Esch.coli*, *Ps. aeruginosa*. These organism reach the lower respiratory tract by aspiration from the pharynx causing necrotising bronchopneumonia.
3. *Wound and skin sepsis*–Infection of surgical wounds and other soft tissues is about 18% of the hospital acquired infections. In the elderly patients above the age to 60, the incidence of post-operative infections. The most important predominant pathogen is *Staph. aureus*, which is followed by *Ps. aeruginosa* and other Gram-negative bacilli.

   Gastrointestinal infections–Food poisoning salmonella infection and neonatal septicaemia in hospitals have been reported. Salmonella infection are associated with poultry or meat.

Prevention–can be achieved by following means :

1. *Administration* of *antibiotics* and antiseptic therapy to the carrier staff or source patient to destroy the pathogenic microorganisms. Before administering therapy, the organism is to be isolated and antibiotic sensitivity test is to be done.
2. An infectious patient is to be isolated.
3. *Proper sterilisation* and disinfection of the inanimate objects in the hospital environment should be done. Thus the source of infection can be controlled.
4. *Disinfection* of excreta and infected material is necessary to control the exit point of infection.
5. The *transmission route* is to be controlled by regular hand washing, disinfection of equipment and change of working clothes.
6. By vaccination e.g. tetanus, gas gangrene and Hepatitis B, the *susceptible* host can be protected.

Infection Control Policy

Effective Hospital Acquired Infection Control Committee (HICC) should be set up in every Hospital for good management of hospital.

Hospital Acquired Infection Control Committee.

Chair-person	Medical Superintendent
Member Secretary	Infection control officer (Microbiologist)
Members	Chief of all clinical Units/Departments, Chief of Blood Bank Service, Microbiologist, Medical Record Officer, Chief of Nursing Services, Infection control sister.
Invited members	Chiefs of all supportive service (OT, Dietetics, Laundry, House keeping etc.)

Meeting should be held at least one a month to formulate and update policy for the whole hospital infection and to manage outbreaks of hospital acquired infections. They should also review :

1. Infection control activities of the hospital,
2. Emergence of drug resistance,
3. Use of different antimicrobial agents,
4. Hospital environment,
5. Sterilisation and disinfectant procedure,
6. Incidence and types of infection,
7. Antimicrobial sensitivity pattern of the prevalent pathogens.

HAICC should have a team of workers, Hospital Acquired Infection Control Team (HAICT) for day-to-day responsibility for the policy.

Hospital Acquired Infection Control (HAICT)

Infection Control Officer (ICO)	Microbiologist
Infection Control Sister (ICS)	Hospital Sister
Clinician	One clinician from hospital.

HAICT should meet weekly one and is responsible for :

1. Surveillance,
2. Control of infections,
3. Monitoring of hygienic procedures,
4. *Advising* HAICC on matters of policy regarding prevention of infection and education of all staff regarding microbiologically safe performance of procedures.

Besides, HAICT is also responsible for :

(a) Sterilisation,
(b) Aseptic techniques,
(c) Cleaning and disinfection,
(d) Skin disinfection and antiseptics,
(e) Prophylactic antibiotics,
(f) Protective clothing,
(g) Isolation of patient so that they cannot spread the infection to others.

80

Infections of Skin, Wounds, Burns, Eyes, Sepsis

Superficial skin infections, wounds infections, burn infection, infection of the eyes, peritonitis abscess are included in pyogenic infections which may be termed as "Sepsis".

Skin and soft tissue infection–Human *intact* skin is a barrier to infection. Certain bacteria (*Tr. pallidum, Brucella abortus*) and certain parasites (*Ancylostoma*) can penetrate the intact skin.

Staph. aureus or *Str. pyogenes* or both gain access to broken skin, produce primary skin infection like impetigo.

Infection of skin

Clinical types–Acne is caused by *Propionibacterium acnes*, anaerobic diphtheroids, coagulase negative staphylococci and micrococci.

Toxin of certain organism and free fatty acids may be responsible for acne.

Staphylococcal infection–Staph.aureus causes boils and carbuncles. These are suppurative lesion, with necrosis at the centre. They discharge a slough with pus. Carbuncle, a large abscess, usually occur in thick collagenous tissue such as back of the neck.

Staph. aureus phage group I and II are main causes of boils, carbuncles, styes and sycosis barbae.

Streptococcal infection

1. *Cellulitis*–Superficial infection of subcutaneous tissue.
2. *Erysipelas*–Spreading infection of dermis.
3. *Erythema and impetigo*–Streptococcal impetigo is less common.
4. *Scarlet fever*–Usually associated with infection of throat.

Gram-negative infections are usually encountered in moist area of groin and axilla. Coliforms, Bacteroides sp and Proteus sp. May cause abscess between thigh and waist related to a preceding trauma :

Table 80.1. Bacterial and Viral Pathogens and different types of skin infections

Organism	Infection
Bacteria	
Staph. aureus	Impetigo, Ritter's disease (toxin epidermal necrolysis) folliculitis, furunculosis, carbuncles, sycosis barbae)
Str. pyogenes	Impetigo, erysipelas, cellulitis, pemphigus
Erysipelothrix	Erysipeloid

Rhusiopathiae	
C. diphtheriae	Cutaneous diphtheria
C. ulcerans	
Propionibacterium	Acne pustules
M. tuberculosis	Lupus vulgaris
Acne	
M. cheloniae	Post–trauma abscess
M. fortuitum	
M. marinum	Swimming pool granuloma
M. ulcerans	Buruli ulcer
M. leprae	Leprosy
B. anthracis	Anthrax (malignant pustule)
H. ducreyi	Chancroid
Treponema sp	Syphilis, Yaws
Viruses	
Herpes virus (types)	Cutaneous warts
Herpes viruses (types 1, 2)	Genital wart.
Herpes viruses (types 1, 2)	Herpes, Whitlow, Eczema, Herpeticum.
Pox virus group	Molluscum contagiosum, O, P

Bacteriological diagnosis

Specimen : Pus, exudate, swabs from lesions

Culture : Inoculated blood agar is incubated — both aerobically and anaerobically.

Identification is done by relevant tests.

Infection of wounds

- Infection may occur in accidental or post operative wound due to bacteria :

Table 80.2. Bacterial infection of surgical wound

Organism	Infections
Aerobic	
Staph. aureus	Can infect any wound.
E.coli	Can infect any wound but nor commonly associated with abdominal, urological and gynaecological wounds.
Proteus sp.	
Klebsiella sp.	
Enterococci	
Ps. aeruginosa	
Anaerobic	
B. fragilis	Common in abdominal, gynaecological wounds.
B. melaninogenicus	
Cl. perfringens	

Pathogenesis, wound infection may be :

(a) *Endogenous infection*–Patient's own bacterial flora i.e. *Staph. aureus,* from skin and anterior nares or coliforms.

(b) *Exogenous infection*–Many organisms are exogenous. Staphylococci from skin and anterior nares, organisms from hospital staff and visitors can be spread directly or indirectly by airborne route.

Gram-negative enteric bacilli (60%) and Gram-positive cocci (30%) are responsible for hospital acquired infection. Gram-negative bacilli may be patient's own flora, or in damp environment. Antibiotic resistant organism (*Ps. aeruginosa*) from the environment may colonise the patient, traumatised skin (e.g. wound, burn, bedsore).

Laboratory diagnosis

Specimen : Pus, exudate and tissue from wound.

Microscopy : Direct Gram-stained smear will reveal the organism.

Culture

1. Blood agar
2. MacConkey agar — for aerobic culture
3. Aminoglycoside agar
4. Robertson's cooked meat medium — for anaerobic culture.

Identification : Isolates can be identified by biochemical and serological tests.

Infections of Burns

Within 24 hours the large moist exposed surface of burns is colonised by bacteria (e.g. bacterial flora of skin, respiratory tract and intestine, streptococci and/ anaerobic spore bearing bacilli).

Staph. aureus is the most common isolate from burn, followed by *Ps. aeruginosa* and various enterobacteria (e.g., *Acinetobacter sp.*) and *Str. pyogenes* group A, B, C and D.

Pathogenesis

The air-borne organisms reach the burnt area and invade directly the burnt tissue.

Laboratory diagnosis is similar to that of wound infection.

Prophylaxis–Local application of antimicrobial agents (silver sulphadiazine cream, silver nitrate solution and chlorhexidine cream) reduce the colonisation of bacteria.

Infection of the eyes

Eyelid infection

1. *Stye*–Staph. aureus causes a small boil or abscess in one of the glands of the lash follicle. They would have originated from anterior nares or implanted from a septic lesion on the body.
2. *Infection of lacrimal apparatus*–Infection of glands (dacryoadenitis) occurs from endogenous sources. Dacryoadenitis may be associated with mumps and gonorrhoea.

Conjuctivitis–Because of flushing action of tears and presence of lysozyme that degrades peptidoglycan of the cell wall of Gram-negative bacilli the conjuctival sac is free from bacteria however, *C. xerosis* and *Staph epidermidis* colonise the conjuctival sac.

Conjuctivitis may occur due to conjuctival sac infection by pathogens.

Clinically, it may be acute type, mucopurulent type, non-purulent type and neonatal.

Aetiology

A. *Bacterial agents*

1. *Staph. aureus* causes acute conjuctivitis
2. *H. influenzae*
3. *H. aegypticus*
4. *Moraxella lacunata*
5. *Chlamydia trachomatis*
6. *Str. pneumoniae*

In newborns, conjuctivitis caused by *Staph. aureus* is commonly observed in "Sticky eyes". In older infants and children, infection due to *H. influenzae* and *Str. pneumoniae* is more common.

C. *Trachomatis* (Serovars D–K) causes inclusion conjuctivitis and trachoma (A, B, C). Endemic area, trachoma is very common amongst children and is a very common cause of blindness in the world.

B. *Viral agents*

1. Adeno viruses (types 3, 7, 8, and 14)
2. Herpes viruses (HSV1)

Keratoconjunctivitis is caused by Adeno viruses type 7, 8 and Herpes virus (HSV1).

Neonatal conjuctivitis

Conjuctivitis in neonates may be acquired either during birth from the mother's genital tract or from some other external sources within 3 weeks of birth.

Aetiology

(a) *From the genital tract*–Infection of eye acquired by the newborn during birth is called *"Ophthalmia neonatorum"* :

1. N. gonorrhoeae
2. C. trachomatis (D–K serovars)
3. Goup B haemolytic streptococci.

(b) *From the external source*–Staph. aureus causes sticky eyes in the newborn.

Keratitis

It is inflammation of the cornea. The infective organisms of conjuctivitis can spread deeper into cornea leading to ulcers or a spreading keratitis.

Causes

1. *Herpes virus*
2. Foreign body with secondary infection due to bacteria or fungi.

Mycotic keratitis

Corneal infection by fungus occur secondarily following injury. Saprophytic fungi, *Aspergillus* and *Fusarium* species are the common causes of infection by opportunistic fungi.

Laboratory diagnosis

A. Bacterial infection except Chlamydial

Specimen : Exudate collected by a sterile platinum loop directly from the patient's eye.

Preparation of smear and culture should be done at the bedside.

In case of delay in transport, swab of exudate should be placed in *Stuart's transport medium* and despatched to the laboratory.

Microscopy

Gram-stained smear reveal the presence of causative organisms.

Culture–Material is cultured on blood agar, and chocolate agar, incubated at 37°C in an atmosphere of 5–10% CO_2.

Identification–Organism are identified by biochemical test and serotyping.

B. Chlamydial infection

Specimen : Scrapings from conjunctiva.

Microscopy–Film is examined by immunofluorescence.

Culture –Tissue culture is performed in cycloheximide treated or irradiated McCoy cells for 2–3 days.

Identification–The organism produce intracytoplasmic inclusion which are identified by Giemsa stain or immunofluorescence.

C Mycotic infections

Specimen : Scrapings from the base or edge of corneal ulcer.

Microscopy

1. In 10% KOH mount, the fungi appear as branched, septate hyphae
2. *Methenamine silver or PAS staining* shows filamentous fungi with hyphae.

Culture : Scraping material is inoculated on Sabouraud's dextrose agar.

Orbital cellulitis

It is serious infection of the cellular tissue of the orbit. It may usually result from spread of infection from adjacent tissue (teeth and sinuses).

Complications are panophthalmitis, brain abscess, meningitis. Painful swelling and protrusion of the eyeball may occur.

Aetiology

Staph. aureus and other pyogenic organisms can cause orbital cellulitis.

Laboratory diagnosis

Specimen of pus collected by surgical incision can be subjected to the laboratory examination which is similar to that of conjunctivitis.

Panophthalmitis

It is an inflammation of whole substance of the eye derived from infections of the outer eyes, foreign bodies and penetrating wounds (traumatic or surgical).

Aetiology

1. *Staph. aureus*
2. Gram negative enteric bacteria (*Ps. aeruginosa*, Proteus sp., Klebsiella sp., E. coli, Enterobacter sp)

Diagnosis–Pus aspirated from the anterior chamber of the eye should be cultured.

Choroiditis and Chorioretinitis

Aetiology : Bacterial, viral, fungal, protozoal infections may cause granulomatous lesion of choroid and retina.

Bacteria : M. tuberculosis, Br. abortus, Tr. pallidum.

Virus : Congenital rubella, CMV

Fungus : C. albicans

Protozoa : Toxoplasma gondii

Helminths. Toxocara canis causes retinitis.

Diagnosis can be done by skin and diagnostic test.

81
Bacteremia, Septicaemia, Endocarditis

Septicaemia

Bacteremia is a condition in which the bacteria are simply present in blood without multiplication.

Septicaemia is a condition in which bacteria circulate and actively multiply in the blood. Pyaemia is primarily septicaemia with metastatic infection.

Endotoxaemia is a condition in which bacterial endotoxin circulates in the blood. Blood in the circulation is sterile.

Bacteria may invade the blood (a) from an infective focus

(b) by introduction of contaminated material into the circulatory system.

The microorganisms are cleared from the blood quickly when the immune system of the host is good. When the immune system is not working the microorganisms persist and multiply in the blood, producing signs and symptoms. "Septic shock" is a condition in which hypotension and signs of inadequate perfusion develop.

Types of septicaemia

Generalised infection–When bacteremia/septicaemia is of greater severity and of longer duration as in brucellosis and enteric fever, there will be generalised infection as basic feature.

Complications of more localised infection

When the organisms spread from localised infective focus into the blood stream, the complications (pyelonephritis, cholangitis, pneumonia, peritonitis, osteomyelitis, abscesses of internal organs) may be observed.

Causative microorganisms of septicaemia

A. *Gram-negative bacilli (60–70%)*

1. Salmonella
   (a) S. typhi.
   (b) S. paratypi A
   (c) S. paratyphi B
   (d) S. paratyphi C
2. Brucella sp.
3. H. influenzae

4. E. coli
5. Klebsiella pneumoniae
6. Proteus mirabilis, Pr. vulgaris.
7. Enterobacter sp.
8. Bacteroides sp.

B. *Gram positive cocci* (20-40 %)

1. Staph. aureus
2. Str. pneumoniae
3. Str. pyogenes.

C. *Gram-positive bacilli*

In pre-antibiotic era, pneumococci and streptococci were most common causes of septicaemia. Now, Gram-negative enteric bacteria (60–70%) are common causes of septicaemia, staphylococci, pneumococci, streptococci are less (20–40%) frequent causes of septicaemia.

E. coli is often isolated from culture at U.K. About 40% Gram-negative bacilli bacteriaemia is complicated by shock, while 10–15% Gram-positive bacteriaemia is complicated by shock. Shock is mediated by various bacterial products in the blood, in particular Gram-negative *endotoxin*. Predisposing factors play a great role in septicaemia.

Table 81.1 : Predisposing factors in Septicaemia

Predisposing causes	Causal microorganism
Abdominal abscess (peritonitis, liver abscess, retroperitoneal abscess)	Coliforms, B. fragilis, Str. faecalis
Infected wounds, burns, abscess	Staph. aureus. Str. pyogenes, Coliforms.
Gynaecological sepsis (puerperal infection, pelvic abscess, salpingitis)	Coliforms, Str. faecalis, Bacteroides, Str. pyogenes, haemolytic group B streptococci
Osteomyelitis, septic arthritis	Staph. aureus
Pneumonia	Str. pneumoniae, H.influenzae
Meningitis	Str. pneumoniae N. meningitids H. influenzae
Meningitis in neonates	Coliform, group B streptococci
Food poisoning	Salmonella sp., Campylobacter sp.
Urinary infection	Coliform, Str. faecalis.

Infective Endocarditis

Endocarditis is mostly causd by bacteria, rarely by fungus.

It can be divided into :

(a) native valve endocarditis,
(b) endocarditis of prosthetic valve, and
(c) endocarditis in drug abuses.

Clinical types

Clinically and pathologically, endocarditis may be (a) subacute (b) acute (c) postoperative.

Table 81.2. Aetiology of infective endocarditis incidence (%)

Microorganism	Incidence (%)
Bacteria	
1. Viridans streptococci (Str. sanguis, Str. mutans, Str. minor, Str. milleri, Stro. bovis)	60–70
2. Enterococcus (Str. faecalis)	60–70
3. Staph. aureus	20–30
4. Staph. epidermidis	10
5. Other bacteria (Diphtheroids, Haemophilus sp. Coliform, Pseudomonas, bacteroids)	10
6. Coxiella, burnetti, C. psittaci	Rare
Fungi	
1. C. albicans	Rare
2. Aspergillus	Rare

The bacteria settle in the previously damaged heart valve. The disease of native valve evolves into two main forms—depending on the type of infecting bacteria. Acute endocarditis is rapidly progressive and fulminating, subacute is mild and runs a chronic course. The correlation between organism and course is not perfect, because infection with *Staph. aureus* can be associated with sub-acute course and viridans streptococci with an acute course.

A. Subacute endocarditis

When damaged or defective valve cups is infected by an organism of low virulence, large firm vegetations comprising of dense fibrin and platelets aggregates with bacteria colonies are formed. Subacute endocarditis is more common and comprises of almost 70% cases of bacterial endocarditis. It does not produce metastatic foci and, if untreated, takes more than 6 weeks and even a year to be fatal.

Causative agents

1. *Viridans streptococci* (most commonly Str. sanguis, Str. mutans, Str. minor) are responsible for 60–80% cases of subacute endocarditis. 2 Other pathogens — Str. faecalis (Syn.Enterococci), *Staph. epidermidis, C. burnetti, Str. milleri, Str. bovis.*

Fungi, C. albicans, Aspergillus are opportunistic pathogens following antibiotic use and immunosuppressants.

B. Acute endocarditis

In this condition, highly virulent pyogenic bacteria (Staph. aureus) affect both normal and abnormal (damaged, defective) valves. The tricuspid valve is more frequently affected. Vegetations are large and crumbling. Valve destruction is greater than in subacute endocarditis. It is rapidly progressive disease and, if untreated, it is fatal in less than 6 weeks.

Causative agents

1. *Staph. aureus* causes about 25% of native endocarditis. It is also an important cause of hospital acquired endocarditis.
2. *Str. pneumoniae* is responsible for about 10 percent cases of endocarditis.
3. Other pyogenic cocci, *Str. pyogenes* and Str. agalactiae (group B) are responsible for 5–6% cases of acute endocarditis.

C. Post-operative endocarditis

Following surgery in which prosthetic valve or other intravascular prosthesis is done, *post-operative endocarditis* develops. Some 5-10 percent cases with prosthetic valves develop this condition due to infection of prosthetic valves.

Causative agents

1. *Staph. epidermidis* is the most common cause organism (27–74% cases).
2. *Staph. aureus* causes 10% cases of prosthetic valve endocarditis.
3. C. albicans (0.5–1.5%).

Endocarditis associated with intravenous drug abuses

In drug abuses most infections occur in tricuspid valve.

Causative agents

1. *Staph. aureus* is responsible for 50% cases.
2. Other organisms–(*Viridans streptococci, fungi, C. albicans, pseudomonas aeruginosa* account for 1–15% cases).

Pathogenesis

Those with pre-existing cardiac diseases are at risk.

Predisposing cardiac diseases are :

1. *Rheumatic valvular disease* (25–30%). Stenosis and incompetence of mitral valve is most common, followed by that of aortic valve.
2. *Congenital valve deformities* (10–20%) e.g. biscupid arotic valve, septal defects, patent ductus arteriosus, coarctation of the aorta.
3. *Intra-cardiac disease* (10–12%) replacement of diseased heart valves with prosthetic valve.
4. *Degenerative cardiac disease* (5%). Calcified aortic stenosis, Syphilitic aortic valve disease.
5. *Drug abuse*–Drug abusers who take drugs intravenously are at risk of endocarditis.

Hospital acquired native-valve endocarditis

Intravascular devices (peripheral-venous, central-venous, pulmonary artery, catheterisation) sometimes lead to endocarditits of normal heart valve. Traumatically induced sterile vegetations may become infected after bacteriaemia.

Staph. aureus (80%) and C. albicans, Aspergillus, Acinetobacter (20%) cause hospital acquired native-valve endocarditis.

Laboratory diagnosis

Blood culture is the important diagnosis before antimicrobial therapy, blood should be as collected.

Specimen : Three to six samples of blood, 10 ml each, are to be collected from antecubital vein over 24 hours. Blood sample should be inoculated into a (50–100 ml) of glucose broth medium. One culture should be obtained from each vene puncture using anaerobic and aerobic techniques. Addition of pyridoxal hydrochloride improves the chances of isolating nutritionally deficient variant streptococci.

Large volume of blood and media

Advantages

(a) Since the number of organisms in the blood may be very few, even one/ml, at least 10 ml of blood is needed.

(b) Large volume of culture medium is also of great necessity to dilute the effect of bactericidal substances present in the patient's blood.

(c) The bactericidal effect of substances detrimental to the growth of bacteria can be inhibited by certain substances like bile salts.

Cultivation : Cultures should be incubated at 37°C and observed daily for growth of bacteria (colony) on the medium, then Gram-staining should be done and subcultured on blood agar aerobically or anaerobically, for at least 3 weeks before cultures are discarded as negative.

Antibiotic sensitivity test

The routine disk diffusion technique with fixed concentration of drug is not adequate for guiding treatment of infective endocarditis. The measurement of the minimum inhibitory concentration (MIC) and minimum bactericidal concentration (MBC) of the antimicrobial agents should be determined. It would be helpful to determine adequate dose of the antibiotic to be used to ensure the serum levels that can penetrate the valves and kill the organisms.

Culture negative endocarditits

Several reasons are suggested for persistent negative blood culture :

1. *Recent antibiotic therapy* : Infective endocarditis are caused by streptococci that are susceptible to a wide range of antibiotics. Some of these cases will recover, while in others the organisms disappear temporarily from the blood. In such cases, repeated blood cultures done after the stoppage of antibiotics may become positive.
2. *Infection by fastidious or slow growing organisms* :These organisms will not grow easily on ordinary media. They require special media with adequate period of incubation (e.g. *Hemophilus influenzae, Bacteroides, Actinobacillus, β–haemolytic streptococci*). When these organisms are suspected, repeated blood cultures should be done by using special media.
3. *Bacteriaemia is intermittent* : In this situation repeated blood cultures are necessary.
4. Infection with *C. burnetti or Chlamydia psittaci*. They will not be isolated by blood culture, the serological tests (CFT) using both phase I and II antigens will give titres above 250.
5. Sometimes laboratory isolates are reported as contaminants, e.g., *Staph. epidermidis* may be causative agent.

Other tests

1. *Electrocardiograms* will show vegetation and valve changes in 75–80% cases of native valve endocarditis.
2. *Leucocytosis,* elevated ESR are common. Measurement of *C–reactive protein* in blood is sometimes more reliable than ESR to assess the progress of the disease.

Treatment

Basically, antibiotic treatment is same in any case of endocarditis.

1. *Combined therapy* : Use of two drugs in combination is preferred and should be bactericidal for the pathogen (Table 81.3). Infecting organism may be very sensitive to antibiotics, but the drug cannot reach the organism within the vegetation in adequate concentration where the bacteria are present in large numbers. Hence antibiotics should be given in high doses where possible and preferably intravenously to eliminate the organisms in vegetation.

Table 81.3. Antibiotic treatment infective endocarditis

Organism	Antibiotic	Period
Viridans streptococci highly sensitive to penicillin	1. Penicillin (1–2gm) Gentamicin (80 mg)	IV, 6 hourly, 2 weeks
	Followed by – 2. Ampicillin (oral) 500 mg.	orally 6 hourly, 2 weeks
Streptococcus less sensitive to penicillin	As above, but continue Gentamicin for 4 weeks	
Staphylococcus	Flucloxacillin 2 gm	I.V. 6 hourly, 6 weeks
	Fusidic acid–500 mg	I.V. 8 hourly, 6 weeks
Staphylococcus in patients allergic to penicillin	Vancomycin 500 mg	I.V. 6 hourly
	Fusidic acid 500 mg	I.V.
Anaerobic streptococci	Benzyl penicillin 1–2 gm.	I.V., 6 hourly, 4–6 weeks,
	Metronidazole–500 mg	Oral/I.V., 8 hourly
C. burnetti, Chlamydia psittaci	Tetracycline 500 mg–1gm	I.V. 12 hourly, 4 weeks

2. *Prolonged therapy*–Treatment should be done for a minimum period of 4 weeks. With intravenous antibiotics and for certain organisms 4 to 8 week may be needed.

Laboratory monitoring of therapy

While treating a case of endocarditis minimum bactericidal concentration (MBC) of the antibiotic is estimated in European countries, particularly when there is switch over to oral therapy.

Prevention : (1) Good dental health, (2) Prophylactic antibiotic cover before dental extraction and other surgical procedure can be useful in the prevention of endocarditis.

82
Hospital Acquired Infections (nosocomial infections)

Since antiquity, the hospitals were regarded as *source* of infections to patients after admission. There was necessity to isolate patients with infectious diseases and it was a great success to bring a dramatic reduction in infection rate by the introduction of handwashing with chlorinated lime. Surgeon Joseph Lister introduced (1865) his antiseptic surgery by the use of carbolic acid. After discovery of pathogenic bacteria in the early 20th century, *Str. pyogenes* infection in burn and post-operative infection has become important. In a survey by WHO (1992) the prevalence of *hospital acquired infection* was reported as 3–21% with a mean of 8.4%. The hospital infections have a mortality of about 1%.

Hospital acquired infections are also called as *nosocomial infections* (from *nosocomion*, meaning hospital) are defined as infections developing in patients after admission to the hospital. The infection may manifest during their stay in the hospital or after the patient is discharged.

Factor influencing infection

1. *Age* : Neonates and elderly of extreme ages may acquire hospital infection because of their long stay in hospitals and inefficient immunity.
2. *Infected patients* : Patient with community acquired or non-hospital infection due to pathogenic microorganisms may enter the hospital and spread the infection to close contents (susceptible patients and attending staff).
3. *Drug resistance* : The drug resistant organisms (*Coliforms*, and *Staph. aureus*) may show increased virulence or transmissibility as well as limiting the choice of therapy.
4. *Susceptible patients* : Hospitalised patients with pre-existing diseases (diabetes, immunosuppression, patients in special care units or with prosthetic implants are at risk and more susceptible to hospital infections. Groups of microorganisms previously regarded as non-pathogenic have now emerged as pathogens. These opportunistic organisms are *Staph. epidermidis*, viridans streptococci.
5. *Surgical procedures* : The natural defence mechanisms of the body surface may be bypassed by injury or by a diagnostic or therapeutic intervention such as insertion of a urethral or intravenous catheters. These are *iatrogenic infections.*

Sources

A. *Endogenous* : Many opportunistic infections are caused by the patients own flora "which are not pathogenic under normal conditions but only when there is underlying disease". This is called as *auto-infection* or *autochthonous infection.*

B. *Exogenous* : Hospital infection is mostly exogenous from other people or immediate objects in the environment.

Exogenous sources

1. *Contact with other patients or staff* : Besides patients and hospital personnel suffering from infections or asymptomatic carriers, people are more important sources or reservoirs.
2. *Environmental sources* are inanimate objects, air, water, and food in the hospital.
   (a) *Inanimate objects* : Bedpans, urinals, light, table, blankets, medical equipments (endoscopes, catheters, needles, spatula, and other instruments), floor, food, water (contaminated by kitchen and other hospital staff or visitor). Coliforms are most common in moist environment (fluids in which they can survive for long time and sometimes multiply).
   (b) *Hospital air* : Hospital over-crowding is responsible for an increase in the bacterial count in the hospital air. Hospital air harbours Gram-positive bacteria.
   (c) *Surface* : Surfaces contaminated by patient's excretions, secretions, blood, and body fluids, animals, insects are sources of hospital infections.

Mode of transmission : There are four main routes of infections :

1. *Contact route* is the principal means of transmission of hospital acquired pathogens.

(a) *Hands or clothings* of hospital staff may get contaminated by microorganisms from their own body or other patients. The important vehicle of transmission of hospital infection is the hand of hospital staff. *Staph. aureus, Str. pyogenes, Esch. coli, Klebsiella,* and *Candida albicans* are spread by hand contact. The hand washing by hospital personnel is a significant contribution to control the nosocomial infections.

If patients susceptible to infection are housed in the same ward where the same staff looks after both infected and non-infected patients, there is a great chance of transmission of microorganisms from one person to another by direct contact of hands and clothings of the same hospital personnel.

(b) *Inanimate objects* are reservoirs of pathogenic bacteria which may spread without increasing their numbers, but *Ps. aeruginosa* may multiply in moisture and enhance the risk of infection.

Certain instruments (endoscope, bronchoscope, cytoscope) are difficult to be sterilised because they do not withstand heating; if they are not properly sterilised or disinfected, there is possibility of transmission of pathogenic bacteria through these instruments.

2. *Airborne route* : Transmission by aerial route may occur by :

(a) *Droplet* of respiratory infection is transmitted from one person to another by inhalation.

(b) *Dust* from bedding, floors, exudate, dispersed from a wound during dressing and from the skin from natural shedding of skin scales, spread to the susceptible site e.g. *Ps. aeruginosa, Staph. aureus.*

(c) *Aerosols* produced by nebulizers, humidifiers and air-conditioners transmit certain pathogens (Coliforms, Legionella) to the respiratory tract, if water in the instrument becomes contaminated.

(d) *Oral route* : Antibiotic resistant Gram-negative bacilli are mostly found in hospital food (*Ps. aeruginosa, Esch. coli, Klebsiella sp.*). They may not cause gastroenteritis, but they may colonise in the recipient's intestine and become the faecal flora of these patients.

4. *Parenteral route :* Transmission of infection by parenteral route has become less frequent because of the use of disposable syringe and needle. Certain infections are transmitted by transfusion of contaminated blood. Hepatitis B and HIV infections may be transmitted in this way.

83
Sterilisation and Disinfection

Sterilisation and Disinfection : These two terms are used to describe the killing or removal of microorganisms. Sterilisation is an *absolute term* which denotes the complete killing or removal of microorganisms of all kinds, while the disinfection is a relative term indicating a mere removal of burden of pathogenic imcroorganisms on the article.

Sterilisation is the process of freeing of an article from all living organisms, including viruses, bacteria and their spores, fungi and their spores, both pathogens and non-pathogens. Sterility is an absolute state. An article can never be "relatively sterile".

Sterilisation of culture media, containers and instruments is essential in bacteriological work for the isolation and maintenance of pure culture. In nursing practice, surgery and medicines, the sterilisation of the instruments, drug and other supplies is important for the prevention of the disease and it is also required for medical and surgical instruments and materials used in procedures that involve the penetration into the blood, tissues and other normally sterile parts of the body, e.g., surgical operation, intravenous transfusion, hypodermic injections and diagnostic aspirators.

Disinfection is a method of freeing an article or instrument from some or all living pathogens which may produce the infection during the use of the instruments contaminated with the pathogens. This term is relative since the sterilisation procedures are unwanted and impracticable, the disinfection should be adopted, e.g., bedpans, baths, washbasins, furniture, eating utensils, bed clothes, fomites, which may spread the infection in the hospitals, cannot be sterilised, but they can be easily disinfected. Similarly, it is not practicable to apply sterilising procedures to the skin. The non-spore forming bacteria present in the skin mostly infect the surgical wound, hence it is of great necessity to disinfect the operative site as a valuable preoperative precaution to kill the vegetative bacteria.

Sterilisation can be affected by the following methods :

I. Physical methods

(a) Heat

(I) Dry heat (incineration, red hot, flaming, hot air oven, infrared radiation)

(II) Moist heat (pasteurisation, boiling water, steam steriliser, autoclave).

(b) Radiation

(I) Ultraviolet radiation

(II) Ionising radiation (X–ray, gamma ray).

(c) Filtration (Berkefeld, Chamberland, Seitz, Sintered glass, Cellulose membrane filters).

II. Chemical methods :

STERILISATION

- PHYSICAL
  - HEAT
    - Dry (Incinerator, Red hot, Flaming hot air oven)
    - Moist: Less than 100°C Pasteurisation at 100°C (Arnold or Koch steam steriliser) more than 100°C (autoclave)
  - RADIATION (X, gamma)
  - FILTRATION (Berkefeld Chamberland, Seitz filters)
- CHEMICAL

Basic principles of sterilisation by heat

Moist heat is more effective than dry heat by sterilising at a lower temperature in a given time, or in a shorter time at a given temperature. Moist heat kills the microorganisms by *coagulating* and *denaturating* their *enzymes* and their *structural proteins* — a process in which the water participates. *Sterilisation, e.g., Killing of the moist resistant spores requires exposure to moist heat at 121°C for 10–30 minutes.* Dry heat is believed to kill the microorganisms by causing *destructive oxidation of essential cell constituents. Killing of the most resistant spores by dry heat requires a temperature of about 160°C for 60 minutes.*

Factor influencing sterilisation by heat :

(1) The temperature and time of exposure.

(2) The number of microorganisms and spores.

(3) The species, strains and spore producing bacilli.

1. The temperature and the time of exposure for sterilisation are inversely related. At higher temperature, shorter time exposure is sufficient, e.g., the heating must be hot enough. For surgical and bacteriological sterilisation, and exposure of the organisms to moist heat at 121°C for 10–20 minutes is sufficient for killing of all pathogenic spore forming organisms and all saprophytes except some strict thermophiles which grow best at more than 40°C. Sterilising time (holding period) is the time during which the microbes themselves should be held at the given temperature and *does not include* the heating up time. The amount of time allowed for heating up is known as *heat penetration time.*
2. The rapidity of the sterilisation is affected by *the number of microbes and their spores.* In practice, before applying heat for sterilisation, the cleaning of all the articles or instruments should be done to reduce the burden of contaminated bacteria for better and rapid sterilisation.
3. The susceptibility to heat is affected by *species, strains and spore forming ability of the microorganisms.* The amount of heat required to kill a given strain or species of bacteria is related to the temperature and the time of exposure and it is stated that the *thermal death point* when the lowest temperature is required to kill completely the bacteria within 10 minutes or the thermal death time when the shortest time is required to kill

completely the microbes at a particular temperature. The most reliable method of measurement of the thermal death point and the time of is *the decimal reduction time* or *D value* which is the time (in minutes) required to achieve a ten-fold reduction in viability of a bacterial suspension at a given temperature under standard conditions.

Effect of Moist Heat

A temperature of 50°C to 65°C may kill within 10 minutes the vegetative forms of most bacteria, yeasts and fungi and animal viruses, *Treponema pallidum* is fragile and killed at 43°C in 10 minutes *Coxiella burnetti* causing Q fever in man is heat resistant. *Bacillus stearothermophilus* is extremely resistant to heat. Poliomyelitis virus is killed at 60°C for 30 minutes and serum hepatitis virus is killed at 60°C for 10 hours. Bacteriophages are killed at the temperature of 65–80°C for 15–30 minutes. The most resistant forms of spores of actinomycetes, yeasts and fungi are killed at 80–90°C in 30 minutes. The spores of *Clostridium tetani. Cl. welchii* are killed at 100°C for 10 minutes, whereas *Cl. botulinum* in 8 hours.

Effect of Dry Heat

Dry heat at 100°C for 60 minutes kill vegetative bacteria which are susceptible to moist heat at 60°C in 30 minutes.

High content of organic substances protect spores and vegetative forms against the lethal action of heat. The heat resistance of spores is diminished with increased acidity and alkalinity. The effect of alkali is used in the disinfection of metal instruments by boiling at 100°C in water containing 2 percent sodium carbonates but this method is not reliable as autoclaving.

Sterilisation by Moist Heat

Microorganisms can be killed by the moist heat if they come in contact with water or steam; otherwise if the articles are protected from wetting, as by grease or in a relatively impervious container exposed at the same temperature; the moist heat will have the weaker effect than the dry heat.

Method of sterilisation by moist heat

In sterilisation, moist heat can be used :

(a) at temperatures below 100°C.

(b) at a temperature of 100°C (either boiling water or in free steam) or

(c) at a temperature above 100°C (in saturated steam under increased pressure) which ensures the complete sterilisation and killing of the most *highly resistant* spores.

Basic principles of moist heat sterilisation

Because of its greatest lethal effect on microorganisms, quicker heating up effect on the exposed articles and its penetrating power through porous materials (paper, cloth wrapper, bundles of surgical instruments, wool stoppers, cotton), saturated steam is a more efficient sterilising agent than the hot air.

When the cooler surface of the articles comes in contact with the steam, the steam condenses into a small volume of water and liberates its large latent heat to that cooler surface of the article (e.g. 1,600 ml. of steam at 100°C condense, at atmospheric pressure into 1 ml of water at 100°C liberating 518 calories of heat). The contraction in volume causes immediate suction of more steam to the same site and this process continues till the temperature of the article is raised to a temperature of the steam. The condensed water provides moist conditions of killing of the exposed microbes, since the penetration by the steam is hindered by the air, the air should not be trapped inside the autoclave; only pure steam is used. The loss of water by evaporation by heating is prevented by the saturated steam. Hence, culture media (both solid and liquid) can be sterilised by the steam under pressure. In the autoclave or steamer, the cotton wool stoppers can be drenched, this drenching can be avoided by covering the stopper with kraft paper. If a wire basket containing test tube is used, it can be covered with a sheet of paper folded down the edges of the basket.

Moist heat at temperatures below 100°C

The process which kills all non-spore forming pathogens (*Mycobacterium tuberculosis, Brucella abortus, Salmonella)* in milk by subjecting the milk to a temperature of 63°C for 30 minutes (the holder method) or 73°C for 20 seconds (the flash method) is known as *"Pasteurisation of milk"*.

Serum or body fluids containing coagulable protein can be sterilised by heating for 1 hour at 56°C on several successive days in water bath. Care must be taken not to allow the temperature to rise above 59°C, which may cause inspissation. Vaccine can be prepared in a vaccine bath at a temperature of 60°C for 1 hour.

Moist heat at a temperature of 100°C

Boiling at 100°C : Boiling at 100°C for 5–10 minutes does not ensure the complete sterility, but it is enough to kill all non-sporing organisms and few spore-forming bacilli (e.g. strains of Cl. tetani may survive boiling for 1–3 hours. Sometimes in microbiology and medicine this boiling method is used, when the absolute sterility unwanted for pipettes, measuring cylinder, rubber stoppers, instruments (scalpels, forceps, scissors, metal or glass syringe) which do not withstand higher temperature. If the supplied water is hard, the instruments, after removal from boiling water, may become covered with a film of calcium salts; to avoid this effect, distilled water should be used. Addition of 2 percent sodium bicarbonate may promote the sterilisation.

Long handed forceps, kept immersed in 3 percent lysol to a level approaching the finger grip, can be used to remove the articles and instruments from boiling water. If the instrument was taken into the hand, while it is wet, its working end (e.g. scalpel blade or syringe needle) may get contaminated with skin bacterium flowing from the fingers in the film of water.

However, boiling water can generally be used for contaminated dishes, bedding and bedpans, because these articles do require neither sterility nor the destruction of spores. Only disinfection is necessary for these articles. At altitude over 5,000 feet (1,500 metre), the boiling time should be increased by 50 percent, because the water boils at this altitude at a temperature of 95°C or below.

Boiling (at 100°C) for 10 minutes kills the vegetative and actively multiplying cells of pathogenic bacteria, rickettsiae, all viruses except hepatitis and poliomyelitis viruses, if these microorganisms are not protected by the blood, food, faeces, mucus, etc. It also kills or damages the cysts of protozoa, ova of helminths, ascospores of pathogenic yeasts, conidia of moulds. Since the spores of *Clostridium tetani, Cl. welchii* and *Bacillus anthracis* and hepatitis virus are resistant to boiling, even for 10 minutes boiling at 100°C for 10 minutes is not effective. Spores present in soil, faeces, dust on instruments and bandages contaminated with blood, dust may be a risk of infection. Whereas Anthrax spores occur only in areas where the infected animals died of anthrax.

Boiling at 100°C for 10 minutes is a sure means of disinfection (not sterility), if the spores and viruses are not present, of instruments and glasswares, if they are not soiled with blood, faeces, food etc. The margin of safety can be increased by boiling for 30 minutes.

Summary

(1) Vegetative forms of all bacteria and fungi pathogenic to man; rickettsiae pathogenic to man, helminths and their ova; many viruses (except hepatitis virus); bacterial toxin (except staphylococcal enterotoxin) are killed or inactivated by boiling at 100°C for 10 minutes.

(2) Bacterial spores; Hepatitis virus; ascospores of fungi, conidia of some fungi pathogenic to man; staphylococcal enterotoxin are not killed or inactivated by boiling at 100°C for 10 minutes.

Steaming at 100°C is commonly used in the microbiological laboratory to sterilise the culture media (both nutrient broth and nutrient agar). It is not as effective as autoclaving. *Koch* or *Arnold steam steriliser* or "Steamer" is a vertical metal cylinder with a removable lid having a small outlet for the steam to escape and at its bottom it contains water which is heated up. Above the water level, a tray bears the articles to be sterilised. Frequent opening of the steamer should be minimised, because the air permitted inside the steamer ultimately interferes with sterilisation.

Sterlisation is carried out as follows :

(a) By a single exposure at 100°C for 90 minutes.

(b) By intermittent exposure at 100°C for 20–45 minutes on each three successive days.

(a) Single exposure at 100°C for 90 minutes–is not suitable as the spores of thermophilic and some mesophilic bacteria can survive this exposure.

(b) Intermittent exposure at 100°C for 20–45 minutes for three successive days is also known as 'Tyndallisation". In this method one exposure will destroy all the vegetative organisms between the heatings, the spores in favourable nutrient medium become vegetative forms which are killed during the subsequent heating. This method is suitable for the medium containing sugars which may be decomposed at higher temperature and for gelatin medium which after prolonged heating, may not solidify on cooling.

III. Moist heat at temperature above 100°C

Sterilisation in the autoclave

Principle employed in the autoclave–water boils when its steam pressure equals atmospheric pressure or it can be interpreted the water boils at 100°C at normal atmospheric pressure (i.e. 76 mm Hg; 14 per square inch pressure). So when the water is boiled within a closed vessel at increased pressure, the temperature at which the water boils and that of its steam will rise above 100°C. The most effective method of sterilisation of culture media (in the bacteriological laboratory) and surgical materials or supplies (in the hospital) is Autoclaving.

The steam should penetrate all parts of the articles to be sterilised in the autoclave and should be hot saturated (i.e. point of condensing to liquid water) and dry (i.e. free from particles of liquid water). This dry saturated steam affects the sterilisation because of its high temperature (latent heat). The ideal minimum holding time is 15–30 minutes at 121°C (15 lb per square inch gauze pressure).

Air discharge : To expose all articles in the autoclave to the pure steam during sterilisation, it is necessary to remove all the air from the autoclave, because (a) the mixture of steam and air results in a lower temperature at a particular pressure, (b) the penetration of steam in the interstices of porous materials (e.g. surgical dressing), syringes, etc., may be interfered by the air, and (b) the air, being denser than the steam from a cooler layer at the bottom of the autoclave, which prevents the sufficient heating of the articles at the lower level.

There are two types of autoclaves :

(a) The simple non-jacketed laboratory autoclave.

(b) Steam-jacketed autoclave with automatic air and condensate discharge.

(a) The simple non-jacketed laboratory autoclave is also called "pressure cooker type". It is made up of a vertical or horizontal gun metal or stainless steel cylinder of about 18 inches in diameter and 30 inches in length with a supporting stand. The lid (door) is tightened by screw clamps and is rendered airtight by means of an asbestos washer. The water level inside the cylinder should be up to 3½ inches for a vertical cylinder of 19 inches internal length. The autoclave is heated by gas burner or electric heater from below the cylinder. The articles to be sterilised are placed on a perforated tray situated above the water level. The lid of the autoclave is provided with a discharge tap for the air and steam, a pressure gauze and a safety valve which is adjusted to blow off automatically at any desired pressure.

Operating of the simple autoclave. Inside the autoclave, the water should be up to required, level i.e., below the perforated tray. The materials to be sterilised are placed on the tray and the heater should be turned on. The lid should be placed in position and fastened by screw clamps, the discharge tap should remain *open* and the safety valve is to be adjusted to the required pressure. In some autoclaves, the pressure has been predetermined and adjusted by the manufacturers. When water boils inside the cylinder of the autoclave, the steam rises, mixes with the air in the chamber and expels out this air through the discharge tap. The operator should allow *the steam and air mixture to escape freely till all the air is completely removed from the autoclave,* which can be adjusted by connecting a rubber *tube from* the discharge tap into a container of cold water into which the steam condenses and the air rises as bubbles to the surface. This procedure can be followed by an inexperienced operator for his own satisfaction, when there is no trained nurse.

When the air has completely escaped, the discharge tap should be closed. The steam pressure rises till it reaches the desired level, e.g. 15 lb per square inch for 121°C, when the safety valve opens automatically and allows the excess steam to escape. From this point, the *holding time* begins and continues for 15 minutes. The heater should be turned off, the discharge tap should be opened gradually and the autoclave should be allowed to *cool* till the inside pressure equals to the atmospheric pressure (0 lb per square inch) which may take about 1 hour; when the chamber pressure is still high, if the discharge tap is opened, there is possibility of danger of explosion of autoclave lid, culture media will boil and spill from the container. An excess amount of water will be evaporated and lost from the media if the discharge tap is not opened until the pressure has fallen much below the atmospheric pressure. It is necessary to have surgical linen and dressing wrapped in paper or cloth for quick drying of the materials after sterilisation. These wrapped articles are moistened by the condensation of the steam; when damp even several layers of paper and cloth wrappings could not check the entry of contaminating bacteria into the sterilised articles. Therefore, *the sterilised articles* should not be kept in contact with unsterilised objects until their wrappings are dry.

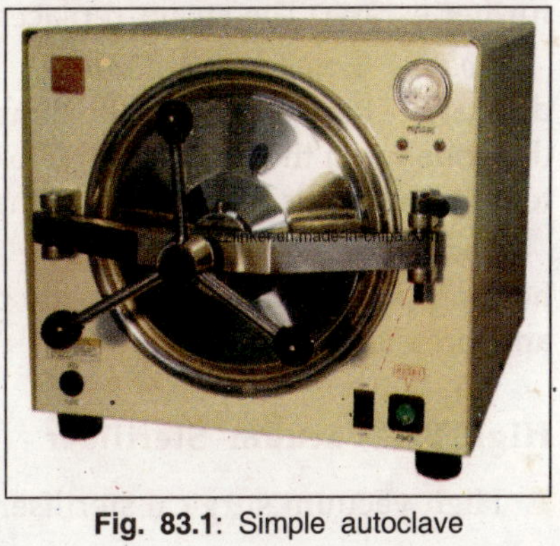

Fig. 83.1: Simple autoclave

(b) Steam-jacketed autoclave (Fig. 83.1) is mostly used in the hospital to sterilise the linen, surgical materials etc.

It is a horizontal cylinder. At the front, there is a swing door which is tightened by screw clamps or by a "capstan head" with its radial bolts and it locks automatically while the chamber pressure is raised. This safety door locked automatically by pressure can prevent the possibilities of a dangerous explosion, if the operator opens early the autoclave by mistake.

The autoclave consists of (1) a steam supply from outside (e.g. an independent boiler), (2) a steam jacket which heats the side walls of the autoclave, (3) a channel discharging air from the bottom of the chamber, (4) a thermometer in the discharge channel, indicating the temperature above the lowest and coolest part of the chamber, vacuum system to assist drying the load. (6) an air intake with a self-sterilising filter for introducing warm sterile air in the chamber, (7) a cooling system to hasten the cooling of the liquids without violent boiling, (8) an automatic control system for heating up, holding, cooling and drying.

Steam supply : The steam supplied to the autoclave should be dry, i.e., free from excess of water, and *saturated*, i.e., not superheated.

Wet steam : The steam released from the boiler at a long distance may become "wet" and inefficient sterilising agent because of (a) cooling and condensation, (b) soaking of porous materials which prevents further penetration and (c) the particles of water possess no latent heat. This, the pressure of the main steam supply should be usually 55 lb. per square inch. The reduction in pressure dries the steam.

Super-heated steam is not satisfactory because it abstracts the water from the exposed materials, may cause the less lethal effect and is still more destructive as dry heat.

Operating of steam jacketed autoclave : A space between the double side walls of the chamber (jacket) is filled throughout the day with the steam at 121°C introduced from the boiler. Water of condensation from the steam is drained off through the jacket discharge channel which is thermostatically controlled. The operator should ensure that there is no obstruction of this discharge channel.

Loading of the chamber : The articles to be sterilised should be arranged loosely so that the steam circulates freely and the air is displaced.

Heating up and air replacement method : The swing door should be closed systematically. The steam from the jacket should enter through a baffle at the back of the chamber. The pressure and temperature should be maintained in the chamber as in the jacket. The cooler and denser air should be displaced by the steam under pressure. If more steam is introduced under pressure, it displaces the air downwards through the articles to be sterilised and the air is discharged out through the chamber discharge channel situated at the bottom of the chamber. At the same time the water of condensation on the cool load and the door of the chamber should be drained off through the same channel. As soon as all free air is eliminated, the inflow of pure steam raises the trap's temperature to 121°C, it closes automatically and it prevents further escape. The steam replaces the air in about 5–10 minutes.

Holding period of sterilisation : Holding period will start when the thermometer in the discharge channel reaches the temperature of 121°C. The exact duration of the holding period depends upon the nature of the load. A "near to steam" trap is essential as it opens when the temperature falls by 1°C below that of the pure steam.

Cooling and drying period : The steam supply to the chamber is dropped at the end of the holding period. The steam inside the chamber starts to cool by loss of heat through the door and pressure falls slowly.

High Pre-Vacuum Steriliser

High vacuum surgical steriliser is the only method of sterilisation that can overcome the effects of bad packing or overloading of the steriliser. Tightly packed load is heated rapidly and uniformly to the sterilising temperature for a shorter time, e.g., 35°C for 3 minutes. The damage to heat sensitive materials is avoided by greatly shortening the time. The steam, admitted to the chamber, heats the whole load to 135°C within 2–3 minutes. The holding period is maintained for 3 minutes, the temperature reaches 135°C. The load is then dried within a few minutes by exhaustion of the chamber to a high vacuum.

Temperature record : Recording thermometer can help the operator to avoid the errors in timing the holding period.

The overall efficiency of the autoclave can be judged by the following two methods : Chemical indicator and spore indicators :

(a) *Chemical indicators,* which show a change of colour or shape after exposure to a sterilising temperature, may be placed under the load, for example, (i) a sulphur pellet kept in a small glass tube will show a change of shape by melting when exposed to 120°C for a few minutes. (ii) Browne's control tubes contain a red solution which turns green when heated at 115°C for 25 minutes (type 1); or 15 minutes (type 2) or at 160°C for 60 minutes. These tubes should be stored at less than 20°C to avoid the deterioration and premature change in colour. (iii) Browie-Dick tape, applied to packs and articles in the autoclave develop diagonal lines when exposed to sterilising temperature for the correct time. (iv) *Sterilisation* in a cellulose tape having on it a chemical indicator which changes its colour when properly heated in the autoclave.

(b) *Spore indicator* : *Bacillus stearothermophilus* grows best at 55°C–60°C. But a preparation of its dried spores is killed at 121°C in 12 minutes when placed within the load in the autoclave. After autoclaving, it can be tested for its viability on the culture media.

Nurse using the autoclaving should be sure that

(a) all the air is allowed to escape and is replaced by the steam.

(b) the pressure of the steam reaches at least 15 pounds to the square inch and remains there;

(c) the thermometer reaches at least 121°C for 20 minutes.

Sterilisation by Radiation

Non-ionising radiation : Ultraviolet rays of sunlight have the bactericidal effects which depends upon the wave length. It is bactericidal when it reaches a wave length of 330 μ (3300A° or Angstrom units). Angstrom is unit of measurement of wavelength. Thus, as the wavelength decreases, the effectiveness of the ultraviolet light increases as sterilising agent. The shortest ultraviolet rays of sunlight reaching the surface of the earth have a wavelength of more than 20 μ, however most commonly used mercury vapours can emit even more effective radiations of 240–280 μ.

The intensity of ultraviolet radiations applied with precautions to protect the skin to the side of operations to check out operative sepsis. Ray from ultraviolet lamps can reduce the bacterial load in the atmospheric dust. Pathogenic microorganisms on the floor and furnitures in rooms can be destroyed by the daylight passing through ordinary glass windows.

Ionising radiation : In practice, sterilisation by radiation is achieved by the use of high speed cathode rays (electrons), X-rays and short X-rays (gamma rays) from an apparatus (linear accelerator) or gamma rays from an isotope source (cobalt 60). This method is very costly for hospital use, but it is used commercially only for the sterilisation of prepacked disposable plastic syringes, transfusion sets and catheters which cannot withstand the heat.

Sterilisation by Filtration

In this process, the fluids (bacterial fluid cultures) can be freed from bacteria by passing through special filters. This method of sterilisation by filtration is specially useful to prevent toxin from bacterial growth and to sterilise the liquids (sugars, serum, antibiotic solutions) which are liable to be damaged by heat. These sterilising filters should be considered as rendering a liquid bacteria free, but not virus free and are satisfactory for laboratory purposes, but in clinical practice, such fluids (e.g. glucose, serum) sterilised by Seitz filtration are not safe.

Types of filters : For bacteriological work, the following types of filters are used :

Sinternware candles (e.g. Berkefeld, Chamberland filters, Asbestos, Asbestos paper disk (e.g. Seitz filter) Fig. 4.2. Sintered glass filters; Cellulose membrane filters.

1. (a) *Berkefeld filters* : They are made from a fossil diatomaceous earth found in deposits in Germany and other parts of the world and are of three grades of porosity, e.g., V(Veil) the coarsest, W (Wening) the finest, and Normal (N) intermediate. Berkefeld V is often used. A small organism (*Serratia marcescens*) should pass through this filter.

   (b) *Chamberland filters* : They are made of unglazed porcelain of various grades of porosity. The finer grades will pass only certain viruses of extreme minuteness (e.g. Foot and Mouth Disease virus). The most porous grade L_1, clarifying filter, allows many microorganisms to pass. The next three L_{1a}, L_2, L_3 are comparable with the Berkefeld V, N, and W candles, respectively. These filters can also be used to obtain bacterial toxin.

2. *Seitz filters* consist of asbestos disk through which (Fig 4.2) the fluid is passed. The disk is inserted into a metal holder which is jointed tightly by screw clamps. The whole filter is wrapped in kraft paper and sterilised in the autoclave. The asbestos disk is discarded after each filtration and is replaced by another new disk for fresh filtration. The disks are available in three grades : Clarifying (K), normal and "special Ek." The normal and "special Ek" do not allow the ordinary test bacterium *Serratia marcescens* to pass through.

3. *Sintered glass cylinder* : They are made of finely ground glass attached to the filtering apparatus and sterilised as in case of Seitz filter. After use they should be washed with running water in reverse direction and cleaned with warm sulfuric acid to which potassium nitrate is added.

4. *Cellulose membrane filters* : There are two types of cellulose membrane filters :

   The gradacol membrane (older type) consists of cellulose nitrate and the modern membrane filter is made of cellulose acetate. The size of many viruses can be determined by these cellulose membrane filters; these filters can retain *Serratia marcescens*.

   Advantages of cell membrane filters are :

   (a) They are much less absorptive and the rate of filtration is much greater,

   (b) Bacteria retained on the surface of this filter can be cultivated by placing this filter on culture media.

Chemical Agents of Disinfection

Chemical sterilising agents are widely used as disinfectants and antiseptics.

Disinfectants are :

(a) chemical agents which are capable of destroying pathogenic microorganisms, but not resistant spores;

(b) potent and toxic;

(c) suitable only for application to *inanimate* objects.

Antiseptics are :

(a) chemical agents which kill microorganisms or prevent their growth;

(b) non-toxic;

(c) suitable for superficial application to *living* tissues.

Volatile antiseptic, e.g., Chloroform. In the sterilisation and preservation of serum for culture media. Chloroform used in the proportion of 0.2 per cent and later it may be removed by heating at 56°C.

Alcohol (Isopropyl alcohol, ethyl alcohol) are bacteriocidal in 70–75 per cent concentration Chlorhexidine or Iodine is superior to alcohol alone for skin disinfectant before venepuncture or hypodermic injection.

2. *Antiseptics of the phenol group* : Lysol (liquor cresolis saponatus) and cresol (black and white fluid) are powerful disinfectants, they are used for sterilising surgical instruments, discarded cultures and killing cultures accidently spilt on the floor or table. Lysol is generally used in a 3 per cent solution and phenol in 0.5 per cent for preserving sera. Sudol is less toxic substitute for Lysol. Dettol is less toxic, irritant and also less active. Hexochlorophane is an even blender agent and is incorporated in various antiseptic preparations. It is effective against Gram-positive and Gram-negative bacteria. It is potentially toxic and should be used with care.

3. *Metallic salts or organic compounds of metals.*

   Mercuric chloride (1:1000) is used as disinfectant. Merthiolate, a proprietary name for sodium ethyl-mercuri-thio-salicylate, is used in a dilution of 1 : 10000 for preservation of antisera or sera, A drop of *silver nitrate* (1 per cent) solution is used for prophylaxis of gonococcal ophthalmia in newborn babies. It is replaced by chlorhexidine (modern antiseptic).

4. *Formaldehyde* is an irritant water soluble gas which is highly lethal to all kinds of microbes and *spores*, killing bacterial spores as readily as the vegetative forms.

   It is cheap and non-injurious to cloth, fabrics, wool, leather, rubber, paints and metals. So it can be used to disinfect the rooms, furniture, and a wide variety of articles which are liable to be damaged by heat (e.g. woollen blankets and clothing) shoes, gum elastic catheters). It can be applied as an aqueous solution or in gaseous forms.

   Disinfection with aqueous formaldehyde solution : A 40 percent (W/V) solution of formaldehyde in water containing 10 per cent methanol to inhibit polymerisation is known as "Commercial formalin." Formaldehyde diluted in water (5-10 per cent) is a powerful and rapid disinfectant when applied directly to a contaminated surface. Bacterial cultures and suspensions are also killed by this disinfectant.

   Cleaned metal instruments may be sterilised overnight immersion in a borax-formaldehyde solution.

   Sodium tetraborate 50 g

   Formaldehyde, 4 per cent in water, 1000 ml.

Glutaraldehyde is bactericidal sporicidal, more effective and less toxic. It is used to sterilise cystoscope anesthetic equipments, plastic materials and thermometers.

Disinfection by Formaldehyde gas : The articles which can be damaged by wetting or cannot be wetted completely with formaldehyde solution can be disinfected by formaldehyde gas provided that the conditions suitable for the action of gas are maintained. The atmosphere must have relatively high (80–90 per cent) humidity and the temperature should be 18°C. Since the penetration of the gas into the porous fabrics is slow, the materials should be arranged in such a way the gas can have access to all contaminated surfaces.

Spraying, heating formalin or heating solid of paraformaldehyde can liberate the gas, when spraying cold, formalin, its polymerisation can be prevented by adding in equal volume of industrial-spirit to cold formalin. Formalin diluted with sufficient water can be boiled to produce an adequate atmospheric humidity. This is a best method, because of the tendency of the gas to polymerise to paraformaldehyde and a maximal vapour concentration attainable at 20°C is 2.0 mg per litre of air, which is a desirable concentration. Higher concentration obtained at high temperature may be explosive. After disinfection, the articles may contain paraformaldehyde emitting irritant vapour for a long period which may be neutralised by exposure to ammonia vapour.

Exposure for at least 3 hours to formaldehyde gas in an airtight metal or painted wooden cabinet is sufficient to disinfect small articles (instruments, shoes, a hair brush). The gas is introduced inside the cabinet by boiling formalin in an electric boiler to the extent of 50 ml 40 percent of formaldehyde per 100 cu ft of air space. Similarly, blankets and the surfaces of mattresses are disinfected in a large cabinet where they are hung *unfolded* so that the fabric can absorb formaldehyde gas (e.g. 500 ml of formalin can be used for 100 lb, fabrics). Finally, the vapour is vented to the open air, *folded* blankets and clothings can also be disinfected only if some heat is applied. They are packed in the chamber of steam jacketed autoclave, then 100 ml formalin per 100 cu ft is placed at the bottom of the autoclave and the chamber is heated at 100°C for 3 hours by passing free steam through the jacket. At last, the vapour is vented through the autoclave vacuum system.

5. *Ethylene oxide* : It is a colourless liquids boiling at 107°C. It is moderately toxic gas above this temperature and forms an explosive mixture when more than 3 percent is present in air. In non-explosive mixture (10 percent ethylene oxide in CO_2 or in halogenated hydrocarbon) can be used for sterilisation. It destroys bacteria and viruses, and kills the spores almost as easily as vegetative forms.

This is a gaseous disinfectant killing microorganisms and spores. It can diffuse more rapidly into dry, porous materials and is of great importance to sterilise articles which are liable to be damaged by heat (e.g. plastic, rubber articles, blankets, pharmaceutical products, lung heart machine etc.).

Sterilisation Methods in Dental Practice

A. *Sterilisation of Bottled Fluids* : Hydrated fluids used for therapeutic intravenous infusions can be sterilised at 121°C for 12 minutes as the contaminating bacteria are already moist and can be easily destroyed at this condition. Similarly sterile water used in the operation theatre can be sterilised in the autoclave.

B. *Sterilisation of empty bottles and impervious bottles* : Empty and dry bottles can be sterilised in the autoclave, if they are not tightly stoppered so that the steam can enter and displace the inside air and are arranged on their sides in the autocalve to permit a horizontal pathway for the entry of steam and escape of air. If unstoppered, they can be sterilised quickly; if stoppered with cotton wool or loosened screw cap, the displacement of air is slow and the holding period is 121°C for 10 minutes. Since the displacement of air in the stoppered container is not certain, it is always better to sterilise the stoppered empty container in hot air oven. The rubber liner inside the screw cap cannot withstand the high temperature (160°C) of hot air oven. This problem can be overcome by using silicone rubber liner.

C. *Sterilisation of wrapped dry porous goods and surgical dressings* : When dry porous goods (e.g. paper), apparatus wrapped in cloth and surgical linen and dressings are to be sterilised by autoclave, it is essential that a) the steam should displace by gravity completely the air from the autoclave, (b) the sterilised articles should be dry before they are removed from the autoclave. In this method, the load should be carefully packed so that there will be adequate spaces for the circulation of the steam. Glass and metal containers are kept open or covered only loosely. Metal drums and caskets must be provided with ports which must not be obstructed by the contents packed against them and must always be fully open during sterilisation and the steam should flow freely from top to bottom. A wrapping of two layers of good muslin it recommended for surgical packs. A single layer of coarse brown (kraft) paper is also satisfactory.

   Surgical dressing and other cloth articles should be arranged in packs no bigger than 12 × 12 × 20 inches and placed on edge in the autoclave so that the layers of cloth are vertical. Rubber gloves are powdered and packed loosely in muslin cloth to allow access of the steam to all parts. It is customary to autoclave rubber gloves at 5 to 10 lbs pressure for a short time to avoid the deterioration, but this exposure does not guarantee sterility, so that the gloves should be autoclaved at the temperature as few other goods, instruments and syringes must be free from oil and grease, jointed instruments open and syringes disassembled. The chamber of the autoclave should not be overloaded and the perforated tray should not be removed.

D. *Sterilisation of surgical instruments* : Boiling is effective when 2 per cent sodium bicarbonate or a germicide is added to the water. There is the risk of recontamination when the instruments are washed before use to remove these substances.

   Heat can blunt the sharp instrument, this effect is mainly due to oxidation, but the pure steam cannot damage. Ethylene oxide and formaldehyde are the only established chemical sterilising agents and can be used to sterilise the instruments (scalpels). Pasteurisation at 75°C or treatment with chlorhexidine in 75 per cent ethanol is recommended to sterilise the instruments (Cystoscopes).

Sterilisation of syringes : In hospital wards and in microbiological laboratories, the syringes are very important in day-to-day use, therefore much heed need be paid to their use, care and sterilisation; sterilisation by chemical agents are not satisfactory, but the sterilisation by heat is the best method.

All glass syringes have many advantages over the glass metal type of syringes; the glass metal syringe is more difficult to clean and is more likely to break on heating due to the differences of expansion of glass and metal, it cannot be sterilised when assembled and it is difficult to keep sterile until ready for use. The solder uniting the glass and metal may melt in hot air oven and autoclave, syringes with cement at the glass metal junction which withstands 200°C are available. The mounts of the stainless steel needle of good quality must fit accurately the nozzle of the syringe.

All glass syringes : All new syringes must be well washed in soap and water with test tube brush according to their sizes. After washing in clean warm water, barrel and piston should be dried. The syringes should be assembled, wrapped, sterilised and ready for use. If this facility is not available, all gas syringes should be sterilised just before use by boiling in a fish kettle saucepan. Distilled water is preferable if the tap water is hard. The syringes should always be dismantled, the barrel and piston are placed in cold water which is brought to boil and kept boiling for 5–10 minutes. When *cool* and *dry*, the barrel and piston should be assembled with sterile forceps or clean, dry fingers, touching only outside of the barrel and the top of the piston. The sterile syringes should be used immediately. The needle should also be boiled at the same time and affixed to the nozzle by means of sterile forceps. It is always better to sterilise all glass syringes in the hot air oven after they are wrapped with kraft paper or the syringe with fitted needle should be accommodated in a test tube with cotton wool plug and the whole unit should be wrapped in kraft paper and sterilised in hot air oven at 160°C for 1 hour. It is sterile indefinitely and is ready for use and also sterilised in the test tubes plugged with cotton wool.

Syringes used for blood culture or aspiration etc. should be immediately washed in cold solution of 2 per cent lysol. If the blood is clotted in the syringe, it is difficult to remove the piston. Hot water should not be used as it will coagulate the protein and the piston will stick. The syringe is cleaned with soapy water with a brush, washed in clean warm water dried and sterilised.

84

Microbial Pathogenicity : Sources and Spread of Infection in the Community

Pathology is the ability of the microbes to initiate the infection. It requires three tributes :

(1) *Transmissibility* or *communicability* — from one host or reservoir to a fresh host;

(2) *Infectivity* — the ability to breach the new host's defences;

(3) *Virulence* a variable factor that may enchance or reduce the capacity of the pathogen to cause overt infection.

Pathogens (Pathogenic microorganisms) cause diseases and they may be (a) opportunistic or (b) true pathogens.

Opportunistic Pathogens : Many commensal or non-pathogenic may be transmissible from person to person or derived from the environment and are present, in large numbers, on the skin, in the upper respiratory tract, in the intestine and lower urinogenital tract, hence they are normal microflora of the body and sometimes they may act against invading pathogenic microorganisms and are unable to invade the tissues as they cannot overcome the healthy body defences. Sometimes, when the body defence mechanism is lowered and when these commensals leave their natural habitat and reach other parts of the body e.g. coliform bacilli (*Escherichia coli*) are mostly harmless commensals in the intestine, but they may cause infection in the urinary tract; similarly *clostridium welchii*, an intestinal commensal, can cause gangrene in locally damaged tissues; *streptococcus viridans* is the commensal of the mouth, after tooth extraction they may invade the blood stream and settle on previously damaged heart values as opportunistic pathogens.

True pathogens : They are those microorganisms which are able to overcome the normal body defence mechanism and initiate the infection.

Several properties are essential for pathogenicity of microorganisms :

(a) *Transmissibility* : The ability of a pathogen to grow profusely in the body and to be shed in large numbers in body fluids or secretions which are capable of dissemination and reach new host after surviving in the adverse conditions, e.g., dessication in the dry dust.

(b) *Infectivity* : Pathogenic microbes are able to initiate the infection by penetrating the healthy body's first line of defence, that is skin, mucous membranes to which they readily gain access. To infect a person, only a few of the pathogens can cross the protective barriers in the respiratory and alimentary tracts. The pathogen may initiate a localised lesion at the site of infection, e.g., staphylococcal boil on the skin or streptococcal pharyngitis in the throat.

The capacity of the microbes to initiate the infection is mostly related to the dosage of the pathogen, its phase of growth and its virulence factors. In salmonella family, the infecting dose of *Salmonella typhi* is very small, whereas large number of *S. typhimurium* (food poisoning salmonellae) must be ingested to produce acute vomiting and diarrhoea. Microorganisms which are in logarithmic stage of growth are more likely to overcome host resistance than those in the latent phase : *Streptococcus* pyogenes is more infective when transferred directly from a person with a sore throat than when it is inhaled after drying in dust particles, because *Strept. pyogenes* has the capsular M protein (antiphagocytic component) during the active phase of sore throat infection.

(c) *Virulence* : The virulence of a pathogen is the ability to kill susceptible animal (mouse, guinea pig etc.). The tubercle bacillus isolated from Indian patients with tuberculosis are often less virulent to the guinea pigs than strains isolated in Britain. The assessment of virulence for animal is not necessarily applicable to virulence of man. *Shigella dysenteriae* causes much more severe infection than *Sh. sonnei*. Similarly, the *gravis* strain of *Corynebacterium diphtheriae* causes more deaths than the *mitis* strain. Type 1 polio virus is more likely to initiate epidemics of paralytic poliomyelitis than is Type 2.

Pathogenesis

Pathogenic bacteria produce diseases by virtue of one or both of the main attributes : Toxigenicity, and Invasiveness.

Toxigenicity

Toxins may be (a) exotoxins, or (b) endotoxins.

(a) *Exotoxins* : German and French workers were first to prove that the products of the diphtheria bacilli, diffused from the local infection or injected as bacteria free filtrates of cultured diphtheria bacilli could produce widespread systemic damage in guinea pigs. The toxin produced by diphtheria bacilli in the throat is carried by the blood stream (toxaemia) throughout the body. When the bacteria grow actively in broth culture, apparently they secrete the poison which is called "exotoxin." Other bacteria which secrete highly potent toxin are tetanus bacilli and *clostridium botulinum*. 1.0 mg of tetanus and botulinum toxin can kill more than one million guinea pigs and it is estimated that 3 kg of botulinum toxin can kill the world population (6.9 billion = 690 crores).

Exotoxins are mainly produced by Gram-positive bacilli (except Shigella bacillus neurotoxin and Cholera enterotoxin) and have special affinity for specific tissues; for example, tetanus, botulinum and diphtheria toxins all affect different parts of the nervous system, tetanus toxin affects control mechanisms that govern motor cells in the anterior columns of the spinal cord, botulinal toxin paralyses cranial nerves by blocking the transmission of effector messages from their endings, and diphtheria toxin has affinity for peripheral nerve ending as well as for specialised tissues like heart muscle.

Exotoxins behave like enzymes : alpha toxin of *Cl. welchii* is a phospholipase (lecithinase C) which acts on phospholipids of cell membrane; diphtheria toxins depress the formation and or release of acetylcholine in different parts of the nervous system.

Endotoxins : They are complex phospholipid polysaccharide protein macromolecules. Most of the endotoxins are lipopolysaccharides and additional endotoxin released by few Gram-negative pathogenic bacteria (*Yersinia pestis* and *Bordetella pertussis*) is protein in nature and is present in the bacterial cytoplasm. They are released only after natural autolysis or artificial disruption of bacterial cells and, therefore, they are called *endotoxins*. Typical endotoxins are particularly associated with Gram-negative bacteria (Salmonella, Shigella, Escherichia, Neisseria) and are distinguishable from exotoxins by the following properties :

(1) they are present in the outer layer of the bacterial cell wall;
(2) they are heat stable;
(3) they are much less toxic and specific in their cytotoxic effects than exotoxins;
(4) they cannot be converted into toxoids.
(5) homologous antibodies cannot render them non-toxic, if combined.

The complex antibodies cannot render them non-toxic, if combined;

The complex phospholipid-polysaccharide-protein molecule can be separated by phenol extraction into :

(a) lipopolysaccharide moiety;
(b) protein fraction;
(c) phospholipid fraction.

The lipopolysaccharide moiety can be split further into different sugars including those that determine the antigenic specificity of the endotoxin and lipid which is mainly responsible for the toxicity.

Pyogenic effect (fever) is the toxic effect produced by the smallest amount of endotoxin 0.002 µg endotoxin per kg body weight is injected intravenously into rabbit or man, it causes within 15 minutes an elevation of body temperature which lasts for several hours.

Invasiveness : It is the other main attribute of pathogenic bacteria. It is its capacity to invade and multiply in the healthy tissues e.g. pneumococcus produces the disease depending entirely upon the quality of invasiveness just as botulinus bacillus depends entirely on its toxigenicity. Thus, the diphtheria bacillus must be initially invasive in order to establish itself in the tissues of the oropharynx, where it manufactures its toxin; the *gravis* strain of diphtheria bacillus has the greater capacity to invade and multiply in the tissues with a consequent greater production of toxin than *mitis* strain. *Strepto. pyogenes* is mainly an invasive pathogen. It also produces an erythrogenic toxin which is responsible for the rash of the scarlet fever. The invasiveness of *Staph. aureus*, *Strepto. pyogenes* and *Cl. welchii* is due to their production of keratolytic and loculicidal toxins which enable them to breach tissue barriers and protect themselves against phagocytosis.

Pathogenic bacteria which are predominantly invasive are :

(1) The *first category* : The pathogenic Gram-positive cocci initially attract phagocytes by chemotactic mechanisms, resist phagocytosis, but ultimately they may be engulfed and destroyed by phagocytes.
(2) The *second category* : Tubercle bacilli, typhoid, brucella bacilli, though they are readily phagocytosed, are more resistant to destruction when within phagocytes and become intracellular parasites which are disseminated by phagocytes throughout the body. There is fight between phagocytes and antiphagocytic bacteria, when specific antibody acting as opsonins come to the aid of the phagocytes in destroying the antiphagocytic bacteria, then these bacteria are destroyed by phagocytes and there is a dramatic fall in temperature–the crisis–as observed in pneumococcal pneumonia. In infection with intracellular parasites there is clinical illness that persists for some week with low fever.

Capsules and Pathogenicity : The bacterial capsule plays an important role in conferring the virulence on bacteria by enabling them to resist phagocytosis and bactericidal, substances in body fluids, therefore the capsulation is important for the virulence of pneumococci, streptococci of Group A and Group C, the anthrax bacillus, the plague bacillus, *Klebsiella pneumoniae* and *Haemophilus influenzae*.

It has been observed that the non-capsulate bacteria are rapidly phagocytosed and, within a few hours, are mostly destroyed, whereas the capsulate bacteria remain free and soon multiply to large numbers. The mechanism of the antiphagocytic property of capsulate bacteria is not known, but it may be that the lipid containing cell membrane of the phagocyte's pseudopodia is inhibited from making contact with the hydrated capsule gel because of the surface charge. However, heavily capsulate harmless saprophytic bacteria and some non-virulent strains of bacillus anthracis and plague bacilli are fairly susceptible to phagocytosis.

Aggressin : Other non-toxic protective or aggressive factors that may contribute to the ability of capsulate and non-capsulate pathogens to invade and multiply in the host tissues are :

(1) *Hyaluronidase* or spreading factor, is an enzyme that dissolves the hyaluronic acid or cement-like substances that binds cells together and so allows pathogens (*strepto. pyogenes, staph.aureus*) to permeate through the tissues.

(2) *Coagulase* a thrombin–like enzyme produced by all pathogenic staphylococci may help to protect the pathogen from phagocytosis into two ways :

(a) by forming fibrin barriers around staphylococci and staphylococcal lesions, and

(b) by inactivating the bactericidal substance present in the normal blood serum.

(3) *Streptokinase* secreted by *Strepto.pyogenes* may promote the spreading of streptococcal lesions.

(4) *Collagenase*, produced by *Cl. welchii* , may play some part in the pathogenesis of gas gangrene.

(5) *Neuraminidase* produced by some bacteria and viruses, acts on mucoproteins of cell surface and may facilitate attacks on the cell.

Organotropism : The affinity of many pathogenic microbes for specific tissues or organs is known as organotropism. Pneumococcus and meningococcus both have the natural habitat in the nasopharynx, but the virulent pneumococcus has a predilection for lung tissues and the meningococcus for the meninges of the brain, whereas gonococcus mainly affects the mucosa of urethra. *Brucella abortus* localise in the uterus of cows because of the presence of erythritol, a growth factor for *Br. abortus,* in the bovine placenta. However, *Coxiella burnetti* and chlamydiae localise in the uterus but they do not use erythritol.

Comparative Characteristics of Toxins

Exotoxins	Endotoxins
1. Composed of proteins, have the properties of enzymes, some have been obtained in crystalline state.	1. Composed of phospholipid. Polysaccharide protein complexes.
2. Easily diffuse from the cell into the surrounding medium.	2. Firmly bound within the bacterial cell.
3. Highly toxic, characterised by the selective affection of certain organs and tissues.	3. Less toxic, selective action poorly expressed.
4. Thermolabile.	4. Thermostable.
5. During parenteral injection, they produce highly active antibodies (anti toxins).	5. During parenteral injection, they produce precipitins, lysins, opsonins, agglutinins and complement fixing antibodies.
6. Under influence of 0.3–0.4 per cent formalin and a temperature of 38–40°C change to anatoxin (Toxoid)	6. Under the influence of formalin and temperature are rendered partially harmless.

HOST FACTORS CONTRIBUTING TO INFECTION

Various host factors, affecting an individual or a community, contributing to the occurrence of the infection are :

1. Very young children and very old individuals are susceptible to infection, because of inadequate body defence mechanism.
2. Malnutrition favours the incidence and severity of infection in poor community.
3. Metabolic diseases like diabetes and hormonal upsets due to corticosteroid therapy predispose to the infection.
4. Haematological disorders like leukaemia, neoplasm and renal diseases may reduce host resistance to infection.
5. Factors such as age, obesity, size of wound, wound drainage, duration of operation and length of stay before or after operation may affect the *nosocomial* infection (hospital acquired infection) caused by staphylococci and Gram-negative bacilli.
6. Acquired immunodeficiency syndrome (AIDS) patients are highly susceptible to various infections.
7. Community factors affecting host resistance are the complex components of poverty (overcrowding, inadequate food, clothing and housing, hypothermia and poor personal hygiene).
8. Drug addiction and alcoholism may predispose to infection.

Sources of Infection for Man

The term *infection* (Latin *inficiere–infectum*–to infect) signifies the sum of biological processes which take place in the human or animal body upon the penetration of pathogenic microorganisms in the host's body by injuring body tissues and producing a reaction on the part of the host, *Source of infection* is defined as the normal growth habitat of the microbes, e.g., a site in the body of the human or animal host. Objects contaminated with live or temporarily inactive microbes may be called as *vehicles* or *reservoirs* of infection, not source of infection.

Man acquires the infection:

(a) From outside sources, which is known as *exogenous* infection, e.g., from human patients with clinical infections, healthy human carriers of the pathogenic microorganism.

(b) Within the patient's own body, the infection is said to be *endogenous.*

Exogenous infection

1. *Patients* : Some microbial infections are acquired from sick patients with active infections (pulmonary tuberculosis, leprosy, whooping cough, syphilis, gonorrhoea, measles, smallpox, mumps and influenza).
2. *Healthy carriers* : Healthy persons, though they carry many species of pathogenic microbes, sometimes show a subclinical infection and are commonly capable of disseminating these pathogenic microbes to other persons who will manifest the signs and symptoms of illness; they are then termed as *carriers*, thus they are potential sources of infection; some infectious diseases are contracted from carriers much more frequently than from patient's, e.g., streptococcal, staphylococcal, pneumococcal and meningococcal infection, diphtheria, typhoid fever, bacillary dysentery, and poliomyelitis.
3. *Convalescent carriers* are persons in whom a limited, localised infection continues for a period of weeks or months after clinical recovery from a manifest infection.

4. *Contact carriers* are those persons who acquire the pathogen from a patient.
5. *Paradoxical carriers* are those who acquire the infection asymptomatically from another carrier. If the carriage persists for more than an arbitrary period of time, e.g. one year in the case of typhoid infection, the person is called a chronic carrier.

(A) Endogenous infection

Endogenous infection may occur in carriers of potentially pathogenic organisms, when these previously harmless bacteria invade. Other surfaces or tissues in the carrier, e.g. Escherichia coli derived from the bowel, where it is harmless, may cause acute suppurative infection in the urinary tract, Staph. aureus from the nostrils may cause boil in the skin infection in a wound; and pneumococci from the naso-pharynx may cause bronchitis and bronchopneumonia. The source of endogenous infection is thus the site in a patient body (e.g. colon, skin or nasopharynx) where the organisms grows harmlessly as a commensal.

Staphylococcal sepsis of the skin and wounds, which is mainly endogenous, may—under certain circumstances—become transmissible, as in hospital, where conditions may favour *cross- infection* between patients. Thus, the *cross-infected* patients suffer from exogenous infection. However, patients with endogenous infections caused by organism of low virulence are not likely to infect other persons, e.g., patients with bronchopneumonia due to pneumococci of less virulence are not a danger to relatives, nurses or other patients and there is no need to isolate them from other patients in hospital.

Modes of spread of Infection

A variety of mechanism can spread respiratory and alimentary infections from host to host, while single mechanism, for which the parasite is specially adapted, can spread venereal and arthropod-borne blood infection :

(1) *Respiratory infection* : The causative microbes are disseminated into the environment in masses of infected secretion, e.g., secretion transferred from the nose or mouth on fingers, handkerchiefs, cups, spoons or secretions expelled in spitting or blowing the nose; they are also discharged to a less extent in the droplet spray produced by sneezing, coughing and speaking, but in normal breathing, they are very rarely disseminated. The secretion contaminates handkerchief, clothing, bedding, floors, furnitures, and household articles (fomites) which may act as vehicles or reservoirs of infection. It dries in dust, most kind of respiratory microbes may remain alive for several days, even for several months, if protected from direct sunlight, e.g., tubercle bacilli, diphtheria bacilli, streptococci, staphylococci and smallpox virus.

(a) Infection may be passed to the recipients by contact, either 1) *direct contact* i.e. touching of bodies as in hand-shaking, kissing and contact of cloth, or ii) *indirect contact* e.g. contaminated eating utensils, door handles, towels; the recipients may transfer the microbes from contaminated finger to his sore or mouth.

(b) Infection may be *dust borne* by inhalation of air borne infected dust particles. The infected numerous dust particles are disseminated into the air from the skin and clothing during normal body movements; from dried contaminated handkerchieves during use, from bed sheets while bed making, from floor during sweeping and walking, and from furniture while dusting. The larger infected dust particles may settle within a few minutes on the floor and other exposed surface, e.g. skin, clothing, wounds and surgical supplies; whereas the smaller dust particles remain air-borne for up to 1 to 2 hours and may be inhaled into the recipient's nose, throat, bronchi, lung alveoli. Within the room of its origin, air-borne infection is very common and dangerous; but its spreading to other rooms in the same building is rare.

(c) The third least important means of respiratory infections is droplet spray, except in the case of the pathogens that are rapidly killed by drying, e.g., meningococcus, whooping cough bacillus, measles and common cold viruses, sneezing, coughing, speaking and other forceful expiratory activities expel a spray of droplets derived from the saliva of the anterior mouth which is infected with small numbers of pathogenic microbes from the nose, throat, lungs. Numerous droplets are expelled, but only a few are infected. The large droplets (over 0.1 mm in diameter) fly forwards and downwards from the mouth to the distance of a few feet, they reach the floor or body sources (eye, face, mouth and clothing) or the persons standing in front of the other person producing the spray, within a few seconds. These particles cannot be inhaled. Measles, chicken pox and dog distemper are common viral infections spread by the larger droplets. The *small droplets* (below 0.1 mm in diameter) evaporate immediately to become minute solid residue or "droplet nuclei" (mainly 1 to 10 μm in diameter), which remain air-borne and may be inhaled into the nose, throat, lung. Few of the droplet nuclei are infected with pathogenic microbes. Measles, chicken pox, and dog distemper are common viral infections spread by the droplet nuclei.

(2) *Mucous membrane, skin wound, discharges and burn infection*

Gonococcal ophthalmia caused by gonococci and inclusion blennorrhea caused by sub-group A of chlamydia may be acquired from the infected genital tract of the mother, when the mucous membrane of eyes of newborn infants gets infected as the infant passes down the infected birth canal.

Leptospira excreted in the urine of the infected animals enter the human body through the skin, similarly larvae of Schistosoma and Ankylostoma penetrate the skin.

The superficial infections may be acquired by (a) contact with infected hands, clothing or other articles, (b) by exposure to the disposition of contaminated droplet spray. Pathogenic streptococci and staphylococci derived from respiratory tract are important.

Causes of wound and burn infection; if pathogenic staphylococci are disseminated from pus discharge, they may cause infection of broken skin and burn wound.

(3) *Venereal infection* : The diseases transmitted exclusively by sexual intercourse are called as venereal diseases, since the causative agents e.g. *Treponema pallidum* and *Neisseria gonorrhoeae* are highly susceptible to lethal effects of drying, they are to be transmitted only by sexual contact. Gonococcus—which causes vulvovaginitis in young girls—may be acquired, under unhygienic conditions, from the common use of towels and bathing facilities. This is non-venereal spread of infection in young girls. Sub-group A of chlamydia (*Lymphogranuloma venereum*–LGV) infection is transmitted by sexual contact. Acquired immuno deficiency syndrome (AIDS) caused by Human immuno deficiency virus (HIV) can be transmitted through sex commonly by homosexuality.

(4) *Alimentary tract infection* : Persons with intestinal infection may disseminate the pathogenic microbes in excreta. These microbes are transmitted in various ways, the so-called *faecal oral routes*, leading to their ingestion by the recipient, e.g., *Salmonella typhi*.

Most of the intestinal pathogens are not much resistant to drying, they may die within a few hours, they may survive on cloth, or in dust for several days. They are more likely to be spread by moist vehicles (*water* or *food*) in which they may survive for several weeks.

(a) *Water-borne infection* may occur when faeces contaminate a water supply, e.g., river or well, which is used without purification for drinking purpose. In typhoid and cholera, water is the common vehicle of infection and the infecting doses may be small. Water is supplied to the citizen by the municipality after purification. Purification, which renders the water non-infective, is carried out on a large scale by storage, filtration and chlorination. Small amounts of water required for drinking purpose may be treated by boiling or by the addition of hypochlorite tablets.

(b) *Hand infection* : The hands of the nurses can get infected while attending the patients and touching the bedpans. Similarly, the hands of the carrier can be contaminated with bacteria contained in the faeces. Such persons may contaminate the foodstuffs, eating utensils, wash hand basins, towels, door handles and other fomites (inanimate objects). A recipient may eat contaminated food or put in his mouth the contaminated utensils or may pick up the microbes on his fingers and then transfer them into his mouth.

(c) *Food-borne infection* may occur through :

(i) a carrier handling the food (food as a vector of disease) :

(ii) preparation of the food in utensils contaminated by handling or washing in contaminated water;

(iii) flies alighting on the food after feeding on infected faeces. Enterotoxins may be produced on the food contaminated by bacteria during their growth in favourable conditions e.g. *Staph. aureus* and *Clostridium botulinum.* These preformed enterotoxins are prerequisites for bacterial food poisoning, whereas food-borne infection may result from the ingestion of only a few pathogenic microorganisms, e.g., *Sh. dysenteriae* which liberate enterotoxin.

(5) *Urine* : Typhoid bacilli are excreted in the urine and faeces, similarly leptospirae are excreted by animals through the urine and enter the mucous membrane and skin.

(6) *Arthropod-borne infections* : In systemic infection, the causative microbes are present in large number in blood, so they may be transmitted to other individuals by blood-sucking arthopods such as mosquito (malaria, filaria, yellow fever), flea (plague), louse (epidemic typhus fever); mite (scrub typhus) and tse-tse fly (trypanosomiasis).

(7) *Laboratory infection* : Laboratory workers may occasionally become infected from artificial cultures or infected diagnostic or necropsy materials collected from patients or experimental animals. Brucella, rickettsia and *Pasteurella tularensis* especially cause laboratory infection; while other organisms (tubercle bacilli, anthrax bacilli, pathogenic leptospiral, Borreliae, freshly isolated typhoid, dysentery bacilli, psittacosis organisms and serum hepatitis virus) should be handled very carefully. The pipetting of infected liquids by mouth leading to their accidental ingestion is certainly a danger of laboratory infections. Accidental self-inoculation with a syringe may take place or the conjuctiva may be sprayed when the needle become loosened from a syringe during an injection. Many laboratory procedures (the expulsion of liquid from a pipette or the use of the mechanical blenders, the centrifugation of tubes bearing traces of liquids on their rim) or drop separated from an inoculation loop may cause laboratory infections, when working particularly with pathogens which may cause air borne infection such as tubercle bacilli, thus it is necessary that all these procedures should be carried out with in an especially ventilated protective cabinet or inoculation hood.

(8) *Congenital transmission* : Serum hepatitis virus can be transmitted from the infected pregnant mother through placenta to the foetus. Similarly, human immune deficiency (HIV) can be transmitted through placenta to the newborn.

Congenital malaria is comparatively rare. The intrauterine transmission of malaria is well-established. The congenital malaria is very common in non-immune infected mothers. It is also believed the passage of the parasite to the foetus occurs only when the placental barrier has been injured.

Congenital toxoplasmosis results from the congenital infection in infants and young children. It usually appears as a form of encephalitis, accompanied by chorioretinitis, hydrocephalus or microcephaly, mental retardation and convulsions. The infection passes from the mother through the placenta late in pregnancy when neutralisation of antibodies cannot take place. The child is usually born jaundiced with purpuric or maculopapular rash; enlarged liver and spleen.

Congenital trypanosomiasis in man is possible and is rare; a case was reported in a child born of an infected mother, in Germany, who died less than three months after birth, because of proven trypanosomiasis. Later, two more proven congenital infections in infants were reported.

Congenital filariasis : The microfilariae of *Wuchereria bancrofti* may pass from the infected pregnant mother to the newborn through the placenta filter.

Basic Principles of Disease Transmission

Portals of entry and portals of exit are two basic principles of disease transmission :

1. Portals of entry

Normally, microorganisms enter the body through *certain routes* and cause the infection; but they cannot gain entrance through other abnormal portals of entry.

(a) Cuts or abrasions of the skin (e.g. bites of arthropods or animals); (b) mucosa of respiratory tract (nose, throat, lungs), eyes and mouth, gastrointestinal, genitourinary tracts are the most important common portals of entry.

Abnormal portals of entry : If harmless saprophytic microorganisms are introduced parenterally into the brain or into the peritoneal cavity by a hypodermic needle, they set up the rapid fatal infection.

Many organisms can cause the infection if they enter only through their *obligate* portals of entry. Thus, dysentery bacilli can produce severe bacillary dysentery, if they are consumed through water or food; but if they are rubbed into the skin wounds, they will not initiate any infection. Severe, even fatal infections (abscess, boil, carbuncle) can be produced if staphylococci are rubbed in the skin; but if swallowed, they are ineffective. Some organisms can enter through any portal.

Path of organism in the body : From the sites (portals of entry) of infection, organisms may pass into the blood stream, initiate a secondary (metastatic) infection in internal organs (i.e. in the meninges of the brain and spinal cord–meningitis).

When the *enteric pathogens* (typhoid bacilli, dysentery bacilli, *vibrio cholerae*) are swallowed, they enter the stomach unaffected temporarily by gastric juice (especially in the presence of food), they set up ultimately gastrointestinal infection. The *respiratory pathogens* locate in or on tonsils, throat (Streptococci, diphtheria bacilli, whooping cough bacilli) may cause the infection, if they pass down into the lungs, they may produce pneumonia (pneumococci) and tuberculosis (tubercle bacilli). The organisms (*Treponema pallidium*, gonococci) find their portals of entry through genital mucosa.

(2) Portal of exit

The pathway by which organisms leave the body of one patient to another patient or healthy individual to initiate the infection is known as portals of exit (Fig 84.1).

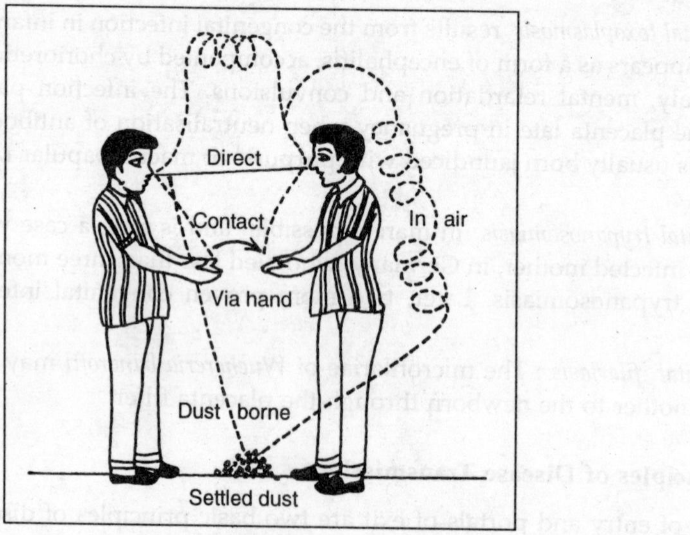

Fig. 84.1: Portals of entry and exit

Vectors

Vectors may be animate of inanimate :

(a) *Inanimate vectors* may be the food, discharges (faeces, saliva, pus), water, bandages, dressing, instruments, bedding, eating utensils and other inanimate objects (fomites) contaminated with infectious discharges.

(b) *Animate vectors* are generally arthropods or mammals : female anopheles mosquito is the vector for malaria; vectors of rabies are dogs or other mammals. Other animate vectors are the *hands* (very common) of the patients, nurses, doctors and patient's relatives coming in contact with an infectious patient or his fomites. Since man cannot be eliminated with Dichloro Diphenyl Trichloroethane (DDT) or muzzled and put on a leash, he himself may be regarded as one of the most dangerous vector of the diseases (e.g. man is the only significant living vector of AIDS, poliomyelitis, measles and syphilis and he is the most frequent live vector of human tuberculosis).

Application

An intelligent well trained professional nurse should know how to deal with the pathogenic microorganisms leaving the patient body to the environment. While attending the patient she should protect herself and the environment from these pathogens. The transmission of most infectious agents should be stopped by her at the portal of exit by immediate collection of and proper disposal of all body excretions, secretions, discharges, tissue likely to contain the pathogens (faeces, urine, saliva, mucus, pus, tissue drainage, used bandage etc.). In case of malaria, infected blood sucking female anopheles mosquito must be destroyed by Dichloro Diphenyl Trichloroethane (DDT) spray.

If the most probable portal of entry is intelligently understood by the nurse, she can adopt the appropriate methods of protection. For example, the respiratory portals of entry can be covered by the masks; cut or abrasions on the hand can be protected by bandage or surgical gloves. The alimentary canal is protected by appropriate selection and disinfection (as by pasteurisation of milk, chlorination of water and cooking) and sanitary preparation of food. The skin must be protected from the biting arthropods by clothing, fly repellants. Tissues and blood can be protected from the infection by vaccination or by prophylactic use of antibiotics and chemotherapeutic.

The Influence of Environmental Factors on the growth of Microorganisms

Chemical, physical, environmental and biological factors influencing the growth of microorganisms are :

Nutrition, moisture, temperature, presence or absence of oxygen, osmotic pressure, pH etc.

(A) *Chemical factors* : 1. Nutrition, 2. Oxygen, 3. pH, 4. Surface, 5. Phenols, Cresols and derivatives, 6. Dyes, 7. Salts of heavy metals, 8. Oxidising agents, 9. Formaldehyde, 10. Antiseptics.

(B) *Physical factors* : 1. Moisture, 2. Temperature, 3. Dessication, 4. Light, 5. High pressure, 6. Osmotic pressure.

(C) *Biological factors* : 1. Symbiosis; 2. Metabiosis; 3. Satellism; 4. Synergism; 5. Antagonism.

(A) Chemical factors

1. Nutrition of microorganism

(a) Metabolism means the digestion and utilisation of food to (i) synthesize the proteins, facts, carbohydrates and other substances of which living cells are made up, and to (ii) furnish the energy necessary for living and reproduction. The protoplasm (cell substance) of all living cells is therefore identical. All living cells utilise and metabolise all foods by means of enzymic mechanism. There are slight differences among different species of bacteria.

Foods of microorganism : Since Carbon (C), Hydrogen (H) , Oxygen (O), Nitrogen (N), Phosphorus (P) and Sulfur (S) with smaller amounts of Magnesium (Mg), Iron (Fe), Copper (Cu), Sodium (Na), Potassium (K) and other elements are the main components of protoplasm and other structures of all living cells; the nutrients of all cells must contain all these elements. In addition, the growth factors, such as nicotinic acid (niacin), thiamine, riboflavine are utilised by bacteria in much the same manner as those cells of human body do. The composition and metabolism of human cells are similar to those of many microorganisms.

Organic compounds : Proteins, carbohydrates, fats.

Inorganic compounds : Sodium chloride, water, carbon dioxide, sulphur, iron, hydrogen.

Carbon source for growth : Like plants, some non-parasitic bacteria are able to utilise carbon dioxide (CO_2) as the main source of carbon and are called *autotrophs* (*autos*–self, *trophe*–nutrition) or *lithotrophs* . Energy is obtained in these organisms by the oxidation of inorganic compounds (Chemosynthetic autotrophs) or from the sunlight (Photosynthetic autotrophs). The majority of bacteria require organic nutrients, such as carbohydrates, amino acids, peptides or lipids to serve as the source of carbon and energy. These organisms are called heterotrophs (Gr. *hetero*–another, *trophe*–nutrition) or organotrophs and they obtain their energy by breakdown of the organic carbon source. They differ in the utilisation of organic compound. Thus some species of the genus Pseudomonas can utilise any one of a hundred organic compounds (sugars, acids, alcohol etc.) as the sole source of carbon and energy. On the other hand, many bacteria are much more specific in their requirements.

Nitrogen source for growth : Bacteria differ widely in their ability to synthesise the main nitrogenous structural units–amino acids and nucleotides. Some are able to grow on ammonium salts as the sole source of nitrogen, while others require a variety of amino acids and nucleotides preformed in the medium.

2. Influence of oxygen and redox potential

Majority of bacteria are able to grow either *aerobically* i.e. in presence of air and free oxygen or *anaerobically*, in the absence of oxygen and they are called as *facultative anaerobes* (e.g. *Salmonella typhi, Staphylococcus aureus* and *Streptococcus pyogenes)*. Certain other bacteria will grow only in the presence of air or free oxygen and are described as *obligate aerobes* (e.g. tubercle bacilli, *Bacillus cereus;* common saprophytes of the soil). Still others will grow only in absence of free oxygen and are usually killed in its presence, they are known as *strict* anaerobes (i.e. *Clostridium tetani*). In the latter case, the ultimate determining factor is the state of oxidation of the environment, this being described in terms of oxidation-reduction or "redox" potential. A sufficiently low redox potential for the growth of strict anaerobe is usually provided by placing the culture media in an atmosphere of hydrogen with the complete exclusion of oxygen (e.g. McIntosh and Fieldes anaerobic jar). It has been suggested that, in the presence of oxygen, a strict anaerobe is liable to produce toxic peroxides which it cannot destroy owing to lack of catalase, an enzyme present in most aerobes and facultative anaerobes. Finally, there is a group of organisms which grow best in the presence of a trace of free oxygen and often prefer an increased concentration of carbon dioxide (CO_2), these are called *microaerophilic.*

3. Influence of hydrogen ion concentration

Hydrogen ion concentration : Hydrogen atoms, when dissolved in water, immediately assume a positive electrical charge they are called hydrogen ions and the acidity of any solution is due to them. Acids such as hydrochloric or acetic acid, possess the property of acidity because they give off hydrogen ions (i.e. they ionize) in aqueous solutions. If a solution contains a large number of these ions, it is very acidic and it is said to have a high hydrogen ion concentration. If it is only slightly acidic or alkaline, it is said to have a low hydrogen ion concentration.

pH hydrogen ion concentration is expressed by numbers used in the symbol of pH , which stands for hydrogen ion concentration. pH is an essential factor in bacterial metabolism and growth. The majority of commensal and pathogenic bacteria grow best at a neutral or very slightly alkaline reaction (pH 7.2 to 7.6). Some bacteria flourish in the presence of considerable degree of acidity and are termed acidophilic, e.g., *Lactobacillus.* Others are very sensitive to acid, but tolerant to alkali, e.g., *Vibrio cholerae.*

Most of the bacteria are rapidly killed by strong acid or alkali solutions e.g 5 per cent hydrochloric acid or sodium hydroxide but the mycobacteria (e.g tubercle bacilli) are resistant to them.

According to their effect on bacteria, bactericidal chemical substances can be divided into surface active substances, phenols and their derivatives, salts of heavy metals, oxidising agents and the formaldehyde group.

4. Surface active substances

Change the electrical charges. Bacterial cells lose their negative charge and acquire positive charge which impairs the normal function of the cytoplasmic membrane.

Bactericidal substances with surface active action include fatty acids and soaps which harm only the cell wall and do not penetrate into the cell.

5. Phenol, Cresol and related derivatives

First of all injure the cell wall and then cell proteins. Some substances of this group inhibit the function of coenzyme (diphosphopyridine nucleotide) which participates in the dehydrogenation of glucose and lactic acid.

6. Dyes

Dyes are able to inhibit the growth of bacteria. The basis of this action is the marked affinity for the phosphoric acid groups of nucleoproteins. Dyes with bactericidal properties include brilliant green, acriflavine etc.

7. Salts of heavy metals

(Lead, copper, zinc, silver, and mercury) cause coagulation of the cell proteins, silver, gold, copper, zinc, tin, lead etc. have an oligodynamic action (bactericidal activity). Thus, for example, silver plated objects, sliverware in contact with water may render the metal bactericidal to many species of bacteria. The mechanism is that the positively charged metallic ions are absorbed on to the negatively charged bacterial surface and alter the permeability of the cytoplasmic membrane. Thereby, the nutrition and reproduction are, possibly, disturbed. Under the influence of the salts of heavy metals, viruses may become irreversibly inactivated as they are very sensitive to these salts.

8. Oxidising agents

Chlorine is commonly used in decontaminating water, because chlorine acts on dehydrogenase, hydrolase, amylase, proteinase of bacteria; chloride of lime and chloroform are used as disinfectants. In medicine, iodine is used successfully as antimicrobial substance in the form of tincture iodine which oxidises proteins of bacterial cytoplasm and causes their denaturation. Potassium permanganate and hydrogen peroxide are other oxidising agents.

Many species of viruses are resistant to heat, chloroform, ethyl and methyl alcohol and volatile oils. All viruses are resistant to 50 per cent glycerine, except Rinderpest virus, sodium hydroxide, chloride of lime and chlorine can destroy viruses as they are oxidising agents.

9. Formalin

(40 per cent formaldehyde) has bacteriocidal effect, because it possibly unites with the amino groups of proteins and brings out denaturation of proteins. Formaldehyde destroys both the vegetative forms and the spores of bacteria. It is also used to decontaminate diphtheria and tetanus toxins and, at the same time, it detoxifies the toxins transforming them into *anatoxins* (toxoids). Phage and tobacco mosaic virus inactivated by formalin can sometimes renew their infectivity.

(B) Physical factors

1. Moisture

Since the bacterial cell consists of water, moisture is essential for its growth. Drying in air is injurious to many microorganisms, it may prevent the growth of microorganisms and may not kill them. One method adopted by microbiologist to keep certain microorganisms alive for long period (20 years or more) to dry them and store them in a refrigerated vacuum. Even delicate, non-sporing organisms may survive drying for many years if they are desiccated a high vacuum (0.01mm Hg) or less in sealed glass ampoule which is stored at room temperature in the dark. This is the basis of lypholisation or freeze drying process of preserving bacterial cultures or vaccines and viral vaccines in the laboratory or also during long distance transport. Quick freezing of bacterial and viral suspension at a very low temperature provokes conditions at which crystals do not form and subsequent disruption of the microorganisms does not occur.

Certain fragile microorganisms — *Neisseria gonorrhoeae* (gonococci) causing gonorrhoea, *Treponema pallidum* causing syphilis, Entamoeba histolytica causing amoebic dysentery — die almost at once when subjected to drying, while tubercle bacilli, Staphylococcus aureus and smallpox virus may survive for several months in sputum, pus, crust, respectively.

2. Temperature

Low temperatures halt putrefying and fermentative process. The process of metabolism is inhibited, as a result bacteria die and the cells are destroyed under the influence of the formation of ice crystals during freezing. *Vibrio cholerae* looses its viability at a temperature of –32°C. Some species of bacteria remain viable at a temperature of liquid air (–190°C) and of liquid hydrogen (–253°C). Diphtheria bacilli are able to withstand freezing for 3 months and enteric fever bacteria (*Salmonella typhi*) are able to live long in ice. Bacillus spores withstand a temperature of –253°C for 3 days. Many microorganisms remain viable at low temperature and viruses are especially resistant to low temperature. Thus for example Japanese encephalitis virus in 10% Brian suspension does not loose its pathogenicity at –70°C for a year; the causative agents of influenza and Trachoma at –70°C for 6 months and Coxsackie virus at –40°C for 1½ years.

Only certain species of pathogenic bacteria are very sensitive to low temperature (e.g. meningococci, gonococci.) During short periods of cooling, these species die quite rapidly. This is taken into account in laboratory diagnosis and the specimens for the presence of meningococci or gonococci should be sent to the laboratory protected from cold. Some microorganisms can grow best at a low temperature (4° to 10°C) are said to be psychrophilic, whereas those bacteria growing best at temperature (from 20°C to 37°C) are called mesophylls.

Most of the pathogenic non-sporing bacteria are killed at 58°C to 60°C for 30–60 minutes. Bacillus spores can withstand boiling (100°C) from a few minutes to 3 hours, but under the effect or dry heat at 160°–170°C in 60–90 minutes. Heating at 121°C (15 Ibs per sq. in gauge pressure) kills the bacteria and their spores within 20–30 minutes.

Some microorganisms will grow only at high temperature ranging from 45° to 75°C and are called as thermophilic e.g. *Bacillus stearothermophilus.*

The bactericidal action of high temperature is due to the inhibition of the catalase, oxidase, dehydrogenase activity, protein denaturation and an interruption of the osmotic pressure. High temperature causes rapid destruction of viruses, but some of the viruses (viruses of serum hepatitis, poliomyelitis) are resistant to environmental factors. They remain viable long in water, in the faeces of patients or carriers and are resistant to heat at 60°C and to small concentration of chlorine in water.

3. Dessication

Dessication is accompanied by dehydration of the cytoplasm and denaturation of bacterial proteins. Gonococci, meningococci, treponema, leptospira and phages are sensitive to dessication.

Vibrio cholerae persist for 2 days on exposure to dessication, dysentery bacteria for 7; plague bacilli for 8, diphtheria bacilli for 30; bacilli for enteric fever for 70; staphylococci and tubercle bacilli for 90 days. The dry sputum of tubercular patients remain infectious for 10 months.

Dessication in a vacuum at a low temperature does not kill bacteria, rickettsiae, viruses. This method of preserving cultures is employed in the manufacture of stable long storage or live vaccines against tuberculosis, plague, brucellosis, small pox, influenza.

4. Light

Direct sunlight has the greatest bactericidal action. Different kinds of light have a bactericidal or sterilizing effects. They are ultraviolet rays (electromagnetic rays with a wave length of 200–300μ, X-rays (electromagnetic rays with a wavelength of 0.005–1mu); gama rays (short wave X-rays); beta particles or cathode rays (high speed electrons); alpha particles (high speed helium nuclei) and neutrons. Rays of short waves used for the disinfection of wards, infectious material, for the conservation of products the preparation of vaccine, treating operation and maternity wards, have a high bactericidal effect. Viruses are very quickly inactivated under the influence of ultraviolet rays with a wavelength of 20–300 mu. These waves are absorbed by the nuclei acid of viruses. Longer waves are weaker and do not render viruses harmless. Viruses in comparison to bacteria åre less resistant to X-rays and gamma-rays. Beta rays are more markedly viricidal.

5. High pressure and mechanical injury to microbes

Bacteria withstand easily atmospheric pressure. Some bacteria, yeasts and moulds withstand a pressure of 3,000 atmospheric pressure. The movement of liquid media has a harmful effect on microbes. The movement of water in rivers and streams, undulations in stagnant water are important factors in self-purification of reservoirs from microbes. *Ultrasonic oscillation* (Waves with a frequency of about 20,000 hertz per second) has a bactericidal activity and it is used for the preparation of vaccines and disinfection of various objects.

6. Osmotic pressure

Like other living cells, bacteria have a semi-permeable cytoplasmic membrane which is subjected to osmotic pressure. Bacteria are very tolerant of changes in the osmotic pressure of their environment and can grow in media with widely varying contents of salts, sugar and other such solutes because of the thickness and mechanical strength of their walls. For most species, the upper limit of sodium chloride concentration permitting growth lies between 5 to 15 per cent. Though halophilic (or osmophilic) species occur which can grow at higher concentration up to saturation. Sudden exposure of bacteria to solution of high concentration (e.g. 2–25 per cent sodium chloride) may cause plasmolysis (i.e. temporary shrinkage of the protoplast and its retraction from cell wall due to osmotic withdrawal of water), this occurs much more rapidly in Gram-negative than in Gram-positive bacteria. Sudden transfer from a concentrated to a weak solution or to distilled water, may cause plasmolysis i.e. swelling and bursting of cell through excessive imbibition of water.

C Biological factor

1. Symbiosis is an intimate mutually beneficial relation of organisms of different species. They develop together better than separately. Sometimes the adaptation of two organisms

become so close that they lose their ability to exist separately (symbiosis of the fungus and blue green algae).

2. *Metabiosis* is one type of relationship in which an organism continues the process caused by another organism, liberating it from all its life activities and thus creating conditions for its own further development (nitrifying bacteria).
3. *Satellism* a symbiont known as the favourable microbe, accelerates the growth of the other (some yeasts producing amino acids, vitamins etc.), enhance the growth of microbes which are very specific regarding their nutrient requirements.
4. *In synergism* there is an increase in the physiological function of microbial association (Borrelia and fusobacterium).
5. In *antagonism* there is struggle for oxygen, nutrients and a habitat (antibiotics).

Application to Nursing

The bacteriologist, nurse will use the methods of the control of the microorganisms by the knowledge of the relation of microorganisms to their environmental factors.

For example, high temperature affect the living cell structure causing death; pathogenic bacteria are capable to produce infection or toxin according to the presence or absence of oxygen. The inhibition or destruction of microorganisms depends upon the removal of food, water and oxygen. In nursing practice, the microbial growth can be controlled by altering the temperature and subjecting the microorganisms to disinfectants.

In nursing situation (operating rooms, nurseries, communicable disease units, isolation wards, intensive care units), microorganisms can be destroyed by physical environmental factors (X-rays, gamma rays etc). Introduction of antiseptics in surgical practice prevented the access of microbes into the wounds. Aseptics are attained by disinfection of the air and equipments of the operating room, by sterilisation of surgical instruments and materials and by disinfecting the hands of surgeon and the skin of the operating field.

Modern methods of aseptics have been well perfected, by which almost all operations are accompanied by primary healing of wounds without suppuration and the post-operative septicaemia has been completely eliminated.

Dental microbiologist would be able to adopt the suitable method of control the growth of microorganisms according to their relationship with the environment. The growth of microorganisms can be slowed down or completely stopped by altering the environmental growth factors. The high temperature can affect the structure of the living bacterial cells, so that they may be completely destroyed. Anaerobic bacteria can grow very well in absence of oxygen and elaborate the toxin which is responsible for the pathogenic effect. In the presence of oxygen, the same bacteria cannot produce such toxin and, hence, they are not pathogenic. It may not be always possible to inhibit or destroy microorganisms by simple removal of food, oxygen, water. In nursing practice, the microbial growth can be controlled primarily by subjecting the microorganisms to the sterilization and disinfection. Ultraviolet rays can be sometimes used to kill the microorganisms in nursing situations (operation rooms, nurseries, communicable diseases).

85

Control of Microorganisms

(Removal, Inhibition and Destruction of Microorganisms)

History : When it was assumed that the communicable diseases were caused by microorganisms, the methods of sterilisation, disinfection and sanitation were adopted in the daily practice. In early nineteenth century, the hospitals were dirty buildings accommodating the patients on the mats spread on the floor, overcrowded together, died and dying in the same beds. Surgeons wore black coat with linen thread, wound around the button of his coat, which was used as suture material. His scalpel, kept attached to his breast pocket, was used periodically for the incision and was sharpened on the heel of his boot. The doctors washed their hands when they were soiled with pus and blood. The sleeve of the coat was rolled back to prevent from getting it spoiled, as these unhygienic conditions prevailed in those days in the hospital.

During this century came, Louis Pasteur (1863) who proved that the microbes caused the diseases. Robert Koch (1865) described many microbial diseases and isolated the causative microbes in pure culture. Later, Lister (1867) advocated in surgery the use of dilute carbolic acid as disinfectant. In obstetric and gynecology practice, the hand washing before delivery and operation was made compulsory. The practice of antisepsis and disinfecting started from 1867.

Napoleon Bonaparte ordered to serve better food for his armies. In order to obey his order, a French scientist, Nicholas Appert developed a process which was called as " Appertizing" which involved steam, heat, and pressure–as in autoclaving–this principle is even now adopted in the modern method of sterilisation in every hospital. Later Pasteur advocated a method to check spoilage of beer by subjecting it to a temperature of 50°–60°C for a few minutes and named it as "Pasteurisation" which is used in our day to day practice, i.e., *Pasteurisation* of milk.

Koch sterilised the culture media by a method of intermittent heat and 100°C. Tyndall modified, perfected the method and called it as "Tyndallisation".

In 1880, Pasteur constructed a miniature early autoclave similar to the modern pressure cooker. In 1890, for the first time in the world, an autoclave was installed in Rochester City Hospital, New York.

It is well-established that the microorganisms (both harmful and harmless) are ubiquitous in nature. The pathogenic (harmful) bacteria should be killed or eliminated completely particularly in surgery, surgical environment, hospital and public health. This procedure can be accomplished by the professional trained nurse by her skillful intelligent application of her Nursing microbiology knowledge in the medical and nursing practice.

In bacteriological laboratory, mostly *pure cultures* grown on nutrient media are dealt with. Therefore, the disinfection and sterilisation methods advocated for pure cultures were followed in the diagnostic laboratory, whereas in nursing practice, the situations are different unlike laboratory, so the ingenious professional nurse has to deal with *mixed cultures*, e.g., resistant forms and vegetative forms of microorganisms living in tissues, exudates, discharges, faeces mucus, pus, blood, Therefore the intelligent, well-trained nurse must exercise her own judgement after evaluating each situation to adopt the best methods to remove, disinfect, inhibit or destroy completely the pathogenic microorganism. The following are the best possible procedures :

(1) Removal by
  - (a) Passing the fluids through very fine filter which retains bacteria;
  - (b) High speed centrifugation.

(2) Inhibition by
  - (a) Low temperature (dry ice);
  - (b) Dessication (drying process)
  - (c) Combination of low temperature and dessication,
  - (d) High osmotic pressure (brine);
  - (e) Microbiostatic chemicals and drugs
    - (i) dyes–eosin, methylene blue, cyrstal violet;
    - (ii) chemical agents–sulfonamide, antiseptics.

(3) Destruction by
  - (a) Heat-dry (hot air oven); moist (autoclave);
  - (b) Chemical agents (disinfectants);
  - (c) Radiation (x-rays, ultraviolet);
  - (d) Mechanical agents (crushing).

Inhibition of Microorganisms : Antimicrobial Agents

Antimicrobial agent is a chemical which inhibits the growth and causes the death of organisms. The agents can be grouped accordingly :

1. If the substance merely causes a cessation of growth of microorganisms, which is reversed when the chemical removed. It is called *static* agent, if the substance kills the bacteria, it is called *cidal* agent. A static agent may become cidal if the concentration is increased. The disinfectants have cidal action, while chemotherapeutic agents are often static at the concentration used.
2. Agents acting on bacteria are *bacteriostatic* or *bactericidal*, those acting on fungi are fungistatic or fungicidal.
3. In practice, chemotherapeutic agents can be distinguished.

(a) *Disinfectants* are chemicals used to kill potentially infective organisms normally present on inanimate objects, surface, water etc. They are potentially toxic to man, when they come in direct contact with man.

(b) *Antiseptics* (mild disinfectants) are relatively non-toxic and non-irritant, antimicrobial agents which may be used for the topical application on the body surface to kill or inhibit the pathogenic microorganisms.

(c) *Chemotherapeutic agents* are chemicals used to inhibit or kill bacteria already established in the body tissues and are used for the therapeutic purposes in the treatment of microbial infections.

Chemotherapeutic agents should act at a concentration that can be tolerated by the tissues of the host and, therefore, they must have a selective toxicity for the microorganisms compared with the host cells. The most widely used chemotherapeutic agents are *antibiotics* which are naturally occurring antimicrobial agents produced by the microorganisms. The most common groups of antibiotic producers are actinomycetes and fungi.

Sulfonamides : The discovery of sulfonamides in 1935, by Dmagk, German chemist, began with the finding that the red dye, Prontosil, was capable of inhibiting infection with *Streptococcus pyogenes,* Prontosil itself had no effect on streptococci in *vitro;* but to be effective it has to be broken down in the animal to sulfonamide. Sulfonamide itself is effective in non-toxic doses. By substituting different organic groups (represented by R group in the formula below). For example, the addition of a pyridine groups gave sulphyridine, a thiazole gave sulphathiazole and so on. In this way, thousands of derivatives called sulfonamide were produced and many of them were found to be effective antimicrobial agents. Because of the development of newer antibiotics, relatively few sulfonamides have found a practical therapeutic use. It was observed that yeast and meat extract had the property of overcoming the inhibitory effect of sulfonamides on bacteria *in vitro.* The sulfonamide " antagonist" in the extracts was isolated and was shown to be para (p)–amino benzoic acid (PABA). It was also shown that PABA is an essential metabolite in any organism and was converted by them to dihydrofolic acid then to tetrahydrofolic acid, which act as a cofactor in reaction leading to the synthesis of nucleic acids and proteins required for cell growth.

It was found that the sulfonamides inhibit the first stage of the synthesis of dihydrofolic acid from para–amino benzoic acid. This drug, trimethoprim, which was later discovered and introduced into the medicine at much later date, inhibits the conversion of dihydrofolic acid into tetrahydrofolic acid.

Summary

P–amino benzoic acid (in the organism or environment)

↓

Sulfonamide

inhibits

↓

dihydrofolic acid

↓

trimethoprim

inhibits

↓

tetrahydrofolic acid

↓

(is a cofactor in the synthesis of nucleic acids and proteins)

Cell growth

↓

Fig. 85.1

Since p-amino benzoic acid and sulfonamide have similar chemical structures (Fig 85.1), there is *competition* between sulfonamide and PABA for the active site on the surface of the enzyme initiating the conversion of PABA to dihydrofolic acid. To inhibit the conversion of one molecule of PABA into folic acid, a large number of sulfonamides molecules are required in the *competitive* inhibition (Fig. 85.2).

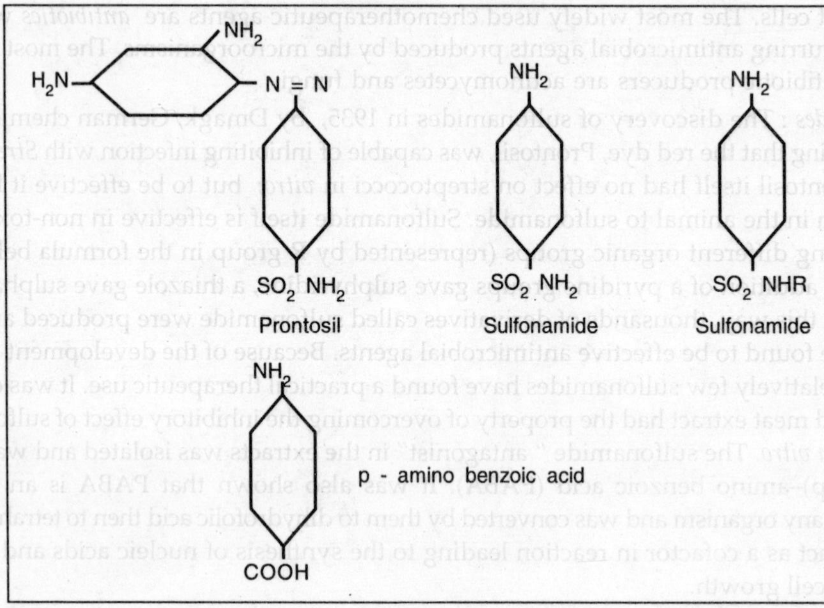

Fig. 85.2

Antibiotics inhibiting cell wall synthesis

Mucopeptide of the bacterial cell walls is responsible for their mechanical strength. If the synthesis of mucopeptide is inhibited, while synthesis of other cell components continue, then the cell can be expected to be lysed rapidly in normal osmotic environment. Penicillin inhibits the conversion of a complex nucleotide (uridine diphosphate UDP–N–acetyl muramic acid pentapeptide) into mucopeptide (Fig. 85.3).

Precursor– UDP–N–acetyl muramic acid pentapeptide —|— Mucopeptide

Penicillin inhibits

Fig. 85.3

Penicillin was discovered by Alexander Fleming in 1922.

Antibiotics affecting protein synthesis : A number of antibiotics (Streptomycin, Kanamycin, Tetracyclines, Erythromycin and Puromycin) are known to inhibit protein synthesis. Streptomycin, discovered by Waksman, was the first antibiotic to be introduced clinically after penicillin.

Antibiotics affecting nucleic acid synthesis. Few antibiotics combine withstand, alter the functioning of nucleic acids though they are generally toxic for therapeutic use. Ribonucleic acid (RNA) synthesis is prevented by Actinomycin, because it forms a complex with double stranded Deoxyribonucleic acid (DNA), but not with single stranded DNA; however, at higher concentrations, DNA synthesis is inhibited. On the other hand, mitomycin links complementary strands of DNA resulting into blockage in DNA synthesis.

Antibiotics action on the cytoplasmic membrane : Polymyxin acts on the cytoplasmic membrane as a cationic detergent binding to the membrane, as a result the semipermeable properties are lost and essential low molecular weight intermediates and coenzymes pass into the environment causing the death of bacteria. Polymyxin should be used with caution as it binds also with the membrane of the host cells.

Source of Antibiotics : Unlike synthetic sulphonamides, most of the antibiotics are produced in the culture media during the growth of certain microorganisms (Streptomyces, Bacillus, Penicillium, Aspergillus). New antibiotics found in plants and animals, terrestrial and marine (Table 87.1).

Manufacture of antibiotics : The desired antibiotic producing organism is cultivated in large tank of suitable liquid medium for a predetermined length of time. The culture is then centrifuged and filtered to remove the microorganisms. The filtered fluid, containing the antibiotic is then subjected to purification and concentration process. These at length yield crystals of the pure antibiotics which are then tested for purity, sterility, then packed and distributed.

Classes of Antibiotics : Antibiotics may be grouped as :

Group I : (Penicillin, Streptomycin, Bacitracin, Polymyxin B) can be used together, they are often synergistic; never antagonistic. For example, when penicillin and streptomycin combined they are valuable in endocarditis. The combination is more effective than the sum of both.

Group II : (Tetracyclines, Chloramphenicol, Erythromycin, Carbomycin, Neomycin, Oleandromycin, Novobiocin) is neither antagonistic nor synergistic. This sometimes works well in combination with antibiotics of first group. This second group is generally of the "broad-spectrum type". There are many other broad-spectrum antibiotics. The usual response to antibiotic therapy and antibiotic resistance or drug fastness are two important properties of organisms.

86
Uses and Preparations of Disinfectant or Antiseptic Lotions

Phenol Group Antiseptics

Lysol (*liquor cresolis saponatus)* and cresol (black and white fluid) are general powerful disinfectants.

Lysol, in 3 per cent solution, is generally used for sterilising discarded cultures; Sudol is less toxic substitute for Lysol.

Phenol (0.5 per cent solution) is effective in preserving sera; Chloroxylenol (Dettol) is less active toxic and irritant.

Hexachlorophane is incorporated in various antiseptic preparations and reduces the skin flora, if it is used repeatedly as detergent containing 2-3 per cent hexachlorophane.

Metallic salts

Mercuric chloride (1 :1000) is an useful disinfectant; merthiolate (1:10,000) can preserve antisera; silver nitrate (1 per cent) is employed for prophylaxis of gonococcal ophthalmia. Chlorhexidine (Hibitane–modern antiseptic) replaces silver nitrate and is effective against both Gram-positive and Gram-negative bacteria.

Formalin (40 per cent solution of formaldehyde in water) is a powerful and rapid disinfectant to decontaminate the surface and disinfect the bacterial cultures.

Borax–formaldehyde solution (sodium tetraborate –5 gm. Formaldehyde, 4 per cent in water, 1000 ml) can be useful to sterilise the cleaned metal instruments.

Tincture of iodine or 5 per cent phenol solution or stronger solution of chloroxylenol (Dettol) can be used as a single application for preparing the skin of the patient for incision or puncture.

Recently the addition of 0.5 per cent chlorhexidine in 70 per cent ethyl alcohol improves the action of 70 per cent alcohol and is also as effective as 1 percent iodine in alcohol and also to be free from irritation.

Cetrimide (Cetavion). This solution has pronounced surface tension lowering properties and on shaking it produces a prolific form. It is incompatible with soap and similar anionic detergent. It has both powerful detergent and bactericidal properties. It is more effective against Gram-positive bacteria and to a lesser degree against Gram-negative bacteria. Aqueous or alcoholic solution of cetavlon do not kill spores. It is specially useful to remove tar, oil or grease.

For all practical purposes, it is highly active against bacteria in concentration as low as 0.1 per cent; one per cent solution can be used for its full detergent power. 0.1 per cent solution of cetavlon in 10 per cent alcohol is sufficient to effect a satisfactory degree of sterility within 2 minutes; for a more rapid sterilisation, higher concentration should be used.

A one per cent aqueous solution of cetavlon has been found to be efficient preparation in the preoperative "scrub up" of the hands. If soap and water are first used, the hands can be finally rinsed with a 0.1 per cent solution of cetavlon to give the necessity of persistent bactericidal film.

One per cent solution of cetavlon can be used in preliminary cleaning dirty, contaminated wounds, oils, grease can be removed.

One per cent solution of cetavlon is very useful to clean dog bite wound, adjunct to routine antirabic vaccination. Basins, bowels, tables can be readily cleaned and disinfected by rinsing with one per cent aqueous solution. Surgical instruments can be effectively cleaned by rinsing with one per cent aqueous solution of cetavlon in a closed container. To prevent rusting, sodium nitrate is thoroughly mixed in the proportion of 4 gm per litre of solutions used for storing instruments should be changed at weekly intervals. The instruments should be rinsed and dried when removed from the solution after use.

Preparation of cetavlon : Aqueous solution of cetavlon is rapidly and simply prepared by adding the concentrate to water. When solutions are being prepared for the storage of sterilised instruments, it is preferable to used boiled or distilled water.

Cetavlon concentrate 20% : It contains 20% cetavlon in aqueous solution distinctly coloured with a non-staining yellow dye. A 1% solution of cetavlon is prepared by mixing 35 ml of the concentrate with about 7 liters of water.

Cetavlon tincture : An alcoholic solution contains 0.5% cetavlon coloured. by adding a harmless red dye. When applied to the skin, its eliminates bacteria and stains the area so that the site of operation is clearly defined. The dye may be removed by washing and will not harm the dressings.

Cetavlex cream : Contains 0.5% cetavlon in an emollient cream base, it can be used in treatment of wounds and burns during emergency.

Savlon concentrate combines the advantages of two outstanding antiseptics of proved value it contains the new antiseptic "Hibitane" (Chlorhexidine gluconate, 1.5% W/V) together with "Cetavlon" (cetrimide, 15% W/V).

87

Antibiotics in Common use

Table 87.1. Antibiotics in Common Use

Antibiotics Common name	Trade name	Source	Characteristics
Penicillin		*Penicillium notatum*	Gram-positive bacteria, Treponema, Neisseria
Paromomycin	Humat	*Streptomyces rimous*	*Entamoeba histolytica*
Streptomycin		*Streptomyces griseus*	*Myco.tuberculosis*
Dihydrostreptomycin		*Streptomyces. sp*	Gram-negative bacteria.
Tetracyclines	Archomycin	Chlortetracycline	Broad-spectrum
Oxytetracycline	Terramycin	*Streptomyces rimosus*	Broad-spectrum
Chlortetracycline	Aureomycin	*Streptomyces aureofaciens*	Broad-spectrum
Chloramphenicol	Chloromycetin	*Streptomyces venezualae*	Broad-spectrum
Erythromycin	Althrocin	*Streptomyces erythreus*	Broad-spectrum (not Enterobacteriaceae)
Carbomycin	Magnamycin	*Streptomyces halstedii*	Broad-spectrum (not Enterobacteriaceae)
Oleandromycin	Matromycin	*Streptomyces sp.*	Broad-spectrum (not Enterobacteriaceae)
Neomycin B	Flavomycin	*Streptomyces fradiae*	Mycobacteria
Viomycin	Viocin	*Streptomyces funiceus*	Gram-positive bacteria, Treponema
Amphotericin B	Fungizone	*Streptomyces nodosus*	*Candida sp.*
Kanamycin	Kantrex	*Streptomyces kanamyceticus*	Broad-spectrum
Nystatin	Mycostatin	*Streptomyces noursei*	Pathogenic fungi
Cycloheximide	Actidione	*Streptomyces griseus*	Saprophytic fungi
Griseofulvin	Grifulvin	Streptomyces griseus	Pathogenic fungi
Bacitracin		*Bacillus subtilis*	Gram-positive bacteria, *Treponema*
Polymyxin B		*Bacillus polymyxa*	Gram-positive bacteria
Pyocyanin*		*Miscellaneous*	Pseudomonas aeruginosa

* One of the first known antibiotic substances. Not used medicinally.

Use of Antibiotics : Some of the antibiotics can be used only by oral route; some in oinment only; others are suitable for intravenous or subcutaneous injection. Some are effective chiefly against Gram-positive organisms and some against Gram-negative organisms. Others have a wide range of activity. They are known as *broad-spectrum.*

Antibiotics, Drug Resistance or Drug-Fastness : Microorganisms often undergo genetic mutations. These mutations generally result in alterations in enzymic equipment in the mutant cells. If mutation occurs in few cells of a species of microorganisms (e.g. *Staphylococcus aureus)* altering the enzymatic equipment of these cells which are multiplying in a patient treated with penicillin. These mutated few cells will produce penicillinase or beta lactamase enzyme acting on beta lactam ring of penicillin become resistant to penicillin and grow in presence of penicillin. They are called as antibiotic resistant or drug-fast. These resistant cells may grow and finally predominate in spite of the drug. The predomination is very dangerous to the patient and for every one around him who may acquire the organisms (e.g. sulphonamide-resistant gonococci). The sufficient quantity of the chemotherapeutic drug in the blood stream affecting organism before it can start growing, can be maintained by using adequate doses. This blood level maintenance can stop the development of such drug-resistant microorganisms.

Blood levels maintenance : The amounts of drug in the blood can be maintained by repeated doses at proper intervals of time. If delayed administration of drug dosage occurs, it may fail to combat a drug-fast infection and the patient may succumb to the infection. Therefore, the nurse responsible for giving repeated dose of such drugs should be very careful that the patient receives the drug *on time* so that his blood levels may not decrease to dangerous low levels.

Microorganism Response to Antibiotics

Microorganisms	Usual response for proper antibiotic treatment	Frequency of appearance of resistance in strains in patients
Pneumococcus		
Meningococcus		
Gonococci	Rapid	Rare
Beta streptococci		
Shigella		
Treponema		
Staphylococcus	Rapid	Very frequent
Alpha and gamma		
Streptococci		
Coliform	Slow or incomplete	Frequent
Proteus		
Pseudomonas		
Tubercle bacilli		
Brucella	Rapid frequent relapses	Rare (once),
Salmonella typhi	require repeated treatments	Frequently (recently))
Rickettsiae		

88
Containers and Swab for Collection of Specimens

Containers used for microbiological investigations should be sterile, leak-proof and strong. Each container should bear the name of the patient, from whom the specimen was collected and his case register number. The investigation requisition form should also accompany the specimen indicating the investigation required alongwith the probable clinical diagnosis and current chemotherapy. Details of previous immunisation should be furnished for serological investigation.

Glass tubes and universal containers : Specimen of exudate, pus, blood, cerebrospinal fluid, urine and faeces should be collected in strong, sterile, corked glass test tubes (4×3/8 inch). Before collection of samples, tests tubes with loosely fitted from plug or bark corks can be sterilised in hot air oven and then the corks should be pressed in.

Universal container or screw-capped bottle is a strong moulded glass bottle (3¼ in height × 11/8) in diameter of one oz (28 ml) capacity with a flat base and wide mouth. It is sterilised with loose cap and then tightened. It cannot be sterilised in the hot air oven as the rubber washer will not withstand the temperature.

The screw-capped universal container has many advantages over the glass test tubes. It is strong, the mouth of the container is sterile because of the screw cap, whereas in case of stoppered glass test tubes, the dust may collect at the rim of the test tube. The content of a container will not leak and will not be contaminated. It is quite stable at the base of the container and it is very convenient for collection of the sample at the bed side and it is very suitable for the collection of serous fluids, e.g., Pleural or peritoneal fluids. The collection of the fluids that may be coagulable on standing can be done in the container to which 0.3 ml. of a 20 per cent solution of sodium citrate is added prior to the autoclaving. This method of collecting fluid may be useful in performing cell count or centrifuging procedures.

Blood may be collected in a sterile universal screw-capped container or test tube fitted with cotton plug for serological investigation. The streptokinase digested or minced blood clot may be cultured in a selective medium e.g. for enteric organisms (Salmonella) or blood for culture may be collected and submitted to the bacteriological laboratory in a special blood cultures bottle containing bile salt broth. Serum from clotted blood can be transmitted to the laboratory preserved in sodium azide or merthiolate (1:10,000) in a sterile polysterin or polypropylene plastic container.

Faeces may be collected in a small bottle of about 2 oz capacity or in a glass specimen tube or by a rectal swab. If the laboratory is situated at a far off place, the container may be transmitted with all precautions by post; the package should be labelled as "Pathological specimen". If there is a delay of some hours before laboratory cultivation can be performed, neutral glycerol saline should be added to the faeces. Rice water stool from cholera patient should be collected on a leaf or paper, but not in disinfected bedpan because disinfectants can kill *Vibrio cholerae*. Specimen should be sent in transport medium, e.g., Alkaline peptone water or Venkataraman-Ramakrishnan (VR) medium.

Urine: For the diagnosis of urinary tract infection, the urine, if required in small quantity, can be collected in a universal container; complete early morning specimens (large quantities of urine) can be collected in a 20 oz screw capped bottles.

Disposable specimen containers

Sterile screw-capped waxed cartoons of 2 oz capacity (such as used for icecream) are suitable for the collection of sputum or faeces. These waxed cartoons cannot be sent through the post because of postal regulations. Plastic polysterene or polypropylene containers of variable size are suitable for urine, feces, pus, blood etc. Recently, disposable plastic specimen containers have become available from various manufacturers. All disposable containers should be destroyed in a furnace after use.

Swab : A swab consists of a piece of wooden (bamboo or broom) stick of about 6½ in long. A round one end of the stick a thin pledget of absorbent cotton wool is tightly wrapped for about ¾ inch. The stick is placed in a test tube (5 in × ½) and the top of the tube is plugged with a cotton wool. This has the advantage that the stick can be broken off short when the swab has to be placed in transport medium in a screw-capped container. Besides collection of specimens, the swab can also be useful in the laboratory for seeding of medium for antibiotic disk sensitivity tests.

A variety of disposable swabs (plain, serum coated, charcoal coated) in plastic tubes are available. They can be destroyed in a furnace after use or sterilised in autoclave before discarding.

Swabs are useful in collecting specimen from :

(i) *Throat* : in cases of suspected diphtheria, tonsillitis;

(ii) *Wound* : specimen from surgical conditions (fistula, sinus) or discharging ears can be collected by swabs;

(iii) *Post-nasal or naso-pharyngeal space* : Specimens from suspected meningococcal carriers and whooping cough can be collected by using sterile post-nasal swab which is made from a flexible copper wire or nichrome (0.51 mm diameter), its terminal end (¼ inch) bent back through an angle of 45 degrees is tightly wrapped with a thin pledget of absorbent cotton wool. For the diagnosis of whooping cough, a pre-nasal swab is preferable to the post-nasal swab.

(iv) *Rectum* : Rectal swabs are very useful in bacillary dysentery in young children.

(v) *Cervix uteri* : A longer sterile stick or wire, 9 inch, is preferable for the specimens in gonorrhoea and purperal infections.

The conditions where delicate pathogens are concerned e.g. meningococcus, gonococcus or *Bordetella pertussis*, it is preferable to place the swab in sterile Bijou bottle containing transport medium, e.g., neutral glycerol saline.

(e) *Infection of Reproductive system* : Coliform bacilli, streptococci, *Mycobacterium tuberculosis*, *Neisseria gonorrhoeae* are pathogens responsible for the infection of female genital tract.

Puerperal sepsis or septic abortions which are acute infections in the female after delivery are caused by *Streptococcus pyogenes*, *Clostridium welchii*, *Bacteroides*, Coliform bacilli.

Cervical swabs should be taken with the help of a speculum under direct vision, put in to Stuart's transport medium and sent to the diagnostic laboratory.

In acute vaginitis, due to *Trichomonas vaginalis* and vaginal thrush due to *Candida albicans,* exudates can be readily obtained by swabing and direct smears can be made on slides for microscopic examination or exudates may be collected by pipette or spoon for wet films.

Acute urethritis and prostatitis in male are due to *N. gonorrhoeae.*, chlamydia or *Mycoplasma hominis.*

Wound infection

F. Wound infection may be

(a) *endogenous* or (b) *exogenous.*

Endogenous infection (autoinfection) are caused by organisms that were commensals elsewhere in the host body, e.g., organisms from large intestine may infect the abdominal surgical wounds after an operation that has involved the incision of the skin.

Cross-infection is an example of exogenous infection where the causative organisms spread from person to person. Infection may occur after accidental or intentional trauma of the skin or other tissues : the latter type is known as " post-operative sepsis".

Specimen collection

Swabs should be well soaked in pus or exudate from infected wounds. Syringe can be used to collect the pus or exudate specimens which can be used to collect the pus or exudate specimens which can be transferred into a sterile test tube. Pieces of tissues removed at operation or curetting or other tissues can be sent immediately to the bacteriological laboratory and they should be homogenised in a tissue grinder before it is used for bacteriological examination. Delay in the transit of specimens to the laboratory must be avoided, particularly in cases of swabs where the exudate may dry in the cotton-wool.

G. Infection of the Conjunctiva

Pseudomonas pyocyanea causes severe conjunctivitis due to the use of contaminated eye drops. Gonococcus (ophthalmia neonatorum), *Staphylococcus aureus* (sticky eye in new born babies), pneumococci, *Moraxella lacunata* and *H. influenzae,* certain viruses (herpes virus, adeno virus,) Tric agent (Trachoma, inclusion blennorrhoea) produce conjunctivitis.

Swabs coated with exudates can be sent to the laboratory in Stuart's transport medium. Purulent exudate from inflamed conjunctiva can be considered as pus. Gonococcus can be shown by direct microscopy and can be grown on heated blood agar medium.

89

Non–Pathogenic (Useful) Microorganisms

Microorganisms may be divided into two groups — according to their activities : (a) the useful, and (b) the harmful.

The first group– the harmless, non-pathogenic microorganisms to man live mostly in the environment. They are called as *Saprophytic* or *Autotrophic* (yeasts, molds and bacteria) and are very useful to the industries for the manufacturing of alcohol, lactic acid, butter, cheese, solvents of paints and antibiotics etc. and to the agriculture to improve to soil fertility.

The second group– the harmful, may be called *pathogenic* microorganisms, damages the host and produces diseases in man, animals and plants. Bout of 1,700 groups of bacteria, about 70 groups are pathogenic to man and can live only in human body, but they may die in external unfavourable conditions.

The activities of useful microorganisms :

Decay, Putrefaction and **Fermentation.**

Decay is the term used generally to denote the gradual decomposition of organic matter (dead animals, plants and their wastes) on or in the soil.

Putrefication is the decomposition of proteins (animal matter) under anaerobic conditions and of carbohydrates (vegetable derivatives starch or sugar). These two processes transform organic matter into useful plant foods. When dead animals and plants are buried in the ground, the soil microflora and the intestinal microflora of dead animal enter into the tissue of the animal or plant. Because of their lipolytic, proteolytic and saccharolytic activities. The microbes break fats, proteins and sugars, respectively. The gases (carbon dioxide, ammonia, hydrogen sulphate etc.) liberated and water formed enter in the air, soil. Besides, nitrogen, phosphorus, sulfur, produced from dead animal body combine with water and become soluble and suitable as food for plants. Ultimately, the dead animal disappears. Later, the living animals and men use the plants as food. In this way, the recycle of the elements is continued. Thus, the life would be impossible on earth without microbial activity and the microbes are useful or essential for animal or human life. The colibacillus and other species of microbes in the healthy human intestine produce vitamins (B_1, B_2, B_{12}, K) essential for the human body. Acidophilic microbes are beneficial to the human body as they interfere with the development of pathogenic bacteria which enter the intestine alongwith food or drink.

It is well known that human beings cannot digest directly the cellulose of the plants and utilise it for their nutrition; but the rumen (stomach) microflora of ruminants (cattle, sheep, goats) can only digest it anaerobically and convert into easily digestible end products like glucose, amino acids, volatile fatty acids, which are excreted through milk or incorporated in animal tissue or muscle. Man drinks milk containing proteins, fatty acids and lactose which are derived from the cellulose of plant or green fodder digested by the rumen microflora as the rumen of cattle is devoid of digestive enzymes. So the rumen microflora are quite useful for human welfare without which milk or meat cannot be obtained from the animal for the human consumption.

Microorganism in food

Moistless acidic foods (milk, cooked cereals, custard, soup) are suitable media for the growth of saprophytic and pathogenic microorganism at warm room temperature and thus we consume large number of saprophytic microorganisms alongwith the foods every day with no harmful effects. The growth of certain microbes in some kinds of food is useful. Certain harmless streptococci added to cheese and butter may produce good flavours in them. Therefore, "starters" (materials containing the desired bacteria) are added to the cream before it is churned into butter and they are also added to milk that is used for making the cheese. Flavour producing bacteria (Lactobacillus) can ferment pickles.

Putrefication is the anaerobic digestion and decomposition of proteins, muscle, egg white, fish) by microorganisms. It is usually accompanied by bad odour due to formation of ammonia, hydrogen sulfate and other volatile odoriferrous substances. Mostly, putrefied materials are not agreeable, but we consume the putrefied milk in the form of cheese and they are dangerous if contaminated. If foods are contaminated with excessive growth of saprophytic microbes, they are *spoiled* foods. This process is known as *Spoilage.*

Fermentation : Under anaerobic conditions, the microorganisms (bacteria, yeasts, moulds) decompose, by their saccharolytic activities, the carbohydrates (sugars) into different kinds of acids, such as lactic acid, alcohol, and gases like carbon dioxide. One of the most familiar type of fermentation is the production of alcohol by yeast from the sugar of fruit juices as in wine manufacture. Certain streptococci (*Streptococcus lactis*) ferment sugar of milk (lactose) into lactic acid which causes souring of milk. This harmless streptococcus alongwith other saprophytic bacteria enters into the milk from the dust, splits the milk if it is not refrigerated. The yeasts, multiply in the dough and decompose the starch (sugar of the flour) and form alcohol and carbon dioxide. The gas bubbles entangled in the dough, raise (leaven) the bread. The bread dries and becomes firm due to the evaporation of alcohol during baking.

The *decomposition* of fat by microorganisms is known as *hydrolysis.* When fats containing butyric and similar volatile fatty acids are decomposed, these acids are liberated and are responsible for the odour and rancidity taste.

Pathogenic (harmful) bacteria may contaminate the foods or milk products, grow and liberate toxin (preformed toxin of *Staphylococcus* aureus *and Clostridium botulinum)* causing food poisoning. *Salmonella typhimurium* is pathogenic to mice, which, when consumed alongwith the food, may also cause food poisoning in man in whom the illness takes the form of gastroenteritis.

The food should be thoroughly cooked, *kept closed in a* vessel or should not be allowed to stand unrefrigerated and should not remain moist, as moist food is a suitable medium for the growth of bacteria.

Application of nursing : Nurse must understand that the food should be protected from microbes and should serve her patients and her own family with clean food.

Microorganisms of water

In ancient times and even now in some backward modern community, the people throw the wastes of household out of window in the streets. These wastes and faeces may contaminate the community water supplies and thereby there will be great epidemics due to pathogens of intestinal tract : typhoid, cholera, gastroenteritis, hepatitis etc. Modern microbiology utilises concept of purifying sewage by the activities of certain saprophytic soil and water microbes is of great importance to the community health in supplying purified water. The microorganisms utilise the organic substances of the sewage as food and turns them into harmless, inoffensive materials which are used as food by plants.

Municipal sewage : Method used for purifying municipal sewage first straining out extraneous objects by passing the 'raw' (untreated) sewage through metal screens or racks, then allowing it to flow very slowly through large tanks. In such tanks, the solid matter in suspension settles to the bottom. This solid material is slowly decomposed through the hydrolytic action of microbial enzymes of *anaerobic and facultative anaerobic* bacteria. It eventually forms sludge (sort of mud) rich in plant food, which is pumped out, dried and used as fertilizer in garden. This sludge is sterilised before packaging.

The fluid part of sewage is sprayed on the surface of large beds (trickling filters) of coarse gravel. During this process, it becomes fully aerated. On the surface of gravel or sand a slimy film develops. This film consists of the growth of aerobic microorganisms, which get their nourishment by decomposing and oxidising offensive materials in the sewages. The sewage trickles slowly through the gravel. As solid matter (humus) is collected in the final tank it is pumped onto the open sludge drying beds. The deodorised, cleaned fluid is collected in drains under the gravel and run out in fields for irrigation.

Activated sludge : In modern activated sludge process, aeration of the sludge is accomplished by violently agitating the sewage with large volumes of air. Solid matter is torn into small granules or particles. These particles contain millions of active aerobic microorganisms which use the air to oxidise and decompose rapidly the offensive matter in the sludge. *Aeration* is the key objective in any form of sewage disposal.

Drinking water : The water of rivers, lakes, springs, oceans contain many saprophytic microorganisms; and these saprophytes are often present in drinking water and are harmless, since they cannot invade the human body. Man consumes large number of these saprophytes with food, water and milk every day. They are harmless. However, water polluted with sewage usually contains pathogenic microbes (typhoid or dysentery bacilli, cholera vibrios, polio, hepatitis virus, amoebae etc.). The only safe way is to boil all water or treat it with chlorine a few hours before use. Tablets of hypochlorite or other chlorine compounds are available for this purpose. The nurse who is faced with the problem of disinfection of water at home can very well remember this method.

Microorganisms of air

Under ordinary conditions, the spores of numerous microorganisms may be found in air all around us. Many of these are spores of molds, yeasts, useful conidia of streptomyces and spores of bacteria of the genera clostridium and bacillus. Spores and conidia are excellently adapted to survive floating about on dust in the air for weeks or years. All these spores are harmless except those of clostridium and bacillus which are pathogenic to man. The number of microorganisms in the air usually depends on the amount of dust since most of the microorganisms are riding around on dust particles. They are usually of the harmless types found in soil and soon die in the dry air and sunlight. However, the air of badly ventilated dark room may contain many pathogenic organisms which are disseminated by the occupants who are carriers of such microbes in the nose and mouth.

In recent years much attention has been paid to the air as means of disease transmission —especially in hospitals. It is known that every drop of saliva and nasal exudate, even from healthy persons, nurses and doctors) contain microorganisms capable of causing disease. Among these are staphylococci, pneumococci, streptococci of scarlet fever, puerperal sepsis, and septic sore throat, diphtheria bacilli, tubercle bacilli and numerous viruses (polio, influenza, adenovirus etc.).

Droplet infection : The air of classroom, theatres and street cars are loaded with microorganisms, especially in winter; sneezing and coughing sprays of saliva and mucus are added to the general population of the atmosphere laden by bacteria and viruses. Transmission of disease by droplets of saliva and mucus is often called droplet infection. These sprays infect the dust and, when dry, this dust carries the bacteria.

Droplet nuclei : The droplets of saliva and dry mucus and the bacteria contaminated in the dried particles float in the air and are inhaled like dust. Such dried particles are spoken as "droplet nuclei". These land on the floor, furniture, lips, hands, surgical wounds.

Application to nursing : Knowledge of microorganisms in the air will be useful to take precautionary measures, to protect herself and her patients from the microorganisms which sometimes may be pathogenic to man.

Industrial Microorganism

It is well established that the microorganisms produce alcohol, lactic and acetic acids during fermentation of carbohydrates; besides these products many other substances of equal importance are also formed. So, the microorganism are widely used in industry.

The skill and knowledge of microbiologist, engineer and chemist are pooled together in the industrial fermentation to produce the large quantity of butyl alcohol, glycerin, antibiotics, vitamins and other substances of great importance, depending upon the species of microorganisms. In the manufacture of rubber, coffee, cocoa, tobacco, linen, spices, leather, pickles, drug and other products the fermentative, putrefactive, synthetic and other enzymatic powers of microorganism are utilised. Thus, it can be concluded that the microorganisms have entered in the business and became very useful to mankind.

Nitrogen fixing microorganism and life

Nitrogen is the component of the cytoplasm of the cell and is essential for the life. Though eighty per cent of the atmosphere contains nitrogen, the atmospheric nitrogen cannot be directly utilised by the living cell, but this nitrogen can be prepared from the atmosphere by the microorganisms by combining it with other elements, mainly oxygen, hydrogen and carbon of the atmosphere. The process of combining nitrogen of the atmosphere with other elements is called nitrogen fixation.

The nitrogen of air can be fixed by certain soil microorganisms by two methods : non-symbiotic and symbiotic (living together for mutual benefit) nitrogen fixation.

Non-symbiotic nitrogen fixation : The direct combination of atmospheric nitrogen as part of the protoplasm of a living cell without the cooperation of any other organism, e.g., atmospheric nitrogen can be built up directly into the protoplasm by the bacteria of the genus Azobacter (Azo= nitrogen), the genus *Clostridium* and other microorganisms. These useful microorganisms are plenty in all the fertile soils. Therefore, a farmer permits the Azobacter, Clostridium and other microorganisms to accumulate nitrogen from the air by allowing a field to lie fallow or unplanted–Nitrogen of the commercial fertilisers are very costly.

Symbiotic nitrogen fixation : The nodules on the roots of leguminous plants (i.e. clover, beans, peas, alfalfa) contain bacteria belonging to the genus Rhizobium. While growing together with the plants this genus Rhizobium collects nitrogen from the air and combines it into substances essential for the growth of both the bacteria and the plants. The process is known as symbiotic nitrogen fixation method.

Nitrification : Nitrogenous compounds released into the soil by leguminous plants may be taken up by other plants and partly decomposed by putrefaction yielding ammonia (NH_3).

As ammonia, nitrogen is generally useless to most green plants. Ammonia is also produced in small amounts by lightning flashes and is also washed into the soil by the rain. To be most readily available to plants, the nitrogen of ammonia must first be oxidised to nitric acid (HNO_3). This important function is carried out by the soil bacteria of the family Nitrobacteracae. The nitric acid they form immediately combines with various substances to form nitrates. The process of changing nitrous acid into nitric acid is called *Nitrification*. These nitrifying bacteria and nitrogen fixing bacteria are of great importance to agriculture. The nitrogen of the air is useless to many organisms. At a depth of four feet, bacteria become less numerous and at 10 to 12 feet, there are usually no bacteria.

Microorganisms in and on human beings : The healthy human body harbours millions of microorganisms on the skin, in the mouth, eyes, genitourinary tract and in the intestine and on every surface of the body which comes in contact with the outside of the world air, food). Under normal conditions, most of the microorganisms do not produce the disease, but under certain conditions (e.g. in wound or after surgery) gain entrance to the deeper parts of the body and produce the disease.

The skin carries large number of bacteria. *Staphylococcus aureus* found in the hair follicles and sebaceous ducts causes the boils, carbuncles, breast abscess, infantile impetigo. The organisms lodged in the deeper layer of the skin cannot be removed by thoroughly scrubbing and then by the application of antiseptics, therefore sterile gloves are worn during operation.

Microorganisms found on and in the human body

Skin

Staphylococus aureus
Staphylococcus albus
Corynebacterium acnes

AXILLA

Mycobacterium smegmatis
Mycobacterium phlei
Staphylococcus albus

SCALPS

Staphylococcus albus
Corynebacterium acnes

EARS

Mycobacterium phlei
Staphylococcus albus
Corynebacterium sp.

CONJUNCTIVA

Corynebacterium xerosis
Staphylococcus albus
Haemophilus sp.

NOSE, MOUTH AND PHARYNX

Streptococcus pyogenes
Streptococcus salivarius
Streptococcus faecalis

DIPHTHEROIDS

Corynebacterium diphtheriae
Corynebacterium xerosis
Neisseria meningitidis
Haemophilus influenzae
Borrelia vincenti
Fusobacterium fusiforme
Trichomonas tenas.

Intestine

Escherichia coli, coliform bacili
Shigella
Salmonella
Clostridium
Clostridium welchii
Streptococcus faecalis
Klebsiella
Pseudomonas
Proteus
Lactobacillus bifidus
Polio virus

PERIANAL AREA

Mycobacterium smegmatis
Escherichia coli and coliform bacilli
Enterococci
Clostridium sp
Staphylococcus epidermidis

GENITALIA

Mycobacterium smegmatis
Lactobacillus acidophilus (vagina)
Trichomonas vaginalis
Corynebacterium sp.

HANDS

Variable (commonly microorganisms of skin, respiratory tract, faeces, and perianal region)

90
Pathogen from the Soil

Bacterial pathogens of the soil (spore forming bacilli).

Most of the spore forming bacilli of human or animal intestine are excreted through their faeces and contaminate the soil and form the spores under adverse conditions. In the human or animal tissue, these spores germinate into infectious bacilli. And produce disease.

GRAM-POSITIVE SPORE FORMING BACILLI

↓

Anaerobic	**Aerobic**
↓	↓
Spore bulging (Clostridium) e.g. *Cl. tetani, Cl. welchii; Cl. botulinum*	Spore central within the bacillus (e.g. *Bacillus anthracis*)

TETANUS, caused by *Cl. tetani*, occurs in man and animals. When a wound is infected with *Cl. tetani* under conditions that allow the organism to multiply and produce the toxin, absorption of the toxin leads to hyper-excitability of voluntary musculature. The disease is characterised by increased muscle tonus and exaggerated muscular response to simple stimuli. *Trismus* occurs as early sign of tetanus in man, when jaw muscles are affected and the disease is called as "lock jaw".

Cl. tetani are Gram-positive rod-shaped bacilli. They are motile with numerous peritrichous flagella. Their spores are spherical, terminal, larger than the diameter of the bacillus producing a typical "drumstick" appearance.

Cl. tetani are obligate anaerobes, grow best at 37°C in cooked meat medium.

The spores may be highly resistant to adverse conditions. They resist dry heat at 150°C for 1 hour. 5% phenol, Iodine in watery solution and hydrogen peroxide (10 volumes) kill them within a few hours.

Tetanus toxin : It is an exotoxin and has two components : (a) neurotoxic constituent (tetanospasmin) is the essential pathogenic constituent and has been separated as pure crystalline protein which can kill mouse in dose of 0.0000001 mg. It is an extremely powerful toxin, second in potency only to the exotoxin of *Cl. Botulinum.*

Tetanolysin is another constituent which causes lysis of red blood cells. It is oxygen labile.

Tetanus antitoxin is often called antitoxin serum (ATS) — can be obtained by immunizing horse with toxoid. This serum is of great value in the prophylaxis of tetanus, when given immediately after wounding. Its use as a curative agent after the development of tetanus is less effective. At the international conference of Tetanus, Mumbai, it was decided that an initial dose of 10,000 units of antitoxin should be adopted in the treatment of adult cases of Tetanus. When intravenous antitoxin is prescribed it should be proceeded by a subcutaneous test dose, followed by an intramuscular test dose at half hour interval. The antitoxin should be diluted, warmed at room temperature and injected slowly into the recumbent patient.

Precautions while injecting antitoxin : Routine precautions should be taken before an antitoxin is administered to avoid the risk of anaphylactic reaction following injection of antitoxin. Informations regarding previous serum injections, any history of asthma, infantile eczema, urticaria and other allergic condition should be obtained from the patient. In the absence of contraindication, the full doses of antitoxin may be injected, but a sterile syringe and needle with adrenaline (1ml of 1 : 1000) solution should be ready. The patient should be kept warm before and after treatment and he should be under observation for at least 30 minutes after the injection.

If the patient has had a previous injection of serum, but gives no history of an allergy, a subcutaneous test dose of 0.2 ml antitoxin shall be given and full dose of antitoxin may be given if no general reactions have occurred after 30 minutes. If the patient gives a history of allergy, the initial test dose should be 0.2 ml of a 1 : 10 dil of antitoxin subcutaneously. If no general symptoms develop within 30 minutes, this may be followed by 0.2 ml of undiluted antitoxin subcutaneously. The full dose may be given if there are no general reactions after a further dose.

Tetanus toxoid : The toxin can be detoxified by the chemical (formaldehyde). During the conversion period the toxin part is destroyed leaving antigenic part intact. Thus the toxoid is an excellent immunising agent.

A course of three 0.5 ml doses of tetanus toxoid (formol toxoid) with intervals of 6 to 12 weeks between the first two doses and 6 to 12 months between the second and third injection is proved valuable in the prevention of tetanus. A reinforcing (booster) dose of 0.5 ml toxoid should be given at intervals of 5 to 10 years to maintain immunity.

Pathogens : Tetanus is usually the result of contamination of a wound with *Cl. tetani* spores from the soil. Deep punctured wounds, wounds associated with devitalised, necrotic tissue and wounds contaminated with soil, ionised calcium salts and silicic acid favour the germination of spores of *Cl. tetani* and multiplication of this organism and production of the toxin. This tetanus toxin is absorbed by the motor nerve endings and spread up the space between the nerve fibres. It seems to act as excitant to the motor cells in the anterior horn of the spinal cord and may diffuse in the CNS. It may also interfere with the normal inhibition of motor impulses, thus producing early increase in tonus and tonic spasms of muscles and also impairs the release of acetylcholine.

Laboratory diagnosis can be done by microscopic examination of Gram-stained films of wound exudate for typical 'drumstick' appearance bacilli. They grow in Robertson cooked meat medium or anaerobically in blood agar medium.

Chemotherapy : A course of systemic penicillin or tetracycline therapy should be given in cases of established tetanus and, at the same time, antibiotics should be applied in and around wound.

Application to nursing : Nurse should invariably disinfect and dispose off all dressings soiled with the wound exudate. She should take all precautions while administrating antiserum to avoid the anaphylactic shock. She should wear gloves while dressing wound and should not delay in treating wound.

GAS GANGRENE, caused by *Cl. welchii,* is characterised by rapidly spreading oedema, necrosis and gangrene of the tissue and gas production. The infection results from the contamination of a wound with soil from manured or cultivated land, dirty clothing, street dust etc. or from skin contaminated with intestinal organisms. The predisposing factors already discussed in detail with regard to tetanus are equally applicable in the case of gas gangrene. In puerperal sepsis cases and especially in case of septic abortion, the organism may gain access via the perineum to necrotic or devitalised tissues and set up a dangerous infection.

Cl. welchii is Gram-positive bacillus, occurring singly or pairs, is non-motile and often capsulated when seen in the tissues. Spores are formed outside the body and are typically oval, subterminal and slightly bulging. They grow best anaerobically at 37°C in blood agar medium and Robertson cooked meat medium. They are saccharolytic and proteolytic; hence in Litmus milk medium, acid clot and gas production result, the gas breaks up the clot and produces the "stormy clot" reaction.

Toxin. Cl. welchii produces 12 types of toxins of which 4 are major lethal toxin and a 8 minor lethal or non--lethal toxins; out of these four major lethal toxins (a, b, g), alpha toxin is produced by all types of *Cl. welchii*, but, notably by type A strain of *Cl. welchii* as the most important of the lethal toxins of the organism and is considered to be the main cause of the profound toxaemia associated with gas gangrene in man. The alpha toxin is lethal, necrotising on intradermal inoculation. It is a relatively heat stable enzyme, lecithinase C. In presence of Ca and Mg ions, it can attack phospholipid constituents of red blood cells.

Laboratory diagnosis : Specimen of exudate should be taken from the deeper parts of the wound surface. The sterile swabs rubbed over the wound surface and soaked in the exudate serve the purpose (one swab for film preparation and another for the culture). If there are necrotic tissues in the wound, small pieces should be placed in a sterile screw-capped bottle and used for microscopic examination and culture.

Chemotherapy : The common antibiotics are used in the following order of the activity, in general, tetracycline, penicillin, chloramphenicol. Severe wounds considered to be the gas gangrene demand intravenous gas gangrene antiserum in addition to *meticulous* removal of dead tissue plus broad and parenteral antibiotics.

Prophylaxis of gas gangrene : A polyvalent serum is available for prophylactic use. The prophylactic dose, given intramuscularly, is 10,000 international units (IU) *Cl. welchii* antitoxin, 5000 units *Cl. septicum* antitoxin and 10,000 units of *Cl. oedematiens* antitoxin. The therapeutic dose, given intravenously, should be at least three times the prophylactic dose and it can be repeated if necessary. Monovalent serum can be used if the causal organism is identified. Reactions to antitoxin administrated intravenously may be severe and precautions should be taken.

Application to nursing : Nurse should be aware that they should use only autoclaving or hot air oven sterilisation or treatment of infected objects by sporicidal gases are necessary to prevent the transmission by fomites. Dressings should be burnt completely. Nurse and surgeon should wear gloves while dressing the oozing wound. Washed and wrapped gloves can be sterilised again.

BOTULISM is a fatal form of food poisoning caused by consumption of preformed toxin of *Cl. botulinum* and characterised by pronounced toxic effects–oculomotor paralysis, pharyngeal paralysis, aphonia. The causal agent is Gram-positive *Cl. botulinum.* It occurs singly or in pair, it is motile, its spore is oval, subterminal and slightly bulging. Its growth characteristic is similar to that of *Cl. welchii* spores of some strains of *Cl. botulinum* withstand moist heat at 100°C for several days. They are destroyed at 120°C (autoclaving). Insufficient heating in the process of preserving foods is an important factor in the causation of food poisoning, a great care should be taken to ensure that sufficient heating is achieved in all parts of the can while manufacturing canned food in canning factories. Home canning of foodstuffs can be done until the spores are ensured to be destroyed by sufficient heat.

Toxin .Toxin of Type A *Cl. botulinum* has been isolated as a pure crystalline protein and is the most potent toxic substance in nature. The estimated lethal dose for a mouse is 0.000000033 mg. i.e. 1 gm toxin is sufficient to kill 1 million individuals if equally dispersed.

Laboratory diagnosis : Suspected food can be examined bacteriologically. The toxin can be demonstrated in the extract of macerated food and in the patient serum.

Application to nursing : Nurse should not allow the patient to eat the canned food if the lids of the tin are bulging at both sides as it indicates the food is contaminated with *Cl. botulinum*. Antitoxin (10 ml) can be given intramuscularly for prophylactic purposes and toxoid in three doses for active immunity.

ANTHRAX is zoonotic disease. It is primarily an infectious disease of domestic animals and is transmitted to man when he comes in contact with them.

Bacillus anthracis is the causal agent of anthrax. It is Gram-positive bacillus arranged in chains or in pairs or singly (Fig 42.1). In the blood and tissue, it exhibits a distinct capsule when stained by polychromemethylene blue. The capsule is stained purplish and bacillus blue. It is called as methylene blue reaction of McFadyean which is very useful to recognise anthrax bacillus in blood films. Its spore, central, oval within the bacillus, can be stained by ordinary staining method.

B. anthracis grows best aerobically at 37°C. Its colonies appear under low power of microscope as lock of hair "medusa head appearance".

Toxin : Anthrax bacillus produces a toxin–"anthrax toxin complex"— which increases the permeability of blood vessels leading to the gelatinous oedema and haemorrhage — particularly in animals.

In man, the infection is acquired from animal source, usually through damaged skin or mucous membrane. The resulting lesion is usually described as "malignant pustule" This starts as papule and becomes a blister within 48 hours and then a pustule with in an increasing area of inflammation — depending upon the resistance of the host.

Infection may also result from inhalation of spores carried in dust or filaments of wool from infected sheep as in wool factories–"Wool sorter's disease." The organisms settle in the lower part of the trachea or in large bronchus and an intense inflammatory lesion results with haemorrhage, oedema, involvement of lungs, spread to the thoracic glands and diffusion into the pericardial and pleural cavities; considerable numbers of organisms are present in the lesion; a septicaemic condition or haemorrhagic meningitis may supervene. Infection of intestinal route is very uncommon.

Laboratory diagnosis. Smears made from the exudate of malignant pustule or sputum of Wool sorter's disease patient are stained with Gram-stain. The finding of bacillus morphologically similar to *B. anthracis* is suggestive but not conclusive.

Chemotherapy. B. anthracis is sensitive to most antibiotics, hence treatment of malignant pustule and Wool sorter disease is successful.

Application to nursing : When taking care of a patient with anthrax, the nurse should wear rubber gloves and a rubber apron. Dressings contaminated with purulent exudates or in fatal cases, fluids exudating from eyes, nose and mouth should be burnt promptly. Autoclaving or exposure to hot air oven at sterilising temperature or exposure to sporicidal gases for sufficient time is effective in destroying the spores. Pulmonary thorax requires the same precautions of respiratory infections. In addition to these, the disinfectant resistant spores of the exudates should be completely destroyed. Besides the public health, nurse should educate in explicit language the community that since the infected animal and dead carcasses are potent source of infection to man the farmers should avoid the contact of infected animals which should be buried very deep with lime. All fomites should be completely burnt.

91
Mycoses

The diseases caused by Fungi are called mycotic diseases or mycoses.

They consist of two groups :

(a) Cutaneous mycoses (Skin, hair, nails affected)

(b) Systemic mycoses (Internal organs affected).

(a) Cutaneous mycoses

Fungi penetrate the skin, hair and nails and grow as branching filaments or hyphae. Only the dead outer layer of these tissues is invaded; whereas the deeper or living layers cannot support the growth of hyphae.

In skin infection, the metabolites of the fungi diffuse into deeper living skin cells. People infected with these fungi become sensitive to these substances, as a result there is skin response with reddened erythematous areas and itching. In the erythematous area, soon appear the little blister. The centre of the lesion becomes scaly and heal, it is then surrounded by an enlarging red outer ring covered with blister. These conditions are known as "ringworm".

In hair infection, the shaft of the hair which is just formed above the living cells in the hair follicles, is attacked by superficial fungi (dermatophytes).

As the living cells continue to form the hair shaft, the infected portion of the shaft is brought upward. The penetration of hyphae of some fungi in the internal structure of the hair shaft may result in easly breakage of the hair within the hair follicle. In this condition, the infected area of the scalp appears *bald*.

In cases where the surface of the hair shaft is only infected by the hyphae of the fungi, the hair breaks often and thereby, the scalp appears as moth-eaten. The fungal infection of the hair of children is very common, compared to adults. Infective nails become yellow, black and brittle.

Tinea (Ringworm)

The medical term"tinea" implies the superficial fungal infection (ringworm) of the skin, hair and nails. Tinea capitis is the fungal infection of the hair of the scalp. When the foot is infected, the condition is called "athlete's foot" or tinea pedis. Fungal infections of the nail and groin are named, respectively, as tinea *unguium* and tinea cruris.

Dermatophytes (derm, skin; phyte, plant) are fungi which are infectious. They are groups of related fungi which embraces three genera and 20 species. Species of fungi occurring in the skin, hair and nail of man and animals are fully responsible for the direct infection from one individual to another and their hyphae in the tissues may directly develop into chains of spores after a long time. Other types of the dermatophytes may live in soil; when they are rubbed on to the skin, they may cause the infection.

The infections caused by dermatophytes are collectively called dermatophytoses or dermatomycosis.

Dermatophytes and their location of the infections

1. Hair, skin, rarely nails.
   Microsporum canis (ringworm, tinea capitis in children)
   M. audouinii (epidemic tinea capitis in children).
   M. gypseum (ringworm, tinea capitis).
2. Skin, hair and nails.
   Trichophyton mentagrophytes (athlete's foot, infection of nails and skin).
   T. rubrum (athlete's foot, tinea cruris, nail infection, sycosis).
   T. tonsurans (tinea capitis), *T. schoenleinii* (favus)
3. Skin, nails, *not hair*
   Epidermophyton floccosum (athlete's foot, tinea cruris, nail infection),

* Sycosis – pustular inflammation of the hair follicle of the face due to dermatophytes (barber's itch).

* Favus–dermatomycosis of the scalp characterised by honeycomb like, itching yellow crusts over the hair follicles.

Application to Nursing : The nurse should have the knowledge that the hyphae and spores of fungi can initiate the infection, if they are lodged on the skin or scalp or another susceptible individuals. Therefore she should take precautions to dispose off scale and stub of infected hair. She should also remember that the infected child can transmit his infection to his schoolmates and even to his pet animal. Dogs and animals should be carefully examined for scaly patches with loss of hair as they may become the source of infection to other human beings. Thus the owners of these animals should be advised to get these animals treated; if not responding to the treatment, they should be discarded.

Systemic Mycoses

The systemic mycoses are caused by fungi which occur in soil as saprophytes. The dust containing spores and hyphae inhaled by man may get logged in the lung, they grow; if they overcome the host defense mechanism, they multiply and produce lesions in the lung; and from these lesions they may be carried through the blood stream to various parts of the body where they setup the infection and lesions are produced. The lesion is limited to a small area of the lung in some people and may heal soon. Wounds of hands and feet are the portals of entry for soil fungi. Only few pathogenic fungi develop the infection.

Coccidioidomycosis

The causative agent, *Coccidioides immitis,* of the disease is commonly encountered in the soil of United States and grows as mould in soil. It is a *diphasic* fungus because it forms *spherule* in the tissue. Most of the people are infected by inhalation of dust laden with fungus; they show only a mild influenza like syndrome with fever.

Erythema nodosum painful red lumps appear on the legs of few patients. Pulmonary symptoms are very severe in some cases resembling to pneumonia and in others they may be suggestive of tuberculosis. If localised, giant cavities are formed in the lung. If the fungus is disseminated to various parts of the body, skin, bone marrow lesions may develop; meningitis is common and the patient will become seriously ill. In addition to the cultivation of the fungus. Skin test, *Coccidioidin* similar to tuberculin test is an useful test for diagnosis (Fig 91.2).

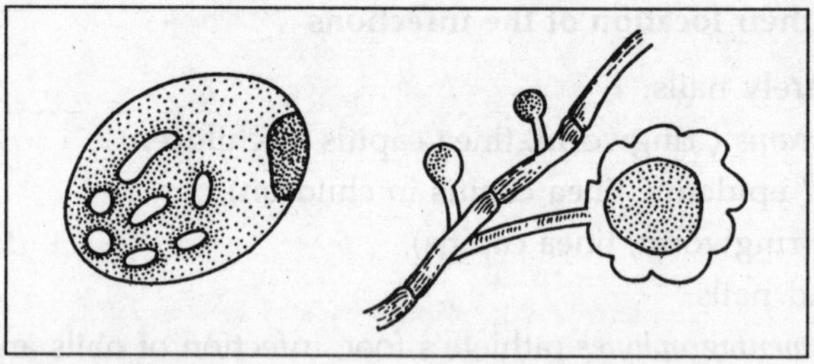

Fig. 91.1: Histoplasma capsulatum: Left—yeast like cell in macrophage. Right—Mycelium from culture bearing microconidia and tuberculate chlamydospore

Histoplasmosis

Histoplasma capsulatum (diphasic fungus) causes histoplasmosis and grows commonly in the soil of United States. The human infection occurs through inhalation of its spore.

Some infected people experience symptoms like influenza or pneumonia or tuberculosis. The prognosis is grave if the pulmonary disease is severe. If the liver or spleen is affected through dissemination the patients are seriously ill.

Skin test with histoplasmin and X-rays can be used for the diagnosis.

Blastomycosis, reported in United States of America and Canada, is caused by *Blastomyces dermatitidis*, diphasic fungus. Lung infections begin with the inhalation of spore or hyphae. Dissemination may be to all parts of the body. Lesions on the skin and in the bones are especially common. Skin test with Blastomycosin can be carried out.

Opportunistic mycoses : They are caused by a large number of soil fungi that are capable of producing infection in man under unusual conditions.

Candiasis : It is caused by *Candida albicans* which is yeast like organism commonly found in the mouth and the genital tract of healthy people, but under favourable conditions they multiply heavily, invade the tissues, and grow into long filaments and in the form of budding yeast like cells.

Diabetes, debility, steroid therapy and prolonged administration of antibiotics are the factors which promote the growth of *C. albicans.*

Candida vaginitis may occur in pregnant women. If the hands are wet for longer period, some people may develop skin lesions of the interdigital webs or of the finger nail.

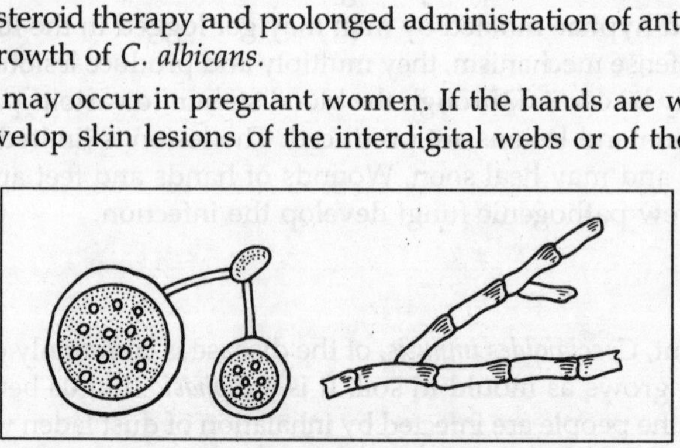

Fig. 91.2: Coccidioides immitis. Left—mature spherule containing endospores and immature spherules as found in tissues. Right—mycelium segmenting form arthrospores

Thrush

Though *C. albicans* (*oral thrush*) is normal flora of the mouth and genital tract, it may invade tissues, may set-up the inflammation and produce pseudomembrane on the lip and the mouth. This condition is called "Thrush". It is also common in neonates who acquire this infection from the infected mothers while passing through the birth canal. Ordinarily the bacteria of the genital tract suppress the growth of *C. albicans*, but if the patients are under antibiotic therapy for a longer period, the antibiotics may inhibit the growth of bacteria. As a result, *C. albicans* is free from the bacteria. Itching or perianal rash may also occur. Besides, if the lung tissue is damaged by tuberculosis or cancer or other diseases, *C. albicans* may multiply in the dead tissue and aggravate the infection. *C. albicans* rarely enter the blood stream; if it invades at all, it may be cause of vegetation of heart valves or lesions in the kidney.

Treatment : Nystatin is the drug of choice for candidiasis. Griseofulvin (oral administration). Betrafen cream and Zole powder (local application) for 21 days are very effective for superficial mycoses.

Application to Nursing : In systemic mycoses, the nurse should take care to dispose off the sputum, pus, dressing and other materials containing the fungus. Otherwise there is every possibility for the spread of the infection to the newly born infants from the mother. *C. albicans* vaginitis should be properly treated.

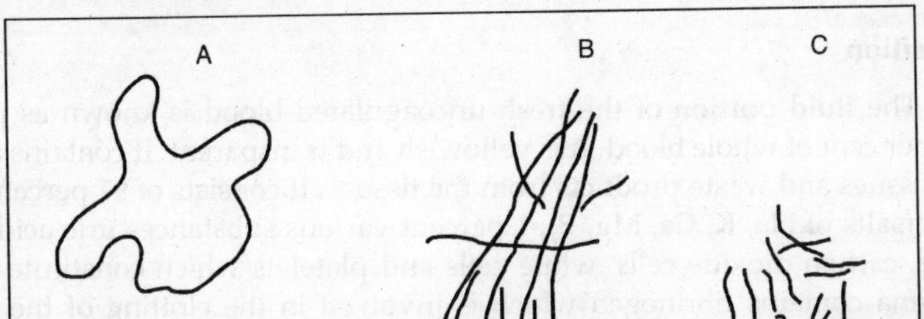

Fig. 91.3: Actinomyces israeli showing granules in pus (A) in broth culture diphtheroid like (B) and branching in brain-heart infusion agar (C)

92
Blood in Relation to Microbiology and Infection

It is well established that the blood supplies food to the various cells and tissues of the human body and removes all waste products from them. It also destroys the invading bacteria and their toxin and disposes them off with the help of living cells and certain substances contained in it. The blood also plays a great role in the production, transmission, prevention, diagnosis and cure of diseases.

Blood composition

Plasma : The fluid portion of the fresh uncoagulated blood is known as plasma which makes up 55 per cent of whole blood. It is yellowish and transparent. It contains proteins, food for the body tissues and waste products from the tissues. It consists of 91 percent water, 1 per cent minerals (salts of Na, K, Ca, Mg, P), 1 percent various substances uric acid, urea, amino acids, glucose, carbon dioxide cells, white cells and platelets which constitute remaining 45 per cent. Plasma contains fibrinogen which is involved in the clotting of the blood, which occurs when the soluble fibrinogen is converted into insoluble fibrin. Other proteins (albumins and various globulins) maintain the water balance of the body. *Gamma globulin* is of the globulin fraction or component. Blood is a rich source of antibodies. These antibodies can be used for treatment and prophylaxis of certain diseases and play an important role in the antibody mediated or humoral immunity.

Red blood corpuscles : Human erythrocytes (Greek, *erythros*, red; *kyotes*, cell) are non-nucleated, biconcave disks. They have a life span of 130 days and are constantly replaced. In adult male, their number is about 5 millions per cubic millimeter and in women, it is about 4.5 million per cubic millimeter. Red blood cells are manufactured in the bone marrow and released into the plasma of the blood. Haemoglobin (respiratory pigment) forms a loose chemical bond with oxygen when exposed to air in the lung, carries oxygen to the tissues of the body and releases it to them. Haemoglobin is released into the surrounding when the red blood cells rupture. The process is known as hemolysis (Greek, *haima*, blood, *lysis* to disrupt or dissolve). *In vivo* and *in vitro*, red blood cells can be lysed by certain bacterial toxins.

White blood corpuscles : They are also known as leukocytes (*Gr. leukos*, white). They are larger and less in number than the red blood cells. They are about 7,000 per cubic millimeter of the blood. They act as scavengers or policemen in the blood. They engulf any foreign particles (dead tissues or bacteria) entering the blood stream, they ingest these particles directly, they move with the help of *pseudopodia* and enter between the tissue cells of the body. If the bacteria enter into the leukocytes through their thin cell membrane, they may be killed and digested by digestive enzymes of the leukocytes. This process is known as *phagocytosis*. Leukocytes can move out of the blood vessels by their amoeboid movement between the cells lining the blood vessels. Leukocytes can be attracted by the chemotaxis to the area of the inflammations caused by foreign particles (bacteria). In the infected spot or boil the white creamy material consists of dead leukocytes (pus cells), dead bacteria, tissue debris, fluid from blood and tissues and is known as "Pus".

Platelets : They are irregular and disk shaped particles of varying sizes and smaller than erythrocytes. They are about 300,000 per cubic millimeter of blood and look like fragments of cells. Their origin is yet unclear and they are also responsible for coagulation of blood. Blood with low platelets may not clot quickly and may cause surgical hazard.

Plasma	Serum
1. Yellowish fluid portion of whole blood;	1. Straw coloured fluid remaining after clotting of blood;
2. It contains fibrinogen, in blood clotting, soluble fibrinogen is converted into insoluble fibrin, the jelly-like substance of the clot.	2. It contains no fibrinogen;
3. It contains antibodies (antibacterial substances and bacterial toxins);	3. It contains antibodies and bacterial toxins;
4. In microbiology (serology), it is used to diagnose some diseases as it may contain antibodies against some infections;	4. It is used in the diagnosis of diseases as it contains antibodies against the diseases;
5. It plays a great role in humoral immunity.	5. It plays an important role in humoral immunity.

Blood circulation

Left ventricle of the heart pushes the blood continuously through the arterial system to the remotest branches–microscopic arterioles, venules or capillary vessels. The wall of the capillary vessels are of one cell thickness. Nutrients and other substances (hormones, oxygen etc.) filter through these thin membranous walls, and diffuse into the fluid (lymph) which is constantly bathing the tissues cells. The nutrients are brought from the gastrointestinal tract and liver by the blood. Waste metabolic products (acids, carbon dioxide etc.) diffuse from the tissue cells into the lymph; then from the lymph into the blood stream of capillary venule and venous system which is in continuity with arterioles. These waste products in the venous (impure) blood are carried to the right auricle of the heart and are pumped to the right ventricle through the lungs when the red blood cells and plasma take up oxygen from the air and give off carbon dioxide. This purified blood returns to the left auricle and then to the left ventricle which pushes again the purified blood to the tissues. In this way, the blood circulates in the body for the benefits of the body (nutrition, metabolism, growth, protection against diseases etc.).

Blood and Diseases : When blood passes through the tissues infected with toxin producing pathogenic microorganisms (e.g. diphtheria, tetanus) carries with it toxin (toxaemia) and if bacteria (Salmonella) enter the blood stream (bacteriaemia). The toxin and bacteria are carried alongwith the blood and are distributed to various parts of the body where they set-up many infections e.g. brain abscess, osteomyelitis (inflammation of bone), otitis media (middle ear infection). Blood borne diseases (malaria, filariasis, yellow fever etc.) can be transmitted by arthropods (mosquitoes) from person to person. The blood carries drugs and antibiotics injected or swallowed to abate the infection.

Blood and Immunity : Cell and antibody mediated immunities against the infection are performed through the circulating blood, leukocytes in the circulating blood are responsible for cellular immunity, whereas the antibodies for humoral immunity. Antibodies (Gamma globulins) are soluble protein molecules secreted into the blood by lymphoid cells which are stimulated by the foreign proteins (Refer to chapter on immunology).

Infection : The term infection is used to designate an entry and the presence of organism, whereas the *disease* to designate the response of the host to the infection.

Host-parasite relationship is a part of science *ecology* where the organisms live together and help mutually. A host-parasite relationship develops during the evolution of many species of living organisms to thrive with each other. *Symbiosis* or *mutualism* is a host parasite relationship; when the organisms are mutually antagonistic they are *antibiosis. Parasitism* or *predation*, when some organisms live at the expense of the others. The infectious disease is an example of *parasitism* relationship.

Commensalism is also an example of host relationship where the organisms thrive side by side peacefully after some struggle for their existence.

During the process of infection, immunity and allergy, many host-parasite relationship and adaptations are established.

Infection is a condition where the microorganisms enter the human body tissues, grow in or on them, may damage them and the host may react to this damage by manifesting symptoms like fever, chills, nausea and headache. Infection may be fatal or serious. A pimple is a simple reaction to the infection of the skin; whereas Typhoid is serious if untreated by antibiotics.

Factors of infection :

(a) Dose of infecting microorganisms;

(b) Virulence of microorganisms : (i) Aggressiveness, and (ii) Toxigenicity.

(a) *Dose of infecting microorganisms* : There is possibility of infection if the number of microorganism entering the body is very large; a million organisms may set up the infection, if the tissue resistance is lowered by fatigue, disease or alcoholism, or after entry into the body, by overcoming the host defence mechanism, whereas a single bacterium (coccus or bacillus) may not be able to establish in the healthy body.

(b) *Virulence of organisms* is the ability of organisms to enter, establish, infect, damage the tissues and produce the disease. The virulence depends upon two factors : (i) aggressiveness and (ii) toxigenicity.

(i) *Aggressiveness* : Skin inhabiting bacteria are not very aggressive as they are unable to penetrate the skin barrier of the body. If they get entry into the skin, they will become aggressive in the favourable environment for their growth. Heavily capsulated organisms (Pneumococci, Anthrax bacilli, Klebsiella) are highly aggressive and dangerous as they cannot be engulfed by leukocytes.

(ii) *Toxigenicity* is the ability of organisms to elaborate the toxin. Bacteria producing toxin may not be aggressive (i.e. invasive), but they damage the body tissues by their toxin; for example, toxigenic strains of diphtheria bacilli lodging on the tonsils or in the throat will produce the toxin which is absorbed in the blood (toxaemia), carried to various parts of the body, and, ultimately, can cause death. Tetanus bacilli are also toxigenic as diphtheria bacilli.

Toxins : Toxigenic strains of organisms produce two types of toxins which are proteins in nature. Toxin may damage the tissues of the body after combining with nerves, heart muscle, liver.

1. *Endotoxins* (Greek, *endon* — inside). They are found in the cytoplasm enclosed by the cytoplasmic membrane. These intracellular toxins, known as *endotoxins*, are released after the death and lysis of bacterial cells (e.g. Gram-negative bacteria, gonococci; typhoid bacilli) produce endotoxin.
2. *Exotoxin* (Greek, *exo* — outside). Toxin producing bacteria liberate toxins through their cytoplasmic membrane. These are known as *exotoxins*. *Corynebacterium diphtheriae*, *Clostridium tetani* produce exotoxins. Few bacteria produce both endotoxin and exotoxin.

Specificity of toxin : Toxins of organisms are specified in their action. Tetanus toxin has an affinity for nerve cells, causing spasm of jaw muscles, i.e., lock jaw. Diphtheria toxin has affinity for heart muscles, death in the severe infections is usually due to acute myocarditis and heart failure. This toxin may lead to such sequelae as post-diphtheric paralysis. In staphylococcal food poisoning, *enterotoxin* of *Staphylococcus aureus* produces vomiting and diarrhoea. This *enterotoxin* is also known as preformed toxin, as this toxin is preformed in the food contaminated by *Staphylococcus aureus* and consumed later.

Application to nursing : Professionals should know that plasma and serum contain antibodies (Gamma globulins) which play a major role by protecting from diseases. She should also be aware of the fact that the patient with low platelet count may be affected by surgical hazards, as his blood may not clot immediately. A knowledge of blood clotting mechanisms is necessary, the soluble fibrinogen is changed into insoluble firbrin which causes clotting. Antibiotics and drugs injected or swallowed are carried by the blood to combat the infection. A sound knowledge of toxin is essential, as the toxins are responsible for many diseases.

93
Sexually Transmitted Diseases (STD)

They are the most common communicable disease transmitted mainly by sexual intercourse. The causative organisms of *STD* are delicate and could not survive outside the body for a longer time.

In recent years, the incidence of *STD* has increased :

1. *Classical venereal diseases*
   (a) Syphilis (Treponema pallidum)
   (b) Gonorrhoea (Neisseria gonorrhoeae)
   (c) Chancroid (Haemophilus)
   (d) Lymphogranuloma *venereum*
   (e) Chlamydia *trachomatis serovars* L1–L3)
   Granuloma inguinale (*Calymmatobacterium granulomatis*)
2. *Other venereal diseases :*
   (a) Non-gonococcal or non-specific urethritis (mainly caused by *Chlamydia trachomatis* serovars D–K)
   (b) Trichomoniasis (Trichomonas *vaginalis*)
   (c) Genital candidiasis (*Candida albicans*)
   (d) Genital herpex simplex (HSV type 1, 2)
   (e) Warts (*Human papilloma virus*)
   (f) Molluscum contagiosum (a pox virus)
   (g) Acquired Immune Deficiency Syndrome, AIDS (HIV 1, and HIV 2) — Table 93.2.

N. gonorrohoea and *C.trachomatis* infect the endocervical canal of sexually mature women. These organisms may be passed to the baby's eyes at the time of delivery resulting in *Ophthalmia neonatorum* (Table 93.2).

Urethritis

Common manifestation of STD in man is urethral discharge. Urethritis due to sexual contact may be of two types :

1. Gonococcal urethritis caused by *N. gonorrhoeae*
2. *N.gonococcal urethritis* is caused by *C. trachomatis, ureaplasma, urealyticum, Trichomonas*

Table 93.1. Causal organisms of urethral discharge vaginitis

Group	Causal agents	Percent
Gonococcal urethritis	N. gonorrhoeae	35–40
Non-gonococcal urethritis	C. trachomatis (types D–K)	30–40
Non-specific urethritis	*U. urealyticum*	1–2
	Herpes simplex virus (types, 1, 2)	2.5
	Trichomonas vaginalis	5–1
	Unknown	20–25

Table 93.2 Incidence of STD in India

Disease	Causative agents	Incidence (%)
Syphilis	Tr. pallidum	7.0
Non–specific Urethritis	C. trachomatis (types D–K) *Ureaplasma urealyticum,* HSV	
Gonorrhoea	*N. gonorrohoeae*	*16.6*
Chancroid	*Haemophilus ducreyi*	32.0
Lymphogranuloma venereum	*Chlamydia trachomatis* (L1, 2, 3)	
Granuloma inguinale	*Calymmatobacterium granulomatis*	1.0
Trichomoniasis	*Trichomonas vaginalis*	3.0
Bacterial vaginosis	*Gardnerella vaginalis,* anaerobes	2.0
Candidiasis	*Candida albicans*	4.0
Genital herpes	*Herpes simplex virus* types 1, 2	1.0
Genital warts	*Human papilloma virus* types, 6, 11, 16, 18, 30, 31, 33, 39, 57	2.0
Molluscum contagiosum	*Pox virus*	0.3
Hepatitis B	*Hepatitis B virus*	0.1
AIDS	HIV type 1, 2	
Genital scabies	*Sarcoptes scabiei*	
Pubic lice (crubs)	*Phtirus pubis*	1.4

* Mixed infection

Gonorrohea

It is caused by *N. gonorrhoeae* (gonococcal).

Clinical features : After unprotected vaginal or anal intercourse, acute onset of purulent urethral or vaginal discharge may occur. Asymptomatic infection is rare in active male but common in females. The incubation period is 2–10 days.

Pathogenesis

Gonococcus is a strict human parasite. The common site for infection is anterior urethra in males and anterior urethra and cervix in female. Mostly urethral mucosa is infected, it may spread to the rectum or oropharynx and eyes.

Complications

(a) *Local spread* : Prostatitis and epididymitis and local infections in male. Gonococci may ascend to the fallopian tubes during menstruation or instrumentation producing salpingitis and pelvic inflammatory diseases which are important causes of sterility in females. Peritoneal spread may occur occasionally and give rise to perihepatic inflammation (*Fitz-Hugh-Curtis* syndrome).

(b) *Huematogenous spread* : Sometimes, bacteria spread by blood producing septicaemia arthritis and meningitis.

(c) *Ophthalmia neonatorum* is a gonococcal conjunctivitis in the newborn that develops from the infected birth canal during delivery.

(d) *Gonococcal vulvo-vaginitis* is a common infection in young girls that results from sexual offences.

Laboratory diagnosis

Specimen

1. Urethral, cervical smears, and swabs.
2. Discharge after prostatic massage may be taken from males in chronic cases and rectal swabs may also be obtained.

In uncircumcised patient, the prepuce is pushed back before making smear. One has to milk urethra, not glans penis. The discharge may be taken by a sterile platinum loop or swab for preparation of smear and culture.

Direct Gram-stained smear will reveal Gram-negative cocci intracellulary. It is diagnostic of gonorrhoea in 95% males, but it is difficult to interpret in females due to this mixed normal flora in females. Asymptomatic carriage of gonococci is common in females but it is less (5%) in males.

Culture

Culture of exudate taken directly from the patient with a platinum loop can be inoculated in (a) Chocolate agar (b) Thayer Martin medium and incubated in 5–10% CO_2 atmosphere at 37°C. Stuart's transport medium can be used in case of delay.

Identification (i) Colonies are translucent and are oxidase positive on addition of tetramethyle-P-phenylenediamine-dihydrochloride. (ii) Produce acid from glucose but *not from* lactose or sucrose.

Other tests

(a) Fluorescent antibody tests to detect gonococci in smears.

(b) Gonococcal complement fixation test (GCFT) is of limited value.

Non–gonococcal urethritis (NGU) (non-specific urethritis)

Certain organisms other than *N. gonorrhoeae* sometimes cause symptomless cervicitis. This infection is called *non-gonococcal urethritis* (NGU).

Symptoms of discharge and dysuria are not clinically distinguishable from gonorrohea.

Post-gonococcal urethritis (PGU)

It is a non-gonococcal urethritis that develops 2 to 3 weeks after antibiotic treatment of gonococcal urethritis in man. *C. trachomatis* is an important pathogen for both NGU and PGU in 30–35% cases.

Aetiology

1. *C. trachomatis* (types D–K) is the most common cause of NGU (30–50%).

2. *Ureaplasma urealyticum* is responsible for a small percentage of cases of NGU.
3. Herpes simplex virus types 1, 2 is responsible for few cases.

The incubation period is from few days to a few weeks, NGU also occur in *Reiter disease* syndrome.

Clinically, NGU is a triad of non-specific urethritis, conjuctivitis and arthritis on exposure to STD. *C.trachomatis* is responsible for 70% *Reiter disease* with associated urethritis.

Diagnosis : 1. Smear from exudate of urethra or cervical discharge can be examined by immuno-fluorescence test with a monoclonal antibody or by ELISA for detection of elementary bodies (antigens) of *C. trachomatis.*

Smear stained with Giemsa stain shows intracytoplasmic inclusion bodies of *C. trachomatis.*

2. *Culture* : Specimen for culture should be collected from urethra, cervix or rectum in the laboratory if possible, and they should be inoculated in McCoy or HeLa cells tissue culture treated with cyclohexamide tissue cultures are incubated for 3 days.

Identification : Intracytoplasmic inclusion bodies in tissue culture are detected by Giemsa stain or immuno-fluorescence.

3. *Serology* : CFT is usually positive Micro immunofluorescence, or ELISA can detect species specific and serovar specific antibody.

Ophthalmia neonatorum is an acute conjunctival infection of the eyes of neonates acquired during delivery from infected maternal genital tract. It is caused by : 1. *N. gonorrhoeae;* 2. *C. trachomatis.*

They cause acute purulent conjuctivitis infection due to *N. gonorrhoeae, has a tendency to involve cornea leading to ulceration and even perforation — Chlamydia conjunctivitis.* Chlamydial infection is less severe than gonococcal ophthalmia with longer incubation period (5–12 days) while gonococcal ophthalmia develops within 36–48 hours of birth.

Table 93.3 Diagnostic points of aetiological agents of urethral discharge

	Characters	Gonococcal urethritis	Non–gonococcal urethritis
1.	*Discharge*		
	Quantity	profuse	Scanty
	Quality	Thick purulent	Mucopurulent/serous
2.	*Symptoms*		
	Type	Acute	Subacute
	Urethral	Self-limiting but may pass on to NGU	Chronic and exasperating
3.	*Incubation period*	2–4 days	1–3 weeks
4.	*Microscopy*		
	(a) Gram-stain Intracellular Gram-negative diplococci	+	–
	Pus cells (polymorphs) per oil immersion field	>5	>5
	(b) *Giemsa/Machiavello stains*		
	Inclusion bodies intracytoplasmic intranuclear	–	+ (*C.trachomatis*)
	Giant cells	–	+ (*HSV*)
	(c) *Hanging drop*	Not required	+ (*T. vaginalis*)
	(d) *Detection of antigen* Immunofluorescence/ELISA (with monoclonal antibody)	+	+
5.	*Cultivation*		
	Artificial	Theyer Martin medium	Tissue culture/Chick embryo
6.	*Serology*		
	CFT with patient's serum	+	+

Diagnosis

A. *Gonococcal infection*

(a) Direct Gram-stained smear of exudate reveals characteristic bacteria in pus cells.

(b) Culture of exudate is carried out in Thayer Martin medium or Chocolate agar and incubated at 37°C in 5–10% CO_2 for 48 hours.

B. *Chlamydia infections*

(a) Direct smear of conjunctival scrapings by immunofluorescence shows inclusion bodies.

(b) Culture is done in irradiated or cyclohexamide treated McCoy cells for 2–3 days.

Giemsa stain shows intracytoplasmic inclusion bodies.

Genital Ulcer

The most common manifestations and earliest clue of STD are *Genital ulcers.*

Causes

1. Hard chancre (Syphilis) by *T. pallidum*
2. Soft chancre (Chancroid) by *H. ducreyi*
3. Herpes progenitalis by Herpes simplex virus types 1, 2
4. Donovanosis by *Calymmatobacterium granulomatis.*
5. Lymphogranuloma venereum C. *trachomatis* (types L1, L2, L3)

Chancroid is the commonest cause of genital ulcers in tropics and subtropics (Table 93.4).

Table 93.4 Characteristics of sexually transmitted genital ulcers

Characters	Chancroid	Primary syphilis	Herpes progenitalis
Number	Multiple	One or few	Multiple
Morphology	Flushy, ulcerated	Well defined	Vesicular eruption
Margin	Undermined flask shaped	Indurated	Superficial erosions.
Pain	Painful	Painless	Burning, itching sensation
Course	Progressive with secondary invaders and purulent	self-healing	Recurrent
Regional Lymph node	Painful fluctuant bubo	Discrete, firm rubber like	Not significant

Table 93.5 Laboratory diagnosis of genital ulcer

	Microscopy	Provisional diagnosis
Exudate		
Gram film	Small Gram-negative bacilli	Chancroid (*H. ducreyi*)
Fontana stain	Slender long spiral organism (12–15μm)	Syphilis (*T. pallidum*)
DGI (dark ground illumination)	Motile spirochaete	Syphilis
Scraping from Ulcer	Intracellular bodies	Donovanosis
Gram stain	(telephone handle appearance)	*Calymmatobacterium granulomatis.*
	Intranuclear inclusion bodies, multinucleated giant cells	HSV types 1, 2

Syphilis

Treponema pallidum causes syphilis, a chronic systemic disease which is transmitted by sexual intercourse.

It is fragile and cannot live outside the body. So it is present in superficial lesions of genitalia and transmitted from one partner to another through intact or damaged mucosa, from infected mother to foetus during pregnancy. The incubation period is 2–4 weeks or 9–90 days.

Clinically there are four stages; the primary and secondary stages are grouped under *early syphilis;* whereas tertiary and quarternary stages are under *late syphilis* which develops mostly two years after the onset of infection and may remain latent throughout.

Early syphilis

Primary lesion : At the entry site, *Tr. pallidum* multiply and within next 3 months the *primary sore* or *chancre* develops on the genitalia.

A small macule appears which soon becomes papular and ulcerates. The flat, dull, red indurated ulcer exudes serous fluid. Regional lymph nodes are enlarged, discrete, rubbery, painless and non-tender. Although the chancre is localised, the spirochaetes are disseminated throughout the body. This chancre may heal spontaneously without treatment in 3 to 8 weeks.

Secondary stage : Six to eight weeks after the appearance of primary chancre, papular rashes of the skin and mucous membrane occurs which are highly infectious and contain large number of *Tr. pallidum*. Rash, condylomata, lymphadenopathy and mucosal ulceration. The secondary changes resolve after several months to be followed by a latent period, which may last for many years.

Late syphilis

Tertiary stage : *Gummata* is a chronic granulomatous nodule of the skin, mucous membrane or bone, it may develop after 3–10 years after initial infection. The lesion contains few *Tr. pallidum* and tissue destruction due to delayed hypersensitivity reaction.

Late or quarternary stage : Ten to twenty years after primary syphilis; there are two main clinical forms :

1. *Cardiovascular syphilis :* aortitis, aneurysm, aortic stenosis, stenosis of coronary ostia.
2. *Neurosyphilis, general paralysis of* the *insane* (GPI) due to degeneration of brain cells and *tabes dorsalis* is destruction of nerve fibres of spinal cord.

Congenital syphilis

T. pallidum can cross placental barrier to infect the foetus. The foetal infection occurs only during primary and secondary stage of disease in mother. There is no primary stage. The infection of foetus may occur from early tenth week to late pregnancy.

Manifestation of Congenital syphilis

1. *In severe infection*, the child is born dead.
2. *In latent infection*, infant is seropositive; but about 50% of infected infants are asymptomatic.
3. *Early manifestations* are skin rash, nasal deformities. They are observed in first few weeks of life.

4. *Late manifestations*, which appear after two years, are keratitis, bone sclerosis, arthritis, joint effusion etc.

Laboratory diagnosis

Specific

(a) Fluid from chancre or scrappings from ulcerated secondary lesions,

(b) Blood for serology.

1. Microscopy

Tr. pallidum can be demonstrated in exudate by dark ground illumination (DGI) or by phase contrast microscopy. Exudate contains both motile and non-motile treponemes. The motile organisms rotate along their long axis, bend and flex along their length and look white spiral against a dark background. Care should be taken to differentiate from the non-pathogenic ones which are shallower and shorter and more angular than *Tr. pallidum* . However, fluorescent antitreponemal antibody test is specific and sensitive.

Serological tests

They will become positive from two weeks after the appearance of the primary sore.

A. Non-specific tests (using cardiolipin antigen) :

1. Wassermann reaction (WR) is a complement fixation test (CFT) and is not in use now-days.
2. Precipitation (flocculation) test

   (a) Kahn–not much used.

   (b) Veneral Disease Research Laboratory (VDRL) test is a routine test nowadays as screening test for the following reasons :

(i) It is cheap, easy to perform and simple.

(ii) It becomes positive two weeks after the appearance of chancre.

(iii) It becomes positive in 70% of primary and 90% of secondary syphilis (but negative in late syphilis).

(iv) Quantitative test of VDRL will show rising VDRL titres in congenital syphilis with passage of time.

(v) Positive test indicates active infection.

(vi) Useful in monitoring the effect of antimicrobial therapy in syphilis.

False positive reaction

Since these tests are non-specific, false positive reactions occur in certain diseases (e.g. malaria, Kala azar, infectious mononucleosis, pregnancy and in some acute infections).

B. Specific tests (using *Tr. pallidum* as antigen). The antigen used against antibodies is derived from the virulent Nichol's strain of Tr. *pallidum*. Hence this antigen will react with antibody produced as a result of the endemic treponemal diseases (Yaws, bejel, pinta).

(1) TPHA (*Treponema pallidum* hemagglutination test) is simple to perform and is specific test. It is now used as routine screening test in advanced countries. Sheep erythrocytes coated with sonically treated Tr. *pallidum* and specific antibody in patient sera causes haemagglutination.

Before performing the test the sera are absorbed with non-pathogenic Reiter treponemes to remove non-specific antibody.

TPHA becomes positive around 4th week of infection and is sensitive in 64% to 87 % cases of untreated primary syphilis.

2. FTA–ABS (Fluorescent treponemal antibody absorption) test : As TPHA assay, sera are pre-absorbed with a non-pathogenic Reiter treponema to remove group specific antibody. Acetone fixed treponemes on slides are incubated with patient's serum. Antibody bound to the fixed organisms are then detected by fluorescein labelled antihuman immunoglobulin by immuno-fluorescent microscope. The sensitivity of FTA–ABS is about 80%, 100% and 95% in primary, secondary and late syphilis, respectively.

3. TPI (Treponema pallidum immobilization) test : Motile virulent *Tr. pallidum* is obtained from testicular syphiloma of infected rabbit and preserved in laboratory. Patient's serum and complement (guinea pig serum) are added to motile virulent treponem and incubated. If *Tr. pallidum is immobilised, it indicates positive result.*

The TPI test is technically difficult to perform, expensive and often negative in primary syphilis. TPI has now been superseded by FTA–ABS test. It is not frequently done now (Table 93.6).

VDRL and TPHA are more useful as routine tests. When these tests are done together, they will become effective screening tests for early and late syphilis.

Table 93.6 : Common serological test for diagnosis of syphilis

Tests	Reactivity % positive stage of syphilis			
	Primary	Secondary	Latent	Tertiary
Non-treponemal test (Reagin tests)				
1. VDRL (Microscopic flocculation) test	59–87	100	73–91	37–94
2. RPR (Rapid Plasma Reagin) test (macroscopic flocculation test)	59–87	100	73–91	37–94
Treponemal test				
1. Immunofluorescence (FTA–ABS)	86–100	99–100	96–99	96–100
2. Haemagglutination (TPI, NHA–TP)	64–87	96–100	96–100	94–100

Chancroid

Haemophilus ducreyi causes Chancroid — a soft chancroid or soft chancre which is sexually transmitted, this disease is characterized by multiple painful ulcerated lesions on corona, glans penis and prepuce in men, and vulva, vagina, and labia in women. Incubation period is 4–7 days.

Clinical features

Chancroid is probably the commonest cause of genital ulcer in tropical countries. The ulcer in chancroid is painful and not indurated and fleshy looking with ragged irregular margins.

Bubo formation

Inguinal lymph nodes are inflamed, painful, tender. The overlying skin becomes erythematous and tense and finally ruptures leading to formation of deep single ulcer.

Diagnosis

Smear examination : Gram-stained smear of exudate shows Gram-negative ovoid bacilli. The bacteria *en masse* have configuration of "Shoals of fish".

Culture : Exudate from an ulcer is directly cultured in 20–30% rabbit blood agar or onto chocolate agar with 1% isovitalex and 5% sheep serum, plus 3 mg/L of vancomycin. Plate is incubated at 20–30°C for 3–5 days, with added moisture and CO_2. Colonies are grey surrounded by a zone of faint haemolysis.

Treatment

Trimethoprim (80 mg) plus sulphamethoxazole (400 mg) tablets is given orally twice daily for 2 weeks. Alternatively, 100 mg doxycycline is administrated orally twice daily for 10 days. A single dose of 2 gm spectinomycin intramuscularly cures the illness.

Lymphogranuloma venereum (LGV)

C. trachomatis serotypes L1, L2 and L3 causes LGV. Serotype L. 2 is most common cause. Incubation period is 3–7 days. LGV is mainly found in tropical and subtropical countries.

Clinical features

The primary lesion is a small, painless vesicle or non-indurated ulcer or papule on the penis in male or on labia, posterior vagina in female. It heals spontaneously in a few days, without any scarring, followed by bubo, 7–30 days later. Inguinal lymphadenopathy is most common. Lymph nodes are initially discrete and later becomes suppurative due to progressive periadenitis.

Diagnosis

Serological test : Rising titres of antibody can be demonstrated by micro-immunofluorescence and complement fixation tests.

Frei-type skin test with LGV antigen shows delayed type of hypersensitivity.

Isolation : Chlamydiae can be cultivated in a variety of cells from chick embryo and mammals. They also grow in yolk sac of 6–8 day chick embryo. They produce small pock-like lesions on Chorioallantoic membrane.

Light microscopy : Chlamydiae are Gram-negative, they stain blue by Castaneda's method and by Giemsa stain. The inclusions, in the cell cultures are better stained by Giemsa; whereas chick embryo yolk sac smears are stained by Castaneda and Machiavello methods.

Treatment : Drug of choice is doxycycline, 100 mg twice daily orally for 2 weeks. Alternatively trimethoprim 80 mg with sulphamethoxazole 400 mg 2 tablets twice daily for 2 weeks.

Granuloma Inguinale

(Syn. Donovanosis, Granuloma venereum)

This diseases is a mildly contagious, chronic granulomatous ulcerative disease involving the skin and lymphatics of the genitalia or perianal areas. It must not be confused with lymphogranuloma venereum caused by *Chlamydia trachomatis.*

The causative organisms of Granuloma inguinale was first recognized by Donovan in 1905. Donovan described the characteristic intracellular bodies in smears made from ulcerated lesions. These organisms are now recognised as capsulate gram negative bacilli; and are called

Calymmatobacterium granulomatis. They measure 1.5 × 0.7 μm and are sexually transmitted. The intracellular organisms present in infected tissues are morphologically identified as "Donovan bodies".

Clinical features

At the site of inoculation, 3–30 days after exposure, the lesion starts as papule or nodule. The papule soon ulcerates to show granulomatous appearance. The ulcer spreads gradually by local extension. It is local — the ulcers are localised on the glans, prepuce or shaft of the penis or peri-anal (area of male). The labia is commonly affected in females, the ulcer is very chronic. The chronicity of the ulcer is of diagnostic importance. The ulcer progresses with extensive involvement and even destruction of the area with mutilation of genitalia. Lymph nodes are not involved. The disease is most common in tropical countries.

Diagnosis

Giesma stain : Donovan bodies can be demonstrated in ulcer smear stained by Giemsa stain. They are rounded coccobacilli, 1-2 μm in size, which are within the cytoplasm of mononuclear cells capsule appears as a dense acidophilic zone around the bacterium, resembling "telephone handle".

Treatment : Doxycycline, in a dose of 100 mg orally twice a day, is administrated for 14 days. Alternatively erythromycin stearate 500 mg orally four times a day is given for 14 days.

Herpes Genitalis

It is caused by *Herpes simplex virus* (HSV) type 1 and 2, the most common one is type 2 strain.

Source : HSV is the aetiological agent in 50% cases of vulvo-vaginitis in young women. Infection is mostly acquired by sexual intercourse; sometimes from lesions of other part of the body; HSV of genital infections has been recorded in 20% male. HSV2 can infect extra-genital sites and throat and breast.

Pathogenesis

Primary genital herpes is characterised by fever, pain, dysuria, vaginal, urethral discharge with enlarged inguinal lymph node. The lesions are bilateral on the external genitalia–vesicles, pustules, ulcers). Both cervix and urethra are involved in 80% of women.

Rectal and peri-anal HSV infections occur in homosexual men and/or heterosexual women practising anorectal intercourse.

Recurrent genital herpes, HSV1 infections have less frequent systemic symptoms and heal faster than HVS2 infections. In 90% patients with HSV2 infection occurrence occurs within 12 months.

About 25% cases of genital herpes are asymptomatic. Both types of HSV are capable of transmission from mother to the foetus, although intrauterine foetal damage is rarely recorded.

Diagnosis : Scrapping from base of the lesion and clotted blood for serology are used in the diagnosis.

Microscopy : Gram/Wright staining shows characteristic intracellular inclusion bodies.

Cultivation : HSV can be cultivated in human diploid fibroblast tissue, culture, growth is rapid. CPE occurs within 24 hours.

Serology : CFT is useful in the diagnosis of primary infection (antibody titres is within 32).

Vaginal Discharge

It is a common complaint of sexually active women and the symptoms are soiling of clothes, pain, pruritus, burning sensation and lower abdominal pain.

Causes

1. Gonorrhoea
2. Infection due to C. *trachomatis*
3. Bacterial vaginosis
4. Tichomonas vaginalis
5. Vulvo-vaginal candidiasis

Pelvic inflammatory disease may result from gonorrhoea.

Diagnosis of the disease and treatment are necessary to control STD. Vulvo-vaginal candidiasis and bacterial vaginosis are not sexually transmitted (Table 93.7).

Table 93.7 : Distinguishing Laboratory tests for pathogens of vaginal discharges

Specimen	Examination	Diagnosis
1. Speculum examination	Microscopic examination.	
Wet mount preparation	1. Motile T. vaginalis	*T. vaginalis*
	2. Yeast cell/Pseudo-hyphae	*C. albicans*
2. Gram-stain of discharge	Gram-negative intracellular diplococci	*N. gonorrhoeae*
	Gram-positive Yeast cells	*C. albicans*
3. Scrapping from vaginal epithelia (Giemsa)	Intracytoplasmic inclusion bodies	*C. trachomatis*
4. Saline preparation of discharge	Microscopic exam shows "Clue cells" epithelial cells coated with cocco-bacilli.	
5. Chemical examination pH	Greater than 45 due to excess amine and production of lactate by Lacto bacilli	Bacterial vaginosis
Amine test	Fluid mixed with 10% KOH leads to emission of fishy odour (due to volatile amines)	Bacterial vaginosis
6. Gram films	Altered vaginal flora Lacto bacilli largely replaced by *G. vaginalis* and other anaerobes	Bacterial vaginosis

Bacterial Vaginosis

This is a syndrome characterised by increased homogeneous white discharge from vagina often described as rotten fishy smell.

Causal organisms :

1. *Gardnerella vaginalis*
2. *Mycoplasma hominis*
3. Several anaerobic bacteria
   (a) *Mobiluncus sp.*
   (b) *Prevotella sp.* (formerly called *Bacteroides*)
   (c) *Pepto-streptococcus sp.*

4. *Trichomonas vaginalis*
5. *Candida albicans*

These organisms are present in large number in vaginal fluid of women with bacterial vaginosis and are probably responsible for the pathogenesis of bacterial vaginosis.

The normal vaginal flora (with *L. acidophilus, L. jenseni*) that play protective role in infection is present only in reduced concentration in bacterial vaginosis which leads to an increase in vaginal pH (more than 4.4).

Transmission : Bacterial — Vaginosis is associated with STD risk factors, such as multiple sex partners and a recent sexual contact with a new partner. However, no single sexually transmitted pathogen has been identified, but there is a massive overgrowth of mixed bacterial flora.

Diagnosis

In a patient with symptoms of abnormal vaginal discharge of white/gray homogeneous material and antibody, the diagnosis is reasonably made by :

(1) Exclusion of trichomonal and candida vaginitis and mucopurulent cervicitis, and absence of *N. gonorrhoeae* and *C. trachomatis* from endocervical specimens.

(2) Chemical examination of vaginal fluids :

(a) pH greater than 4.5, increased pH is partly due to reduced production of lactate by Lactobacilli.

(b) *Amino test* : When vaginal fluid is mixed with a 10% solution of KOH, fishy odour is immediately liberated. The odour is due to volatile amines present in vaginal fluid.

(c) *Saline microscopy* : Vaginal discharge contains *clue cells* (squamous epithelial cells coated with cocco-bacillary organism). Leukocytes are usually absent.

(d) *Gram films :* Gram-stained smear shows altered vaginal flora. The normal vaginal flora of Lactobacilli in vagina is largely replaced by G. vaginalis and other anaerobes.

Treatment : Only women with bacterial vaginosis symptoms are to be treated. Metronidazole in a dose of 400–500 mg orally twice daily is administrated for 7 days. Alternatively, a single dose of 2.0 gm is administrated orally.

Trichomoniasis

Trichomonas vaginalis, a protozoan causes trichomoniasis which is characterised by the production of thick greenish yellow vaginal discharge of low pH (>.5). The vaginal epithelium is inflamed with petechial lesions in the cervix. It is mainly transmitted by sexual intercourse. Metronidazole is the drug of choice.

Diagnosis

Specimen

Swab of vaginal discharge should be collected freshly in Stuart's transport medium.

Microscopy

Motile trichomonads and polymorphs can be seen in direct wet film. Direct microscopy is 80 percent positive as culture.

Culture

Since the diagnosis is more difficult in male, the culture is of great necessity.

Early morning first-voided urine deposit or a urethral swab specimen is cultured in Fineberg's medium and incubated for 5 days and examined for motile protozoa at 2 and 5 days.

Vulvo-Vaginal Candidiasis (Thrush)

It is caused by several species of *candida albicans* but C. *albicans* is common (80 percent) and is a normal commensal of mucous membrane of vagina and bowel. When infection occurs, white membranous patches are formed in the vagina and vulva accompanied by vaginal discharge that may be thick and watery (pH less than 4.5).

Infection is endogenous and precipitate by antibiotic therapy and systemic disease (diabetes). Some cases are sexually transmitted.

Diagnosis

Specimen : Swab from vaginal secretion.

Microscopy

(1) KOH mount, Microscopical examination of vaginal secretions in 10 percent KOH shows yeast cells.
(2) Gram stained smear shows characteristic Gram-positive yeast cell with budding pseudohyphae.

Culture

Specimen is inoculated in Sabouraud's agar medium and incubated for 4–8 hour at 37°C. The colonies are typically wavy. The fungi are identified by the formation of germ tubes in culture in serum and formation of chlamydospores in nutritionally poor medium (corn meal agar).

Treatment : Intra-vaginal nitromidazole (e.g. miconazole) for 7 days. Oral treatment with Ketoconazole is recommended only in severe and recurrent infections.

Genital warts

They are also known as *Condyloma acuminata* and are common in sexually active adults. Now they are considered as one of the most important STDs.

Sites of Occurrence

(a) Women : vulva, vagina and cervix.
(b) Male : Shaft of penis, perianal, skin and anal canal.

Cause

Human papilloma virus (HPV) types 6,11, 16, 18, 30, 31, 33, 39 and 55 are closely linked (and probably a direct cause) to moderate to severe squamous dysplasia, and overt cancer of the cervix, anus, vulva, vagina and penis. Thus the genital wart is associated with high risk of cervical cancer. So women with STD should undergo routine Cervical Cytological screening.

Clinical Picture

Infections are sub-clinical. Warts of vulva and vagina are mostly visible but those of cervix cannot be distinguished from the normal cervical mucosa. Treatment is unsatisfactory. Regrowth after treatment is frequent, probably due to recrudescence of the latent disease as a result of the defective immune system or reinfection.

Diagnosis

(1) Polymerase chain reaction can detect HPV.

(2) Cytological and histological examination of cells in urine for detection of inclusion bodies of HPV.

Pelvic Inflammatory Disease

Pelvic inflammatory disease (PID) is a clinical syndrome in women that comprises of a combination of endometritis, salpingitis, parametritis, oophoritis and pelvic peritonitis due to ascending genital infection (vagina, and cervix) which usually occurs from gonococcal or chlamydial mucopurulent cervicitis/or from bacterial vaginosis. PID affects mostly sexually active adolescent and young women. Ninety per cent disease are sexually acquired.

Cause :

(a) *C. trachomatis*

(b) *N.gonorrhoeae*

(c) *Mycoplasma hominis.*

Diagnosis

Specimen : Endocervical discharge and blood.

(1) Gram and Giemsa stained smears to show the presence of *N. gonorrhoeae* and *Chlamydial* inclusion bodies, respectively.

(2) *Serology*, Chlamydial seropositive women may show tubal scarring, infertility or ectopic pregnancy.

Inguinal Bubo : It is an enlargement of the lymph node in the groin area. As the same can be caused by STD or associated with other clinical syndrome, it is necessary to diagnose the underlying cause of bubo.

Origin

(a) Lymphogranuloma venereum–*C.trachomatis* (L. 1–3).

(b) Chancroid–*H. ducreyi*

(c) Syphilis–*T. pallidum*

Clinical Manifestation

(1) *Inguinal bubo without active ulcer :* In case of lymphogranuloma venereum, there is swelling of inguinal lymph nodes (initially external inguinal and subsequently internal inguinal groups.) The bubo is usually inflamed, tender with redness of overlying skin, as the bubo enlarges, it starts showing softening and fluctuation, if not aspirated, the bubo ruptures with multiple sinuses.

(2) *Bubo with active ulcer.* In chancroid due to *H. ducreyi*, the genital ulcer may be followed by inguinal bubo which is round uniocular and undergoes suppuration.

(3) In *primary syphilis*, genital ulcer is associated with painless inguinal lymphadenitis, whereas secondary syphilis is associated with generalised lymphadenopathy. The lymph nodes are painless, firm, discrete with rubbery consistency and other signs of secondary syphilis such as skin rash, and condyloma are also present.

94
Pyrexia of Unkonwn Origin

Sometimes the cause of a febrile illness (greater than 38°C) remains uncertain in spite of investigations, hence it is called as pyrexia of unknown origin (PUO).

The patient with PUO must have persistent fever at least one week, usually longer, and often three weeks.

Causes : The most common causes of prolonged PUO are (a) Chronic infections; (b) Tumours, (c) Connective tissue disorders; (d) Granulomatous diseases (e) Drug hypersensitivity reactions (Table 94.1) :

Table 94.1. Causes of PUO

Cause		Percentage
Infection	Bacterial, viral, fungal, parasitic disease	35
Neoplasms	Lymphoma (Both Hodgkin's and non-Hodgkin's lymphoma), leukaemia, other cancers (e.g. hypernephroma, hepatoma, disseminated malignancy).	20
Connective tissue disease	Systemic lupus erythematosus, polyarteritis nodosa, temporal arteritis.	20
Granulomatous diseases	Sarcoidosis, Crohn's disease, granulomatous hepatitis.	15
Drug hypersensitivity reaction	Drug induced fevers, cryptic hematoma, pschogenic fever.	10

Infection

Aetiology : As a cause of PUO, infections account for about 35% cases. Without accurate determination of the nature and location of infection, many cases of PUO due to infecting agents, agents are eradicated by blind anti-microbial therapy.

(A) *Bacterial infections* : Due to repeated blood culture and widespread use of antibiotics, bacterial endocarditis due to streptococci is a sure cause of PUO; but antibiotic use or infection by highly fastidious organisms, fungi (Candida, Aspergillus), *Rickettsiae* and *Bacteroides* are important factors in culture-negative endocarditis.

Certain organisms (*S. typhi*, *S. choleraesuis*), *Neisseria meningitidis* and *Brucella* give rise to chronic intermittent bacteriaemia without prominent localised findings.

Sinusitis, mastoiditis, subacute osteomyelitis (particularly vertebral osteomyelitis), retroperitoneal abscesses and secondarily infected organised clot of an aortic aneurysm also present as PUO. Gram-negative bacilli (*E. coli*, *Bacteroides* and *Salmonella* have been recovered from these patients. In such patients, blood culture usually becomes intermittently positive.

(B) *Viral infections*

(1) Infections mononucleosis due to *Epstein–Barr virus*.

(2) *Cytomegalovirus* infection

(3) Hepatitis A

Infected patient with these viral infection may suffer from prolonged febrile illness without prominent localised findings.

(C) *Parasitic Infection*

(1) *Protozoal diseases* Malaria, amoebic hepatitis or liver abscess, visceral leishmaniasis (Kala–azar), toxoplasmosis, and trypanosomiasis.

(2) *Metazoal disease* : Filariasis, particularly during first year of infection.

Laboratory diagnosis

A. Haematology

Rarely specific.

B. Biochemistry

Liver function tests reveal liver damage in relevant cases.

C. Bacteriology

1. Blood culture–should be done
2. Anaerobic culture of pus
3. Mycobacterial culture
4. Urine culture.

D. Serology

Useful in infections mononucleosis (Paul Bunnel test) enteric fever, hepatitis A, B infection, lyme disease, CMV infections and sometimes in amoebiasis.

Table 94.2 Bacterial disease presenting as PUO

Cause	Disease
Sytemic infections	
Infective endocarditis	Infections of heart valves
Tuberculosis	Pulmonary, non-pulmonary (bone, kidney, cryptic miliary)
Atypical mycobacterial Infection	Progressive disseminated infection due to *M. avium–intracellularae*
Enteric fever	with atypical symptoms
Brucellosis	Occupational disease.
Leptospirosis	Occupational disease.
Coxiella burnetii	A fever endocarditis, most common in males in agriculture.
Psittacosis	Infection due to *C. psittaci* may look much like typhoid fever suspected, if the patients keep parrots/pigeons.
Localised sepsis	
Hepatobiliary sepsis	Cholecystitis, Cholangitis, liver abscess.
Intra-abdominal abscess	Arising in spleen or related to a ruptured diverticulum or appendix.
Pelvic abscess	Usually follows gynecological sepsis, sometimes post-operative.
Renal infection	Chronic pyelonephritis, perinephric abscess.
Dental infection	Alypical dental abscess.
Miscellaneous	Sinusitis, prostatitis.

5. *Skin test* : Mantoux test for histoplasmosis, coccidioidomycosis, sarcoidosis (Kvelm-Siltzbach skin test).

6. *Other tests*

(i) Immunologic tests (LE cells phenomenon, antinuclear antibody test in SLE etc.).

(ii) Biopsy of lymph node or other tissues.

95
Laboratory Diagnosis of Bacterial Diseases

Laboratory diagnosis of Infectious diseases can be done as :

1. *Specimen* : should be collected aseptically.
2. *Demonstration* of bacteria and their products.
3. *Isolation* of bacteria by *culture*.
4. *Identification* of bacteria by biochemical tests and serological tests.
5. *Animal inoculation* test.
6. *Serology* : Detection of antibody titre.

Quality control of laboratory reagents should be done regulatory.

1. *Specimens* should be collected aseptically in sterile container, well-chosen and of good quality. Specimen container should be correctly labelled. Special risk of infection associated with handling of the specimen, if any, should be indicated on the label (e.g. *Hepatitis B* or *HIV infection*).

Transport and storage : The specimens should be despatched immediately to the laboratory since some specimens (e.g. *stool*) act as good growth medium for the *commensal* and *non-fastidious* bacteria that outgrow the pathogens. Particularly Gram-negative bacilli. Non-sporing anaerobic bacilli and *Neisseria* sp. are fragile during transport. Therefore, these specimens are to be inoculated immediately after collection. If delay is expected, they should be collected in *transport media*. When the delay is unavoidable, storage at 4°C can be done but bacterial overgrowth is the main problem (e.g. urine) found low temperature kills some bacteria (Table 95.1).

2. Detection of bacterial and their products

Microscopy

1. *Direct demonstration* is a rapid diagnosis method and provides the quality of sample and nature of pathogens. Microscopic examination of (Gram, Ziehl-Neelsen, Albert) stained smears are done.
2. *Immunofluorescence* : Many organisms (*Legionella pneumophila*), *Chlamydia trachomatis*, rickettsial antigen) can be detected in tissues. Immunofluorescence tests using monoclonal antibodies are highly specific.
3. *Periodic Acid–Schiff* (PAS) and *methenamine silver*-staining can detect parasites in tissue (Pneumocystis *carinii*).
3. *Culture :* The specimen is inoculated in suitable media and incubated aerobically and anaerobically. Isolates are identified by a series of biochemical tests and agglutination tests.

4. *Detection of antibody (Serology)* : About 5–10 ml of blood is collected aseptically in a sterile container and allowed to clot. After clotting, serum is separated by centrifugation. Serum is used for serological tests and antibiotic assays. Serum is used for most of the tests, but other body fluids (e.g. pleural, pericardial, cerebrospinal fluid, urine, faecal extracts and saliva) are sometimes used. Haemolysis and bacterial contaminaton of sera are not suitable for tests. " *Paired sera*" (Samples collected at weekly intervals) are to be tested for detection of rising antibody titre. Antibodies against whole organisms or against only one class of antigen can be determined.

Advantage of serological tests over culture

(1) Where causative organisms cannot be cultivated, e.g. syphilis.

(2) When the organisms grow slowly in culture.

(3) When the organisms have disappeared from blood and have taken shelter in internal organs.

(4) It takes few hours to perform the test.

Table 95.1. Collection, transport, storage of specimen

Specimen	Collection	Storage and transport
Urine (Pyogenic organism)	Midstream specimen	Fresh sample preferred, In case of delay, 4°C storage, slide coated with solid medium (MacConkey agar) dipped in urine, transported in a sterile container.
Urine (AFB)	Three first morning, samples of 3 consecutive days.	Refrigeration.
Faeces (Bacillary dysentery)	In sterile container samples collected	Fresh sample are to be plated without delay; faeces, mucus are to be collected in 30% buffered glycerol saline.
Faeces (Cholera)	Do	Samples are transported in alkaline peptone water, Monsur's medium or Venkatraman-Ramakrishnan medium.
Sputum (pyogenes)	Morning sample in a wide-mouthed sterile container.	Specimen to be freshly plated
Sputum (AFB)	Morning sample collected on 3 consecutive days.	Specimen is concentrated before culture.
Serous fluid (Pleural, synovial, ascitic)	Fresh sample in sterile container	Citrate added to prevent clotting.
CSF	Collected by lumbar puncture in to a sterile container	Fresh sample preferred.
Blood culture	6-10 ml sterile blood	Screw-capped. Bottle of 50 ml glucose broth for aerobic culture. (RCM for anaerobic bacilli)
Pus, swab (throat, wound)	Specimen collected by sterile cotton wool swab	Specimen cultured without delay. In case of delay, specimen is placed in Stuart's Transport medium. Delicate bacteria are preserved.

Quality Control

The term " *Quality control*" in health laboratory refers to a set of checking procedures to ensure a reasonable degree of consistency in the findings and results for improvement of the patient care service.

It consists of (1) Internal quality control (IQC) and External quality control (EQC) of reagents and equipments.

(1) *Internal quality control* : The main aim of IQC is to ensure day-to-day consistency (precision) of laboratory observations regarding reagents, media, equipment and staff.

(a) *Equipment* should be properly service, maintained and checked daily and record is maintained.

(b) *Media* and *reagents kits* (commercially available) should be regularly checked for good performance and also checked for standard controls with stock cultures and with current positive specimens.

(c) Laboratory personnel (staff) should be competent to find out possible problems during course of routine work.

(d) Laboratory technician should have uptodate knowledge from the revised laboratory procedure manuals.

(2) *External Quality Control Scheme* : In U.K. there is United Kingdom. External Quality Control Scheme (Central level laboratory). Specimens prepared centrally are sent to participating peripheral laboratories for reporting on the specimen within a given time. Laboratory with poor performance are kept confidential and necessary help is provided to them. Thus the performance of the participating laboratory is assessed continuously. In India, Central and Regional level EQC laboratories should be set up to assess and guide several laboratories. All reagents used in the laboratory should be tested regularly to know whether they give correct positive and negative results with control organisms or sera.

96
Microbial Genetics

Genetics is the study of inheritance, except for RNA viruses, all hereditary characteristics are encoded in DNA. Each bacterial colony consists of descendants of a single cell. The progeny thus formed maintained their character with the parent cell from generation to generation. The chromosomal DNA plays a pivotal role in the maintenance of genetic stability within the organism and the species by providing genetic information to the progeny possessed by the parent. This is accomplished by most accurate replication of its DNA. Occasional inaccuracies result in heritable variations in a small proportion of daughter cells which is about one per 10^4 to 10^{10} cell division.

Nucleic Acid

Nucleic acid is a polynucleotide and nucleotides are linked by means of 3, 5 phosphodiester bonds. They are of two types–DNA (deoxyribonucleic acid), and RNA (ribonucleic acid). RNA is structurally similar to DNA except for two major differences The sugar in RNA is *ribose* instead of *deoxyribose* in DNA and the base *uracil* (instead of thymine present in DNA).

The following products are obtained on hydrolysis of the nucleic acids :

Composition of Nucleic acids

	Basic structures	DNA	RNA
1.	Bases		
	Purines	Adenine	Adenine
		Guanine	Guanine
	Pyrimidines	Cytosine	Cytosine
		Thymine	Uracil
2.	Sugar	D–2 Deoxyribose	D–Ribose
3.	Acid	Phosphoric acid	Phosphoric acid

Structure of Chromosomes

The structure of DNA molecule is composed of two strands of complementary polynucleotide chains wound together in the form of double helix. Bacteria, like other prokaryotic cells, are *haploid* (with one copy of each gene) and its nucleus consists of a circular chromosome of DNA molecules of approximately 1 mm long when straightened. Unlike eukaryotic cell, it is not associated with histone or non-histone proteins and lies free in the cytoplasm of bacteria. Each strand has a backbone of deoxyribose and phosphate groups. One of the four nitrogenous bases are purines; adenine (A) and guanine (G) and the pyrimidines: Thymine (T) and Cytosine (C) is attached to each deoxyribose.

The *Two strands*. These two strands are held together by hydrogen bonding between the bases on the opposite srands in such a specific manner that hydrogen bonds can only be formed between adenine and thymine (A–T), between guanine and cytosine (G–C).

Replication of DNA

During replication of the DNA molecule, the two strands separate at one end, each then acts as a template for the synthesis of a complementary strand. The newly formed double stranded DNA molecule from the parent cell DNA are sorted between the two daughter cells. DNA replication is, therefore, *semi-conservative* as each strand is conserved intact during replication. DNA dependent DNA polymerase is the main replicase enzyme in replication of complementary strand of DNA. It is believed that the enzyme of DNA replications is fixed of the specific site of cell membrane, possibly of mesosome, where the replication of DNA begins. Synthesis of DNA occurs in short segments which are late joined together by ligases. There are three DNA polymerase, polymerase III is thought to be responsible for replication of DNA and polymerase I for repair work. Polymerase II is of minor importance.

Repair mechanisms : The incorrect nucleotide sequences are excised by the help of nuclease and replacement is done by the appropriate nucleotides with relegation of the sequence.

Restriction enzymes (restriction endonucleases) : These enzymes provide bacteria with a mechanism to distinguish between their own DNA and DNA from other biological sources, and thereby depend many bacteria against incoming foreign nucleic acids.

RNA

The DNA gene represents a code which is transcribed on m–RNA and then translated as the particular polypeptide. RNA mostly occurs in a single stranded form. There are three distinct types of RNA in a cell — messenger RNA, (m–RNA), ribosomal RNA (r–RNA), and transfer RNA (t–RNA),

Transcription and translation

RNA polymerase attaches itself to the beginning of a gene on the DNA and synthesizes single complementary polyribonucleotide strand, called m–RNA using one of the strand in the DNA–double helix as a template. This process is known as *transcription*. After transcription, m–RNA passes into cytoplasm and the m–RNA and t–RNA comes together on the surface ribosome which contains r–RNA. The triplet base sequence on m–RNA is known as *codon*. The t–RNA molecule has got a triplet at one end the amino acid at the other end. The ribosome moves along the m–RNA carrying the amino acid from t–RNA, the polypeptide growing sequentially until the entire m–RNA molecules has been translated into corresponding sequences of amino acid. This process is called as *translation*.

Plasmids

Plasmids are extra chromosomal DNA molecules and consist of circular double stranded DNA of 1–2000 mega daltons which replicate autonomously in the host cell.

Besides the chromosomal DNA molecule some bacteria such as *Escherichia, Klebsiella, Salmonella, Shigella* and *Proteus* possess extra-chromosomal DNA which is about 1–3% of the weight of bacterial chromosome. These have been described by two different terms. Those situated in the cytoplasm in free state and replicate autonomously (independent replicons) are known as *Plasmids*. DNA molecules that remain attached to the bacterial chromosome are called *Episomes*. It is not possible to differentiate between plasmids and episomes and the two terms are synonymously used. Like chromosome, plasmids contain their own genetic information which control their replication and ensure segregation of one copy into each daughter cell at cell division. Plasmids are not essential for normal function of host bacterium but their presence in bacteria confers properties of drug resistance, toxigenicity, conjugative plasmid and others.

Plasmid types : Plasmids are three main types based on their function :

1, R–plasmid 2, Colfactors 3, F or Fertility factor.

Table 96.1. General properties of bacterial plasmids

1. Physical properties	Double stranded, circular, supercoiled DNA, exist autonomously within a cell.
2. Replication	Contains genes for self replication.
3. Incompatibility	Two members of same group cannot co-exist in the same cell.
4. Transferability	Some plasmids (not all) are self transferable.
6. Recombination	Some plasmids can integrate with host chromosome (epistome).
7. Mobilisation	Self transferable plasmid can mobilise chromosomal gene or other plasmid by integration.
8. Relationship to host	Non-essential for cell survival.

1. *R. plasmid* : R–plasmid (R–factor) consists of two components, One component is *resistance* transfer factor (RTF) which carries the genes that govern the process of intercellular transfer and other component is called *resistant determinant* (R. determinant) carrying resistant genes for each of the several drugs.
2. *Colfactors* : Colcino genic (Col) factors are found in several species of coliforms which produce extracellular colicines. These bactericidal substances are lethal toxins for other strains of the same or closely related species of bacteria. Since similar antibacterial substances are also produce by other bacteria other than coliforms, this group of substances has been named as *bacteriocines*. Colicins are produced by *Esch. coli*, pycocin by *Pseudomonas*, diphthericin by *Corynebacterium diphtheriae*. Composition of bacteriocin varies from protein to lipoprotein–polysaccharide complex. Bacterial strains producing bacteriocid in are resistant to their own bacteriocin which helps inter species typing of organisms.
3. *F* or *fertility factor* : The fertility plasmid, F–factor is transfer factor, that contains the basic genetic information necessary for extra-chromosomal existence, self-transfer and for the synthesis of sex pilus, but it is devoid of other identifiable genetic marker such as drug resistance genes. Though F plasmid is inherited as a stable trait it is not required for normal cell functioning and is lost spontaneously on occasion. Cells carrying F plasmid free in the cytoplasm (F+ cells) have no unusual characters apart from their ability to mate with F cells and renders them F+ by conjugation.

   Cell carrying F factor (F+ cell) possess sex pilus and extrude an extra-cellular protein that attaches donor cell (F+) to recipient cell lacking fertility factor (F–). The sex pilus of male bacteria (F+ cell) is probably responsible for forming conjugation–tube with female (F–) bacteria, through which genes are transferred from F+ to F– Cells.

Cell properties encoded by plasmids

1. Drug resistance.
2. Virulence–toxigenicity and invasiveness.

3. Antimicrobial agents-antibiotics and bacteriocin production.
4. Genes determining metabolic pathways.
5. Specialised recombination system e.g. RTF R determinant association and dissociation.
6. Conjugation foundations (transfer gene).

Genetic Engineering

Genetic engineering is *the recombinant DNA technology* by which any genetic system can be analysed. By genetic engineering, it is now possible to separate and isolate gene virtually from any cell type (bacteria, yeasts and higher forms of life including man) and to insert into bacterial cell in such a way so that it can be expressed in the formation of desired protein. Specified gene can be identified by chemical or radioactive probes containing complementary sequences of DNA so that the DNA sequence can be used as the probe in hybridization reaction. *Hybridization* is the technique in which two single strands of nucleic acid come together forming a stable double stranded molecule.

Separation of DNA fragments

Desired genes or DNA fragments are separated by several techniques :

1. *Gel electrophoresis* : The DNA fragments are separated by gel electrophoresis based on their size, the smaller the fragments, the more rapid the rate of migration.
2. *DNA probe* : Bacteria possess a variety of restriction endonucleases, commonly called restriction enzymes. Certain restriction enzymes protect their host by cleavage of foreign (external) DNA that might be introduced by a virus and therapy protects the host. This property is utilized in gene separation. The enzyme recognizes a specific oligonucleotide sequence in the double stranded DNA and breaks the DNA molecule at this site and produces discrete fragments that can be separated by gel electrophoresis. This technique is generally applied for analysis or manipulation of genes in bacteria. This method is not applicable with DNA of higher organisms, as they contain introns. In higher organisms, messenger RNA, synthesizing desired protein, is isolated from the cell—with the help of reverse transcriptase a DNA copy is prepared from the RNA. Thus a double stranded DNA is prepared using DNA polymerase separated DNA fragments can be used for gene cloning and also can be identified by gene probing by labelled DNA probe. These nucleic acid probes (DNA and RNA probes) can be utilized for various investigation (Table 96.2).

Table 96.2. Diagnostic DNA probes

Group	Diseases
Bacterial	Legionella pneumophilia, Mycoplasma pneumoniae, C. jejuni, H. pylori, M. tuberculosis, M. avium, M.intracellulare, E. coli, (ST and LT toxin)
Viral	HSV types 1, 2 Hepatitis B virus, Rota virus type A HIV 1; HIV 2
Protozoal	Plasmodium falciparum

Application of gene cloning

(1) Genetic cloning in bacteria is now widely used in developed countries for *preparation of many mammalian proteins.* e.g., somatostatin, human growth hormone, insulin, several interferon and tissue plasminogen activators.

(2) *Preparations of some vaccines* are done by making only the antigen against which the antibody is required, e.g. Hepatitis B virus, rabies, and malaria, *B. pertussis.*

Polymerase chain reaction (PCR for DNA amplification.

The development of PCR has made a revolutionary impact in molecular biology from 1983.

Principle : The technique is based on the nucleic acid sequence in a region which, for a diagnostic application, is produced in large amounts in *vitro* from small amounts of complex template.

Procedure : The PCR involves three main stages. The reaction is subjected to a series of temperate variations :

(1) *Melting of DNA*

The double stranded DNA is dissociated to a single stranded DNA at a denaturing temperature of 94°C.

(2) *Hybridisation of primers to target DNA*

In an annealing temperature of 50°–70°C, oligonucleotide primers hybridise to target DNA.

(3) *DNA synthesis*

The synthesis of DNA is carried out at a polymerisation temperature using heat resistant DNA polymerase derived from *thermus aquaticus* (Taq) in the presence of free deoxynucleotide triphosphate — resulting in duplication of starting material.

Melting the product of DNA duplexes and repeating the cycles, typically to 20 to 30 or more, an exponentia increase in the amount of target DNA occurs.

Application

The PCR provides extremely rapid analysis (one day), ease of automatic relative economy and 100 per cent efficiency.

There are many variations and modifications of PCR concept which include :

(a) *Synthesis of C DNA* with reverse transcriptase followed by the amplification of cDNA.
(b) *Single stranded DNA* can be synthesised by later alteration in the ratio of oligonucleotide primers.
(c) *Detection of nucleotide* sequences of infectious agents (Table 96.3).
(d) *Research application* : Recombinant DNA construction, mutagenesis of cloned DNA and detection of rare nucleotide sequences.

Table 96.3. PCR in detection of nucleotide sequences in infectious agents

Group	Organisms
Bacteria	*H. pylori, L. pneumophilia, M.tuberculosis,C. trachomatis, M. pneumoniae*
Viruses	Coxsackie virus, Cytomegalo virus, Herpes simplex virus, Hepatitis B virus, Hepatitis C virus, Human immuno-deficiency virus, Measles virus, Human papilloma virus, Rota virus, Rubella virus
Rickettsia	Rickettsia rickettsiae
Fungi	C. albicans
Protozoan	T. gondii, Pneumocystis carinii, Trypanosoma cruzi

97
Bacteriology of Milk

Milk always contain some bacteria derived from :

(i) *Milk ducts of udder* : Even when best possible precautions are taken, some bacteria are derived from the udder. The number is highest in the pore and lowest in milk obtained by striping. An aseptically drawn raw milk may contain 10 bacteria to several thousand per ml.

(ii) *Milk equipment* : Unsterile milking equipment is a major contribution of bacteria of milk.

(iii) *The milker's* hands also contribute to bacteria in milk, which can be avoided by proper cleaning of hands before milking the animal.

(iv) *Unclean milker* and *dust* in *milking shed* : These are also sources of bacteria in milk.

(v) Water used for cleaning udders and for adulteration also partly contribute to bacteria in milk.

(vi) *Diseased animals* : Pathogenic organisms causing infections in animals (e.g. mastitis, brucellosis, tuberculosis) may be excreted in milk.

(vii) *Carriers* : Carriers of infectious disease (e.g. typhoid, paratyphoid, dysentery, food poisoning bacilli, coagulase positive staphylococci, or haemolytic streptococci) who milk the animal sometimes act as sources of pathogenic bacteria of milk.

Milk-borne diseases

Source	Diseases
1. **Infections primarily from animals**	Tuberculosis, Brucellosis, Streptococcal infections, Enterotoxigenic Staphylococci, Salmonellosis, Q fever, Cowpox, Foot and mouth disease, Anthrax, Leptospirosis, *Campylobacter fetus*, *Yersinia enterocolitica*.
2. **Infections primarily of man**	Typhoid, Paratyphoid, Cholera, Shigellosis, Enteropathogenic *Esch. coli*, Staphylococcal food poisoning, Streptococcal infections, Tuberculosis, Hepatitis.

Bacteria in human milk

(a) *Prior to infant feeding* : *Staph. epidermidis* (100% samples), str. mitis (69%), Gaffkya tetragena (19%), *Staph. aureus* (13%)

(b) *After breast feeding* : Some organisms mentioned above are seen but in large numbers derived from maternal skin and infant's mouth.

Pasteurisation of milk

Pasteurisation of milk eliminates the risk of most infections (90%) including the more heat-resistant tubercle bacilli and Q fever organisms but it does not destroy thermophilic bacteria and bacteria spores.

Pasteurisation is the process in which the milk is heated at a particular temperature for a fixed period required to destroy any pathogens but may be present in the milk while causing minimal changes in the composition, taste and nutritive value.

There are several methods of pasteurisation :

(a) *Holder method* : Temperature employed is 63–66°C for 30 minutes followed by rapid cooling to 5°C. It is useful in smaller set ups.

(b) *Flash method*: Temperature employed is 72°C for 15 seconds and then rapidly cooled to 4°C. It is used for larger quantities of milk.

(c) *Ultra-high temperature* (UHT) *method* : Rapidly heated usually in two stages between 125°–132°C for a few seconds (2–3) only and then rapidly cooled.

Biological standards of milk

Standards of milk is laid down under Milk Regulation Acts of 1965 and 1972 in England and Wales :

(i) *Untreated milk :* Raw milk under most favourable conditions may contain at least 500 bacteria per ml. But under bad conditions, the number may be several million.

(ii) *Pasteurised milk* should not contain coliform in 0.1 ml milk, and on submission to phosphatase test, must give a reading not exceeding 10 µg of p-nitrophenol per ml of milk.

(iii) *Sterilised milk* should satisfy the turbidity.

(iv) *Ultra-heated milk* must contain less than 10 bacteria per 0.01 ml. (i.e. 1000 bacteria per ml).

Bacteriological examination of milk

It consists of :

(a) enumeration of viable bacteria

(b) test of coliform bacilli

(c) chemical tests

(d) examination of specific pathogens.

Sampling

(i) if the milk is contained in retail milk bottles, one unopened is to be sent to the laboratory.

(ii) When the milk is in a large container, sample is collected by a sterile dipper from the depth of milk by a sterile 4 oz screw-capped bottle.

(1) *Viable count* : The plate count method of test is done by serial dilutions of milk sample (1:10, 1:100; 1:1000 in sterile Ringer' solution) incorporating in yeast, extract milk agar in 10 cm. petri dish and then incubated at 30–31°C for 72 hours. Number of colonies multiplied by dilution factor gives colony count in the fixed amount of milk.

(2) *Coliform test*: Varying dilutions of milk are inoculated in 3 tubes of McConkey's fluid medium with Durham's tube and incubated at 37°C for 48 hours. The production of acid and gas is noted. Contamination of milk by coliform bacilli usually occurs from dairy utensils, dust and dairy workers.

(3) *Chemical test*

Methylene blue test : This simple test is an economical substitute of viable count. Viable bacteria reduce the dye in milk when kept in cool dark place. Solution of methylene blue used gives a final concentration of 1/300,000. The milk is decolourised after reduction of methylene blue and rate of reduction is related to the degree of bacterial contamination. Raw or untreated milk is considered satisfactory if it fails to decolourise methylene blue in 30 minutes under standard conditions.

Resazurin test is also dye reduction test similar to methylene blue test. Unlike methylene blue test, reduction of resazurin by bacteria passes through a series of colour changes — blue, lilac, marve, pink to the final colourless state of complete reduction.

Then *Ten Minute Resazurin test* is usually done in Creameries, in which changes of colour of milk containing the dye is noted after 10 minutes and compared with a set of colour standards in a Lovibond comparator.

(b) *Phosphatase test* : This is statutory test for pasteurised milk. The enzyme phosphatase, normally present in cow's milk, is inactivated during pasteurisation of milk. The standard technique of detecting the presence of enzyme is based on its ability to breakdown disodium p-nitrophenyl phosphate and liberate p-nitrophenyl.

The test is done by adding 1ml of milk to be tested to 5ml buffer substrate solution (buffer + disodium phenyl phosphate) in a test tube. The mixture is incubated in water bath at 37°C, for 2 hours. A yellow coloured solution of p. nitrophenyl is produced if the milk contains phosphatase. The colour is compared with standard solution by a comparator or colorimeter. In a properly pasteurised milk, the concentration of p. nitrophenyl is less than 10 μg per ml of milk.

(c) *Turbidity test* : The test for sterilised milk distinguishes between pasteurised and sterilised milk. When milk is heated to at least 100°C for 5 minutes, the soluble protein in milk get denatured and that cannot be precipitated by ammonium sulphate.

4. *Detection of specific pathogens : Tubercle bacilli* : The milk is thoroughly mixed and 50 ml amounts are centrifuged in each of two tubes at 300 r.p.m. for 30 minutes. Part of the deposit is used for ACID FAST BACILLI (AFB) and part is used for inoculation into guinea pigs.

Brucella

Isolation of *Br. abortus* is attempted by inoculating cream on serum, dextrose agar. The cream and centrifuged deposit of milk may also be injected intramuscularly into guinea pigs.

The animals are killed after six weeks, the serum is examined by *Br. abortus* suspension and spleen is used for culture of brucella.

Brucella in animals can be detected by demonstrating antibodies against brucellae in milk by *Milk Ring Test* (MRT) and other *agglutination tests.*

Bacteriology of Air

The immediate environment of man comprises of air on which depends all forms of life. Since a man respires about 500 cft in a day, the content of air is important; particularly so when the air contains pathogenic organisms.

Sources of air pollution

(i) *Human sources* : Man is an important source of spreading bacteria in the environment in the droplet during coughing and sneezing. The air-borne bacteria may be derived by evaporation of droplet by aerosols. The bacterial content in air increases with increased density of human and animal population. Pathogenic organisms do not multiply in air and are seldom carried from more than short distance infections that spread by droplets include tuberculosis, Q fever, psittacosis and coccidioidomycosis etc.

(ii) *Environmental sources* : Soil and vegetations contains organisms which also become air–borne. Majority of these organisms are non-pathogenic such as *Achromobacter, Sarcina, Micrococci,* sometimes coliform bacilli, spores and fragments of moulds.

Pollution of different types of air

(i) *Outdoor air pollution* : Outdoor air bacteria depends on types of soil and vegetation, humidity of air and density of population. The air in ocean is almost bacteria-free. However, outdoor air contains much less bacteria than indoor air and the organisms present are non-pathogenic e.g. *Achromobacter, Sarcina, Micrococcus, Bacillus subtilis* and spores and segments of moulds. The upper air contains much less bacteria. Pathogenic bacteria usually do not survive in outdoor air.

(ii) *Indoor air* : Indoor air also contains droplets of organisms dissimilated by man and animals or skin scales carrying infective organisms.

Hospital air may contain droplet nuclei or skin scales carrying infectious organisms.

Bacteriological examination

Bacteriological examination is necessary for operation theatre, some store house of food, pharmacy, and hospital wards. There are two methods :

1. *Sediments method* : Petri-dish (9–10 cm diam) containing nutrient agar and blood agar is exposed to air for half to one hour and the plates are then incubated at 37°C for 24 hours colonies are then counted.
2. *Slit sampler method* : The number of bacteria in a measured amount of air is determined by this method. A known volume of air is directed into a plate of culture medium through a slit of 0.25 mm wide. The plate is rotated mechanically so as to allow the organisms to spread out in the medium. One cubic foot of air is made to pass through the slit. In the same way, 10 cubic feet is tested. The culture media are incubated and colonies counted which gives the number of bacteria present in the air.

Interpretation

Most bacteria found in the air are harmless saprophytes, or commensals and even in the wards of hospital and other closed rooms occupied by the patients and carriers. Approximately 1% of the air-borne organisms in the wards or closed rooms are pathogenic. *Staph. aureus* is predominant air-borne organisms., about 0.1 to 10 organisms are present in one cubic foot air.

Streptococcus pyogenes may be found in large in the air (10/cu ft, air) in rooms occupied by patient with scarlet fever and streptococcal tonsillitis.

2. It is not definitely known what should be the minimum size dose of organisms that may cause infection following inhalation. This depends upon the type of pathogenic organisms and the best immune response. It has been found that as little as 0.000008

tubercle bacilli per cubic foot air is sufficient to cause infections. Thus, a man may be infected even when the inhalation is only a single pathogen in 500 or so cu ft air that he respires during 24 hours.

3. The following limits of air pollution may be acceptable :
   (a) Factories, offices, homes etc. 50 per cu ft;
   (b) Operation theatre 10 per cu ft.
   (c) Dressing room operation theatre for neurosurgery–1 per cu ft.

98
Bacteriology of Water, Milk and Air

Bacteriology of water

Soft water should be free from microorganisms and chemical substances and drinking water in particular should not only be safe but also pleasant to drink.

Drinking water is liable to contamination with sewage and other excreted materials which may cause intestinal and systemic infections. Much of the ill-health in developing countries is attributable to lack of drinking water.

The hazards of water pollution are classified into two broad groups :

(1) Biological, and (2) Chemical.

Chemical pollutants of diverse nature (e.g. detergents, solvents, cyanides, heavy metals, minerals, sulfides, ammonia, toxic compounds) derived from industrial and agricultural wastes are increasingly finding their way in the public water supplies.

Biological hazards of water supplies

Faecal pollution of water supplies may lead to introduction of a variety of intestinal pathogens that comprise water-borne diseases.

The object of microbiological study of water supplies is to detect whether water has been polluted by pathogenic organisms such as shigella, salmonella, cholera vibrios, etc. Though it would be ideal to demonstrate the possible pathogenic organism in water, but, if present, they are usually few and for outnumbered by non-pathogenic organisms. As a result their detection is not only technically difficult but also costly in time and money. Therefore we rely on tests that detect indicators of human/animal pollution in water, the presence of commensal bacteria of intestinal origin. The organisms most commonly used as indicators of pollution are *Esch. coli* and coliform group.

Bacteriological indicators

These are based on organisms indicative of pollution of water by human/animals faeces such as :

(1) Esch. coli and coliform group as whole.

(2) Faecal streptococci (Str. faecalis), and

(3) Clostridium perfringens.

Table 98.1. Water-borne Diseases

Group	Diseases
A. **Caused directly by infective agents**	
(a) Viral	viral hepatitis (Hepatitis A, E) poliomyelitis, rota virus diarrhoea in infants.
(b) Bacterial	Cholera, typhoid, paratyphoid, Esch. coli diarrhoea, bacillary dysentery, *Yersinia enterocolitica*, Campylobacter jejuni and *C. coli* diarrhoea.
Protozoal	Amoebiasis, Giardiasis, Balantidium coli diarrhoea.
Helminthic	Round. Whip worm, Thread worm, Hydatid disease.
B. **Diseases due to aquatic host**	
(a) Cyclops	Guinea worm, Fish tapeworm.
(b) Snail	Schistosomiasis.

While evaluating faecal pollution of water supplies, one has to keep in view the bacteriological flora in water as natural water almost always contains a few harmless organisms.

Bacterial Flora of Water

Sources	**Organisms**
(A) *Without faecal contamination*	
(1) **Natural water bacteria (mainly derived from air by rains)**	***Microbes, Pseudomonas, Serratia, Flavobacterium, alcali genes, Acinetobacter***
(2) **Soil bacteria (washed in water)**	**Bacillus subtilis, B. megatorium, Klebsiella**
(B) *After faecal contamination*	
(1) Intestinal bacteria (through sewage)	Esch. coli, Klebsiella, Str. faecalis, Cl. welchii.
(2) Sewage bacteria proper	P. vulgaris or sporogenes, filamentous bacteria (e.g. Nocardia)

1. Coliform

Lactose fermenting coliforms : *Esch. coli, Klebsiella, Enterobacter.* Coliform groups include both faecal and non-faecal organisms. *Esch. coli* is the typical example; *Klebsiella* sp is an example of non-faecal groups. All coliforms are assumed to be of faecal origin unless a non-faecal origin can be proved.

For the following reasons, coliforms are chosen as indicators of faecal pollution :

(i) *Commensals. Esch. coli* are present in great abundance in intestine of man—about 200–400 billion of these organisms are excreted by a man per day and their presence in water is an indication of faecal contamination.

(ii) *Detection. Esch. coli* and other coliforms can easily be detected in cultures, even one bacterium in 100 ml water.

(iii) *Survival. Esch. coli* can survive longer for days or weeks, while the pathogens tend to die out more rapidly.

(iv) *Resistance.* Coliform offers greater resistance to purification process (e.g. chlorination) than pathogens.

Thus when *Esch. coli* are present in sample of water, the assumption is the probable presence of intestinal pathogen in the water supply.

2. *Faecal streptococcus (str. faecalis)* are regularly found in faeces though their number is much less than *Esch. coli* . Their presence in water are not regarded as confirmatory evidence of recent faecal contamination of water in doubtful cases.
3. *Cl. perfringens* also occurs in faeces regularly. They are also excreted in much smaller number than *Esch. coli*. Presence of spores indicate faecal pollution.

Bacteriological diagnosis

I. **Collection of samples :** Samples are to be collected in sterilised glass bottles of 230 ml with ground glass stoppers protected in kraft paper :

1. *Sampling from tap pump outlet* : Before collecting sample the mouth of the tap or hand pump should be flamed with a blow lamp or spirit lamp. A tap is turned at maximum rate and the water flows for 5 minutes, bottles are then filled with water.
2. *Samples of water from reservoir (stream, rivers, lakes and tanks)*. The stopper is removed carefully by one hand and with another hand the bottle is held at the base and submerged in a depth of about 20 cm with the mouth upwards. If there is a current, the bottle should be faced to the current.
3. *Sampling from a dug well.*

   A stone of suitable size is attached to the sampling bottle with a string. Then a clean cord of suitable length is tied with the bottle and lowered to the required depth and filled with water. The bottle should not touch the sides of wall any time, water-filled bottle is then quickly raised to the surface and stoppered.

Transport: The sample should be examined within one hour and up to 3 hours; where delays for more than 3 hours are expected the bottles should be kept on ice or in an icebox.

Neutralisation of Chlorine : When a sample is collected from a chlorinated water supply the chlorine should be neutralised immediately by sodium thiosulphate.

II. **Methods of analysis :** Standard tests usually employed in water bacteriology are :

(a) Presumptive coliform test and differentiate or confirmatory tests for *Esch. coli, Str. faecalis.*

(b) Detection of Str. faecalis and *Cl. perfringens.*

(c) Colony count–enumeration of viable bacteria (also known as *plate count*).

Presumptive coliform test

Two methods are in use for estimation of probable number of coliform bacilli in water, multiple tube method and membrane filter (MF) method. The multiple tube method is widely used.

Multiple tube method : By this test the most probable number (MPN) of coliform organisms are detected in 100 ml water.

Media : Double strength and single strength modified MacConkey fluid medium containing bromocresol blue sterilised in bottles tubes containing Durham tube of indication of gas production.

Procedure : Measured amounts of sample of water are added by sterile graduated pipettes as :

(i) 50 ml of water to 10 ml double strength medium.

(ii) 10 ml water to 10 ml double strength medium.

(iii) Five 1 ml quantities to each 5 ml double strength medium.

(iv) 0.1 ml quantities of water to each single-strength medium.

The bottle/tubes are incubated at 37°C for 48 hours. An estimated coliform count is made from the tubes showing acid and gas production by the help of a *Statistical table*. The reaction may occasionally be due to combination of organisms or due to other organisms.

Differential coliform test

Eijkman test is usually done to confirm whether coliform bacilli detected in the presumptive test are *Esch. coli* or not. *Esch. coli* produces gas when grown in bile salt lactose peptone water at 44°C but a typical coliform bacilli tube is subcultured in two tubes of single strength — MacConkey's medium with inverted Durham tube at 44°C in water bath for 24 hours. Those yielding gas in Durham's tube contain *Esh. coli.* Confirmation of *Esch. coli* may be made by test for indole production as shown in the following table :

Table 98.2. Differentiating features of typical and atypical coliform bacilli

Gas at 48°C	Indole production at 44°C	Organism
+	+	Typical coliform bacilli
+	–	Irregular type of coliform bacilli
–	+	Other coliform bacilli
–	+	Other organisms (e.g. *Cl. welchii, Str. faecalis*)

Sometimes spore bearing bacilli may give false positive reactions in the presumptive test, hence the presumptive positive tubes should preferably be placed on solid medium to confirm the presence of coliform.

Membrane filter (MF) *method* : The membrane filter technique is used in some countries for the presence of coliform as standard test. A measured volume of water is filtered through a membrane specially made of cellulose ester. Bacteria are retained on the surface of membrane. The membrane is inoculated (face up-wards) in suitable medium for 15–20 hours and the number of colonies are counted directly. An advantage in that the bacterial colonies can be counted in 20 hours but it is not suitable for turbid water.

B. *Detection of faecal streptococci and Cl. welchii*

Their presence in water provides useful confirmatory evidence of their pollution of water in doubtful cases. Str. *faecalis.* Subcultures from presumptive positive bacteria bottles in coliform test are made into tubes containing 5 cc of glucose azide broth and incubated at 45°C.

Production of acid in the medium indicates presence of *Str. faecalis.*

Cl. welchii : The water in question is inoculated in litmus milk medium and incubated anaerobically at 37°C for 5 days and looked for stormy fermentation.

C. *Colony count* : One ml. test sample of water is placed in petri dish (10 cm diameter) and then 10 ml. melted yeast agar (45°C–50°C) is poured on the water, mixed thoroughly and allowed to solidify. One more plate is prepared. One plate is incubated at 22°C and other at 37°C for about 18–24 hours. After incubation the colonies are counted using hand lens. Each colony represents one viable bacterium in the original specimen. Colony count provides an estimate of total numbers of viable bacteria present in 1 ml specimen. Sample may be diluted when it is tubed and total count is made by multiplying the number of colonies with the dilution factor.

Interpretation of total count

(i) Growth at 22°C indicates the amount of decomposing organic matter present in water. Organisms growing at 22°C are usually non–pathogenic and however, in the presence of excess organic matter the sample is likely to be contaminated by parasites and potentially pathogenic organisms.

(ii) Growth at 37°C is more important index of contamination of water sample. A high count of bacteria at 37°C is undesirable for water consumption purpose. It also causes spoilage of food and drink at home and also in factory.

Biological examination of water

Sometimes water may contain microscopic organisms such as algae, fungi, yeast, protozoan, minute worms, etc which are collectively known as *plankton.* These plankton organisms are index of pollution and produce objectionable taste in water.

Interpretation of results : It is not possible to lay down a rigid bacteriological standard to which all drinking water supplies should conform. As already mentioned, bacterial flora of water differs widely to different sources such as well, river, lake or reservoir. On the basis of repeated tests of water a standard has been suggested by pioneer workers in the field into Class 1, Class 2, Class 3, and Class 4 types — based on presumptive coliform count per 100 ml sample shown in below table.

Table 93.3. Classification of drinking water according to bacteriological tests

		Presumptive Coliform Count per 100 ml.	Each Count per 10 unit
Class 1	Excellent	0	0
Class 2	Satisfactory	1–3	0
Class 3	Suspicious	4–10	0
Class 4	Unsatisfactory	More than 10	1 or more

Throughout the year, 50% of samples should fall into Class 1, 80% should not fall below Class 2 and the remainder should not fall below Class 3.

(ii) With deep tubewell or other pure waters that are normally into Class 1, sudden deterioration in standard even to Class 2 is to be considered as significant.

Bacteriological examination of sewage and sewage effluents

Method is same as for water :

1. *Viable bacteria* : It is estimated by plating and counting colonies. A small amount of specimen of water is used for testing coliform bacilli. Amount of water to be tested depends on the likely extent of pollution of the effluent. Bacterial count in sewage water varies between 1 million in 100 million per ml crude sewage.
2. *Enteric pathogens* : Sewage water for membrane filter technique is employed during isolation of salmonellae from communal sewage.

Isolation of pathogens from water and sewage

Sometimes water may have to be examined for presence of specific pathogens (e.g. *Salmonella, Shigella, Vibrio cholerae,* etc.).

1. *Concentration* of the organisms in the sample yields better result. Sample may be concentrated by membrane filter technique. Pathogenic bacteria retained on the surface of membrane are transferred into a suitable differential medium and incubated.
2. *Dilution method* : As the number of pathogenic bacteria present may be scanty, larger volume of multiple samples may have to be examined for isolating the organisms. A volume of 10 ml of enrichment and selective media (selenite broth for salmonella, alkaline peptone water for *Vibrio cholerae*), is mixed with nine times its volume of water and incubated for 24 hours and then subcultured in suitable media. Isolated organisms are identified by biochemical test and serotyping.

SECTION VI
MEDICAL MYCOLOGY

99
Medical Mycology

General Introduction to Mycology

Fungi (Lat. *fungus*—mushroom) are eukaryotes with a distinct nucleus and rigid chitinous cell wall and were formerly regarded as plants without chlorophyll and are now grouped with protozoa, slime moulds and most algae as Higher Prostita. Mycoses are infections caused by true fungi.

Eumycetes contains more than 80,000 species and can be classified morphologically into :

(1) **Phycomycetes** are fungi with an unicellular, non-septate mycelium (500 species). The spores (endospores) are enclosed in special sporangia. Reproduction is sexual and asexual.

Atypical representative of Mucor (bread mould) is **Mucor mucedo.** Pathogenic species of this Mucor (mould) may cause infection of lungs, middle ear and general severe infectious process in man. The mould (filamentous) or mycelial fungi grow as long filaments (hyphae) and reproduce by formation of spores. The major part of the mycelium the vegetative mycelium grows and penetrates into the substrate absorbing nutrients for growth; other hyphae form aerial mycelium and protrude from the **vegetative mycelium** into the air. They form various kinds of spores and disseminate them in the air.

(2) **Ascomycetes** of sac fungi (35,000 species) have a multicellular mycelium. They reproduce sexually by means of ascospores (spores which develop in spherical spore cases), **asci—ascus (Gr. askos**—sac) and asexually by conidia (exospores which have the function of asexual reproduction in many fungi).

(Oral thrush; Polyps in mouth)

The genus **Aspergillus** belongs to the class **Ascomycetes.** These fungi have divided separate mycelium and an unicellular conidiophore which terminates in a **fan-like row** of short sterigmata from which the spores are pinched off in chains-conidia (Gr. **konia**—dust). The fruiting part of the aspergillus resembles a jet of water from a watering can and hence the name "Sprinkler" mould. **Aspergillus** niger is a representative of Aspergilla and is widespread in nature, certain species may cause aspergillosis of the lungs, ear and eye of man and may infect the whole body.

The genus **Penicillium** belongs to the class **Ascomycetes.** The mycelium and conidiophore are multicellular. The fruiting body is in the shape of a brush. The conidiophore branches towards its upper part and terminates into sterigmata from which even-rowed chains of conidia are pinched off (Fig. 99.1). This genus of fungi is widespread in nature (fodder, milk products, moist objects, old leather, ink, jam). The type species is **Penicillium glaucum.**

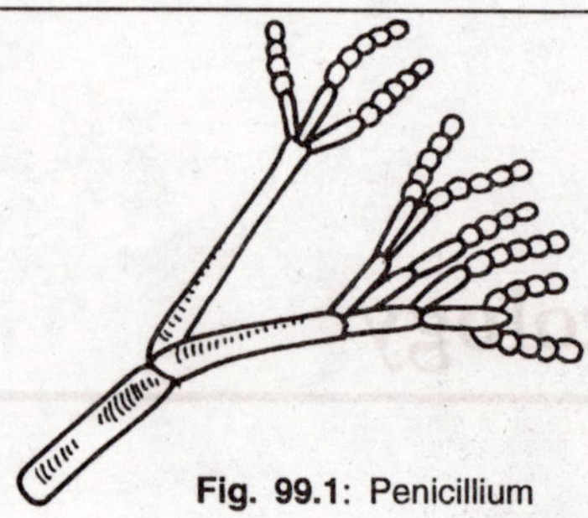

Fig. 99.1: Penicillium

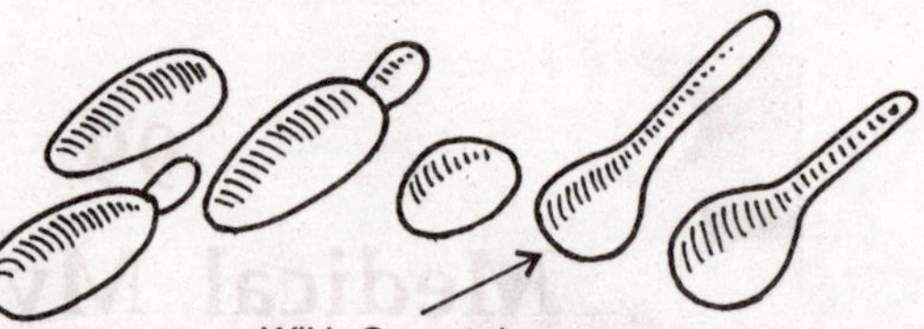

Fig. 99.2: Candida albicans

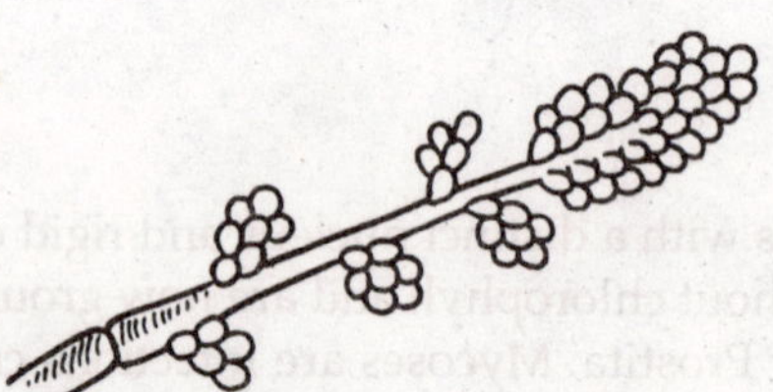

Fig. 99.3: (a) Microconidia (grape–like clusters)

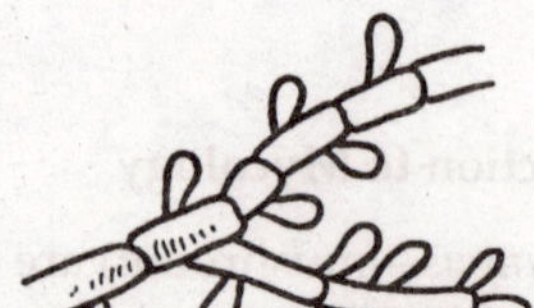

Fig. 99.3: (b) Microconidia of Vegetative hyphae

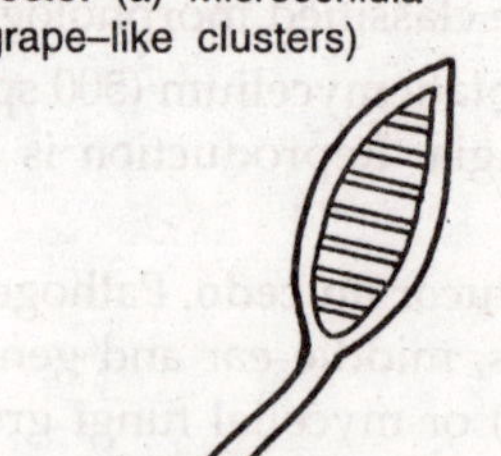

Fig. 99.3: (c) Macroconidia of Microsporum

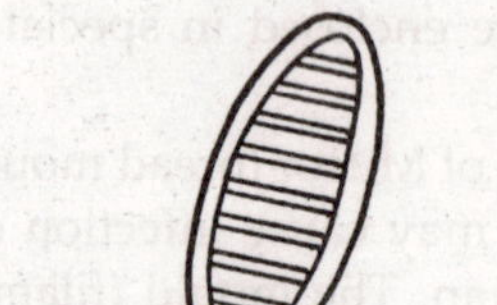

Fig. 99.3: (d) Macroconidia of Trichophyton

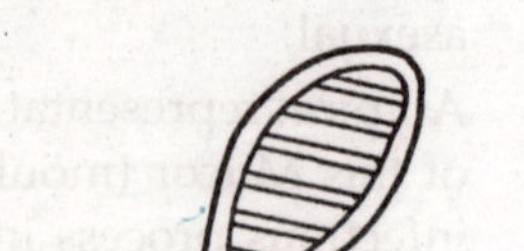

Fig. 99.3: (e) Macroconidia of Epidermophyton

Certain species (**Penicillium notatum, Penicillium chrysogenum**) are used for the production of penicillin which is widely used in the treatment of many infectious diseases. Some species of this genus of fungi are pathogenic and cause infection of the skin, nails, upper respiratory tract, lungs and other organs of man.

Yeasts belong to the class Ascomycetes. They are large, oval, round, rod shaped cells. They have a double cell wall and well defined nucleus. The cytoplasm is homogeneous—sometimes of a fine granular structure. It contains inclusions (glycogen, volutin, lipid) and also filamentous bodies-chondriosomes which are responsible for synthetic process of the cell.

Yeasts multiply by budding, fission, sporulation and some of them reproduces asexually. Daughter cells produced by budding from the parent cell transform into independent individuals. The yeasts can also reproduce by sporulation. When there is lack of nutrition, 2, 4, 8 or 16 endospores are formed inside the cells of some species of yeast. Yeast cell forming the ascospores is called the ascus (sac), while sporulating yeasts are known as Ascomycetes, since the yeasts ferment various carbohydrates, they are widely used in brewing beer, in wine making and in baking bread. Saccharomyces cerevisiae, S. elipsoides are typical representatives of the yeasts.

Among the asporogenic yeasts (family **Saccharomycetaceae),** there are species pathogenic to man; they are called as **Candida** (Fig. 99.4) which cause grave disease known as candidiasis. They occur as a result of the growth inhibition of the normal microflora by antibiotics used for treating a number of infectious diseases and inflammatory processes.

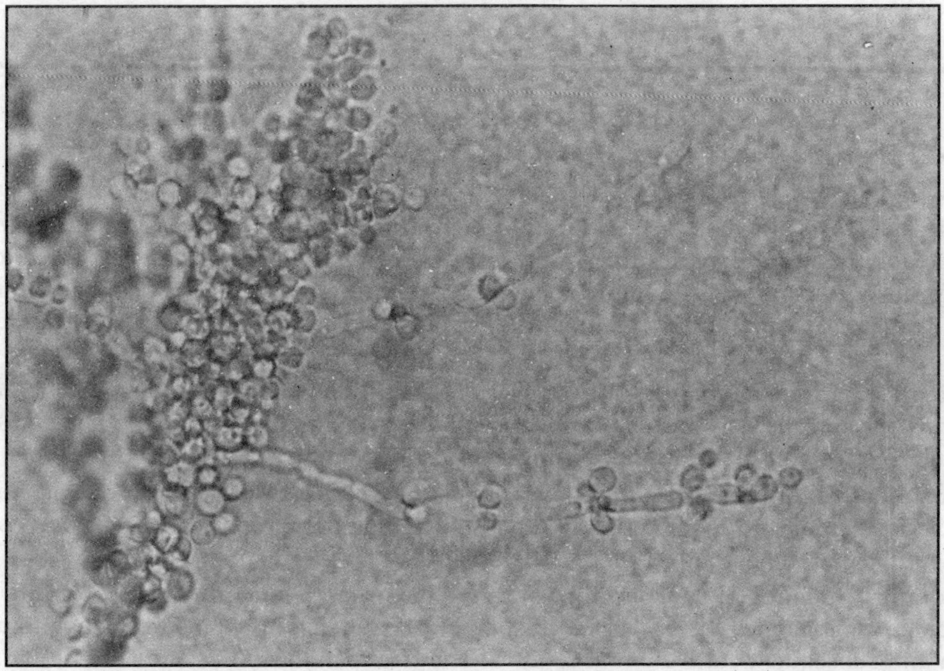

Fig. 99.4: Candida albicans with germ tube 400X

(3) **Basidiomycetes :** Fungi with a multicellular mycelium. These organisms predominantly reproduce asexually by basidiospores (basidia reproductive organs) in which a certain number of spores develop, usually 4. Certain species are free parasites. Two hundred species of mushrooms are used as food. Twentyfive species of mushrooms are poisonous.

Smut fungi invade grains crops causing disease known as smut. Rust fungi affect sunflowers and other plants producing orange coloured spots on infected plants.

Imperfect fungi (Fungi imperfecti) are a rather large group of fungi consisting of a multicellular mycelium without either asco- or basidio-sporangiophore, but only with conidia. Reproduction is asexual; but the sexual reproduction is unknown. To this class belong the orders **Hyphomycetes, Melanconiales** and **Sphaeropsidales.**

Among the **hyphomycetes,** which may be of great interest to the physicians are : **Fusarium graminearum** causing intoxication in human (drunken bread), and **Fusarium sporotrichioides** causing intoxication in man and domestic animals who had eaten the grain crops which had remained in the fields during the winter.

Pathogenic species of imperfect fungi are causative agents of dermatomycoses (**superficial mycoses)** : favus (**Achorion schoenleini);** trichophytosis **(Trichophyton violaceum),** microsporosis **(Microsporum lanosum)**, epidermophytosis **(Epidermophyton inguinale).**

100

Pathogenic Fungi

Aspergillus : The pathogenic species are : **Aspergillus fumigatus, A. roseus, A. flavus, A. niger.** More than forty species have been recovered from patient suffering from various clinical forms of Aspergillosis. In human beings, they are responsible for lesions in the lungs, bronchi, cornea, ear canal and other organs and tissues. The diseases is prevalent among millers.

Penicilli : There are more than thirty species of **Pencillium** pathogenic to man. They cause penicilliosis affecting the skin, nails, ears, upper respiratory tract and lungs (pseudotuberculosis). Pathogenic species are : **P. minutum, P. linguae, P. glaucum and P. albumb** (Fig 99.1)

Mucor fungi : More than fifteen species of **Mucor** fungi cause mucormycosis characterised by lung lesions similar to tuberculosis in their clinical manifestations; keratitis, otomycosis, vulvovaginitis, granulomatous leison of the skin.

Laboratory diagnosis of **aspergillosis**, **penicilliosis** and **mucormycosis** is made by microscopic examination of the pus, its inoculation into common nutrient media or Sabouraud's medium and subsequent cultivation at 25-28°C. The treatment is by nystatin.

101
Imperfect Fungi

Many imperfect fungi have septate hyphae and asexual conidia resembling those of Ascomycetes, but sexual or "perfect" state has not yet been described for these fungi—hence they are called as **Fungi imperfecti.** A majority of the pathogenic moulds, yeasts, yeast-like fungi (candida) and dimorphic fungi (Histoplasma, paracoccidioides) belong to this group—**Fungi imperfecti.**

Sporotrichum has a septate mycelium. Lateral branches extend from the hyphae bearing single conidia or clusters of conidia at their sides or ends. The **Sporotrichum** grows on common nutrient media (pH 6.5) producing the best growth on Sabouraud's medium at 25 to 28°C. Growth is slow. The colonies are leathery, fluffy, smooth or folded and quite frequently pigmented.

This causative agent enters the subcutaneous tissue and the lymph nodes through abrasions of the skin; as a result gumma similar to that in syphilis and tuberculosis are produced in the pharynx, larynx, muscles and synovial membrane. It may also cause abscess of the bones, joints and internal organs. Antibiotics and sulphonamides have no effect.

Candida : They are unicellular organisms (Fig. 99.2) which reproduce by budding. Neither conidia nor ascospores are produced. They possess **no true mycelium;** the pseudo-mycelium is devoid of a membrane and septa and develops by successive or terminal budding (Fig. 99.2).

Candida albicans (Fig. 99.2) and **C. tropicalis** are most important in human pathology. About 20 species of the genus candida are human pathogens and are present on the skin and mucous membrane of the mouth, gastrointestinal tract and urinogenital organs of man. They occur on fruit, vegetables and other foodstuffs, in bath sewage, washing from catering establishments, and on dishes.

The infection is acquired when body is weakened and in the presence of unfavourable conditions (increased moisture, skin maceration, long term occupational contact with sugar containing fruit and vegetables, inadequately disinfected baths). Debilitated children, bath-house attendants, confectioners are susceptible to candidiasis.

Candidiasis associated with the long term use of antibiotics (penicillin, chlortetracycline etc.) have become of great importance. They cause profound disturbances of symbiotic relationship among normal microflora resulting into a condition of dysbacteriosis which enhances intensive multiplication, spread into the buccal, intestinal and vaginal mucosa (Fig. 99.2) and their transformation from the saprophyte state into conditionally pathogenic and pathogenic forms. As a result, local and general lesions develop.

The yeast like fungi affect the skin between the fingers and toes in the inguinal and axillary folds, the nails and nail folds, the mucous membrane of the lips and mouth corners, the tongue, fauces, oesophagus, and sometimes the vagina with the development of white films. Infection of the mucosa is known as "Thrush".

The gastrointestinal, respiratory, urogenital and nervous system, liver, biliary tract, pancreas, bones, kidney are also involved in candidiasis. The most common candida infection is vaginitis or **vaginal thrush** which is characterised, in pregnant women, by a whitish discharge with a pH below 5.2, and, microscopically, some pus cells and many yeasts, including pseudomycelium, can be seen. In infection due to trichomonas and bacteria, the discharge is more purulent and less acid.

Oral thrush occurs in debilitated or bottle fed infants. Creamy white patches are found covering red, raw areas of mucous membrane and tongue. It also occurs in adults in angular cheilitis, in sore mouth caused by ill-fitting dentures and all too frequently, after prolonged courses of oral antibacterial therapy.

Infections of the skin are common in diabetes and skin lesions are characterised by erythema, exudation and desquamation and occur most commonly in the axilla and groin, on the vulva and glans penis. It also affects the interdigital clefts, the skin folds round the nails and sometimes nail itself.

Infections of the intestine occur in infants, the aged, and those on long courses of oral antibiotics. Symptoms are pruritus ani or diarrhoea. The organism survives well in exudate collected on swabs and may even multiply if there is delay in transmission to the laboratory. It may be demonstrated microscopically in wet preparation or Gram-stained smears and grows readily at 25 to 28°C (room temperature). The incorporation of antibiotics in medium may inhibit the growth of other bacteria.

Characteristic of **C. albicans** is the production of curved, elongated germ tubes (Fig. 99.2) within three hours when it is transferred from peptone water to mammalian serum at 37°C. Chlamydospores of **C. albicans** grown on corn meal agar (Gram-stain).

On Sabouraud's medium, after two days, **C. albicans** produces high convex, off-white colonies 1.5 mm in diameter. It ferments carbohydrates; but it **fails to split urea;** which is used in differentiating it from other yeasts, PCR is rapid and sensitive method to detect **C. albicans** and other yeasts in blood.

Before undertaking the treatment, it is always advisable to correct the underlying disturbances (diabetes or poor hygiene). The usual treatment is to give the polyene nystatin locally. Nystatin is very poorly absorbed from the gut so that the systemic infection must be treated with amphotericin B. Another polyene, trichomycin, is often used in vaginitis as it effective against trichomonas and candida.

Blastomyces dermatitidis and Cryptococcus neoformans cause Blastomycosis.

Blastomyces dermatitidis is a large budding cell which is microscopic, its mycelium is segmented, branching and with conidia protruding laterally. On blood agar at 37°C, the fungus produces white, moist, waxy, soft, wrinkled colonies of the yeast only. On Sabouraud's medium at 25°C it produces fluffy white colonies which turn brown. The disease becomes chronic with skin lesions on the face, hands and buttocks. Internal organs are rarely affected.

Cryptococcus neoformans is round and oval yeast like cell, with one or two buds, which is frequently surrounded by a capsule. On Sabouraud's medium, it forms mucoid, white colonies which later become brown and creamy in colour. This fungus causes in man a deep-seated, systemic chronic blastomycosis—commonly in agricultural workers and animal breeders. The lungs, intestine, skin, subcutaneous tissue, lymph nodes, brain, meninges and bones are involved, and the mortality is very high. Laboratory diagnosis is by microscopic examination. The use of ineffective broad spectrum antibiotics is banned. The physical condition of the body should be strengthened. Special antibiotics (nystatin, neomycin, candicidin) are prescribed for blastomycosis and candidiasis.

102
Dermatophytes

Common (superficial) dermatophyte infections (ringworm or tinea) of skin, hair and nails are caused by the members of a group of thirty to forty related filamentous fungi that can digest keratin. These fungi are called "dermatophytes". The saprophytic members of this group—which normally live in the soil and from which the human and animal pathogens have probably been derived—play an important role in breaking down the keratinised tissue of dead animals. From 1843 till recently, only the asexual forms of the fungi were known and were placed under fungi imperfecti in three genera—**Epidermophyton, Microsporum** and **Trichophyton**—distinguished by the morphology of their large asexual spores or "macroconidia". Recently, however, the sexual forms of perfect states of about half the Microsporum and Trichophyton species have been identified. They belong to genera of the Ascomycetes. The species whose perfect states have been identified are mostly soil organisms but include some common pathogens. The following species are responsible for ninety per cent of the dermatophyte infections of man. **Microsporum audouinii; M. canis; Trichophyton rubrum** (Fig. 99.3d); **T. mentagrophytes** (Fig. 99.3e); **T. verrucosum and Epidermophyton floccosum; Drechslera helminthosporidium.**

Their **morphology** consists of hyphae and arthrospores formed by segmentation of a hypha into a row of separate thick-walled cells. In artificial culture, two kinds of asexual spores, microconidia and macroconidia are also formed. The microconidia (Fig. 99.3b) are unicellular small (2 to 5 μm), round or pear shaped, borne laterally or terminally singly or in clusters. The macroconidia (Fig. 99.3c, d ,e) are multicellular and their shape, size and surface are used to differentiate the genera. In **Microsporum,** they are usually numerous, **spindle-shaped,** with a rough surface and 5 to 15 segments and measure 40 to 150 μm in length. In Epidermophyton, they are **pear shaped** with a smooth surface and measure about 30-40 μm. Two or three often arise from the same hypha. In **Trichophyton,** they are usually scanty and often irregular in shape; characteristic ones are smooth; cylindrical, with 2 to 6 segments and 10 to 50 μm long.

At room temperature (26 to 28°C), Sabouraud's medium is suitable for isolation and is improved by adding cycloheximide which inhibits many common contaminants but does not affect dermatophytes.

Their spores are not killed by the mild wet heat of laundering so their destruction in clothings may require boiling or formaldehyde vapour. The benzoic and salicylic acids of Whitfield's ointment are fungicidal. (Griseofulvin is fungistatic to treatment with it). Cyclopiroxolamine (Batrafan) cream, Miconazole nitrate (zole) dusting powder are recent antifungal drugs.

Diseases due to dermatophytes : The usual name given to these infections is ringworm or tinea and this name is qualified by the name of the site affected, e.g., tinea capitis or tinea pedis, but special names are also used in dermatology for particular manifestation, e.g., kerion, favus.

When the skin is infected, the fungus spreads radially in the dead keratinised layer in the form of branching hyphae with occasional arthrospores. The inflammatory reaction from living tissue below may be very mild and only little dry scaling or hyperkeratosis is seen. More commonly, here is irritation, erythema, oedema and some vesiculation, especially at the spreading edge and this irregular pink periphery gives rise to the name "ringworm". The species that commonly attack the skin are Trichophyton sp. **E. floccosum** (groins and feet) and **M. canis.**

Infection of the nails renders them irregular, discoloured and friable. The fungs grows deep into the substance of the nail. The species usually responsible are **T. rubrum** and both human and animal strains of **T. mentagrophytes.**

When the scalp is infected the fungus grows in the horny layer of the epidermis and down into hair follicles. The hyphae surround and invade the hair shaft and, once within it, they grow outwards. The hair continues to grow and the hyphae break up into long chains of arthrospores, in some species within the shaft (endothrix infections) but more commonly mainly on the outside (ectothrix infections). After two or three weeks growth the weakened hair breaks off, leaving either a black dot at the follicle mouth as in endothrix infections.

Ectothrix infections are caused by **Microsporum** sp., and **T. mentagrophytes,** whereas endothrix infections are due **T. violaceum** and **T. schoenleinii.** The last is the normal cause of favus.

Laboratory diagnosis of ringworm is based on direct microscopic demonstration of hyphae arthrospores in the keratinised tissue and on colonial appearance and hyphal and conidial morphology in culture. Genera are distinguished according to the morphology of macroconidia and species by a combination of microscopic and colonial features.

The specimens of the nails should be collected after cleansing with 70 per cent ethyl alcohol. From skin lesions, scales of 2 to 3 mm in diameter should be scrapped outwards with a blunt scalpel from the active periphery of the lesion and the vesicles should be sniffed off.

Good material from nails can be obtained by scraping from the nail with a scalpel. The dusty stumps of ectothrix infections can be recognised by the naked eye, the hairs when located can be plucked with fine forceps. Specimens should be folded up in black paper.

In the laboratory, the specimens are "cleared" with 20 per cent KOH and examined. The hyphae appear greenish, branching, running across the outlines of the colourless cells of skin or nail. In nails, arthrospores are easy to see than the hyphae and their position within or outside the hair shaft may allow a presumptive diagnosis of the species.

Culture is carried out an Sabouraud's medium with added cycloheximide at 28°C (room temperature). Colonies of dermatophytes may be visible in two to three days. Cultures are usually reported as negative until after three weeks.

Oral griseofulvin is the treatment of choice for hair infection and those due to **T. rubrum.** It may be less effective for infections of the skin and nails, particularly those of the feet and those due to human strains of **T. mentagrophytes** for which Whitfield's ointment should be tried first.

103
Infections of Deeper Tissues

These infections are mainly in warm climates in people whose bare skin is exposed to soil, dust or recurrent trauma. **Mycetoma** is the commonest and most widespread syndrome which is caused by filamentous fungi or higher bacteria under aerobic actinomycetes. **Chromoblastomycosis** and **subcutaneous phycomycosis** are two other syndrome caused by more than one fungus.

These infections are chronic, localised and acquired by the traumatic inoculation of opportunistic organisms normally present in the soil or on thorns.

Madura foot is characterised by a swelling often with sinuses discharging pus which may contain granules of varying size (0.5 to 2 mm) and colour (black, red buff). The main actinomycetes responsible for this condition are : **Nocardia brasiliensis, N. asteroides, Streptomyces madurae.** They destroy soft tissue, bone, tendon and nerve.

Grains (colonies of the organisms) in the pus may be collected into the surgical gauze. Their size and colour suggest the species responsible.

After crushing the granules, wet preparation and Gram-stained smears should be made. The size of the hyphae is more than 2 μ in width in fungus whereas, in case of actinomycetes, it is less than 1 μm.

Sabouraud's medium (without cycloheximide) at 26°C can be used to cultivate the fungi and Lowenstein Jensen medium at 37°C for actinomycetes. Some are sensitive to antibiotics **in vitro** but none is sensitive **in vitro,** Nocardia sp. may be semi acid fast and are sensitive to many antibacterial antibiotics, sulphones and sulphonamide-trimethoprim mixtures—both **in vivo** and **in vitro.** The only effective treatment for fungal mycetoma is the surgery, nocardial and streptomyces infection respond to long course of dapsone and cotrimoxazole.

(a) Chromomycosis is a chronic warty dermatitis caused by traumatic inoculation of one of five closely related pigmented fungi : **Phialophora pedrosoi, P. compacta, P. verrucosa, P. dermatidis** and **Cladophialophora carrionii.** Microscopically, the hyphae are brown and several types of spores are produced. Treatment is not satisfactory.

(b) Subcutaneous Phycomycosis can be caused by Absidia sp. and Rhizopus sp. by infecting and penetrating the mucous membrane of the nose, sinuses and stomach when patients are **in extremis.**

Dimorphic fungi : The majority of fungi are filamentous, some exist as yeasts and other change from one form to other depending upon the conditions of growth. The last are called dimorphic fungi and include a number of pathogens; **Sporothrix schenckii, Blastomyces dermatitidis, Paracoccidioides brasiliensis, Histoplasma capsulatum.** Another pathogen, **coccidioides immitis** is dimorphic in different way. The infections they cause are not communicable from man to be acquired by inhalation. The process is slow with cellular granulomatous reaction.

Infection with S. schenckii, usually follows injury to the hands with the contaminated splinters or thorns but may be acquired from infected animals. A local "chancre" forms and small subcutaneous abscess, develop along the line of inflammed drainage lymphatics, **Paracoccidioides brasileinsis** causes "South American blastomycosis" which is chronic, progressive pyogenic, granulomatous disease with a predilection for lymphatic tissue. Its main lesions are common in mucous membranes, lymph nodes, skin, spleen and intestine. It is fatal if not treated. It is acquired by inhalation. Treatment is not yet satisfactory.

Histoplasma capsulatum is a dimorphic fungus found in many parts of the world in soil enriched with the droppings of certain birds and mammals. When its spores are inhaled by a mammalian host they develop into yeasts which set up an intracellular infection of the histiocytes. The clinical manifestations in man vary from an asymptomatic pulmonary infection to fatal generalised disease. There are many parallels with tuberculosis. The usual outcome is a small calcified peripheral focus in lung.

Coccodioides immitis is a dimorphic fungus. Its infection is acquired by inhalation and is normally asymptomatic. It has many parallels with tuberculosis and histoplasmosis. The treatment is by **amphotericin B. Rhinosporidium seeberi** causes the development of polyps in the submucosa of the nose, mouth, conjunctiva, in the skin. Natural infections occur in man, horses, mules and cows in most parts of the world, commonly in **India** and **Sri Lanka** (Fig. 103.2).

A portion of polyp may be crushed in water between slide and coverslip. Some large cysts and many small spores should be seen, if it is **Rhinosporidium seeberi.** Treatment is surgical.

In the year 1993 a new species of fungus, **Nodulisporium sp,** was found for the first time to cause Allergic Fungal Sinusitis in a young woman.

SECTION VII
MEDICAL PARASITOLOGY

104
Class Rhizopoda and Ciliata

Medical Parasitology

It is a branch of Medical Sciences which deals with Parasites and their relationship with the host and consists of (1) **Protozoology** (study of protozoa), (2) **Helminthology** (Study of helminths), (3) **Entomology** (Study of insects).

A parasite is an organism which adapts itself to live in or on another organisms on which it is depended for its nutrition or metabolism.

Human parasites belong to animal kingdom protozoa, helminths and arthropods :

1. **Ectoparasite** is the one which lives on the surface of the body, e.g., the human louse.
2. **Endoparasite** is normally found inside the human body, e.g., the roundworm.
3. **Commensal** lives in or on a host for its own benefit but does not produce disease, e.g., **Entamoeba coli.**
4. **Pathogens** are parasites which are pathogenic to man, e.g., **E. histolytica.**
5. **Symbionts** are two organisms which live in close association, so that each derives benefit from the presence of other.
6. **Infection** occurs when a parasite establishes itself within a host; and **Infestation** when a parasite lives superficially on the host.

A **host** is any animal that harbours a parasite. A host may be (1) definite, (2) intermediate, (3) a reservoir.

A **definite** host is one that harbours the vegetative, the adult, or the sexual stage of the parasite. Man is a definite host for **Taenia saginata.** An **intermediate** host is the one which harbours the cystic, larval, immature, or sexual stage. Cattle are intermediate host for T. saginata. A reservoir is an animal which replaces man in the life cycle—Antelope is reservoir host of African trypanosomiasis.

Scheme of study of parasites

1. History of the parasite, 2. Geographical distribution, 3. Habitat, 4. Morphology, 5. Life-cycle; 6. Modes of infection, 7. Pathogenecity and clinical features, 8. Laboratory diagnosis, 9. Treatment and prophylaxis.

Protozoa are microscopic single celled animals. **Helminths** (Worms) are **metazoa** and are provided with tissues and organs derived from three embryonic layers.

Reproduction of Protozoa : May be by (1) asexual multiplication, (2) sexual reproduction.

1. **Asexual multiplication** : (a) by binary fission (e.g. **E. histolytica**) or (b) by multiple fission or **Schizogony** (e.g. Plasmodia in RBCs).
2. **Sexual reproduction** : (i) by conjugation in which there is interchange of nuclear material due to a temporary union (e.g. Ciliata) or (ii) by syngamy or sporogony in which male and female mate to produce zygote which finally divides into sporozoites.

African trypanosomes reproduces asexually in the blood by repeated longitudinal fission. American trypanosomes roll into round shapes in the tissue, then elongate to trypanosome form and reenter the blood-stream.

Intestinal Protozoa

I. **RHIZOPODA – Entamoeba histolytica, E. coli, Acanthamoeba castellani, Naegleria fowleri.**
II. **MASTIGOPHORA – Giardia intestinalis, Trichomonas hominis**
III. **SPOROZOA – Isospora belli, Crypto-sporidium, Toxoplasma gondii**
IV. **CILIATA – Balantidium coli.**

E. histolytica is cosmopolitan, occurs in three forms : Trophozoite (Fig. 104.1) Precystic (Fig. 104.2) and Cystic (Fig. 104.3, 4, 5) forms and passes its life cycle in one host only, i.e., man. When the fully developed cysts containing four nuclei are swallowed by man, they pass down the intestine where the excystation of oocysts takes place at alkaline pH, hence the trophozoites (Vegetative amoebae) are formed and invade the intestinal mucosa, multiply, cause flask shaped ulceration of the intestine, few enter the blood-stream, are carried to other organs (i.e. liver, lung, brain) where they give rise to **amoebic abscess,** some are discharged into the lumen of the gut and are transformed into small **precystic** forms from which the adult cysts are developed and passed in the faeces. Thus the life cycle is repeated.

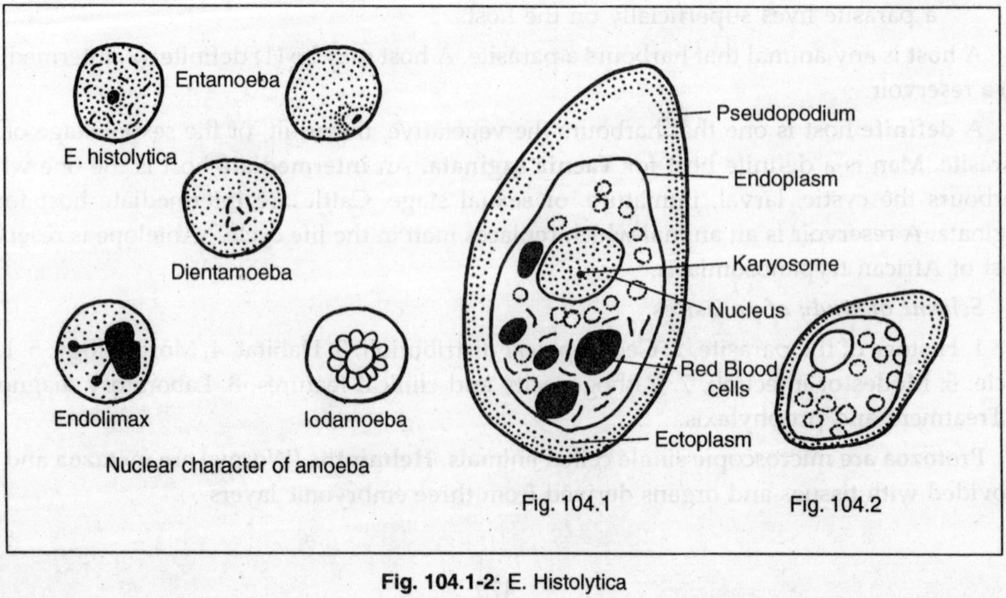

Fig. 104.1-2: E. Histolytica

Clinical features : The incubation period is 4-5 days. **E. histolytica** causes **amoebic dysentery** or amoebiasis which is characterised by the passage of blood and mucus in the stool.

The macroscopic and microscopic differences between the stools of amoebic and bacillary dysentery and described next :

Characters	Amoebic dysentery	Bacillary dysentery
Macroscopic differences		
Frequency	6-8 motions per day	Over 8 motions per day
Quantity	Relatively copious	Small
Odour	Offensive	Odourless
Colour	Dark red	Bright red
Nature	Blood and mucus mixed with faeces	Blood and mucus only, no faeces
Reaction	Acid	Alkaline
Consistency	Not adherent to the container	Adherent to the container
Microscopic differences		
RBC	In clumps; yellow green in colour	Discrete or in rouleaux, bright red in colour
Pus cells	Scanty	Numerous
Macrophages	Very low	Large and numerous
Eosinophils	Present	Scarce
Pyknotic bodies	Very common	Nil
Ghost cells	Nil	Numerous
Parasites	Trophozoites of **E. histolytica**	Nil
Bacteria	Many motile bacteria	Non-motile bacteria
C.L. crystals	Present	Nil

* *Charcot – Leyden crystals. In saline preparation, they appear as diamond shaped crystals, clear and refractile*

In intestinal amoebiasis a definite diagnosis can be done by (1) Stool examination in which the cysts (in formed stool), and the trophozoites (in diarrhoeal stool) are identified; (2) Sigmoidoscopy, in which scrapings from any lesions in the rectum are examined for trophozoites.

In extra-intestinal amoebiasis, the following procedures are followed :

(1) Clinical diagnosis of amoebic liver abscess (ALA) by (a) hepatomegaly, pain, fever and sweating, which is later confirmed by the presence of cysts and trophozoites in the tissues, (b) X-ray or ultrasonography of the abdomen, (c) Immunodiagnosis tests. The haemagglutination, complement fixation, gel diffusion; recent cellulose acetate precipitin (CAP), Dot immunobinding assay (DIB) and Sandwich Enzyme linked Immunosorbent Assay (ELISA) tests.

Treatment : Amicline plus is a complete current amoebicide used for eradication of extra intestinal and intestinal amoebiasis.

Prophylaxis : Personal prophylaxis consists of (1) Use of boiled drinking water, (2) Protection of food and drink from flies, cockroaches and rats, (3) Avoiding eating unwashed raw vegetables and fruits, and (4) Personal cleanliness while taking food.

Community prophylaxis comprises of (1) Effective sanitary disposal of faeces; (2) Protection of water supplies from faecal pollution; (3) Avoidance of the use of human excreta as fertiliser and (4) Detection and isolation of carriers.

E. coli (Figs. 104.6, 7, 8, 9) are worldwide and live in the large intestine of man. They are similar morphologically and in their life cycle to **E. histolytica** and are commensal. Recently E. dispar is accepted as non-pathogenic.

Trophozoites and Cysts of E. Histolytica and E. Coli

	E. histolytica	E. coli
TROPHOZOITES		
Fresh Preparation		
Size	20-30 microns	20-40 microns
Motility	Very active	Sluggish
Cytoplasm	Clearly defined into cytoplasm seen mixed with faeces	Not defined cytoplasm scarcely seen
Cytoplasmic inclusions	Red blood cells leucocytes and tissue debris but no bacteria	Bacteria and other materials but never red blood cells
Nucleus	Not visible in unstained preparation	Visible in unstained preparation
Stained with iodine		
Nuclear material	Central Karyosome fine chromatin granules line the delicate nuclear membrane	Eccentric Karyosome, coarse chromatin granules line the thick nuclear membrane
CYST		
Fresh preparation		
Chromatoid bodies	Rounded ends	Filamentous, thread-like with square or pointed ends.
Stained with iodine		
Size	10-15 microns	15-20 microns
Nucleus	1-4; central Karyosome	1-8; eccentric Karyosome
Glycogen mass	Visible in uninucleate stage	Large and visible in the binucleate stage.
		(Figs. 104.6, 7, 8, 9)

Naegleria fowleri (Free living amoeba), **Acanthamoeba castellani**, elongated, 10-40 microns, are rapidly motile. Their cytoplasm contains vacuoles and mitochondria (absent in Entamoeba) no red blood cells. They develop flagella after 2-4 hours in distilled water. They can be stained

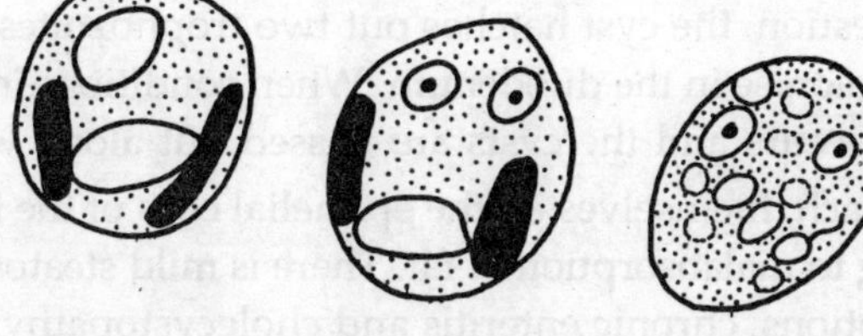

Fig. 104.3 Fig. 104.4 Fig. 104.5

Fig. 104.3-5: E. Histolytica

with Giemsa stain. Though they survive transit through the gastrointestinal tract and passed in stool, they are known to cause primary amoebic meningoencephalitis (PAM). In children, swimming in warm soil-contaminated pools, these amoebae enter via the nose and cribriform plate, into the brain tissue where they cause extensive haemorrhage and damage in the cerebrum and cerebellum; even they may enter from skin ulcers. There is report of corneal ulceration or keratitis from contaminated saline used with contact lenses. **Balamuthia mandrillaris;** a recent free living amoeba, is pathogenic to man.

Microscopic examination of cerebrospinal fluid (CSF) will show the trophozoites and red blood cells but no bacteria.

Treatment with amphotericin B has been successful. Sulphonamide and B-hydroxystibamide have been recommended for Acanthamoebiasis.

Prophylaxis by avoiding swimming in warm soil contaminated water, contaminated saline should not be used with the contact lenses.

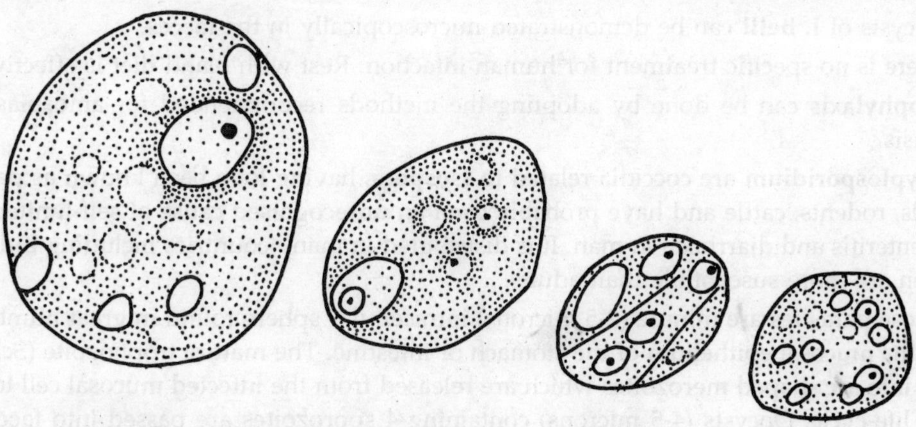

Fig. 104.6 Fig. 104.7 Fig. 104.8 Fig. 104.9

Fig. 104.4-9: Entamoeba coli

Mastigophora (Intestinal Protozoa)

Giardia intestinais : Causal agent of giardiasis has both trophozoite (Fig. 106.14, 15) and cyst (Fig. 106.16) stages which can be seen in page 497.

Human infection is brought about by ingestion of food or drink contaminated with cysts. Within 30 minutes of ingestion, the cyst hatches out two trophozoites which then multiply in enormous numbers and colonise in the duodenum. When conditions in the duodenum become unfavorable encystment occurs and the cysts are passed out along with faeces.

Their trophozoites attach, themselves on the epithelial cells of the intestine and disturb the intestinal function leading to malabsorption of fat. There is mild steatorrhoea (passage of stools with excess fat), loose motions, chronic enteritis and cholecystopathy. Recently, 1994, there is a report of giardiasis of stomach.

Diagnosis is by (1) microscopic examination of trophozoites in diarrhoea stools and cysts in formed cysts; trophozoites in the duodenal aspirates; (2) fluoroscopy which may demonstrate the hypermotility of the jejunum and (3) X-ray which may reveal mucosal defects. CIEP can detect G. intestinalis in faeces by using faecal antigen.

Treatment : Metronidazole or **quinacrine** can eliminate the infection. Only by personal hygiene, its spread can be prevented.

Trichomonas hominis found in ileocaecal region, may invade the vagina; but they are non-pathogenic (Fig. 106.11).

Sporozoa

Isospora belli are parasites of the small intestine of man and form oocysts and sporocysts. After ingestion by man, the mature oocysts liberate sporocysts which enter into the cells of the villi of small intestine where they multiply by schizogony (Trophozoite, schizont and merozoites) and ultimately the oocysts develop by sporogony and passed in the faeces. The lesions produced by I. belli is unknown in man; but in calf; there is mucous diarrhoea. In man, the symptoms are anorexia, nausea, abdominal pain and diarrhoea. The infection in man is usually self-limited. In immunocompromised (AIDS) patients, I. belli causes severe complications (diarrhoea).

Oocysts of **I. belli** can be demonstrated microscopically in the faeces.

There is no specific treatment for human infection. Rest with bland diet is effective.

Prophylaxis can be done by adopting the methods recommended for amoebiasis and giardiasis.

Cryptosporidium are coccidia related to **Isospora,** having long been known as parasites of fowls, rodents, cattle and have probably been an unrecognised cause of self-limited, mild gastroenteritis and diarrhoea in man. It is distributed in many countries including India. The children are more susceptible than adults.

Those parasites are minute (2-5 microns) intracellular sphere found in great number just under the mucosal epithelium of the stomach or intestine. The mature trophozoite (Schizont) divide into arc shaped merozoites which are released from the infected mucosal cell to begin a new life-cycle. Oocysts (4-5 microns) containing 4 sporozoites are passed into faeces and become infective agents. If stained by modified Ziehl-Neelsen staining, oocysts in the stool appear faintly blue with reddish or purple corpuscles. Reverse Passive Haemagglutination (RPHA) is a promising technique for the detection of cryptosporidium antigen in human faeces.

Patients infected with cryptosporidium have watery diarrhoea, cramps, upper abdominal pain (exacerbated by food ingestion), weight loss and flatulence, nausea, vomiting, anorexia, myalgia, malaise, dehydration, fever not common. The disease is self-limited. They cause severe intractable diarrhoea in the immunocompromised persons (e.g. those with AIDS) and immunocompetent individuals.

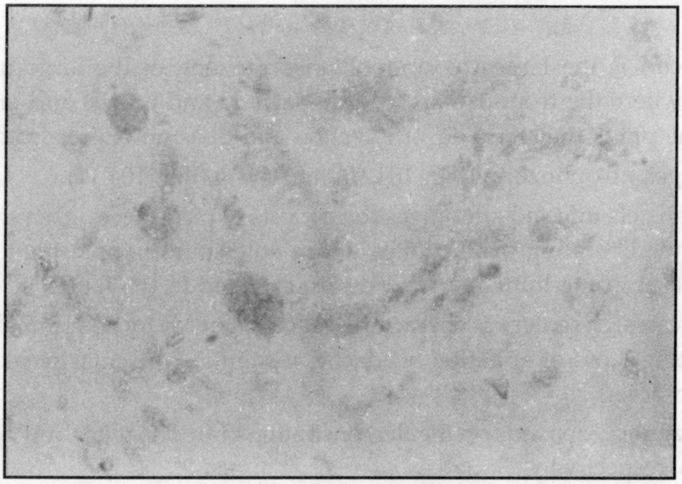

Fig. 104.6-9: Entamoeba coli cysts × 400

Only supportive therapy is available for those with AIDS or congenital immunodeficiency. Spiromycin (Rovamycin) may temporarily be effective.

Prophylaxis : Though initially recognised in animals, cryptosporidial infections is increasingly recognised as important cause of diarrhoea in both immunocompromised and immuno-competent individuals. Previously, it was in animals but the transmission from human to human is possible.

Toxoplasma gondii is distributed all over the world and is an obligatory, intracellular, **coccidial** parasite. It may occur in two forms : **extracellular and intracellular** forms.

The life cycle of **T. gondii** may be (a) enteric and (b) exo-enteric.

(a) **Enteric cycle :** After eating mouse brain containing cysts of **T. gondii,** cycles of schizogony and sporogony develop inside the intestinal mucosa of the cat ultimately liberating oocysts in the infected cat's faeces.

(b) **Exo-enteric cycle** : The oocysts, after ingestion, liberate sporozoites which, in man, penetrate the mucosa of the intestine and are carried by blood and lymph stream to distant organs (brain, eyes, liver, lymph nodes, heart, skeletal muscles and placenta of the pregnant uterus) where they form pseudocysts which multiply causing damage to the central nervous system and musculature.

***Toxoplasmosis** may be congenital or acquired.*

In congenital toxoplasmosis, there is encephalitis, chorioretinitis, hydrocephalus, mental retardation and convulsion. Polymerase Chain Reaction (PCR) test on amniotic fluid is rapid, safe and accurate for prenatal diagnosis.

Acquired toxoplasmosis is very rare in adults, often fatal.

In laboratory diagnosis, complement fixation test of Warren and Sabin; skin test of Sabin and Feldman are often used; ELISA (recent) test is used to assist the diagnosis. Indirect haemagglutination (IHA) test can be used.

Radiological diagnosis is done to show cerebral calcification.

Treatment is unsatisfactory. Sulphonamides and pyrimethamine are currently used.

Class Ciliata

Balantidium coli is the largest cosmopolitan protozoon of the large intestine of man, monkey and pig, where the trophozoites feed on bacteria and mucus and on the cells of the intestinal wall. The pig is the reservoir of infection and does not suffer from the infection.

It has two stages : trophozoite (Fig. 104.10) and cysts (Fig. 104.11).

Life cycle : Man gets infected after ingestion of cysts in pig's faeces. Excystation takes place in the large intestine liberating trophozoites which enter into the intestinal mucosa causing ulceration and encyst in the human and cysts are excreted in the faeces.

In majority of cases, dysentery is characteristic accompanied by abdominal pain, tenesmus, nausea and vomiting. Loss of appetite, headache, insomnia, muscular weakness and loss of weight are also observed.

Laboratory diagnosis depends on the demonstration of trophozoites and cysts in dysenteric and formed stools, respectively.

Treatment : Carbarsone diodohydroxyquin and Tetracycline are used in treating human cases.

Prophylaxis is same as that of amoebiasis.

Microsporidia (New human protozoa) are unicellular Gram-positive organisms with mature spores and are associated with AIDS patients.

Of 4 species (**Enterocytozoon bieneusi, Pleistophora, Encephalitozoon cuniculli** and **Nosema corneum**), E. bieneusi causes diarrhoea. Modified trichrome stain is the standard technique used to detect microsporidia in stool specimens.

Cyclospora (recent parasite) are coccidian-like or cyanobacterium-like bodies (CLB-the name Cyclospora sp. has been proposed). They were found to cause prolonged diarrhoeal disease loss of appetite, fatigue among travellers and foreign residents at Kathmandu, Nepal in 1993. Duration of diarrhoea in those infected with CLB was seven weeks. Antibiotic Trimethoprim is effective. Mode of infection is via contaminated drinking water or unboiled milk. Cyclospora cayetanensis is a recent species.

Leptomyxid amoeba (newly discovered protozoa) was also responsible for primary amoebic meningoencephalitis, granulomatous amoebic encephalitis and keratitis in contact lens wearers. Clotrimazole and bifonazole were amoebostatic rather than amoebicidal on a clinical isolate of **Acanthamoeba polyphage** associated with Acanthamoeba keratitis.

Demonstration

1. A wet saline preparation of fresh loose dysenteric stool from acute amoebic dysentery will show few pus cells, agglutinated red blood cells (RBCs) and trophozoites of **E. histolytica.** This study can be performed only in the ward as the trophozoites are fragile and will be lysed under adverse conditions during transport to laboratory. The trophozoites can be identified by their (a) active motility and (b) presence of ingested RBCs.

   A drawing of such a preparation is kept for the study.
2. A wet preparation with Lugol's iodine from a formed stool of chronic case will reveal cysts of **E. histolytica.** The presence of 1-4 stained nuclei and glycogen mass can be noted (Fig. 104.2, 3, 4).
3. A similar wet preparation will show cysts of **E. coli.** Their larger size and the presence of 4-8 nuclei can be noted.

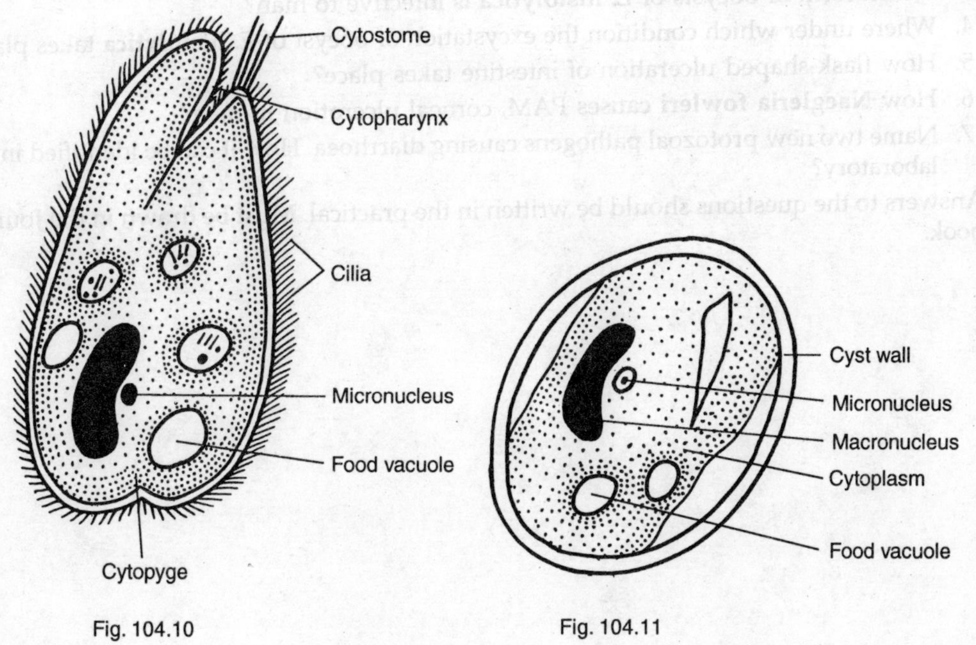

Fig. 104.10-11: Balantidium coli

* 4. A dry faecal smear from a case of acute amoebic dysentery stained with iron haematoxylin, showing trophozoites of **E. histolytica.** The minute chromatin granules of nuclear membrane and the small centrally placed karyosome in the nucleus can be noted.
5. A similar stained preparation with trophozoite of **E. coli.** Their chromatin dots are coarser and the karyosome is large and placed eccentrally.
6. A similar preparation showing immature cysts of **E. histolytica.** Their chromatoid bodies are dark thick rods with rounded ends. The ends of chromatoid bodies of **E. coli** are filamentous (Nuclei of the trophozoites and cysts are morphologically similar in the respective species).
7. A smear of faeces from diarrhoea case stained with modified AFB stain showing cryptosporidium.
8. A smear of faeces from a case of ciliate dysentery stained with iron haematoxylin. Trophozoite of **Balantidium coli** is large (50-200 μ × 40-70 μ). The presence of cilia, cytostome, kidney shaped macronucleus, round micronucleus and vacuoles can be noted. Their cysts are smaller and circular with macro and micro nucleus and vacuoles (Fig. 104.10.11).

Questions

1. Enumerate the causal agents of dysentery and how will you differentiate between **E. histolytica** and **E. coli.**
2. What are the most recent methods of diagnosis of amoebiasis?

3. Which form of oocysts of **E. histolytica** is infective to man?
4. Where under which condition the excystation of oocyst of **E. histolytica** takes place?
5. How flask-shaped ulceration of intestine takes place?
6. How **Naegleria fowleri** causes PAM, corneal ulceration in man?
7. Name two new protozoal pathogens causing diarrhoea. How it can be identified in the laboratory?

Answers to the questions should be written in the practical. Must be drawn in the Journal notebook.

105
Plasmodia (Malarial Parasites)

Plasmodium vivax causes tertian malaria.

Pl. falciparum - malignant tertian malaria

Pl malariae - quartan malaria

Pl. ovale - ovale malaria

They reside in RBCs, are carried to various organs (mainly liver).

Morphology — Table 105.1

Life cycle : Human cycle. Man, intermediate host, gets infected by the bite of infected female Anopheles mosquito. Sporozoites, infective forms, enter directly into liver cells (not in RBCs) for their development. This is (1) **pre-erythrocytic schizogony.** The merozoites are liberated. The micromerozoites enter into RBCs whereas the macromerozoites reenter the liver cells. At this stage, there is no clinical manifestation.

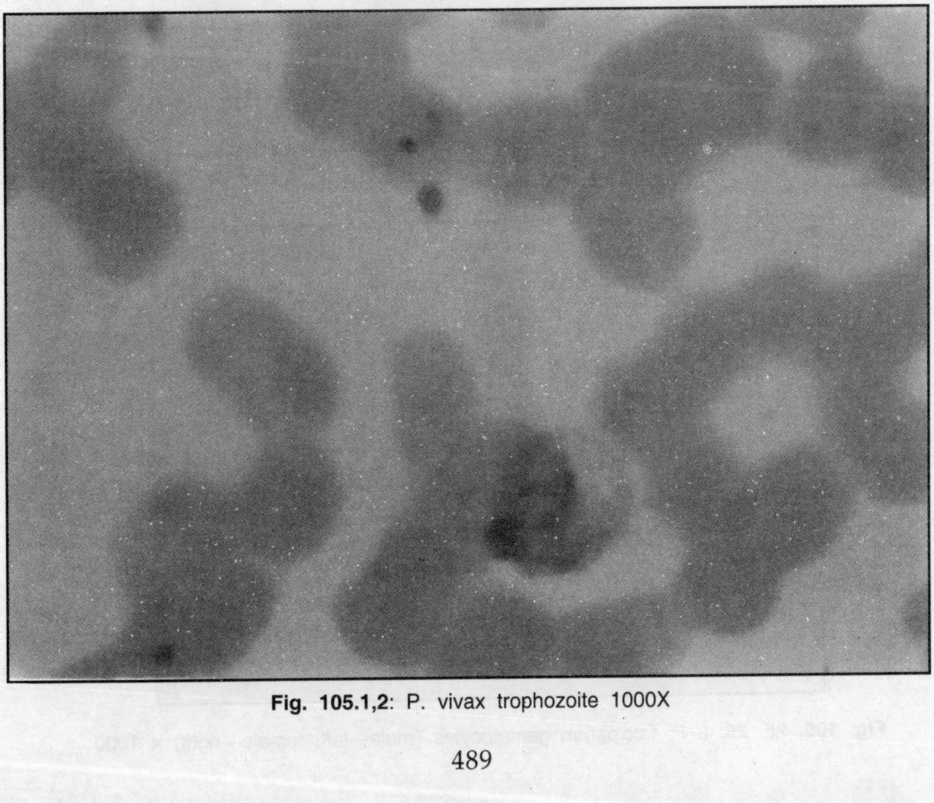

Fig. 105.1,2: P. vivax trophozoite 1000X

2. **In erythrocytic schizogony :** In RBCs, the parasites pass through three stages trophozoites, schizonts, and merozoites. At this stage, there is clinical attack of malaria (overt malaria). (3) **Gametogony.** After the erythrocytic schizogony, the merozoites develop into gametocytes (sexual forms) which sexually reproduce in the mosquito and the individuals who harbour their gametocytes are called "carriers." (4) **Exo-erythrocytic schizogony.** After the micromerozoites infect RBCs the preerythrocytic schizogony disappears completely in P. falciparum—hence no relapse, but there is recrudescence due to improper treatment, whereas in P. vivax, P. ovale and P. malariae, there is relapse (liver cycle).

Mosquito cycle : Mosquito bites and ingests both asexual forms (that die) and sexual forms that transform into micro (male) and macrogametocytes (female), zygote, ookinete (motile zygote), oocysts and, finally, infective sporozoites.

Clinical features : The onset is usually sudden in vivax, shivering, fever, headache, malaise, muscular pain.

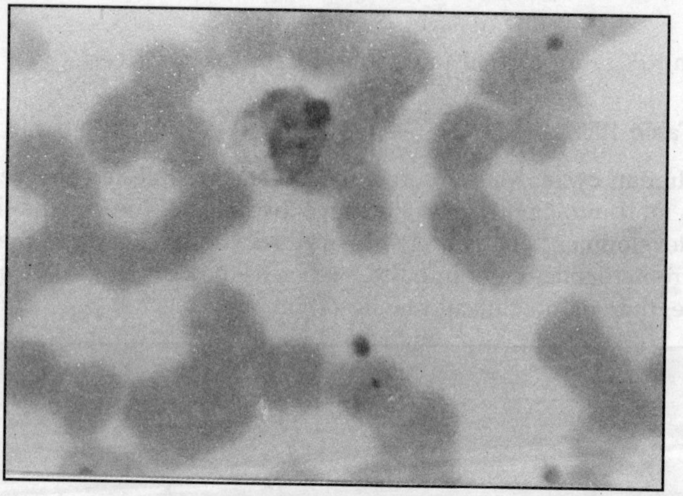

Fig. 105.14,5: P. vivax mature schizont × 1000

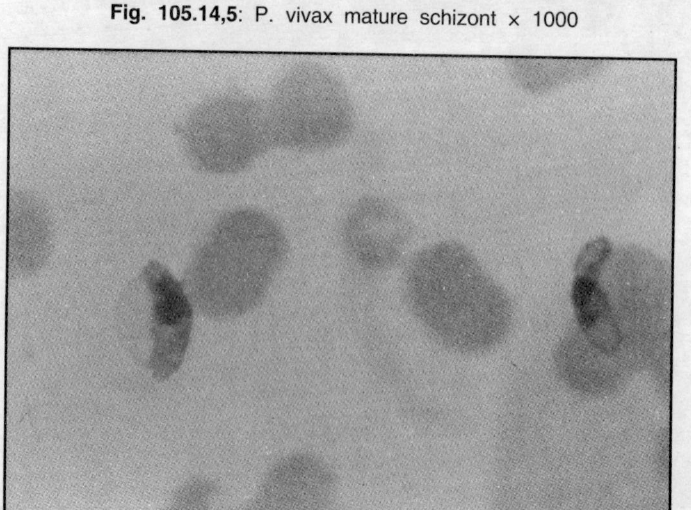

Fig. 105. 25, 26: L P. falciparum gametocytes (male—left; female—right) × 1000

Laboratory diagnosis : (a) Demonstration of Plasmodia in Leishman stained or Acridine Orange (AO) stained blood smear is the method of choice. Magnetic Resonance Imaging (MRI) is most recently used to diagnose cerebral malaria due to P. falciparum. Fluorescence microscopy using Acridine Orange stain can detect P. falciparum ring in smear.

Serology : CFT, slide flocculation, latex agglutination, IHA, FA test are still under experimentation. Genetic engineering method and Polymerase Chain Reaction (PCR) are recent methods. In recent years, ELISA, ABC-ELISA (new test) immunoblot, DNA probes are useful epidemiological tools. A rapid manual test for P. falciparum. Para sight F test is simple, specific, sensitive and rapid (10 minutes) test in a single drop of blood.

Treatment : Chloroquine, quinine, primaquine are commonly used but halofantrine, pyronardine, mefloquine-sulphadoxine, pyrimethamine (Fangimel) are recent drug of choice for treatment of resistant malaria. Recently, Albendazole was found to kill cultures of P. falciparum.

Demonstration

(All smears are from peripheral blood and stained by Leishman stain).

1. A peripheral blood smear showing the early trophozoite form (ring form) of **P. vivax.**

TABLE 105.1 MALARIAL PARASITES OF MAN

Differential characters of Erythrocytic phases (After staining)

SCHIZOGONY	P. VIVAX 48 HOURS	P. FALCIPARUM 48 HOURS OR UNDER	P. MALARIAE 72 HOURS	P. OVALE 48 HOURS
Forms peripheral blood	Trophozoites, schizonts	Rings, crescents only Gametocytes	Trophozoites, schizonts gametocytes	Trophozoites, schizonts gametocytes
Trophozoites Ring form;	Size, 2.5 μm cytoplasm opposite nucleus (Fig. 105.1.2)	Size 1.25 μm-1.5 μm cytoplasm fine, regular accole form (Fig. 105.7, 8)	Same as P. vivax (Fig. 105.13)	Same as P. malariae (Fig. 105.19)
Growing form	Irregular with a vacuole. Actively amoeboid (Fig. 105.3)	Assumes compact form Pigments collect into a single mass early (Fig. 105.14.15)	Band like, Slightly amoeboid. Vacuole disappears early	No ribbon shape, Slightly amoeboid (Fig. 105.20)
Schizont (Mature)	Size, 9-10 μm Regular, completely fills and enlarged red blood cells (Fig. 105.4, 5)	Size, 4.5-5 μm, Fills two thirds of a red blood cell cell which is not enlarged (Fig. 105.10, 11)	Size, 6.5 to 7 μm Regular almost fills a normal sized red blood cels (Fig. 105.16, 17)	Size 6.2 μm Fills three quarters of red blood cell which is slightly enlarged (Fig. 105.21)
Merozoites	12-24 Arranged in an irregular grape-like cluster (Fig 105.6)	18-24 or more arranged in a grape-like cluster. (Fig. 105.12)	6-12, Arranged around a central mass of pigment like a 'daisy' or a rosette (Fig. 105.18)	6-12 Irregularly arranged (Fig. 105.22)
Malarial pigments	Yellowish brown fine granules	Dark brown or blackish one or two solid blocks	Dark brown; coarse granules	Dark yellowish brown; coarser than P. vivax

Contd.

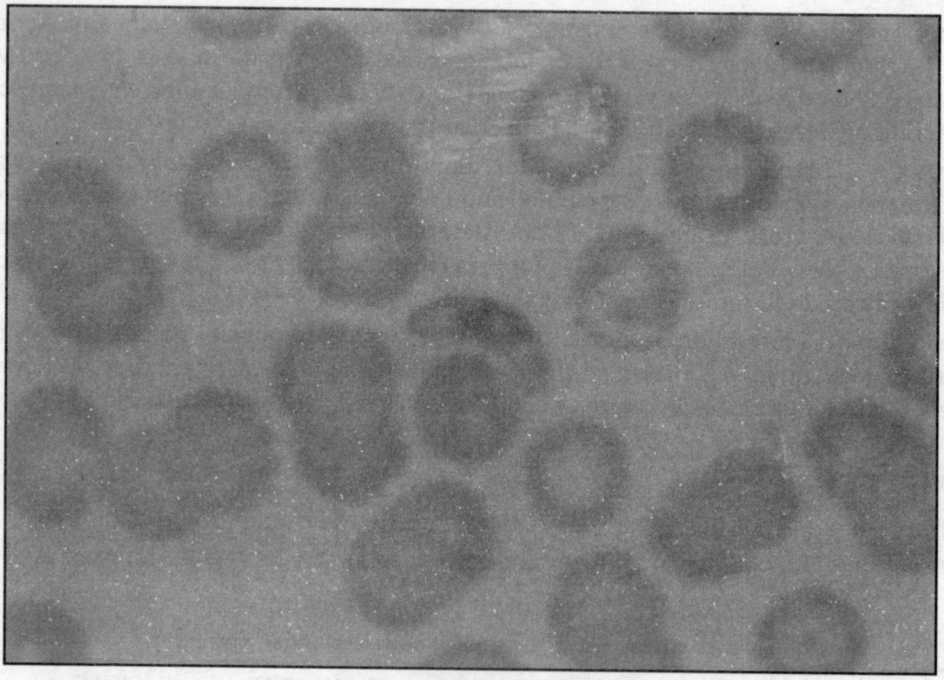

Fig. 105.25: Male gametocyte of P. falciparum × 1000

MALARIAL PARASITES OF MAN

Table 105.1 Differential characters of Erythrocytic phases (After staining)

SCHIZOGONY	P. VIVAX 48 HOURS	P. FALCIPARUM 48 HOURS OR UNDER	P. MALARIAE 72 HOURS	P. OVALE 48 HOURS
Infected R.B.C.	Enlarged, pale Schuffner's dots present.	Unaltered, crenation reddish, violet colour, Maurer's dots.	Not enlarged, not pale and no dots.	Enlarged, oval, James's dots.
Gametocyte	Spherical, much larger than a red blood cell. Schuffner's dots. (Fig. 105.23, 24)	Crescentic larger than red blood cell host cell hardly recognisable (Fig. 105.25, 26)	Round, Oval size of red blood cell (Fig. 105.27, 28)	Oval size of red blood cell host cell slightly enlarged with James's dots (Fig. 105.29, 30)
	Female : Cytoplasm blue; nucleus small and compact Male : Cytoplasm pale blue, nucleus large and diffuse			

Note the large size of the ring and a single red chromatin dot (nucleus) (Fig. 20.1.5).

* 2. A blood smear showing the late trophozoite form (amoeboid form) of **P. vivax.** The red cell is enlarged and contains fine red dots (Schuffner's granules) (Fig. 20.2.3).

3. A smear showing schizonts of **P. vivax.** Note the chromatin dot (nucleus) divided into 12-24 masses (merozoites).

4. Schizont of **P. malariae** in the blood smear. The number of merozoites is less, 6-12, and is arranged in a "rosette" form around the central mass of pigment.

5. Gametocytes of **P. vivax** in the blood smear are spherical, large and have only one chromatin dot, no division is seen.

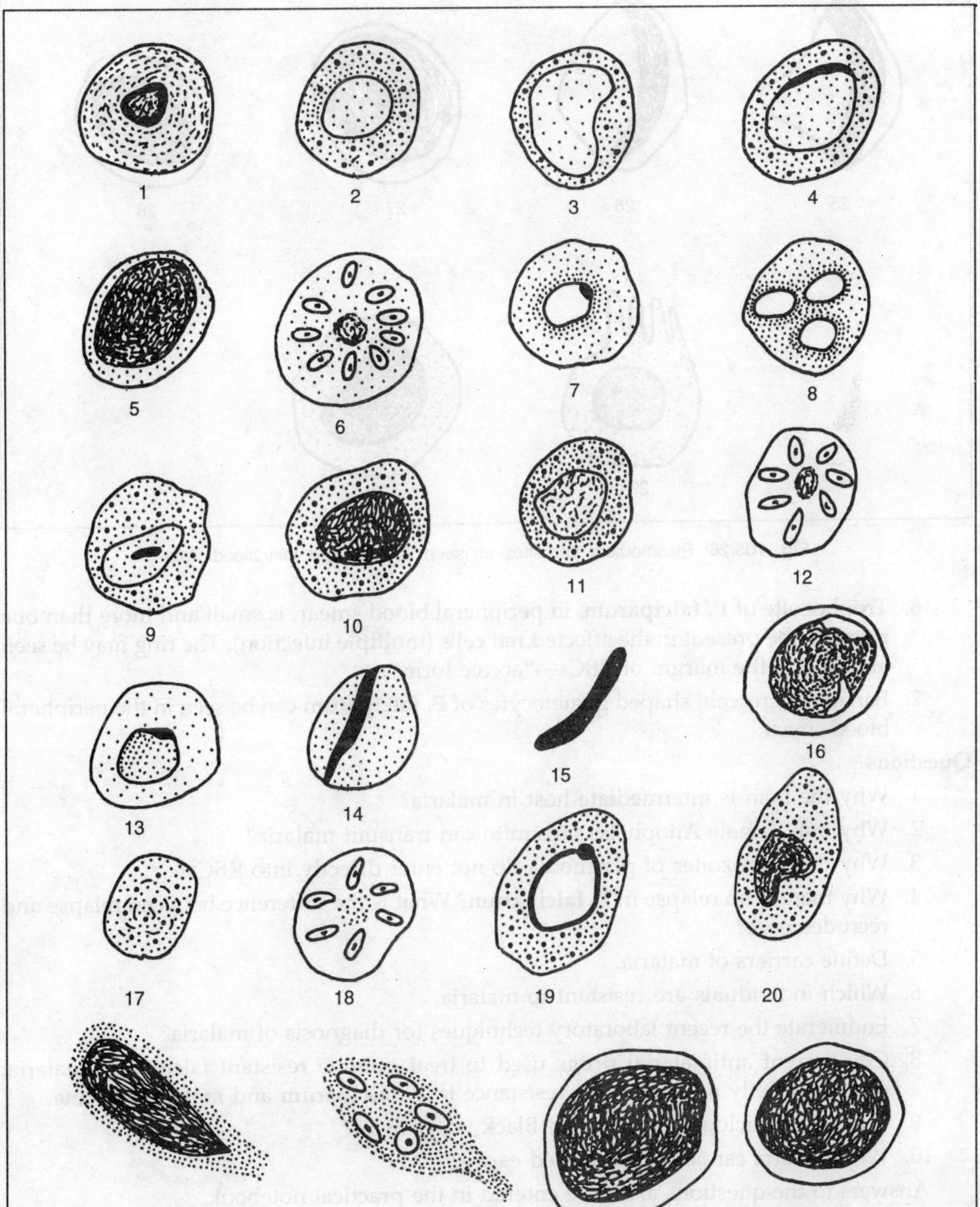

Fig. 105.26: Plasmodium parasites as seen in thick and thin blood films

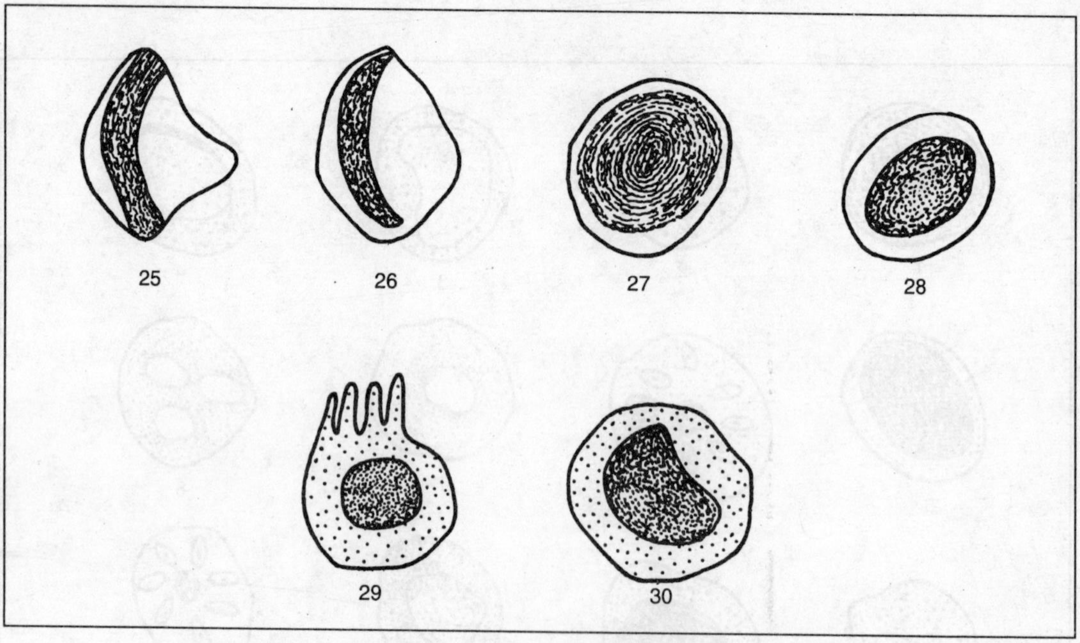

Fig. 105.26: Plasmodium parasites as seen in thick and thin blood films

6. Trophozoite of **P. falciparum,** in peripheral blood smear, is small and more than one ring may be present in the affected red cells (multiple infection). The ring may be seen attached to the margin of RBCs—"accole form".
7. Banana or crescent shaped gametocytes of **P. falciparum** can be seen in the peripheral blood smear.

Questions

1. Why the man is intermediate host in malaria?
2. Why only female Anopheles mosquito can transmit malaria?
3. Why the sporozoites of plasmodia do not enter directly into RBCs?
4. Why there is no relapse in **P. falciparum**? What is the difference between relapse and recrudescence?
5. Define carriers of malaria.
6. Which individuals are resistant to malaria.
7. Enumerate the recent laboratory techniques for diagnosis of malaria?
8. Cite current antimalarial drugs used to treat quinine resistant falciparum malaria; describe briefly multiple drug resistance in **P. falciparum** and malarial vaccine.
9. What is pernicious anaemia and Black water fever?
10. Why malaria cannot be controlled easily?

Answers to the questions are to be entered in the practical notebook.
Must be drawn in the practical notebook.

106

Class Mastigophora (Flagellate)

Blood flagellate (Trypanosoma) Intestinal flagellate (Giardia intestinalis) Atrial flagellate (Trichomonas vaginalis)

Genus Trypanosoma

Trypanosome, blood flagellate protozoon, is an elongated spindle shaped body with tapering ends. Its nucleus is central and anterior to kinetoplast. The undulating membrane is proceeding forward as free flagellum (Fig. 106.1).

Human pathogenic trypanosomes are :

1. **T. brucei — rhodesiense - gambiense** group (Human strain) **T. rhodesiense** (Fig. 106.2) and **T. gambiense** (Fig. 106.3) causes African trypanosomiasis.
2. **T. cruzi** (Fig. 106.4) causes South American trypanosomiasis (Chagas disease).

T. gambiense occus in 3 forms (long, short and intermediate) in blood lymph node, CSF.

Life cycle : T. gambiense multiply in the blood of man (definite host). After ingestion by intermediate host (tse tse fly, **Glossina palpalis**), they reproduce in the lumen of the fly and migrate back to salivary gland (anterior station development). These metacyclic infective forms are introduced into man by the bite of the fly.

Clinical features : An elevated painful "trypanosomal chancre" at the site of bite. After trypanosomal invasion, lymph nodes, spleen, liver are enlarged. If the CNS is invaded, sleeping sickness develops with severe headache, mental dullness and apathy and the sleepiness becomes pronounced and finally death ensues.

In the **laboratory** (A) Trypanosome can be demonstrated microscopically in 1. Peripheral blood; 2. Lymph aspirate; 3. Bone marrow smear and 4. CSF. (B) Cultivation in media. (C) Animal inoculation.

Serology : Gel precipitation test, indirect fluorescent antibody test (IFAT). CFT, ELISA. Besides, ELISA and capillary passive haemagglutination (HA), a Card agglutination test (CATT) has been recently introduced. It is simple, specific and sensitive.

Treatment : Melarsoprol and Berenil are current drugs.

Trypanosoma cruzi

It is a pleomorphic trypanosome, occurs in human blood as typical trypanosome (Fig. 106.1) and in reticuloendothelial cells and tissue as Leishmania. In vectors as Leishmanial (Fig.106.5) Crithidia (Fig. 106.6) and metacyclic trypanosome. It can be cultivated on Novy MacNeal and Nicolle (NNN) medium (Fig. 106.7—Leptomonas).

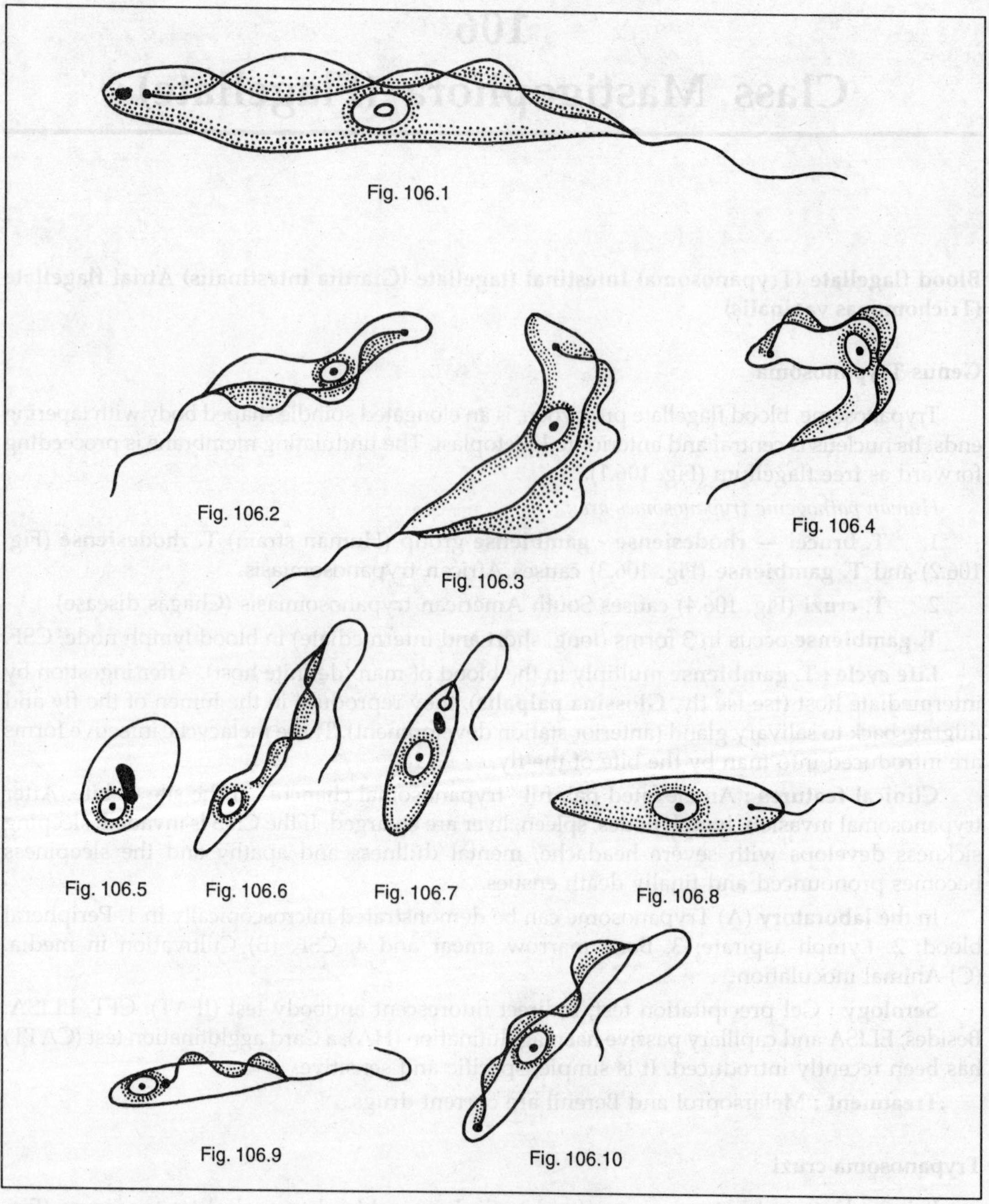

Fig. 106.1-10: Trypanosoma

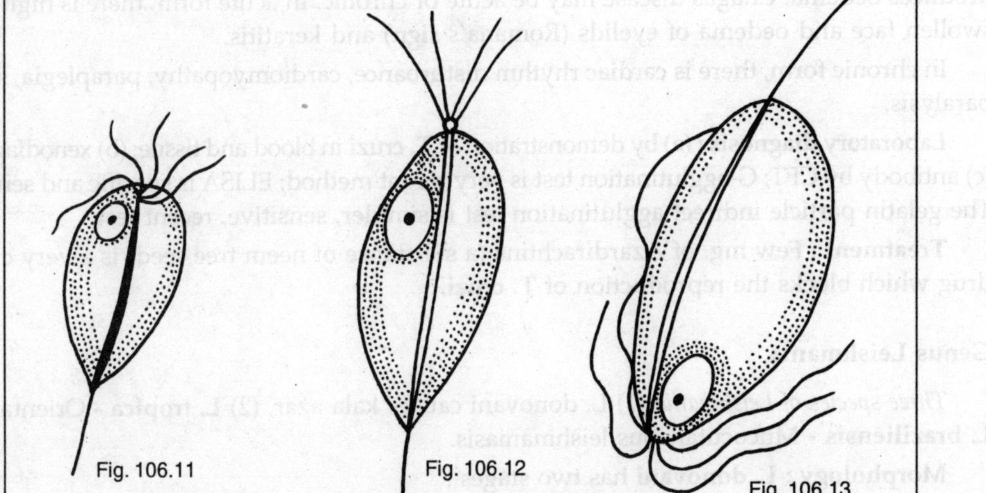

Fig. 106.11 Fig. 106.12 Fig. 106.13

Fig. 106.11-13: Trichomonas

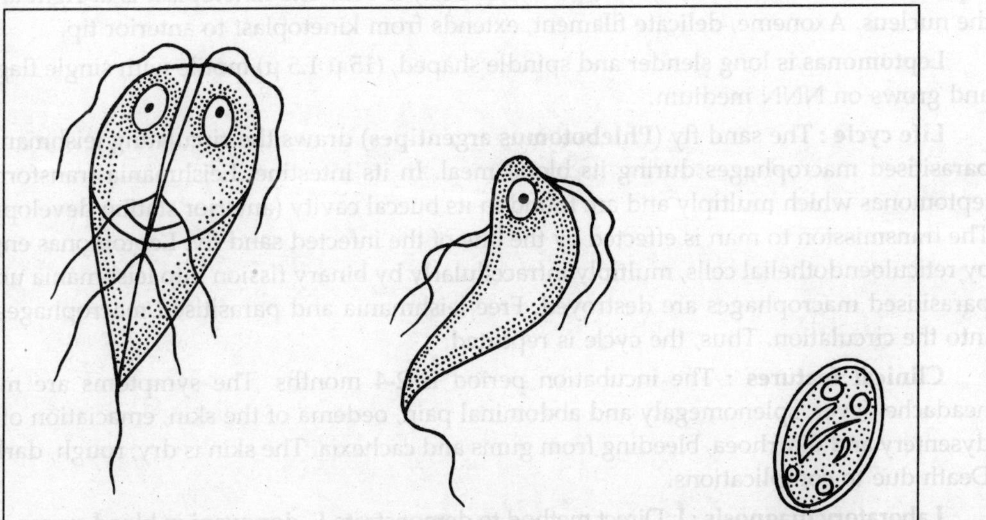

Fig. 106.14 Fig. 106.15 Fig. 106.16

Fig. 106.14-16: Flagellates → Giardia intestinalis

Life cycle : Reduviid bug (**Triotoma infestans**) ingests trypanosomes while biting infected man. In its stomach, they transform into amastigote, (Fig. 106.5), promastigote (Fig. 106.8) epimastigote (Fig. 106.9) and metacyclic forms which are excreted with its faeces (Posterior station development). These infective metacyclic trypanosomes (Fig. 106.10) are rubbed into the scratches made by bug, invade the subcutaneous tissue, transform into amastigote, promastigote and trypomastigote forms which are liberated in the circulation. Thus, the cycle is repeated.

Clinical features : In the skin, primary lesion (Chagoma) blocks the lymphatics and produces oedema. Chagas disease may be acute or chronic. In acute form, there is high fever, swollen face and oedema of eyelids (Romana's sign) and keratitis.

In chronic form, there is cardiac rhythm disturbance, cardiomyopathy, paraplegia, spastic paralysis.

Laboratory diagnosis : (a) by demonstration of **T. cruzi** in blood and tissue; (b) xenodiagnosis, (c) antibody by CFT; G-agglutination test is very recent method; ELISA is specific and sensitive. The gelatin particle indirect agglutination test is simpler, sensitive, recent test.

Treatment : Few mg. of Azardirachtine (a substance of neem tree seed) is a very current drug which blocks the reproduction of **T. cruzi.**

Genus Leishmania

Three species of Leishmania (1) L. donovani causes kala azar, (2) **L. tropica** - Oriental sore; **L. braziliensis** - Mucocutaneous leishmaniasis.

Morphology : L. donovani has two stages :

1. Leishmania (amastigote); 2. Leptomonas in sand fly, and in culture.

Leishmania is an ovoidal body (2, 3 microns), intracellular in the monocytes and polymorphonuclear leucocytes of man. In blood smear stained by Giemsa stain, its cytoplasm is pale blue and the nucleus is red, parabasal body is red. The kinetoplast is at right angle to the nucleus. Axoneme, delicate filament, extends from kinetoplast to anterior tip.

Leptomonas is long slender and spindle shaped, (15 μ 1.5 μ) motile with single flagellum and grows on NNN medium.

Life cycle : The sand fly (**Phlebotomus argentipes**) draws the circulating leishmania and parasitised macrophages during its blood meal. In its intestine, Leishmania transform into leptomonas which multiply and are found in its buccal cavity (anterior station development). The transmission to man is effected by the bite of the infected sand fly. Leptomonas engulfed by reticuloendothelial cells, multiply intracellularly by binary fission into leishmania until the parasitised macrophages are destroyed. Free leishmania and parasitised macrophages enter into the circulation. Thus, the cycle is repeated.

Clinical features : The incubation period is 2-4 months. The symptoms are malaise, headache, fever, splenomegaly and abdominal pain, oedema of the skin, emaciation of chest, dysentery and diarrhoea, bleeding from gums and cachexia. The skin is dry, rough, darkened. Death due to complications.

Laboratory diagnosis : I. Direct method to demonstrate **L. donovani** in blood smear, culture and biopsy of lymph node and sternal puncture. Polymerase Chain Reaction (PCR) can detect L. donovani in impression smear.

II. Indirect method, blood count, old serology — Aldehyde test, Antimony test and CFT. Recent serological techniques — IFAT, CIEF and ELISA and Direct agglutination test (DAT). IFAT is very sensitive; ELISA is specific, sensitive and most practical test. As compared to ELISA and IFAT, DAT is most recent technique and is found to be most specific sensitive and easy to perform and economical.

Treatment : Ketoconazole is effective against **L. donovani.** Amphotericin B intravenously is very effective to multidrug (sodium stibogluconate, allopurinol plus ketoconazole and pentamide isothionate) resistant **L. donovani** and is extremely effective relapse-free.

Leishmania tropica
(Causes Delhi boil or Oriental sore)

In its morphology and life cycle. It is similar to **L. donovani** but it does not invade the viscera.

Clinical features : The incubation period is several months. Lesion on the skin (reddish papule, ulcer with raised edge), Symptoms are fever, chills and inflammation.

Laboratory diagnosis : Microscopic examination of stained smear from the sore will reveal **L. tropica** but blood smear will not. Montenegro reaction (skin test) can also be done.

Leishmania braziliensis

Its morphology, life cycle and laboratory diagnosis are similar to that of **L. donovani** and **L. tropica.**

Clinical features : Ulcer in the mucous membrane of the mouth, and hard and soft palate. Symptoms are fever, anaemia, pain and malaise.

Giardia intestinalis (Fig. 106.14, 15, 16 — see in page 497)

(See also page 484 under intestinal protozoa)

Genus : Trichomonas has been classified according to their habitats into :

(1) **Trichomonas hominis** — lleo — caecal region (Fig. 106.11)
(2) **Trichomonas tenax** — Oral cavity (Fig. 106.12)
(3) **Trichomonas vaginalis** — Vagina and urinary tract (Fig. 106.13)

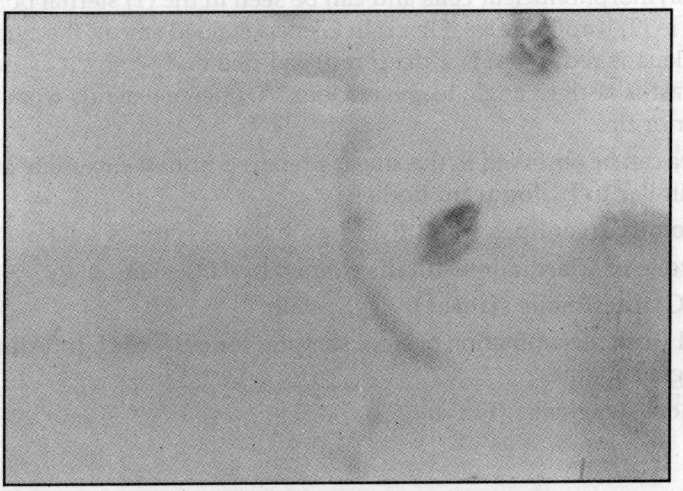

Fig. 106.11: Trichomonas hominis X 400

Trichomonas vaginalis

History : Donne (1836) observed this species in female and male genital organs.

Habitat : This flagellate is mostly found in human vagina and prostate gland.

Morphology : It exists only in trophozoite stage (Fig. 106.13). It is considerably larger (13 microns), its undulating membrane is shorter and its cytostome is much less conspicuous.

Biology and Life cycle: In the female, this parasite feeds on the mucosal surface of the vagina, ingesting bacteria and leucocytes. It grows in the more acid condition than that of the healthy vagina. The infected female is the reservoir of **T. vaginalis** and the infection is acquired by male in extra-marital intercourse.

Pathogenicity and Clinical features : T. vaginalis causes degeneration and desquamation of the vaginal epithelium, followed by leucocytic inflammation of the tissue layer. Very large numbers of trichomonads and leucocytes are now present in the vaginal discharge which is greenish or yellow. The vaginal secretions **diagnosis** can be found in centrifuged urine and vaginal secretion.

Demonstration

(All smears are stained by Giemsa stain)

1. A smear from the peripheral blood of African sleeping sickness showing Trypanosoma gambiense. This organism is fusiform (14 μ 1.5 μ). The nucleus is placed centrally. The Kinetoplast is at the posterior end and from which the flagellum starts and proceeds forward as free flagellum, at the anterior end. It is similar to **T. rhodesiense.**
2. **T. lewisi** in the peripheral blood smear of rat is morphologically similar to other trypanosomes.
3. **Glossina palpalis** (Glossina or tse tse fly) is the insect vector of African sleeping sickness.
4. **T. cruzi** has a characteristic **C shape** and found in the blood of Chagas disease.
5. **Triatoma infestans** (reduvid bug) is the vector of Chagas disease.
6. **Leishmania donovani** bodies or L.D. bodies are ovoidal bodies (2-3 μ) are intracellular in the polymorphonuclear cells and can be seen in the (1) sternal bone marrow smear, and also in (2) Kupffer cells of liver. In Giemsa stained smear, the cytoplasm stains blue and nucleus is red; there is a deep red, rod-like body-known as parabasal body. Its kinetoplast is at right angle to the nucleus. Axoneme extends from the kinetoplast to the anterior tip.
7. **L. tropica** can be observed in the smear prepared from the exudate of the Oriental sore and is similar to **L. donovani** bodies.
8. **Phlebotomus argentipes** (sand fly) is an Indian vector of kala azar.
9. Trophozoite of **Giardia intestinalis** stained by H.E. stain.
10. Cyst of **G. intestinalis** stained by H.E. stain.

    Practical work : Examination of stool samples for cysts of **G. intestinalis** after staining with Lugol's iodine.
11. Trichomonas vaginalis (Fig. 106.13).

Questions

1. When the sleeping sickness stage of infection takes place?
2. How can you differentiate morphologically T. cruzi from T. gambiense?
3. Why **Triatoma infestans** and **Glossina palpalis** are required in the life cycle of **T. cruzi** and **T. gambiense**, respectively. Similarly, why sand fly is needed in the life cycle of **L. donovani?**
4. What is kala azar, Dum Dum fever, Oriental sore, Delhi boil?
5. **Enumerate recent serological tests for the diagnosis of African sleeping sickness and Chagas disease.**

6. Name a very recent drug which is effective against Chagas disease by blocking the reproduction of **T. cruzi.**
7. Which stage of **L. donovani** is infective to man?
8. Give an account of very recent serological tests used to diagnose kala azar.
9. Cite a very recent drug effective to multidrug resistant **L. donovani.**

Answers to the questions should be entered in the practical note book.

Muse be drawn in the practical note book.

Intestinal Helminths

Cestoda : Diphyllobothrium latum, Taenia saginata, T. solium, Echinococcus granulosus, Hymenolepis nana, Dipylidium caninum.

Trematoda : Fasciolopsis buski, Fasciola hepatica, Gastrodiscoides hominis.

Nematoda : Trichinella spiralls, Trichuris trichiura, Strongyloides stercoralis, Ancylostoma duodenale, Necator americanus, Enterobius vermicularis, Ascaris lumbricoides.

107
Class Cestoda

Diphyllobothrium latum (Fish tapeworm) : The adult worm is ivory or yellowish grey in colour, measuring 3-10 metres in length. The head (scolex) is small, spatulated or spoon shaped, has a pair of slit grooves (bothria) ventrally and dorsally and has no rostellum (a beak-like projection on the head) and no hooklets (Fig. 107.1). Scolex is followed by "neck" and 3,000 segments (Proglottids, Fig. 107.2). A single worm may discharge as many as one million eggs (Fig. 107.3) per day.

Life cycle : When the egg of **D. latum** passed out along with the faeces of the infected host (man) comes in contact with water, the ciliated embryo (**coracidium,** Fig. 107.4) escapes from the egg and swims in the water. It is ingested by a cyclops (Fig. 107.5, 6) and transforms into **procercoid** larva (Fig. 107.7). When the infected cyclops is ingested by a fish, procercoid develops into plerocercoid or sparganum (Fig. 107.8) larva in the fish which is infective to man. On consuming insufficiently cooked fish, man becomes infected. The plerocercoid larva develops into an adult worm, ultimately the eggs are excreted in the faeces.

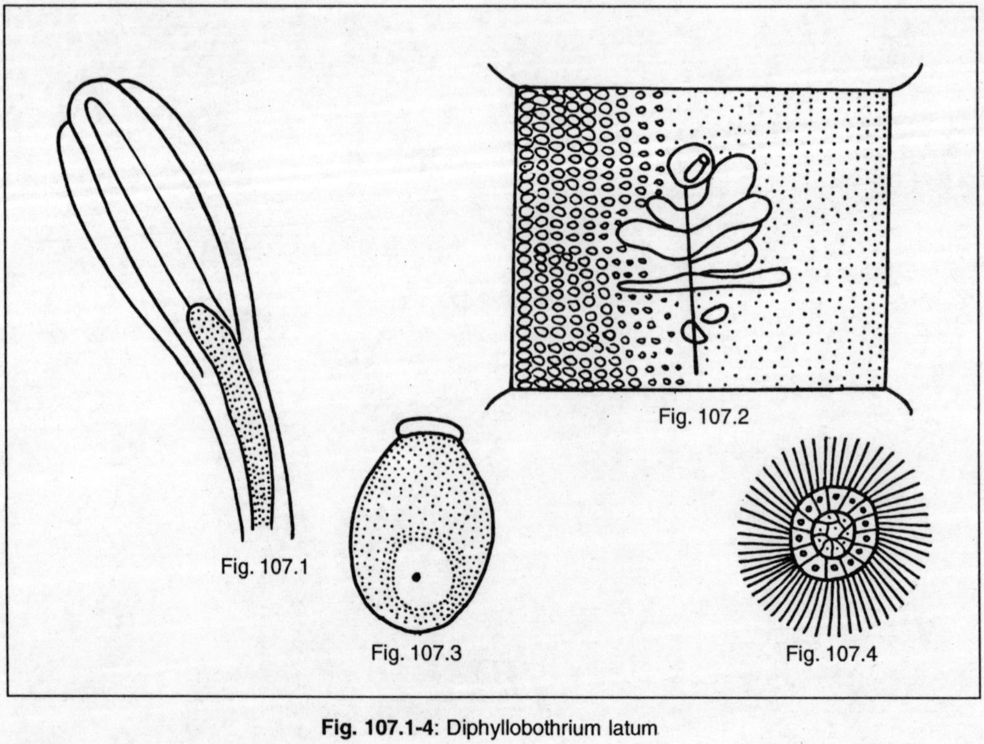

Fig. 107.1-4: Diphyllobothrium latum

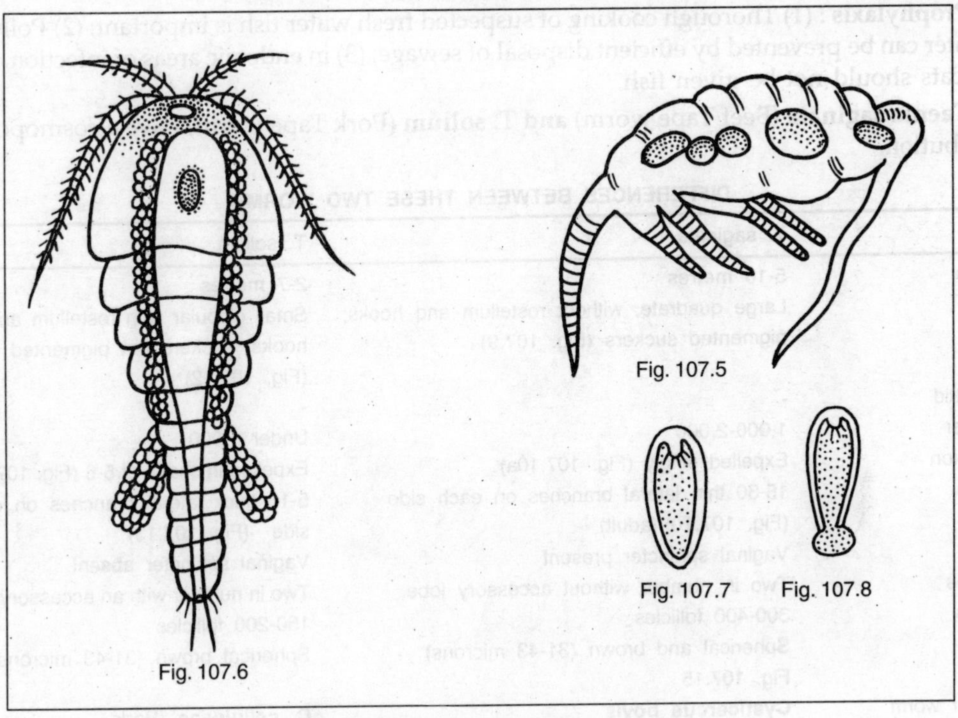

Fig. 107.5

Fig. 107.6

Fig. 107.7 Fig. 107.8

Fig. 107.5-8: Diphyllobothrium latum

Clinical features : The presence of adult worm in the intestinal tract causes no symptom, but sometimes, non-specific abdominal symptoms have been ascribed. If the worms attach themselves to the jejunum, clinical vitamin B_{12} deficiency develops.

In the **laboratory**, mircoscopical examination of the faeces will reveal the eggs; sometimes proglottids can be observed in the stool.

Treatment : Quinacrine hydrochloride, niclosamide and paromomycin are found effective. Pernicious anaemia can be treated with folic acid.

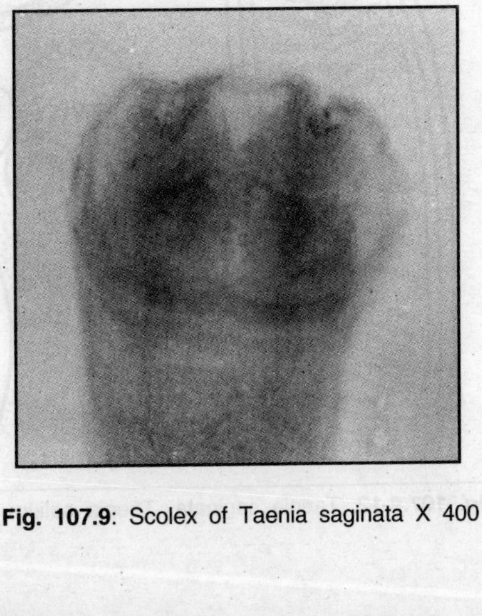

Fig. 107.9: Scolex of Taenia saginata X 400

Prophylaxis : (1) Thorough cooking of suspected fresh water fish is important; (2) Pollution of water can be prevented by efficient disposal of sewage; (3) in endemic areas of infection, dogs and cats should not be given fish.

Taenia saginata (Beef Tape worm) **and T. solium** (Pork Tape worm) have a cosmopolitan distribution.

DIFFERENCES BETWEEN THESE TWO WORMS

	T. saginata	T. solium
Length	5-10 metres	2-7 metres
Head	Large quadrate, without rostellum and hooks; pigmented suckers (Fig. 107.9)	Small globular with rostellum and hooks; suckers not pigmented (Fig. 107.12)
Proglottid	-	-
Number	1,000-2,000	Under 1,000
Expulsion	Expelled singly (Fig. 107.10a)	Expelled in chairs of 5-6 (Fig. 107.10b)
Uterus	15-30 thin lateral branches on each side (Fig. 107.10)/(adult)	5-10 thick lateral branches on each side (Fig. 107.13)
Vagina	Vaginal sphincter present	Vaginal sphincter absent.
Ovaries	Two in number without accessory lobe.	Two in number with an accessory lobe.
Testes	300-400 follicles	150-200 follicles
Eggs	Spherical and brown (31-43 microns) Fig. 107.15	Spherical brown (31-43 microns)
Bladder worm	**Cysticercus bovis** (measly beef), not found in man (Fig. 107.11)	**C. cellulosae** (Pork measle, measly pork) occasionally found in man (Fig. 107.14)
Intermediate host	Cattle	Pig

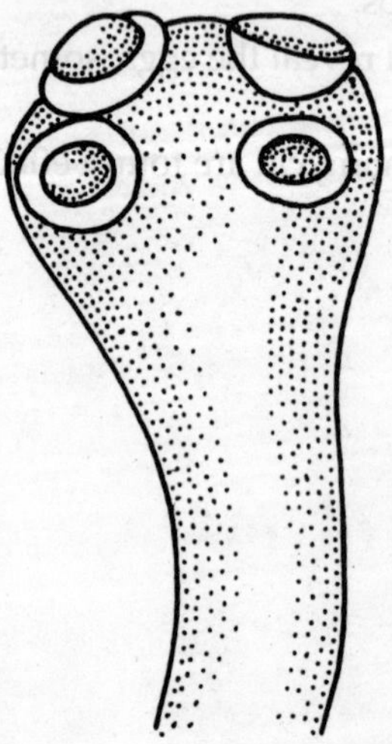

Fig. 107.9

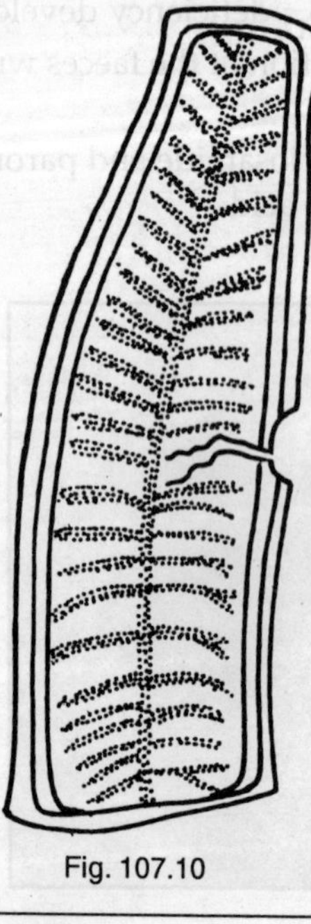

Fig. 107.10

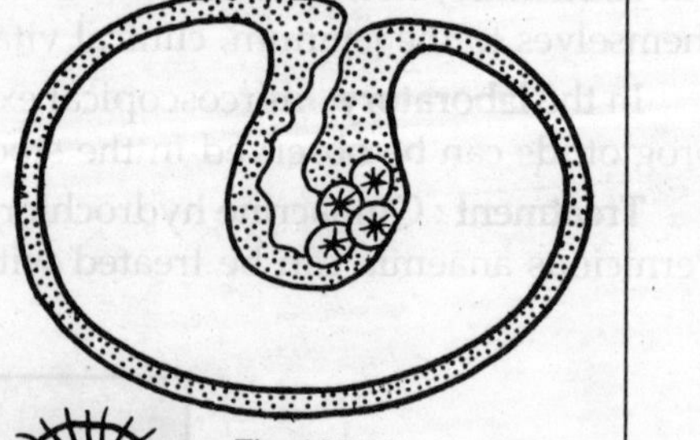

Fig. 107.11

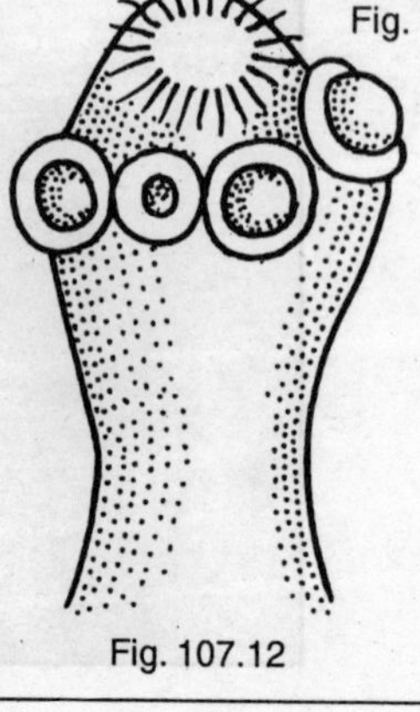

Fig. 107.12

Fig. 107.9-12: Taenia saginata, Taenia solium

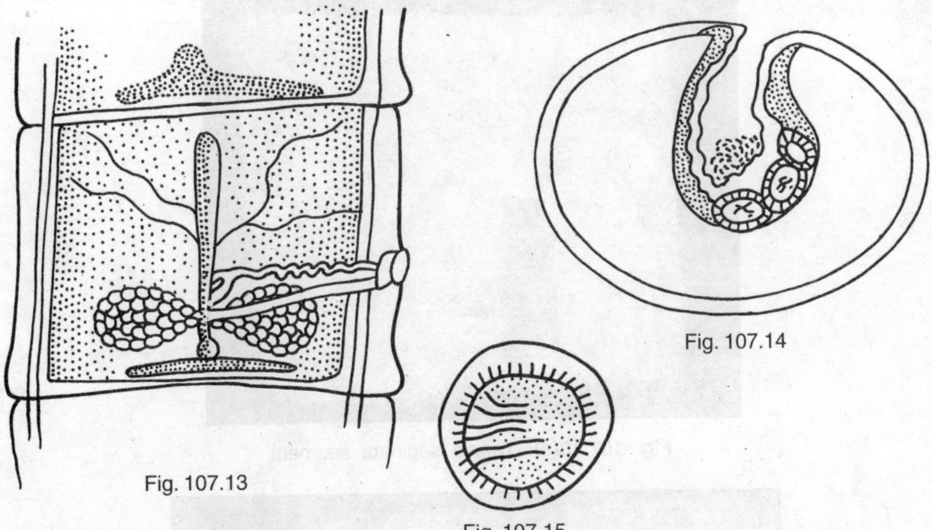

Fig. 107.13

Fig. 107.14

Fig. 107.15

Fig. 107.13-15: Taenia saginata, Taenia solium

Life cycle of T. saginata

While grazing on the polluted ground, the mature eggs are ingested by cattle. The oncospheres are hatched out from the eggs in the duodenum. These embryos penetrate the intestinal wall of the cattle, are carried through blood stream and reach the liver, the right side of the heart, lungs, the left side of the heart and the systemic circulation. These oncospheres are filtered out in the striped muscles and transform into bladder worm (**Cysticercus bovis**). On ingesting infected raw beef, man becomes infected with this bladder worm. The larva is digested out of the beef, the scolex evaginates, attaches itself to the intestinal wall of man and develops into adult worm which liberates eggs. The life cycle of **T. solium** is similar to that

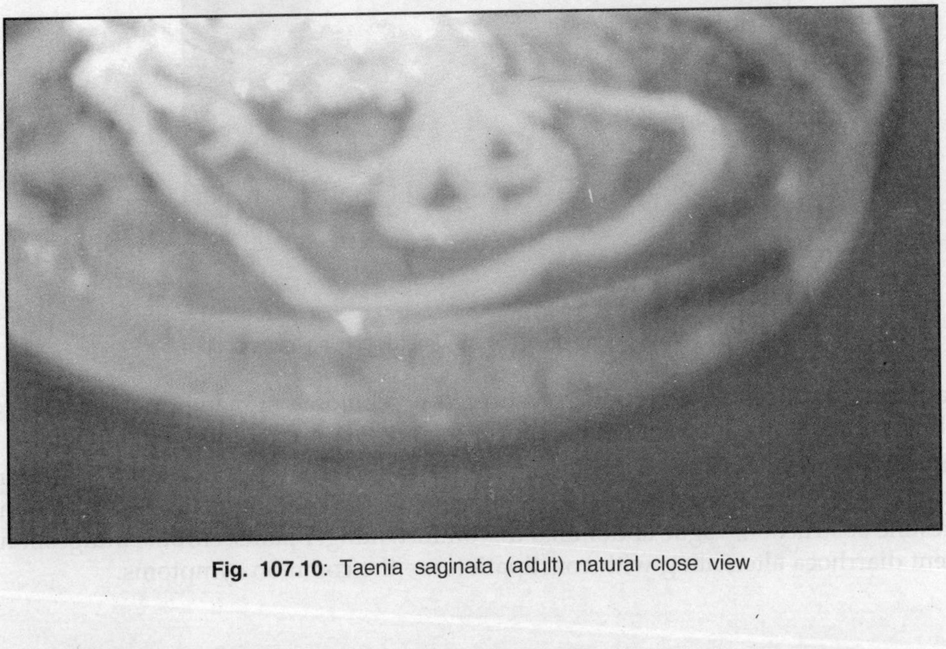

Fig. 107.10: Taenia saginata (adult) natural close view

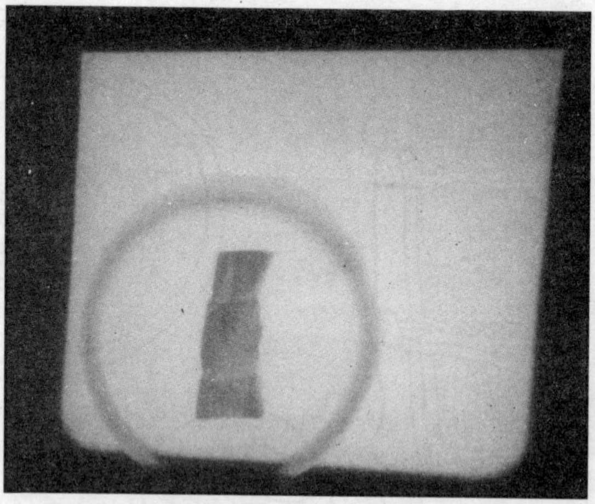

Fig. 107.10(a): Taenia saginata segment

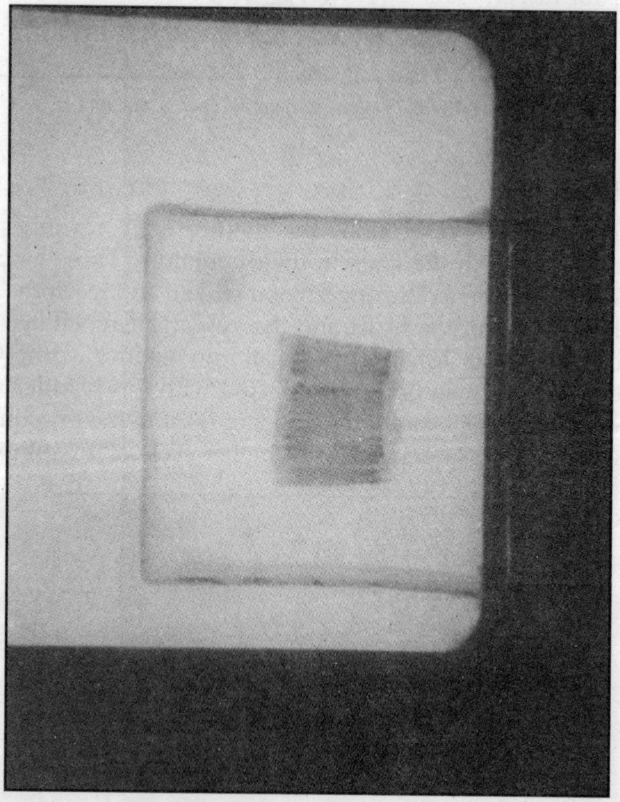

Fig. 107.10(b): Segment of T. solium (dissecting microscope)

of **T. saginata** but **C. cellulosae** produce cysticercosis cellulosae in man or neurocysticercosis in the brain of man, resulting into epileptiform seizures with a rapidly fatal outcome.

Clinical features : Because of its large size, **T. saginata** is responsible for considerable disturbance in the normal function of the intestine; whereas **T. solium** may cause irritation and less intestine obstruction, vague abdominal discomfort, hunger pains, chronic indigestion and persistent diarrhoea alternating with constipation are the common symptoms.

Laboratory diagnosis can be done by demonstration of Taenia egg (eggs of both Taenia sp. are identical), by recovery of gravid segments. A dot-ELISA test can be used by diagnose neurocysticercosis.

Treatment : Quinacrine, niclosamide, bithionol, mebendazole, are effective. Albendazole is effective for neurocysticercosis (T. solium).

Prophylaxis : Consists of : (1) Personal hygiene, (2) general sanitary measures; (3) avoidance of ingestion of raw pork or beef and vegetables irrigated by sewage water; (4) rigid quality inspection of pork and beef in all slaughter houses; (5) avoidance of faecal contamination.

Echinococcus granulosus (Dog Tape worm)

The adult worm (Fig. 107.16) is a minute tape worm, has a scolex, neck and strobila comprising three segments and measures 3-6 mm in length. It has a pyriform scolex provided with four suckers and a protrusible rostellum armed with two circular rows of hooklets. The neck is short and thick. Its egg (Fig. 107.17, 18) cannot be distinguished from that of Taenia and is infective to man, cattle, sheep.

Life cycle : The infected definite host (dog) passes the stool with the eggs onto the ground. While grazing on the polluted ground, the intermediate hosts (sheep, goats and cattle) swallow these eggs, whereas children get infected while playing with dogs. The eggs hatch in the duodenum, the oncospheres migrate through the intestinal wall, enter the mesenteric venules and become lodged in the capillary filter beds in various organs and tissues (liver, lungs, various organs) and develop into a cystic cavity (hydatid cyst — Fig. 107.19, 20). When the organs or tissues containing fertile hydatid cysts are ingested by dog, the cysts develop into adult worms. The eggs are passed out in the dog's faeces.

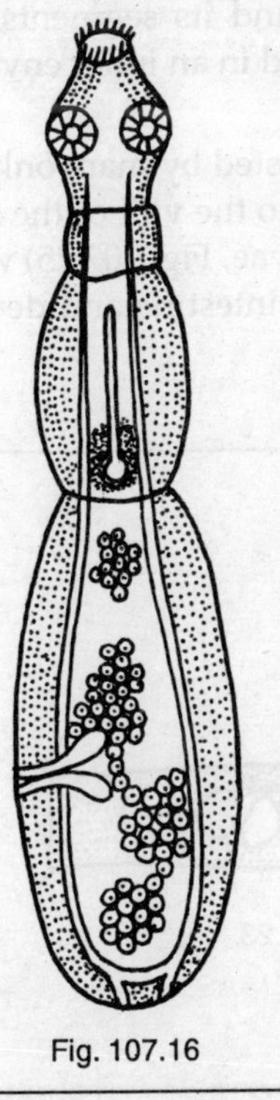

Fig. 107.16

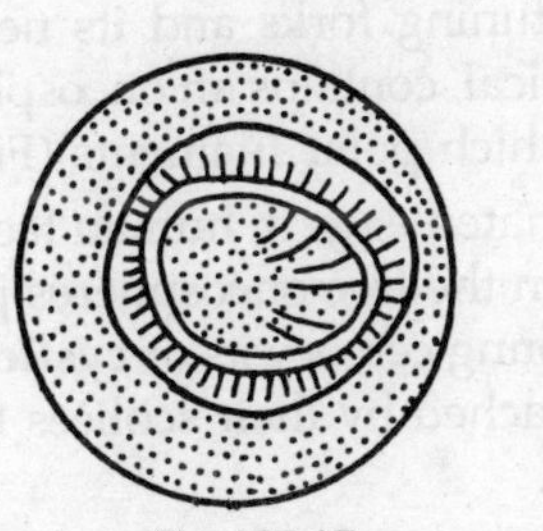

Fig. 107.17

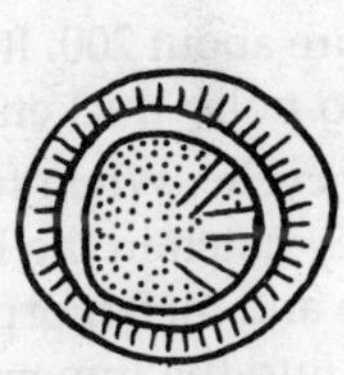

Fig. 107.18

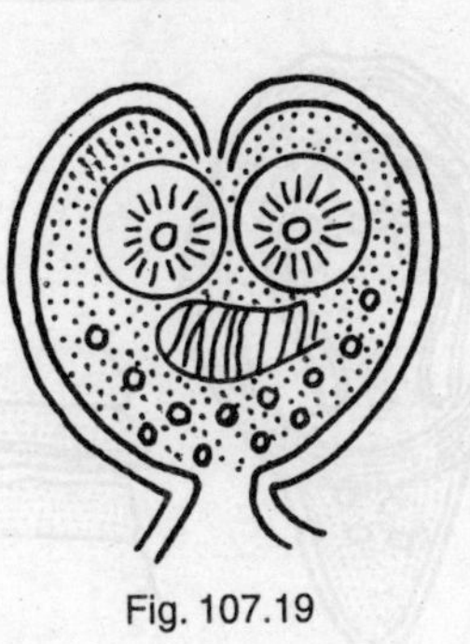

Fig. 107.19

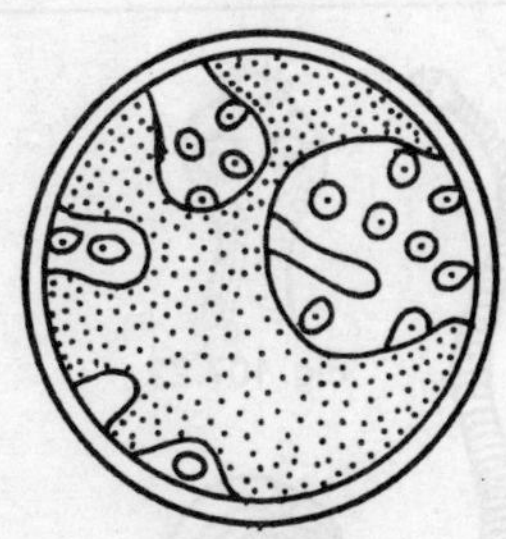

Fig. 107.20

Fig. 107.16-20: Echinococcus granulosus

Clinical features: The damage produced by hydatid cyst of **E. granulosus** is both mechanical and toxic. The young cysts which develop into embryos lodged in the vital centres may interfere with the function of the organs, damage the organ (brain, orbital capillary, heart valve) and even cause death.

Laboratory diagnosis : Casoni's test or intradermal test, precipitin test, complement fixation test; haemagglutination; bentonite flocculation test; latex agglutination test; fluorescent test ELISA; exploratory cyst puncture; roentgenogram and recent Computed Tomography (CT) scan and Magnetic Resonance Imaging (MRI) are techniques used for the diagnosis of hydatid disease. Coagglutination test is very recent sensitive, specific, rapid (within 30 minutes), inexpensive, Dot-blot-ELISA is confirmative test.

Treatment : Albendazole is most effective than thiobendazole and mebendazole. Surgical technique is also helpful. Combination of praziquantel and albendazole is very effective.

Prophylaxis : This consists of (1) avoidance of handling infected dogs; (2) avoidance of ingestion of raw vegetables polluted with eggs; (3) personal hygiene (cleaning hands before eating); (4) preventing dogs from eating the carcasses of sheep; cattle and dogs in infected areas; (5) discarding all infected viscera; in slaughter houses by dumping them into pits inaccessible to dogs and (6) educational propaganda in schools.

Polycystic hydatid disease caused by **E. vogeli** can be treated with albendazole.

Hymenolepis nana

H. nana (Fig. 107.21) is a cosmopolitan parasite. It is small and measures up to 25-40 mm in length by one mm in diameter. Its scolex (Fig. 107.22) is minute, rhomboidal and has four suckers and a short rectractile rostellum armed with 20-30 hooklets in one single row. The rostellar hooklets are shaped like tuning forks and its neck is long and its segments (Fig. 107.23) are about 200. It egg is spherical, contains an oncosphere enclosed in an inner envelope with two polar thickenings from which polar filaments (Fig. 107.24).

Life cycle : When fully embryonated eggs in human faeces are ingested by man, only one host, they hatch in the intestine, then the free oncospheres penetrate into the villi of the small intestine and metamorphose into young cercocysts or **cysticercoids** (larvae, Fig. 107.25) which migrate into the lumen, become attached by their scolices to the small intestine and develop into mature worms which lay eggs.

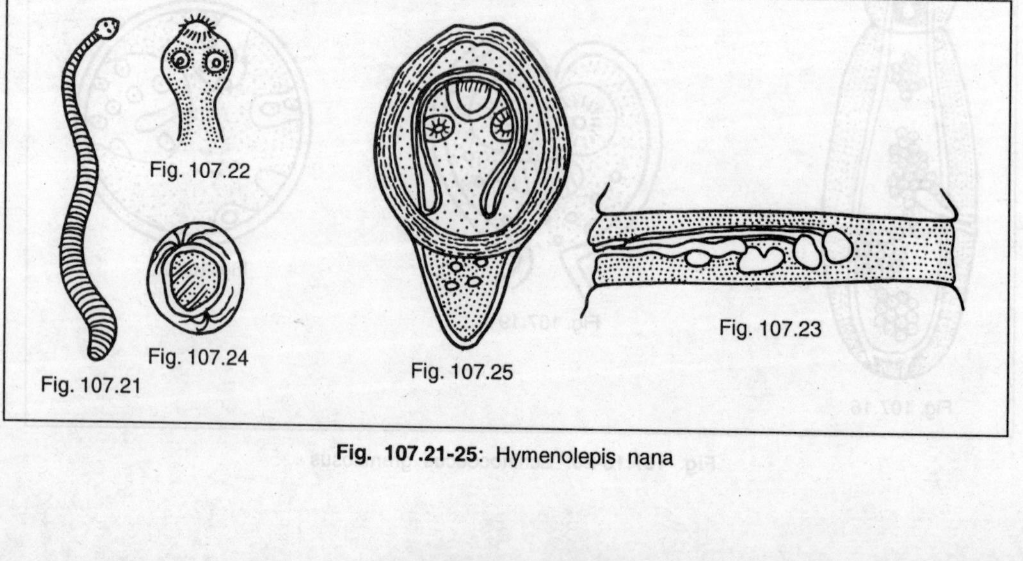

Fig. 107.21-25: Hymenolepis nana

Clinical features : There is generalised toxaemia due to absorption of the metabolic wastes of the parasite. The general symptoms are headache, dizziness, anorexia, pruritus of nose and anus, periodic diarrhoea and abdominal pain.

In the **Laboratory,** the characteristic eggs can be demonstrated microscopically in the patient's stool.

Treatment : Niclosamide, Hexylresorcinal crystalloid. Quinacrine and Mebendazole are very effective.

Prophylaxis : This comprises 1. Avoidance of ingestion of eggs, through contaminated food or drink. Contamination may occur from toilet seats, soiled linen or directly from anus to mouth. 2. Personal hygiene and 3. A well balanced diet which reduces susceptibility to infection.

Dipyllidium caninum

It is common tape worm of dog and cat. The eggs deposited on the ground are ingested by dog fleas. These eggs hatch in the intestine of flea, develop into procercoid and later into cysticercoid larvae. Man or dog gets infected by the ingestion of infected fleas. Clinical manifestations are intestinal disturbances, indigestion, loss of appetite and toxic nervous symptoms. Diagnosis by the demonstration of characteristic eggs in the mother capsule.

Treatment : Quinacrine, Mebendazole and Niclosamide are effective.

Prophylaxis : By avoiding handling of infected dogs and by dusting of dogs with gammexene or DDT.

Demonstration

1. A complete tape worm (**T. saginata**). A large number of proglottids and the globular head can be noted.

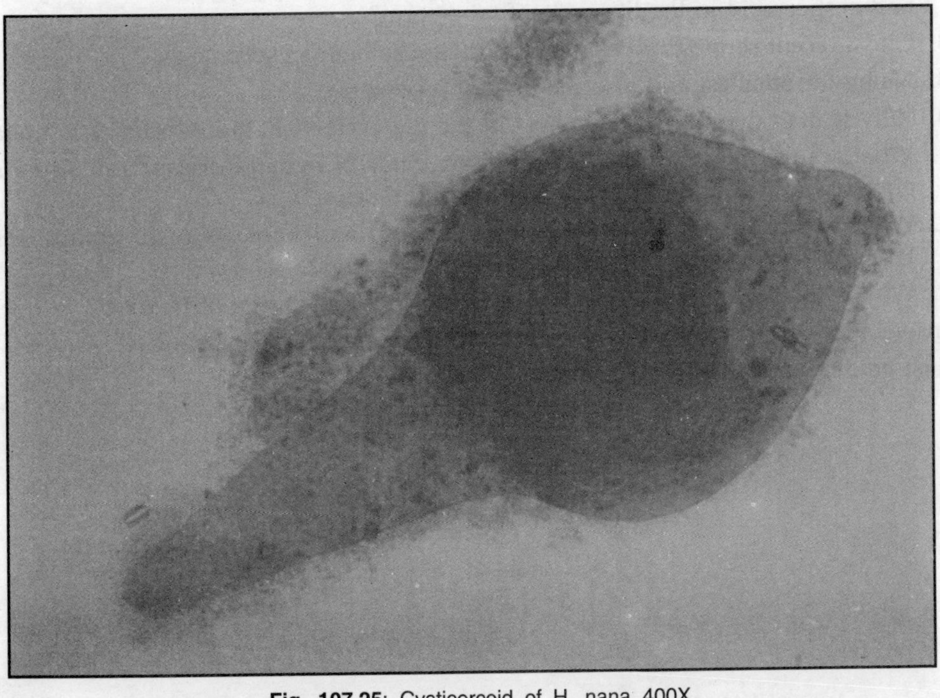

Fig. 107.25: Cysticercoid of H. nana 400X

2. Scolex of **T. saginata** with four suckers.
3. A mature gravid segment of T. saginata is longer than broader with large number of lateral branches (more than 15).
4. Ovum of T. saginata and T. solium is round (31-43μ) thick striated brown embryophore (outside) and oncosphere (inside) with six hooklet (hexacanth embryo). Ova of both species are morphologically similar.
5. Scolex of **T. solium** shows four suckers and rostellum with double row of hooklets.
6. Scolex of **D. latum** has two slit like grooves (suckers).
7. Ovum of **D. latum** is oval and operculated.
8. Ovum of **H. nana.** The space between the egg shell and embryosphere is filled with thread like bipolar filaments.
9. Cysticercoid of **H. nana.**
10. The adult of **E. granulosus** has globular head and only 3 segments. The ovum of **E. granulosus** is similar to that of **T. saginata** and **T. solium.**

Questions

1. Give common and scientific names of all cestodes.
2. How is the word Diphyllobothrium derived?
3. What is coracidium and its importance in the life cycle of **D. latum** and also plerocercoid or sparganum?
4. How is microcytic anemia caused by **D. Latum**?
5. How many hosts are required in the life cycle of **D. latum**?
6. Describe briefly the differences between **T. saginata** and **T. solium.**
7. What are the common names of **C. cellulosae** and **C. bovis** and the role of cysticercus and cysticercoid in the life cycle of tapeworm?
8. Cite a recent serological test used to diagnose neurocysticercosis.
9. Name the smallest and also the longest tapeworm.
10. Why is man the intermediate host in the life cycle of **E. granulosus** as in malaria?
11. What are the latest current diagnostic methods of hydatid disease and also a recent effective anthelmintic drug used in hydatid disease?
12. What is the difference between the rostellum and hooklets of **E. granulosus** and **H. nana** and also the difference between their eggs?
13. Why is the intermediate host not involved in the life cycle of **H. nana**?

Answers to the questions should be entered in the practical notebook.

Must be drawn in the journal practical notebook.

108
Class Trematoda

Fasciolopsis buski (Giant intestinal fluke)

It is an elongated and ovoidal (Fig. 108.1, 2) trematode. The eggs of **F. buski** and **F. hepatica** are large like a hen's egg and are identical (Fig. 108.6).

Life cycle : When immature eggs are discharged in the faeces, they mature in water and hatch out the miracidium (Fig. 108.3) which swims in the water, penetrates into the snail (Fig. 108.4) and develops into sporocysts, first and second generation rediae and cercariae. These cercariae encyst on the seed pods of water caltrop into metacercariae. Man gets infected by swallowing the metacercariae which excyst in the duodenum and ultimately develop into adult worm, which lays eggs in human faeces.

Clinical features : Toxic diarrhoea and hunger pains are the first signs. Heavy infections have symptoms similar to gastric ulcer. Generalised toxic and allergic symptoms appear as oedema of the face, abdominal wall and lower limbs.

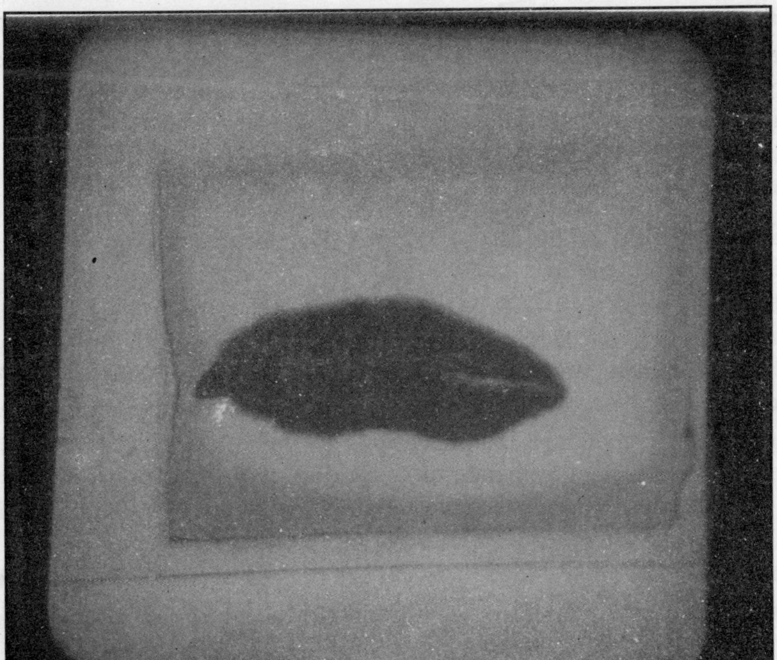

Fig. 108.5: Fasciola hepatica adult

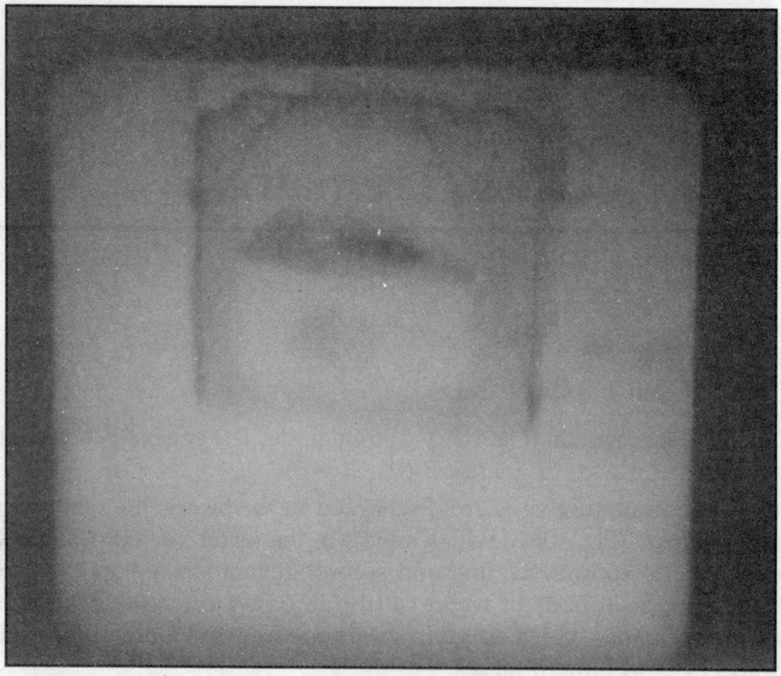

Fig. 108.10: Clonorchis sinensis (dissecting microscope)

Specific **diagnosis** depends upon the recovery of the egg of **F. buski** which is similar to that of **Fasciola hepatica.**

Treatment : Hexylresorcinol crystalloids and tetrachlorethylene are very effective.

Prophylaxis : Destruction of snails by 1 : 50,000 copper sulphate solution, sterilisation of night soil, before it is used as fertiliser and cooking of raw vegetables properly or immersing them in boiling water for few seconds before eating are all effective measures.

Fasciola hepatica (Sheep liver fluke)

It is a fleshy brown fluke (Fig. 108.5). Its eggs (Fig. 108.6) are large, ovoidal, operculated, light yellowish brown in colour.

Life cycle is similar to that of **F. buski,** Cercaria (Fig. 108.7) is also developed but the excysted metacercariae (Fig. 108.8) of **F. hepatica** migrate through the intestinal wall into the peritoneal cavity. From here, they traverse the liver parenchyma to the biliary passages, where they settle down and grow to maturity. Adult worms liberate eggs in the faeces.

Clinical features : The clinical manifestations are hepatic and obstructive jaundice with coughing and vomiting, generalised abdominal rigidity, abdominal pain on pressure, urticaria, irregular fever, persistent diarrhoea, later marked anaemia. Cholelithiasis is a frequent complication.

Laboratory diagnosis is based on the recovery of typical egg of **F. hepatica** in the stool.

Treatment : Emetine hydrochloride, bithionol hexachloroparaxylene, albendazole are effective.

Prophylaxis : (1) eradication of adult worms in reservoir hosts by adequate chemotherapy, (2) destruction of snails by the use of 1 : 50,000 copper sulphate; (4) education of the local population about the danger in eating raw vegetables.

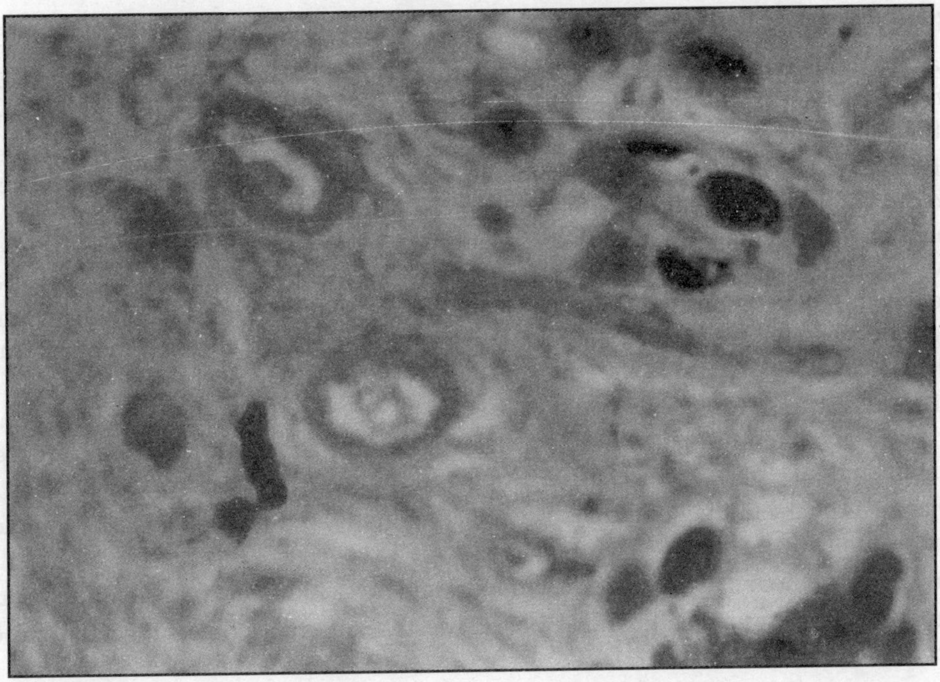

Fig. 108.21: Mature egg of S. haematobium 1000X

Gastrodiscoides hominis

The living worm (Fig. 108.9) is bright pink in colour and pyriform in outline. Its eggs are ovoidal operculate. Its life cycle is unknown. In man, it produces clinically mucous diarrhoea. In the laboratory it can be diagnosed by the demonstration of the typical eggs in the faeces.

Other Trematodes

Clonorchis sinensis (Chinese liver fluke) is flat, transparent, fleshy and spatulate (Fig. 108.10). Its eggs are ovoidal, light yellowish and operculated (Fig. 108.11).

Life cycle : When fully embryonated eggs containing miracidium are ingested by snails, the miracidium hatches out from the egg and transforms ultimately into cercariae (Fig. 108.12) which escape from the snails and swim in the water. On contact with fresh water fish, these cerceriae attach to the fishes and encyst in the skin or in the flesh. Man gets infected by ingestion of infected fish, the metacercariae excyst in the duodenum and enter the common bile duct where they mature and discharge eggs.

Clinical features : There are three stages in the manifestation of symptoms : (1) the mild, symptomless; (2) the progressive stage with irregular appetite, fullness in the abdomen, diarrhoea and hepatomegaly, and (3) the severe stage with portal cirrhosis syndrome. Catarrhal cholangitis occurs due to occlusion of the bile passages of sticky masses of eggs and by tissue proliferation. Symptoms of systemic toxaemia are palpitation of the heart, tachycardia, vertigo, tremor, cramps and mental depression.

Diagnosis can be done by Indirect ELISA; Double sandwich ELISA for mass survey.

Opisthorchis felineus : (Cat liver fluke) is morphologically similar to **C. sinensis** (Fig. 108.13) and also its eggs (Fig. 108.14). Its life cycle is too similar, but the cercariae (Fig. 108.15) attack fish. Clinical features, diagnosis, prophylaxis are similar to those of **C. sinensis,** but there is no specific treatment.

Paragonimus westermani

Paragonimus westermani : (Oriental lung fluke) is a reddish brown, plump, ovoidal fluke with rounded anterior end (Fig. 108.16). The eggs are ovoidal and have a flattened operculum (Fig. 108.17).

Life cycle : Eggs escaping through the bronchioles are coughed up, are swallowed and passed out of faeces. They hatch out miracidia in the water which swim in the water and attack the snails in which redia (Fig. 108.18), cercariae (108.19) produced liberated swim in the water and invade the viscera of cray fish or crab where the metacercariae encyst. Man becomes infected by ingestion of infected crabs. The metacercariae excyst in the duodenum and migrate through the intestinal wall, reach the abdominal cavity and travel through the diaphragm to the pleural cavity and settle in the lungs.

Clinical features : Chest pain, night sweats are common symptoms. Paroxysmal coughing is followed by haemoptysis after physical exertion. The manifestations are severe. Bronchopneumonia, or bronchiectasis with pleural effusion are the physical signs.

Diagnosis by the finding of the characteristic egg in the sputum or faeces. The complement fixation test may be positive.

Treatment : Emetine hydrochloride, bithional and hexachloroparaxylol are found effective.

Prophylaxis : (1) avoid eating raw crabs; (2) destroy the snails; (3) disinfect the sputum or faeces.

Genus schistosoma (Blood fluke)

It comprises – 1. **Schistosoma haematobium** — causing schistosomal haematuria. 2. **S. mansoni**, and 3. **S. japonicum** (intestinal schistosomiasis).

S. haematobium is in the vesical venous plexus. The **male** adult is shorter (10-15 mm × 0.8-1 mm) and stouter, is covered with minute integumentary tuberculations, and has two suckers (Oral sucker Fig. 108.20; ventral sucker is larger, Fig. 108.20a), a **gynaecophoric canal** in which the female is held during copulation (Fig. 108.20b). The female is long (20 × 0.15 mm) and slender (Fig. 108.20c). **Egg** (size 112-170 μ × 40-70 μ) has a distinct terminal spine (Fig. 108.21).

Life cycle requires 2 hosts : (1) man (definite host); 2. fresh water snail (intermediate host). When eggs are discharged in the water during micturition by the infected person; the ciliated larva (**miracidium** first stage larva Fig. 108.27) is hatched out and infects the snail on contact, reaches the liver, develops into sporocyst (second stage larva) and finally into bifid tailed cercaria (Fig. 108.26) which breaks out of the snail. It comes in contact with the human skin, while the man wodes the cercaria infested water, enters the skin, transforms into tailless cercaria (Schistosomule infective form to man) and enters into the circulation in the intra-hepatic portal vessel, there it becomes sexually mature, reenters the blood stream and settles in the vesical venous plexus. The male holds the female within the gynaecophoric canal for mating and the fertilised female lays eggs which work their way through the vessels and mucosa of the urinary bladder and are excreted through urine.

Clinical features : The incubation period is 10-12 weeks. Irritation, minute haemorrhages at the site of entry on the skin followed by anorexia, headache, malaise, pain in the back and limbs, fever, night sweating.

Laboratory diagnosis : (1) Microscopic demonstration of terminal spined eggs in the urine deposit and in biopsied vesical mucosa. Ultrasonography can also be done.

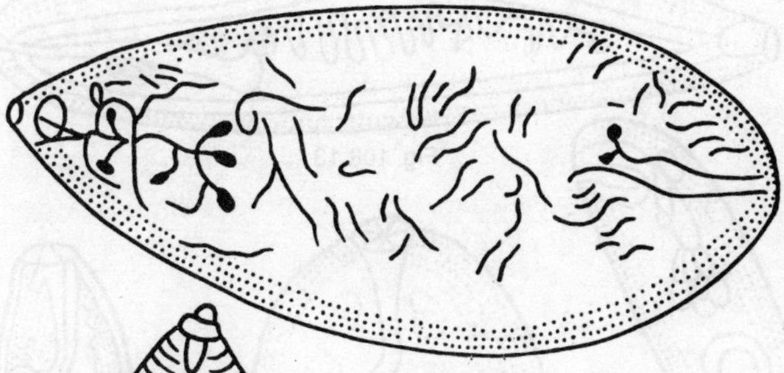

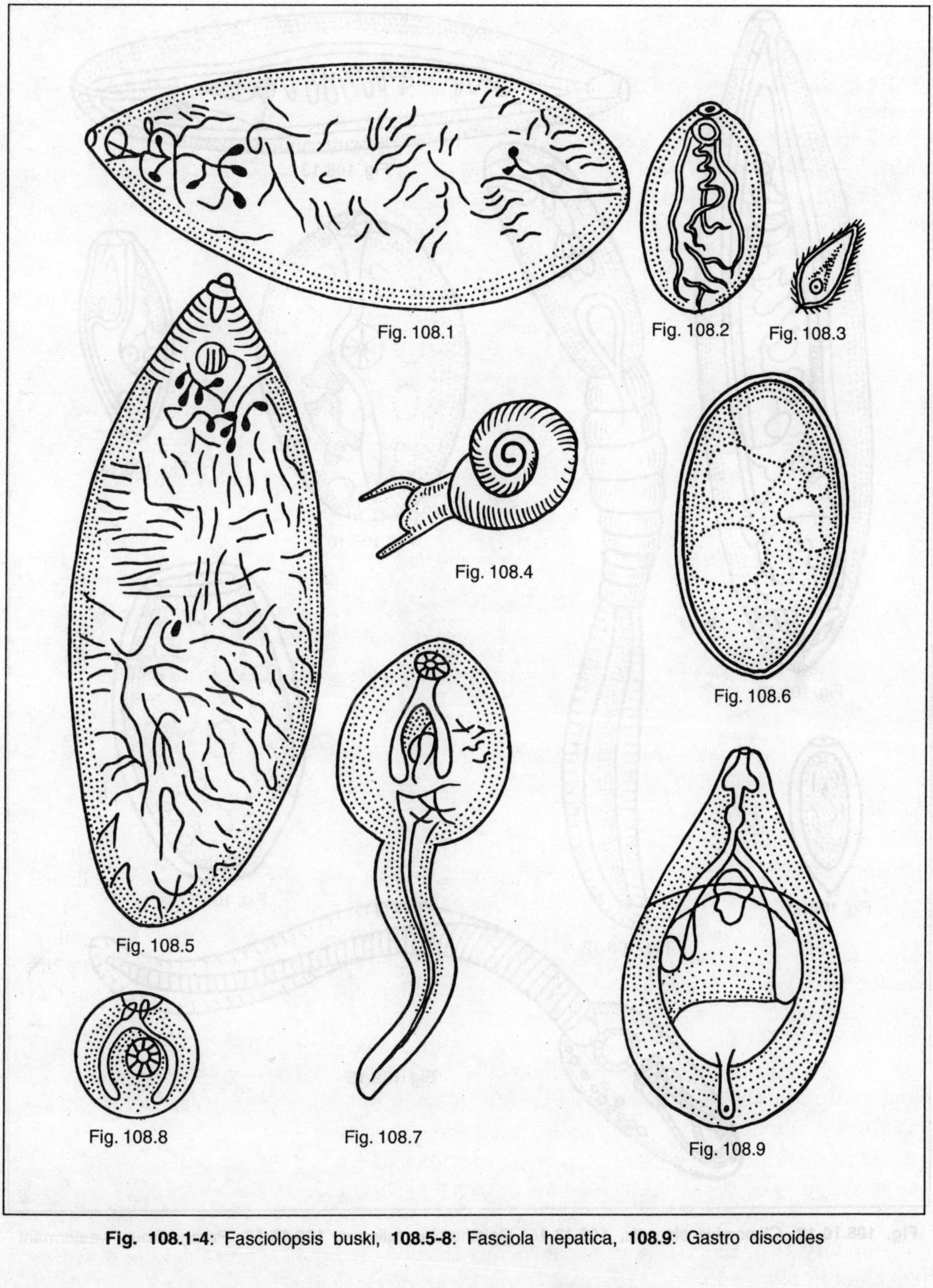

Fig. 108.1

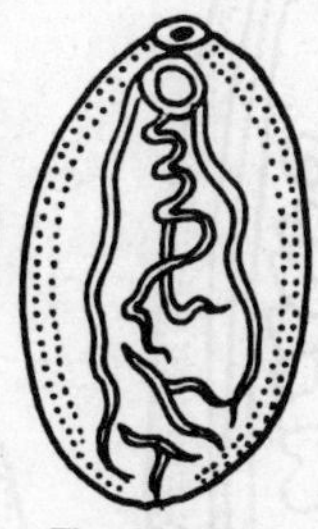

Fig. 108.2

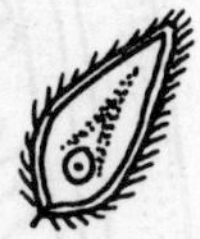

Fig. 108.3

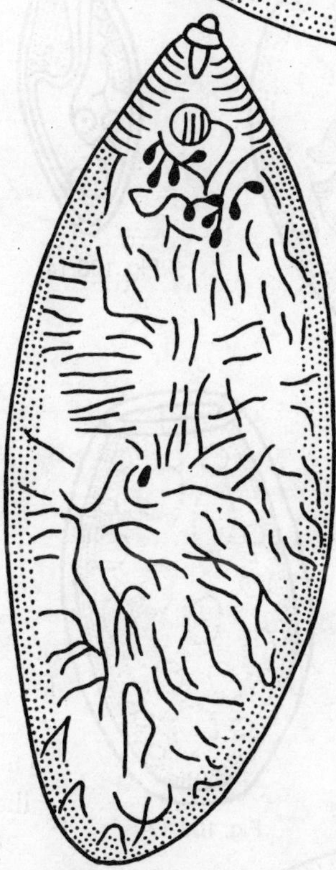

Fig. 108.5

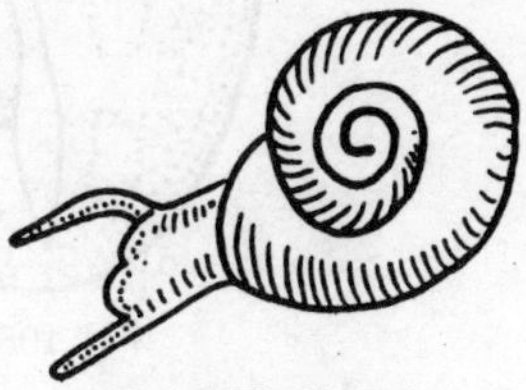

Fig. 108.4

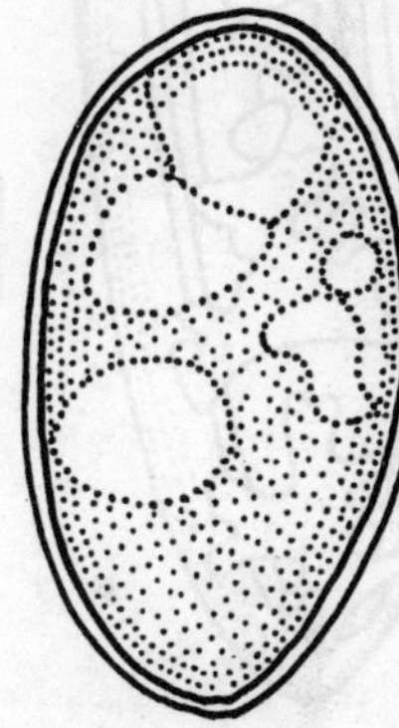

Fig. 108.6

Fig. 108.8

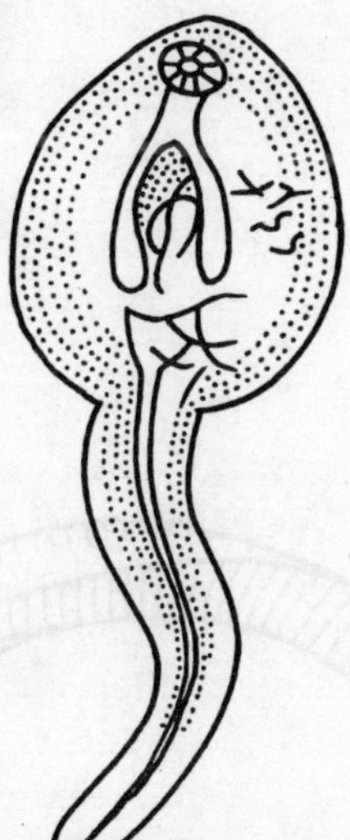

Fig. 108.7

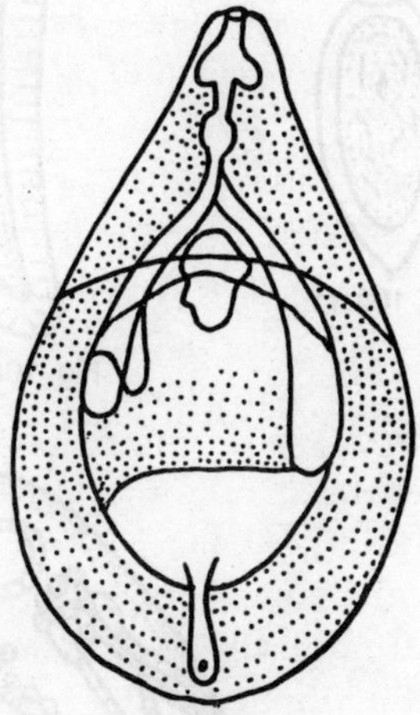

Fig. 108.9

Fig. 108.1-4: Fasciolopsis buski, **108.5-8**: Fasciola hepatica, **108.9**: Gastro discoides

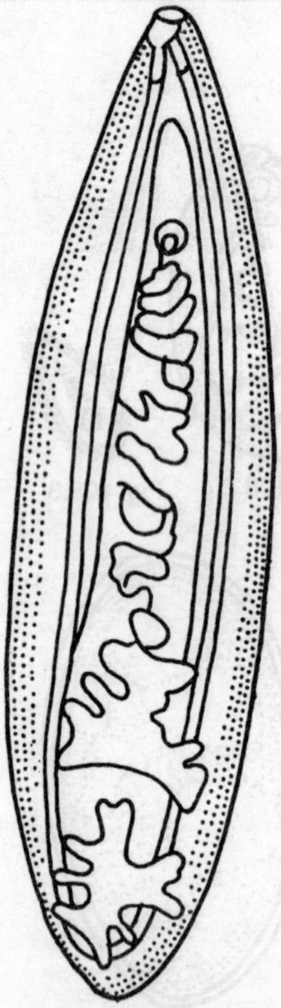

Fig. 108.10

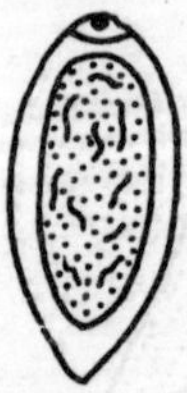

Fig. 108.11

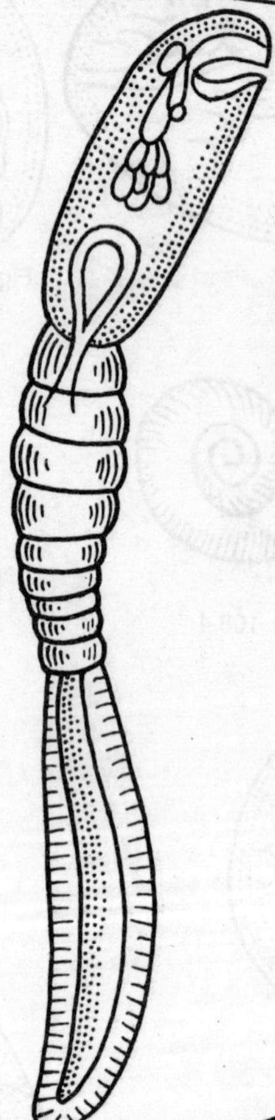

Fig. 108.12

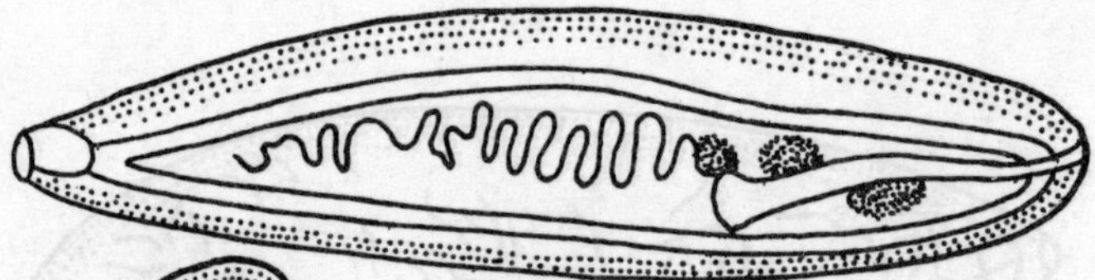

Fig. 108.13

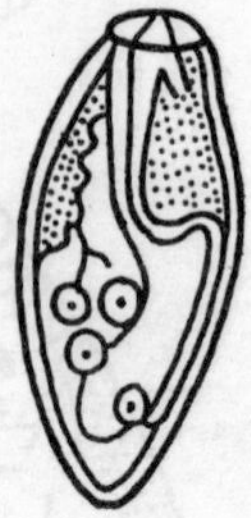

Fig. 108.14

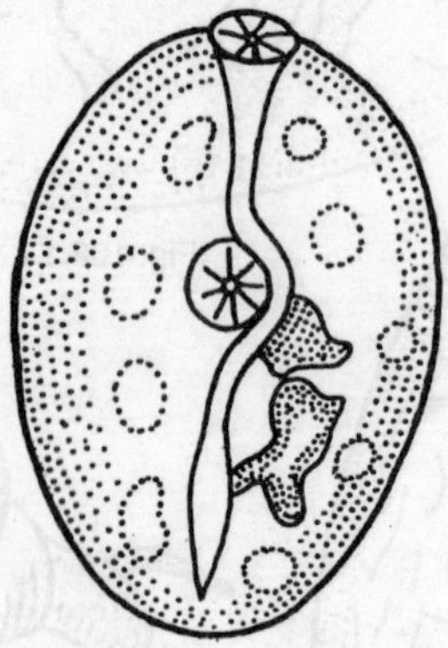

Fig. 108.16

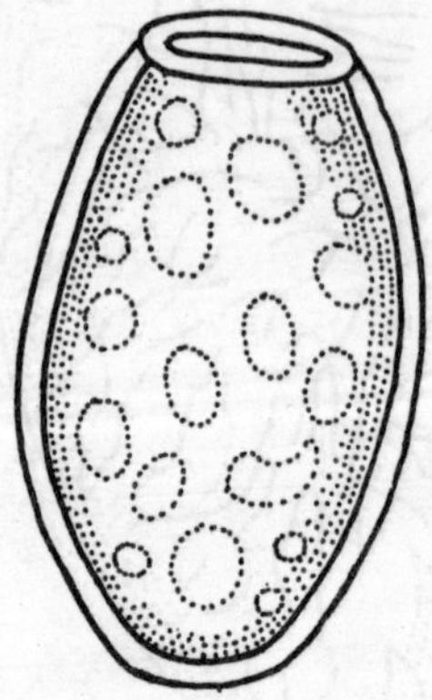

Fig. 108.17

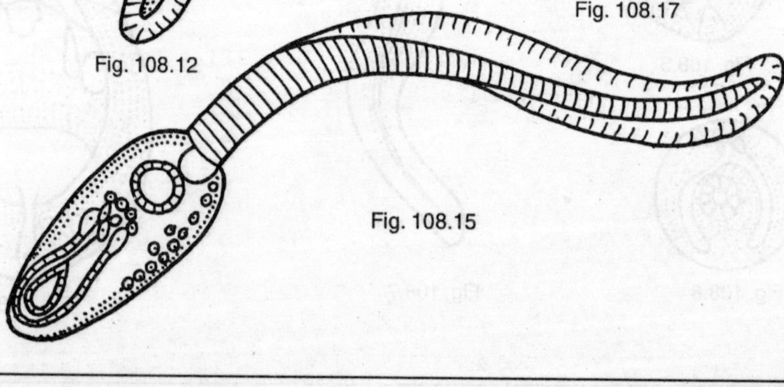

Fig. 108.15

Fig. 108.10-12: Clonorchis sinensis, **108.13-15**: Opisthorchis felineus, **108.16-17**: Paragonimus westermani

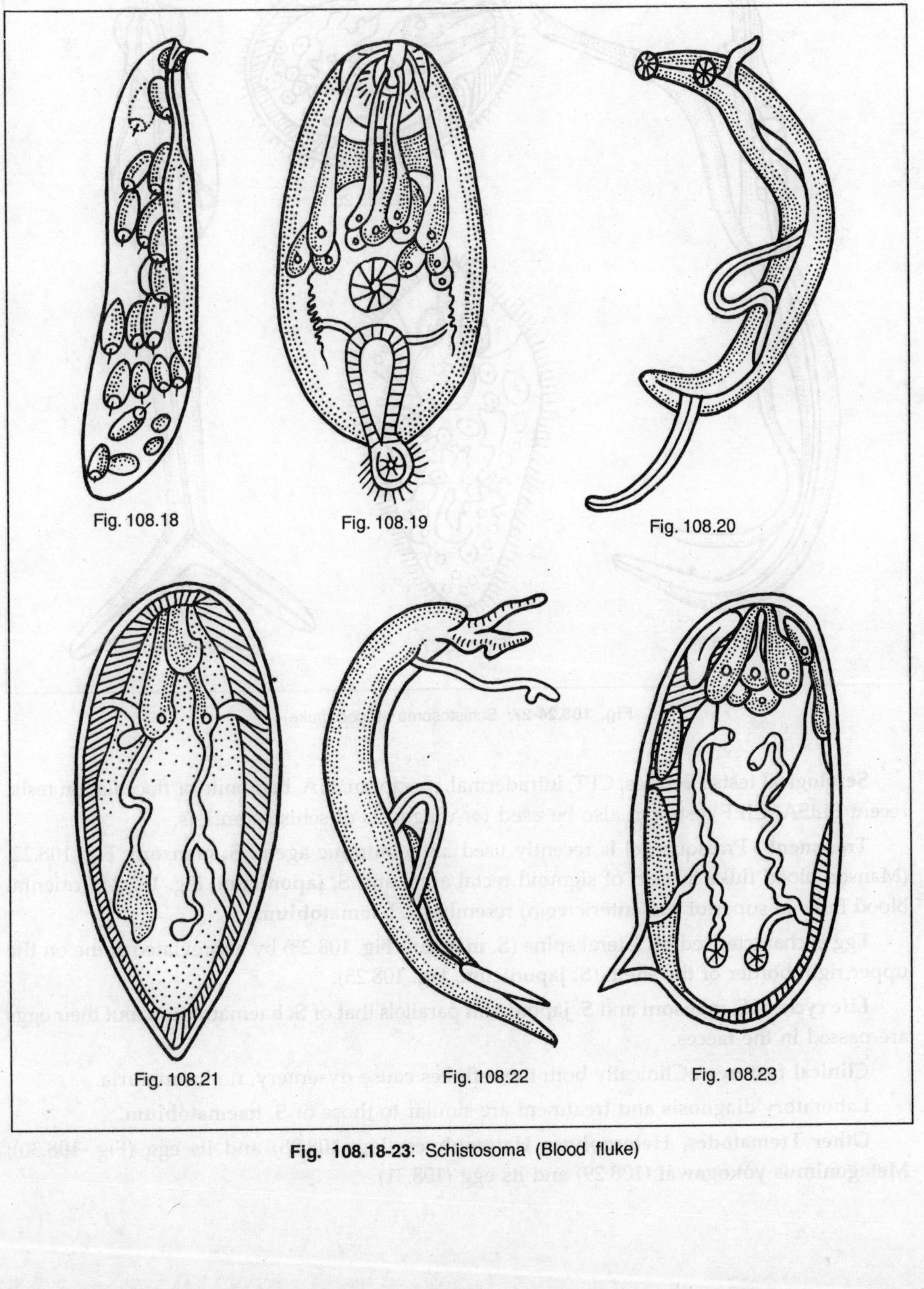

Fig. 108.18-23: Schistosoma (Blood fluke)

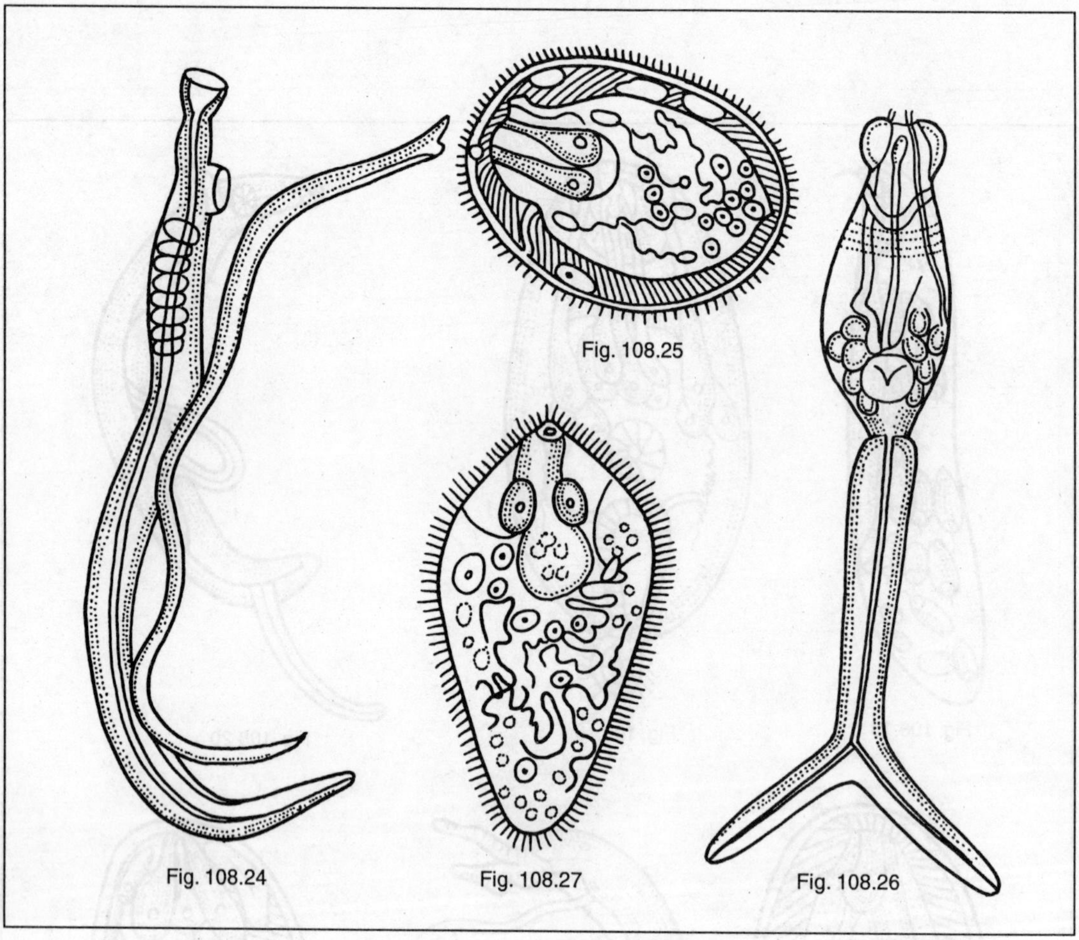

Fig. 108.24-27: Schistosoma (Blood fluke)

Serological tests : Besides, CFT, intradermal, precipitin, HA, bentonite or flocculation tests, recent ELISA, CIEP tests can also be used for diagnosis of schistosomiasis.

Treatment : Praziquantel is recently used anthelminthic agent. **S. mansoni,** Fig. 108.22, (Manson blood fluke in vein of sigmoid rectal area) and **S. japonicum,** Fig. 108.24, (oriental blood fluke in superior mesenteric vein) resemble **S. haematobium.**

Egg is characterised by lateral spine (**S. mansoni** Fig. 108.23) by abbreviated spine on the upper right border of the shell. (**S. japonicum,** Fig. 108.25).

Life cycle of **S. mansoni** and **S. japonicum** parallels that of **S. haematobium,** but their eggs are passed in the faeces.

Clinical features : Clinically both these flukes cause dysentery, no haematuria.

Laboratory diagnosis and treatment are similar to those of **S. haematobium.**

Other Trematodes, Heterophyes Heterophyes (Fig. 108.28) and its egg (Fig. 108.30); **Metagonimus yokogawai** (108.29) and its egg (108.31).

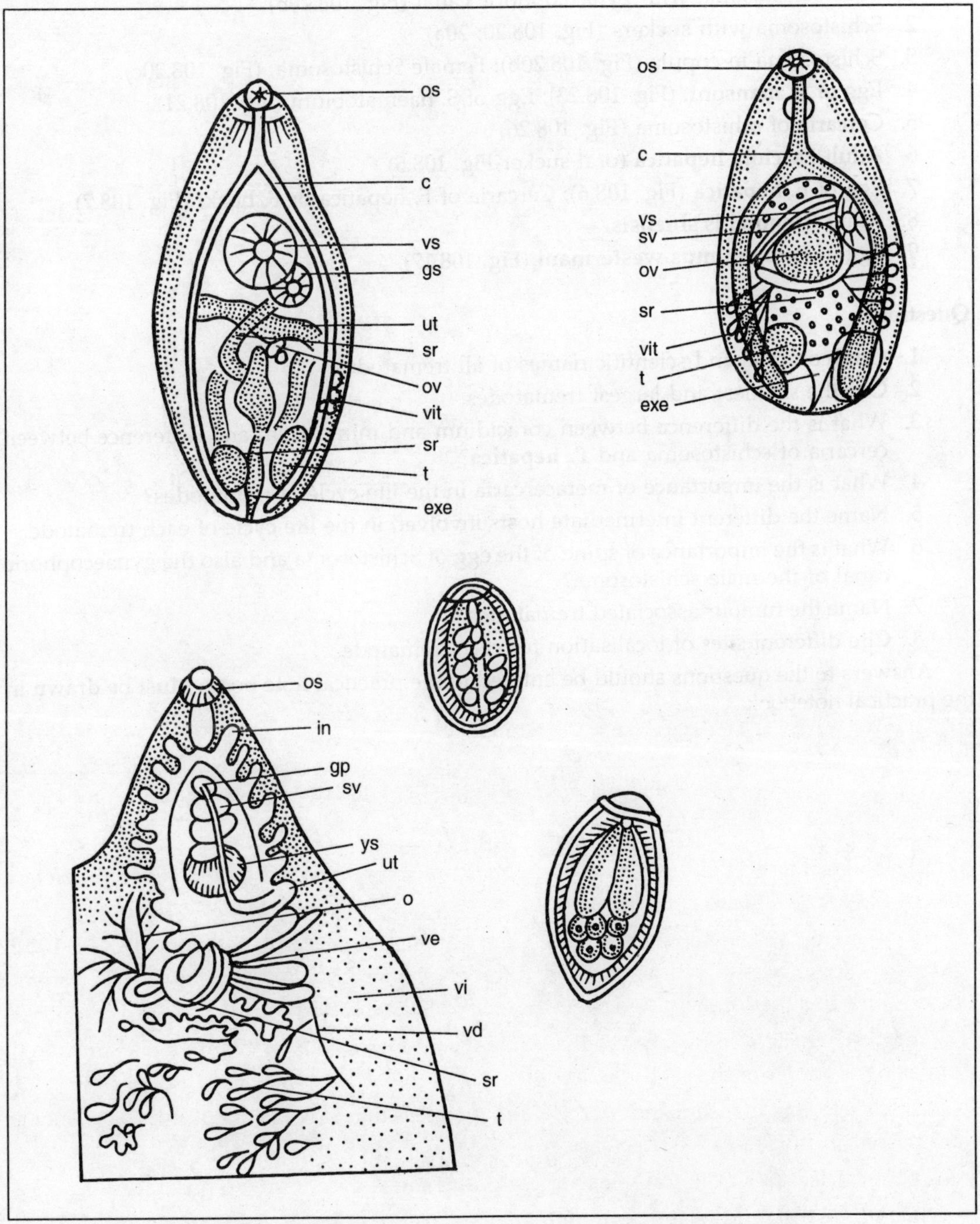

Fig. 108.28,30: Heterophyes **108.29,31**: Metagonimus **108.5**: Fasciola

Demonstration

1. Male schistosoma with gynaecophoric canal (Fig. 108.20b).
2. Schistosoma with suckers (Fig. 108.20; 20a).
3. Schistosoma in copula (Fig. 108.20b); Female Schistosoma; (Fig. 108.20c).
4. Egg of **S. mansoni.** (Fig. 108.23); Egg of S. haematobium (Fig. 108.21).
5. Cercaria of schistosoma (Fig. 108.26)
6. Adult **Fasciola hepatica** (oral sucker-Fig. 108.5)
7. Egg of **F. hepatica** (Fig. 108.6); Cercaria of F. hepatica or F. buski (Fig. 108.7)
8. Adult **Clonorchis sinensis.**
9. Egg of **Paragonimus westermani** (Fig. 108.17).

Questions

1. Give common and scientific names of all trematodes.
2. Cite the smallest and largest trematodes.
3. What is the difference between coracidium and miracidium and difference between cercaria of schistosoma and **F. hepatica**?
4. What is the importance of metacercaria in the life cycle of trematodes?
5. Name the different intermediate hosts involved in the life cycle of each trematode.
6. What is the importance of spine of the egg of Schistosoma and also the gynaecophoric canal of the male schistosoma?
7. Name the tumour associated trematodes.
8. Cite different sites of localisation for each trematode.

Answers to the questions should be entered in the practical note book. Must be drawn in the practical notebook.

109
Class Nematoda
Trichinella Spiralis (Trichina Worm)

It is one of the smallest nematode (1.4-106 mm in length by 40-60 mm in diameter, (Fig. 109.1, 2).

Life cycle : When man consumes raw meat infected (Fig. 109.3) with the cysts (Fig. 109.4) of **T. spiralis,** the cysts are digested out of the meat in the stomach. After excystation, the larvae invade the intestinal mucosa and develop into adults. The males die after fertilising the females which, in turn, discharge larvae (Fig. 109.4). Some of them escape into the lumen of the intestine and the majority enter into the circulation through the mesenteric lymphatics, and settle at last in the striated muscles (Fig. 109.3). Pigs can perpetuate the infection.

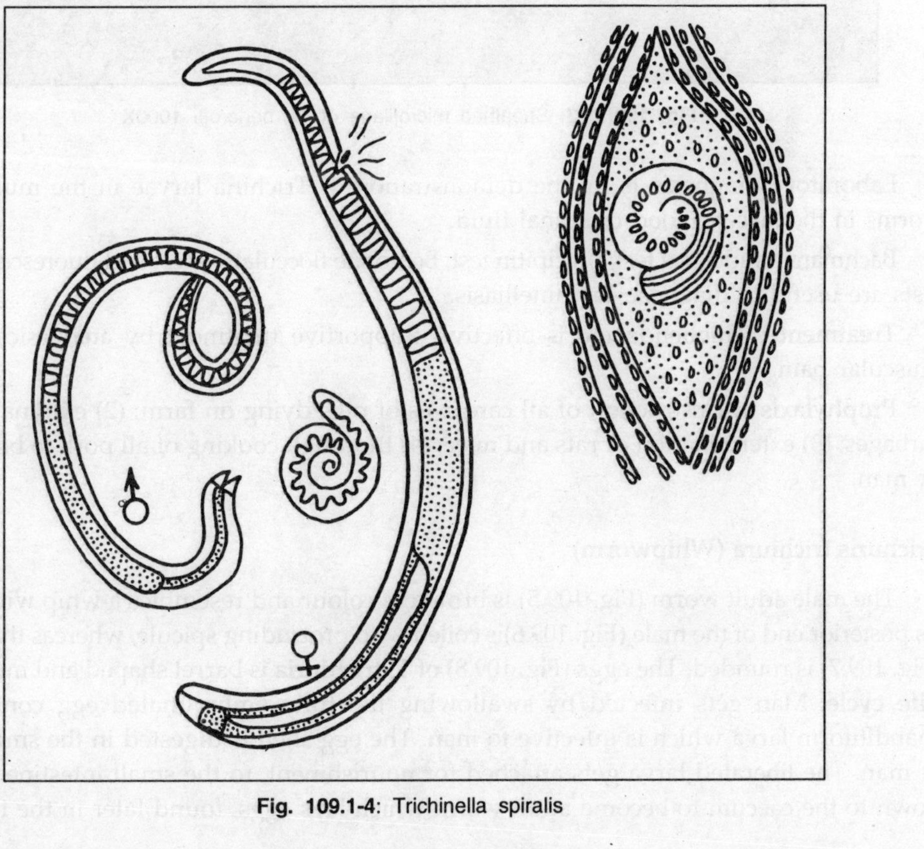

Fig. 109.1-4: Trichinella spiralis

Clinical features : Symptoms of nausea, vomiting, toxic diarrhoea or dysentery, colic, profuse sweating, muscular pain, oedema around eye, nose and limbs, encephalitis, meningitis, deafness may occur.

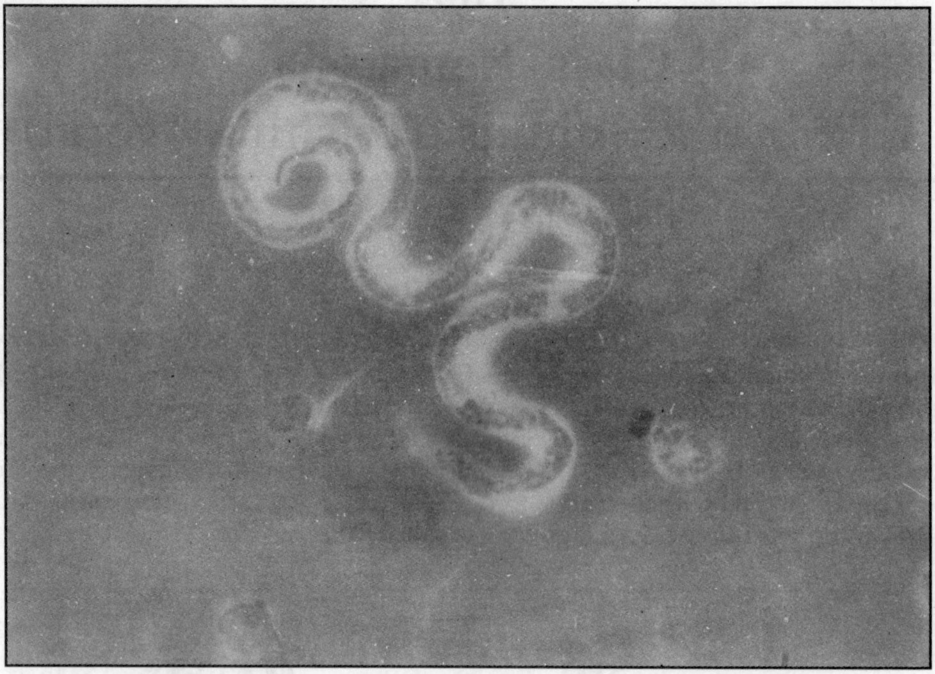

Fig. 109(a) 3: Sheathed microfilaria of W. bancrofti 1000X

Laboratory diagnosis is by the demonstration of Trichina larvae in the muscles, adult worms in the faeces, blood or spinal fluid.

Bachman intradermal test; precipitin test; Bentonite flocculation test and fluorescent antibody tests are useful to diagnose Trichinelliasis.

Treatment : Thiobendazole is effective. Supportive treatment by analgesics to reduce muscular pain.

Prophylaxis 1. Destruction of all carcasses of pigs dying on farm; (2) elimination of raw carbages; (3) extermination of rats and mice; (4) thorough cooking of all pork to be consumed by man.

Trichuris trichiura (Whipworm)

The male adult worm (Fig. 109.5) is brown in colour and resembles a whip with a handle. Its posterior end of the male (Fig. 109.6)is coiled with protruding spicule, whereas that of female (Fig. 109.7) is rounded. The eggs (Fig. 109.8) of **T. trichiuria** is barrel shaped and mucoid plugs **Life cycle.** Man gets infected by swallowing the fully embryonated egg containing the rhabditiform larva which is infective to man. The egg shell is digested in the small intestine of man. The liberated larva gets attached for nourishment, to the small intestine and passes down to the caecum to become adult worm which lays eggs, found later in the faeces.

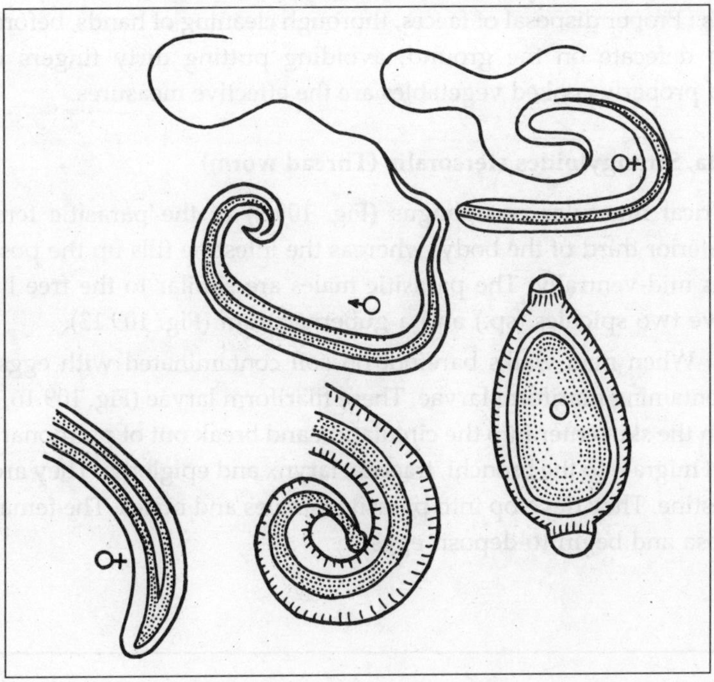

Fig. 109.5-8: Trichuris Trichiura

Clinical features : The common symptoms are abdominal pain, vomiting, constipation, abdominal distension and systemic intoxication. The skin is dry and the patient is emaciated. The clinical picture is similar to that of hook worm disease, apendicitis or dysentery. In the **laboratory,** the characteristic egg of **T. trichuris** can be demonstrated in the patient's stool.

Treatment : Dithiazamine iodide, thiabendazole and mebendazole are effective. Very recent antihelminthic Albendazole (Chewable single dose) is most effective.

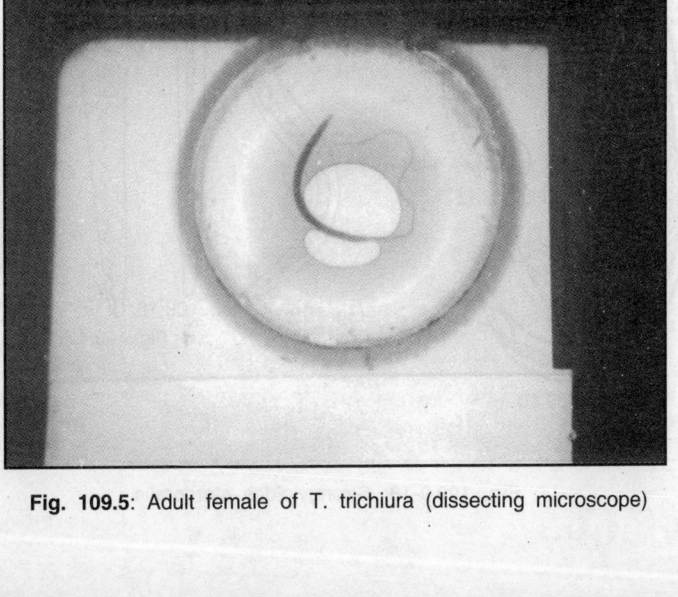

Fig. 109.5: Adult female of T. trichiura (dissecting microscope)

Prophylaxis : Proper disposal of faeces, thorough cleaning of hands, before meals; children not allowed to defecate on the ground, avoiding putting dirty fingers into mouth and consumption of properly cooked vegetables are the effective measures.

Class Nematoda, Strongyloides stercoralis (Thread worm)

The cylindrical muscular oesophagus (Fig. 109.9) of the parasitic female (109.10, 11) occupies the anterior third of the body, whereas the intestine fills up the posterior two-third. The anus opens mid-ventrally. The parasitic males are similar to the free living males (Fig. 109.12) and have two spicules (sp.) and a gubernaculum (Fig. 109.13).

Life cycle : When man walks barefoot on soil contaminated with eggs (Fig. 109.14) of **S. stercoralis** containing filariform larvae. These filariform larvae (Fig. 109.16, 17, 18) penetrate directly through the skin enter into the circulation and break out of pulmonary capillaries into the alveoli, then migrate to the bronchi, trachea, larynx and epiglottis. They are swallowed and reenter the intestine. They develop into parasite females and males. The females penetrate the intestinal mucosa and begin to deposit eggs.

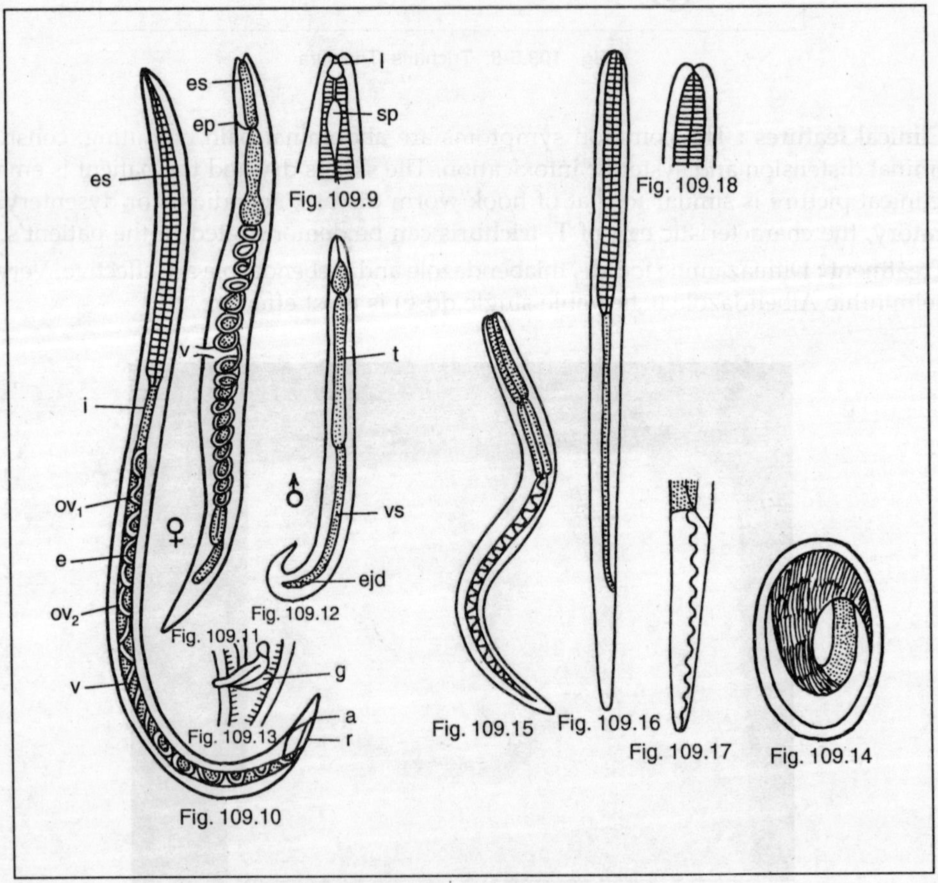

Fig. 109.9-18: Strongyloides stercoralis

Clinical features : There will be petechial haemorrhage at the site of entry of larvae followed by intense pruritus, congestion, oedema and urticarial rash. There will be broncho-pneumonia with consolidation of the lobules. Frequent coughing, pleural effusion and pyothorax are the symptoms.

Three types of enteritis may occur : (a) Catarrhal enteritis; (b) Oedematous enteritis; and (c) Ulcerative enteritis. There is accompanying diarrhoea with mucus and blood which may be very painful.

Laboratory diagnosis is by the recovery of active rhabditiform larva (Fig. 109.15) from the stool, sputum, duodenal washing. Serology is not quite satisfactory. Direct smear (cheapest), modified Baermann techniques agar plate culture (costly) method can be used.

Treatment : Thiabendazole, mebendazole and the current albendazole are drugs of choice.

Prophylaxis (1) The human body must be protected from infective soil and from contaminated faeces; (2) Constipation should be avoided by use of cathartics; (3) Careful cleaning of hands.

ANKYLOSTOMA DUODENALE (Old World hookworm), Necator Americans (New World hookworm, Table 109.1).

TABLE 109.1 : DIFFERENTIAL FEATURES

	A. duodenale	N. americanus
Size	Adult worm, larger and thicker (Fig. 109.19, 20)	Adult worm, smaller and more slender (Fig. 109.21, 22)
Anterior end	Bends in the same direction as the body	Bends in the opposite direction of the body
Buccal capsule	Six teeth, four hook like on the ventral surface and two knob like on the dorsal surface (Fig. 109.25)	Four chitinous plates, two on the ventral surface and two on the dorsal surface (Fig. 109.26)
Copulatory bursa	Dorsal ray is single, total number of rays-13 (Fig. 109.27)	Dorsal ray is split from the base. Total number of rays 14 (Fig. 109.28)
Posterior end of female	A spine is present	A spine is absent
Vulval opening	Behind the middle of the body	In front of the middle, of the body
Pathogenicity	More pathogenic	Less pathogenic

Life cycle : Eggs with four blastomeres (Fig. 109.29) in faeces hatch out rhabditiform larva (Fig. 109.23) in soil which develops later into filariform larva (Fig. 109.23, 24), infective to man, enters the skin, blood circulation, breaks out from the pulmonary capillaries, migrate to epiglottis, oesophagus, intestine where they grow into adult worm which lays eggs.

Clinical features : In the moderate type, the symptoms are heart burn, flatulence, fullness of the abdomen, and epigastric pain. These are relieved by eating clay, mud or earth (which is known as pica or geophagy). There may be low grade, intermittent fever, lassitude, dyspnoea and palpitation of the heart.

In the severe type, there is constipation or diarrhoea. The skin is dry, harsh and pale yellow. Pot belly is a typical physical sign in children. Finally, there is physical exhaustion, cardiac failure and anasarca.

Laboratory diagnosis : Direct demonstration of characteristic egg in the stool; indirectly, blood examination will reveal the nature of anaemia.

Treatment : Supportive treatment for anaemia. Specific treatment by thiobendazole, mebendazole and current albendazole is very effective.

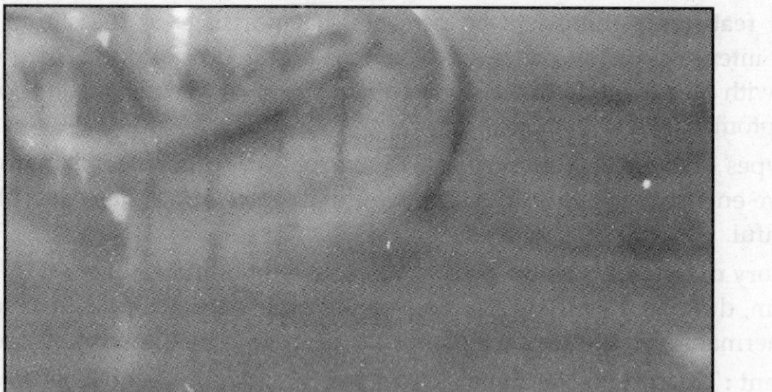

Fig. 109.18: Female adult worm of A. lumbricoides–natural close view

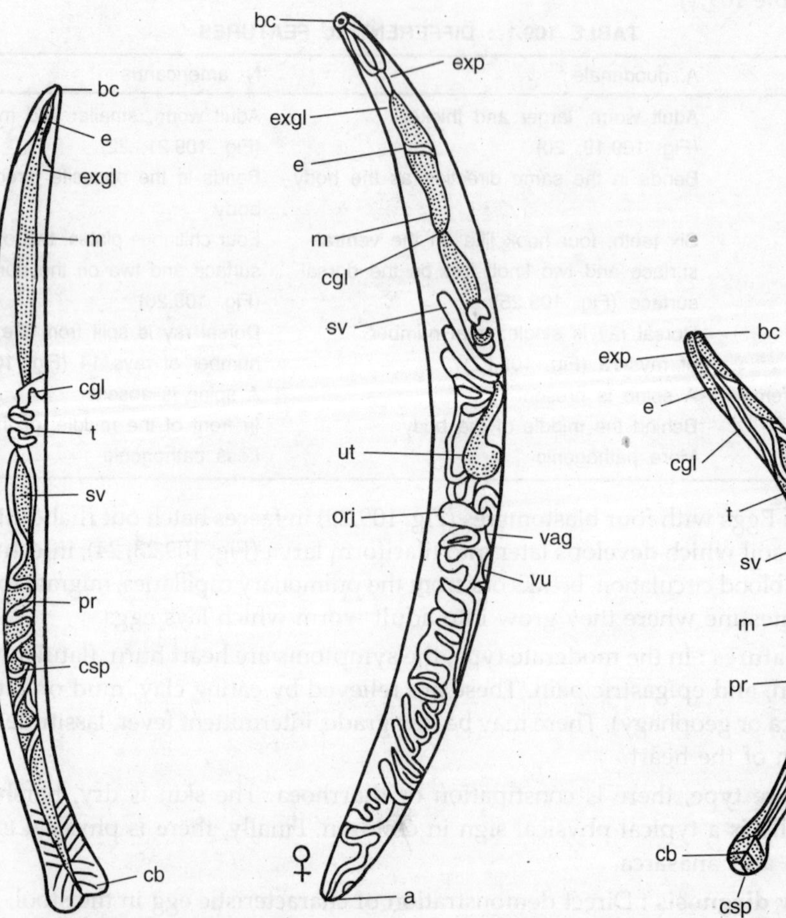

Fig. 109.19 Fig. 109.20 Fig. 109.21

Fig. 109.19-21: Ascaris lumbricoides

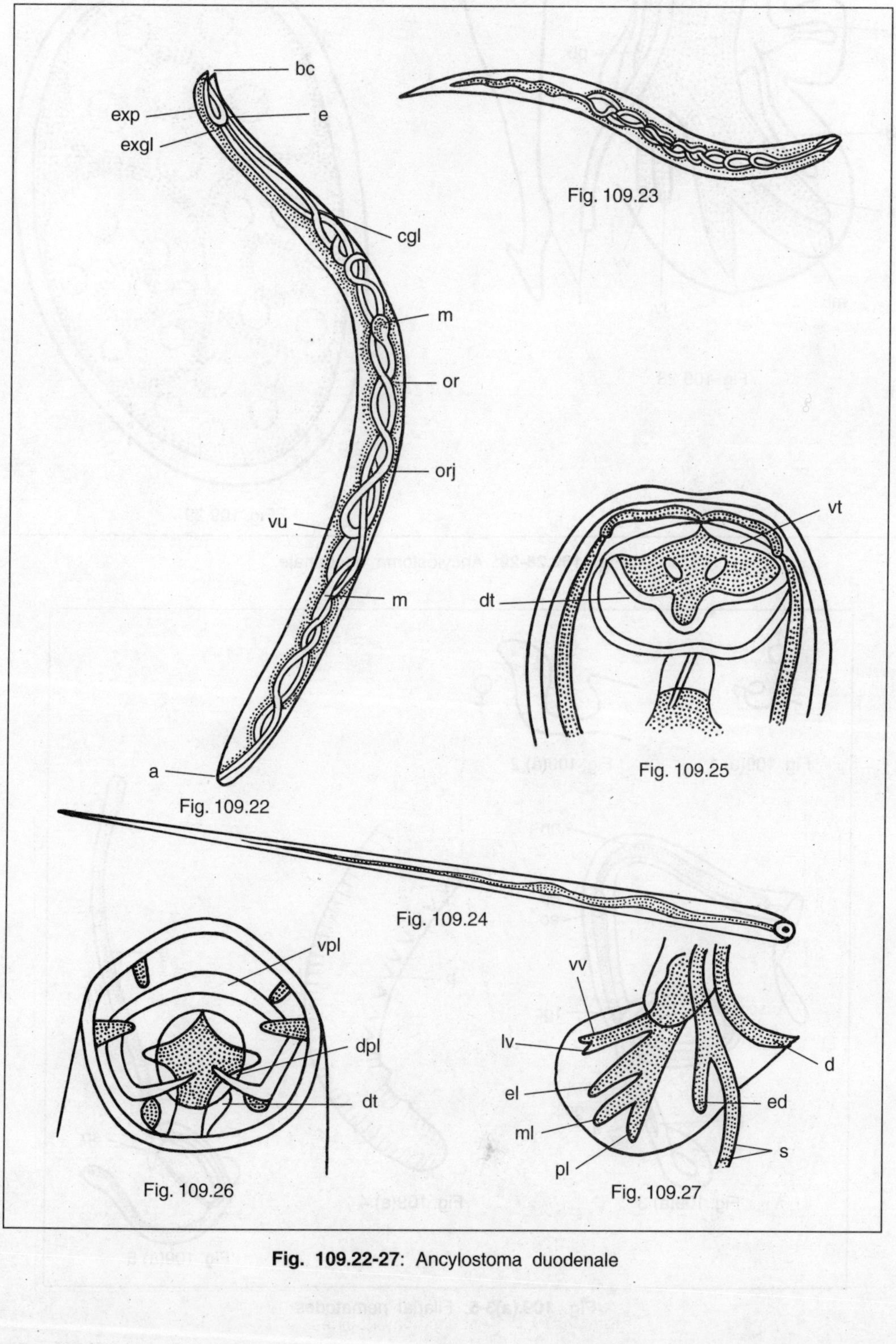

Fig. 109.22-27: Ancylostoma duodenale

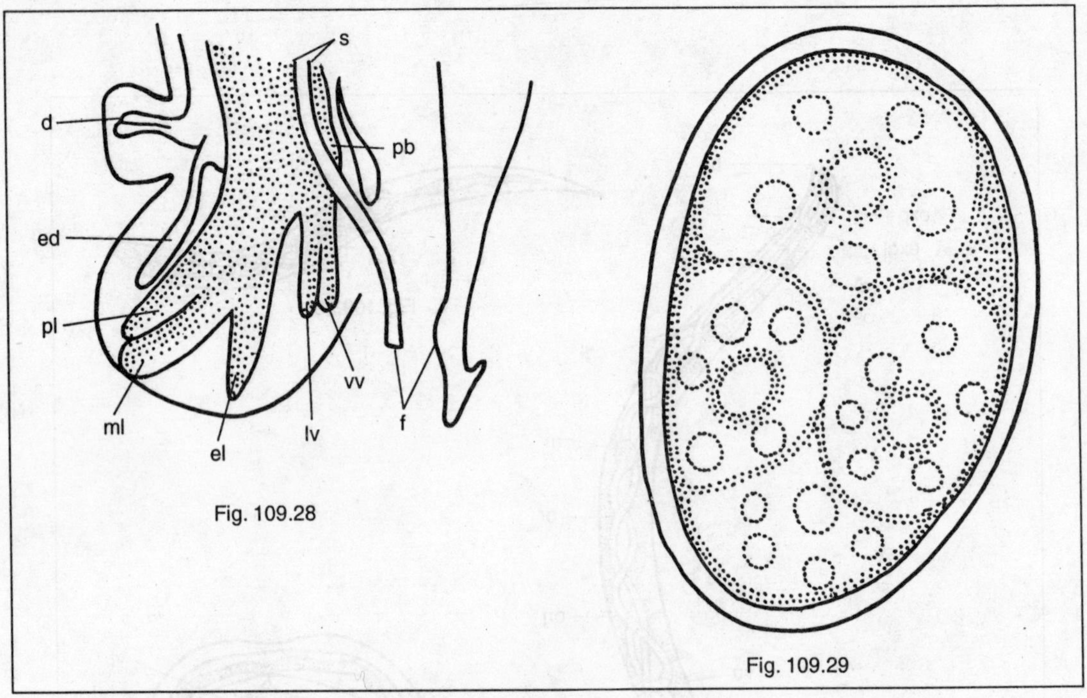

Fig. 109.28-29: Ancylostoma duodenale

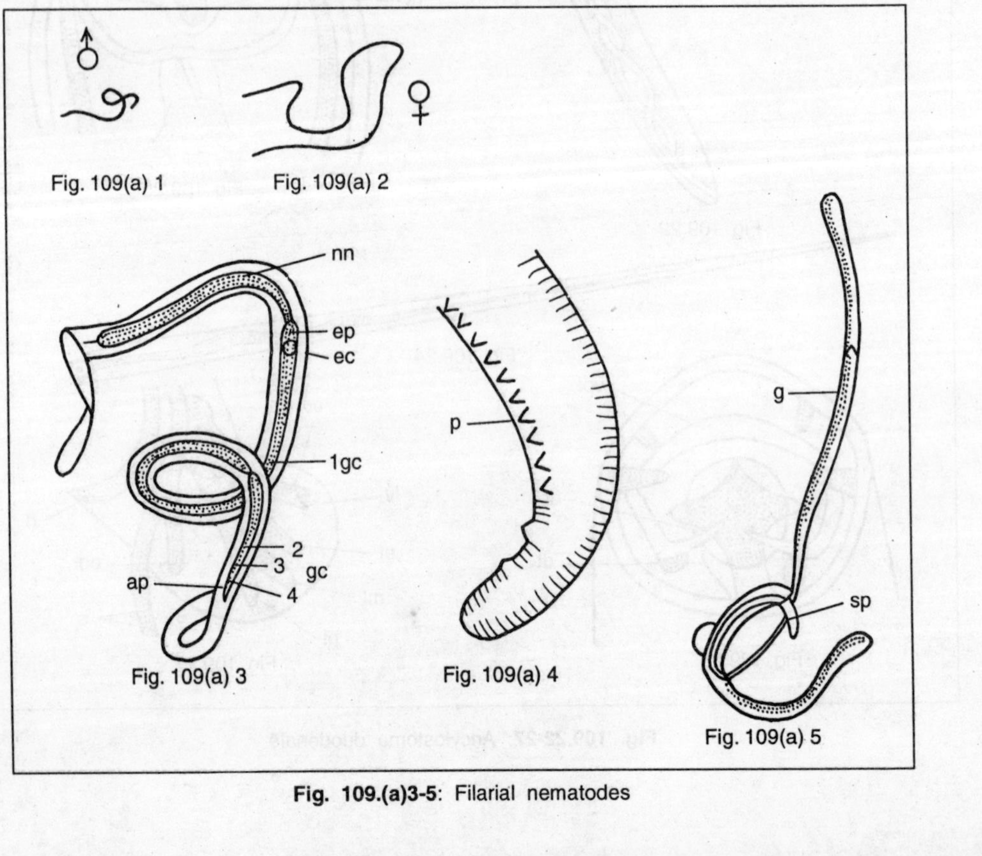

Fig. 109.(a)3-5: Filarial nematodes

Prophylaxis : Personal protection by wearing gloves and boots; disinfection of faeces or soil and prevention of soil pollution; treatment of carrier and whole community is effective prophylaxis.

Enterobius vermicularis (Pin worm or seat worm)

The adult worm (Fig. 109.30, 31) is small, white, and similar to a small piece of thread. Posterior end of male has spicules, papillae, (Fig. 109.32, 33). Anterior end has cervical alae (Fig. 109.34).

Life cycle : When the fully embryonated eggs (Fig. 109.35) infective to man, are ingested by man, they hatch out the larvae in the intestine which grow into adult worms which crawl out of the anus during the night and deposit eggs on the perianal skin. The mode of transmission is by anus to mouth (auto-infection).

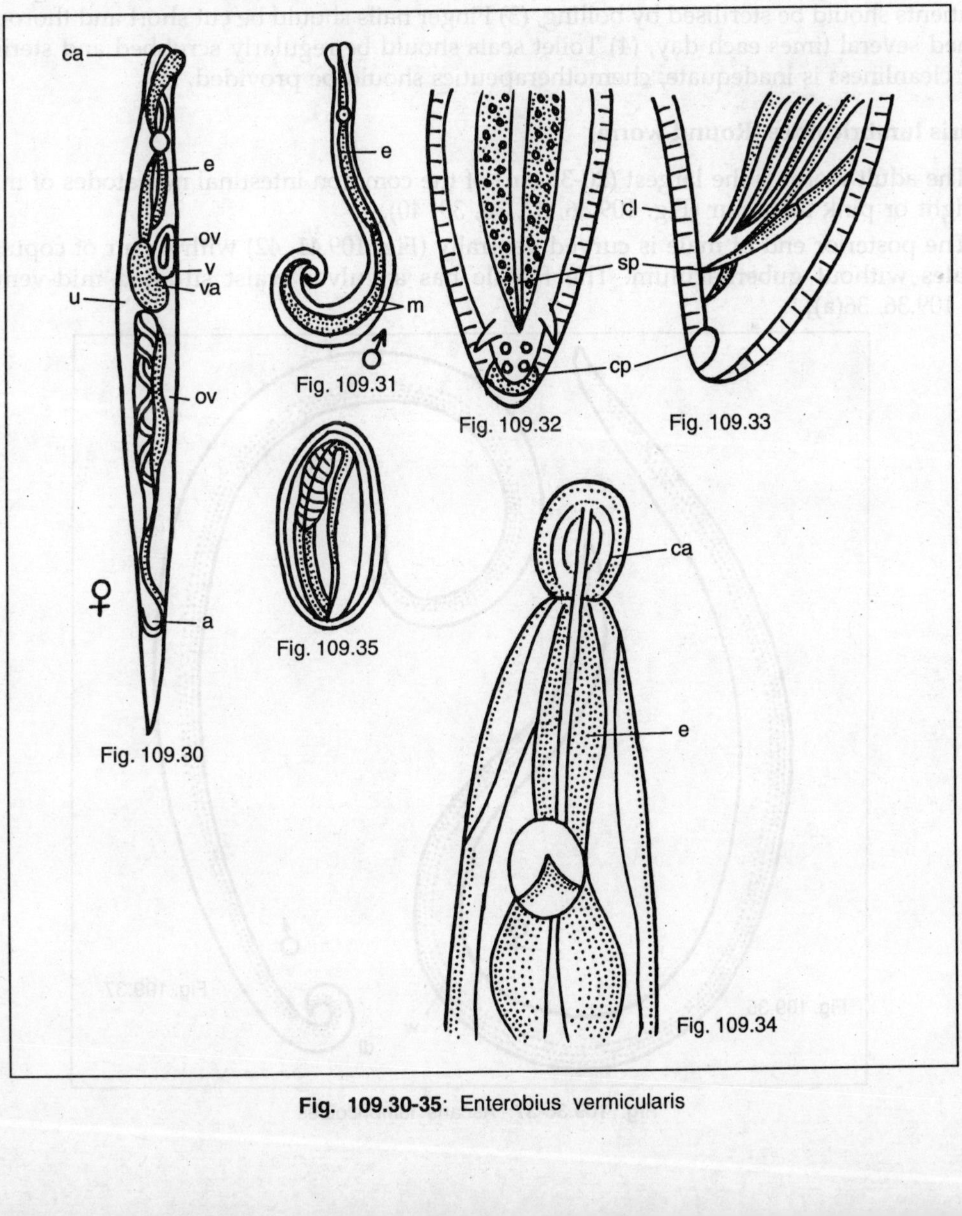

Fig. 109.30-35: Enterobius vermicularis

Clinical features : Absorbed metabolites may cause a characteristic helminthic toxaemia. Gravid females, migrating out of the anus, may oviposit on the peri-anal and perineal skin of the anus and cause severe pruritus with severe scratching which is characteristic of this infection. Sometimes, it may enter the female genital tract causing salpingitis and at last encyst in the peritoneal cavities. There may be urethritis, nocturnal enuresis (frequency of micturition) and masturbation. Loss of appetite, loss of weight, nervousness, insomnia, nightmare, nail biting, nose picking and grinding of teeth at night.

Laboratory diagnosis can be performed by (1) the identification of the recovered adult worm; and (2) the microscopic demonstration of the characteristic egg. Copulatory spicules at posterior end of male (Fig. 109.32, 33), double bulb oesophagus (Fig. 109.34) at anterior end of the adult worm.

Treatment : Piperazine adipate, thiobendazole, mebendazole and albendazole are effective anthelmintic drugs.

Prophylaxis : (1) Personal hygiene should be strictly observed, (2) The clothes and garments of patients should be sterilised by boiling, (3) Finger nails should be cut short and thoroughly cleaned several times each day, (4) Toilet seats should be regularly scrubbed and sterilised, (5) If cleanliness is inadequate, chemotherapeutics should be provided.

Ascaris lumbricoides (Round worm)

The adult worm is the largest (20-35 cm) of the common intestinal nematodes of man. It is bright or pink in colour (Fig. 109.36, 37, 38, 39, 40).

The posterior end of male is curved ventrally (Fig. 109.41, 42) with a pair of copulatory spicules without gubernaculum. The female has a vulvar waist situated mid-ventrally [Fig. 109.36, 36(a)].

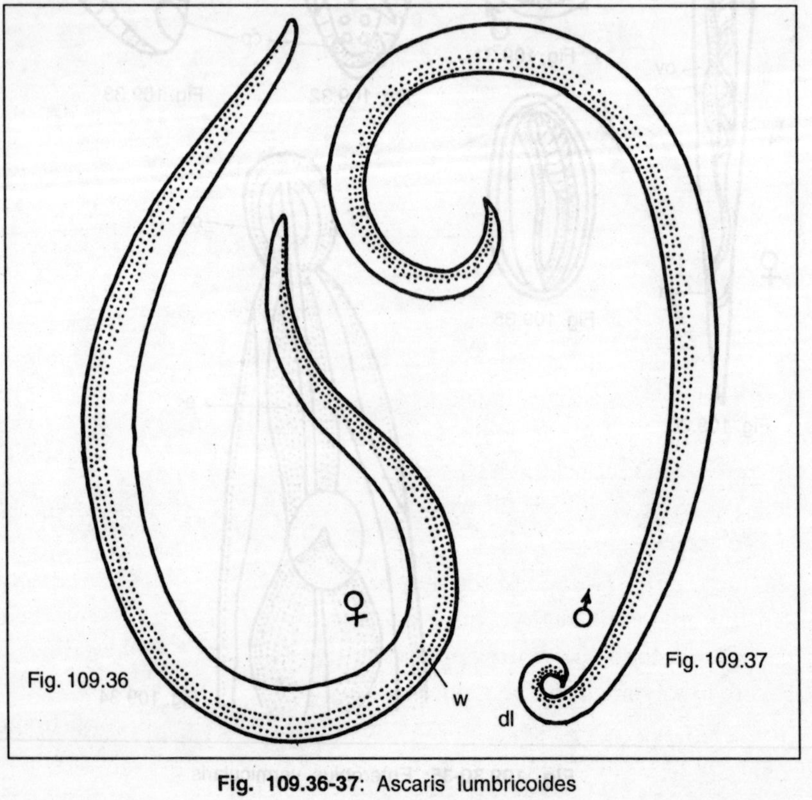

Fig. 109.36-37: Ascaris lumbricoides

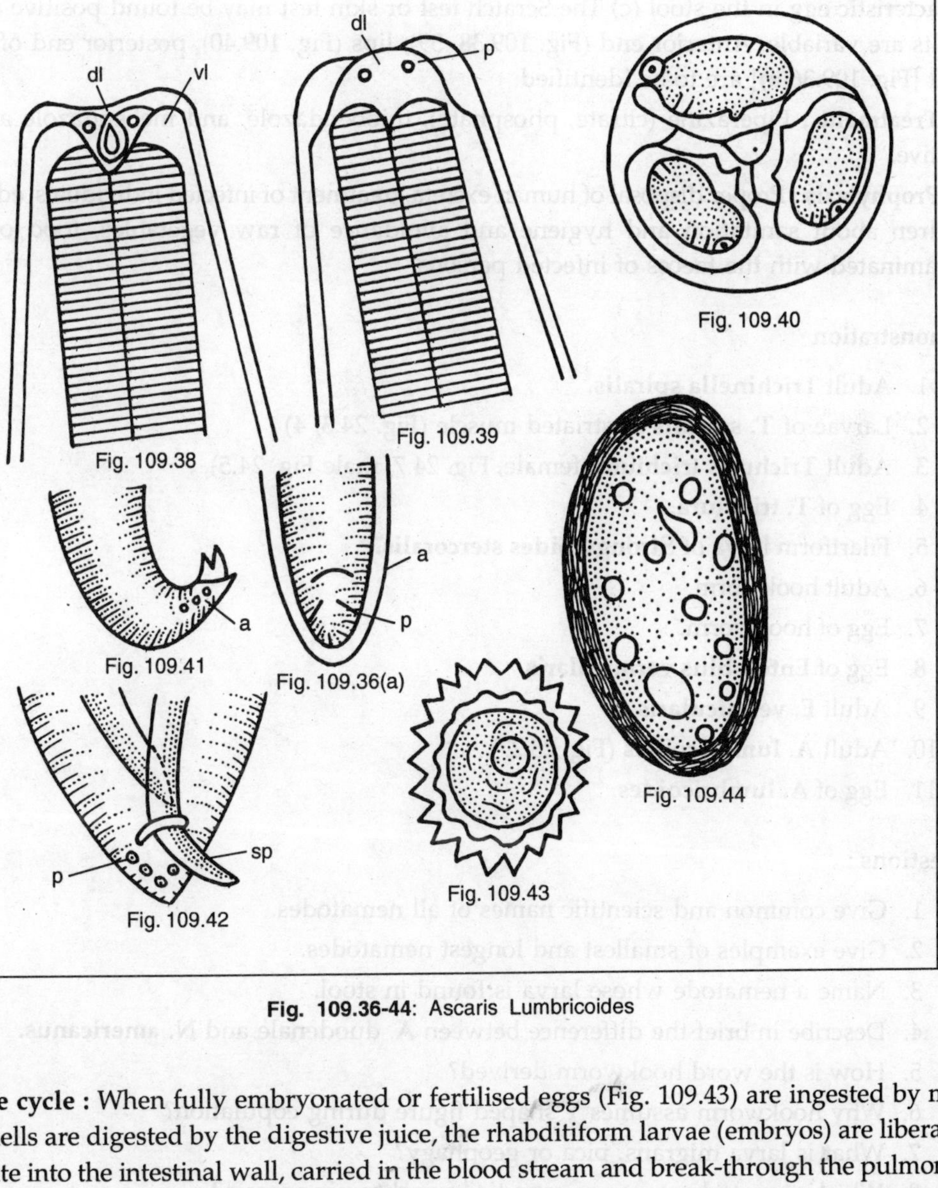

Fig. 109.38 Fig. 109.39 Fig. 109.40 Fig. 109.41 Fig. 109.36(a) Fig. 109.42 Fig. 109.43 Fig. 109.44

Fig. 109.36-44: Ascaris Lumbricoides

Life cycle : When fully embryonated or fertilised eggs (Fig. 109.43) are ingested by man, their shells are digested by the digestive juice, the rhabditiform larvae (embryos) are liberated, penetrate into the intestinal wall, carried in the blood stream and break-through the pulmonary capillaries into the alveoli. These larvae crawl up the bronchioles, epiglottis and are swallowed. In the intestine, they develop into adult worms, the female is fertilised and lays both fertilised and unfertilised eggs (Fig. 109.43, 44).

Clinical features : The most common symptoms are vague abdominal discomfort, acute colicky pain in the epigastric region, poor digestion, diarrhoea and fever. The wandering worms may cause symptoms like acute appendicitis, gastric or duodenal trauma, oesophageal perforation, severe involvement of the genito-urinary tract of males and females; and invasion of the heart. Moreover, the larvae which migrate through the capillaries of the brain and eyeball may produce symptoms of meningitis, epilepsy, retinitis and palpebral oedema.

Laboratory diagnosis : (a) Detection of adult worm in stool or vomit; (b) Demonstration of characteristic egg in the stool (c) The Scratch test or skin test may be found positive and the results are variable. Anterior end (Fig. 109.38, 39); lips (Fig. 109.40), posterior end of female adult [Fig. 109.36(a)] are to be identified.

Treatment : Piperazine (citrate, phosphate), thiobendazole, and mebendazole are very effective.

Prophylaxis : Proper disposal of human excreta, treatment of infected individuals, educating children about sanitation and hygiene and avoidance of raw vegetables, food or drink contaminated with the faeces of infected persons.

Demonstration

1. Adult **Trichinella spiralis.**
2. Larvae of **T. spiralis** in striated muscle (Fig. 24.3, 4)
3. Adult **Trichuris trichiura** (female, Fig. 24.7; male Fig. 24.5).
4. Egg of **T. trichiura.**
5. Filariform larva of **Strongyloides stercoralis.**
6. Adult hookworm.
7. Egg of hookworm.
8. Egg of **Enterobius vermicularis.**
9. Adult **E. vermicularis**
10. Adult **A. lumbricoides** (Fig. 25.27)
11. Egg of **A. lumbricoides.**

Questions :

1. Give common and scientific names of all nematodes.
2. Give examples of smallest and longest nematodes.
3. Name a nematode whose larva is found in stool.
4. Describe in brief the difference between A. duodenale and **N. americanus.**
5. How is the word hookworm derived?
6. Why hookworm assumes Y shaped figure during copulation?
7. What is larva migrans, pica or geophagy?
8. Which nematode causes microcytic hypochromic anemia?
9. Cite a current anthelminthic drug effective against all trematodes.
10. Why **E. vermicularis** migrates out of anus during night?
11. Why NIH swab is desirable for stool collection from anal region?
12. What are the clinical features in children infected with **E. vermicularis**?
13. What is the importance of vulvar waist in **A. lumbricoides** and also its ascarase?
14. Why is the intermediate host not required in the life cycle of **A. lumbricoides**?
15. Why is filariform larva of **S. stercoralis** found in the stool?

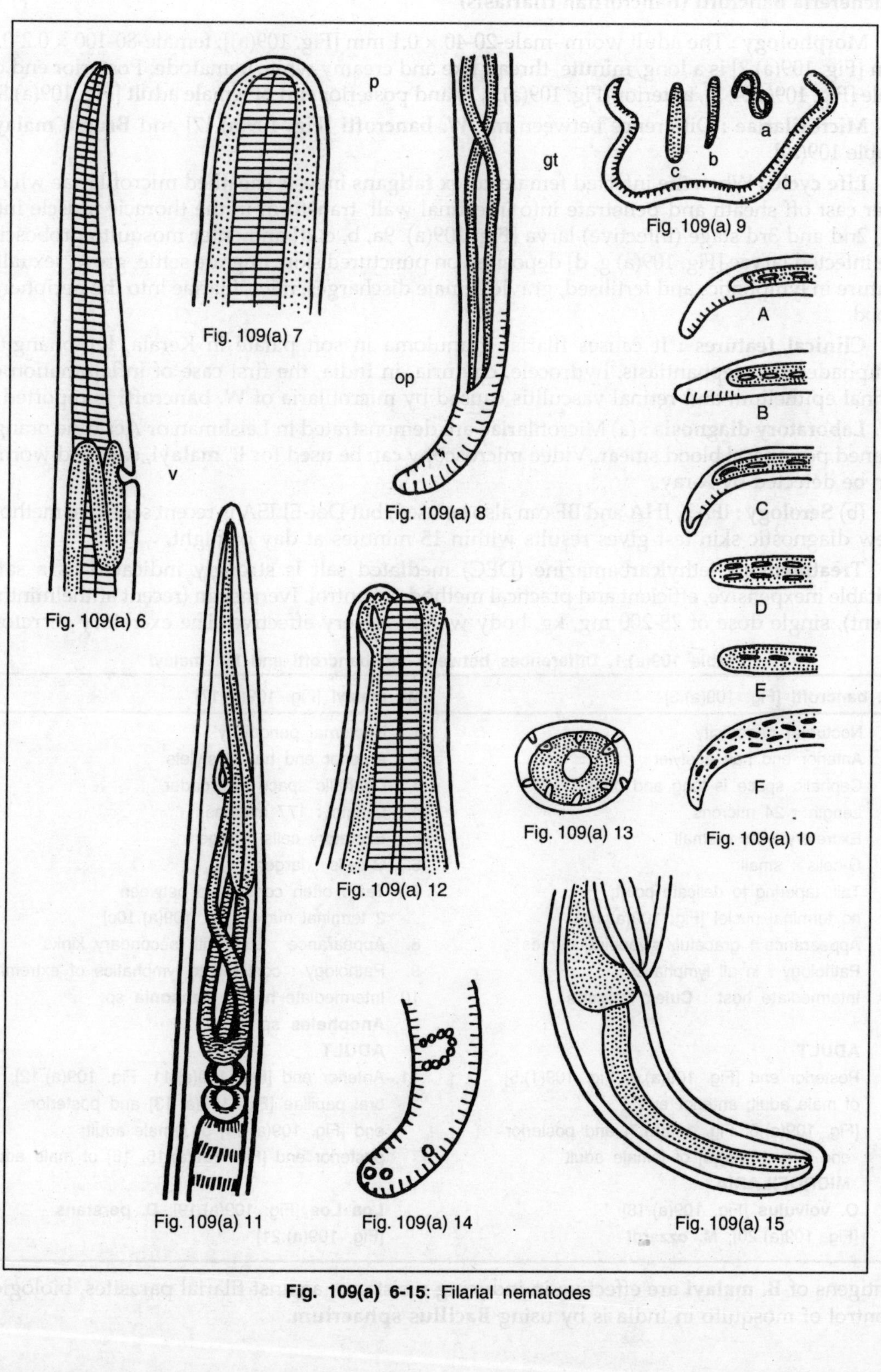

Fig. 109(a) 6-15: Filarial nematodes

Wuchereria bancrofti (Bancroftian filariasis)

Morphology : The adult worm–male-20-40 × 0.1 mm [Fig. 109(a)]; female-80-100 × 0.2-0.3 mm [Fig. 109(a).2] is a long, minute, thread like and creamy white nematode. Posterior end of male [Fig. 109(a).4, 5], anterior [Fig. 109(a).6, 7] and posterior end of female adult [Fig. 109(a).8].

Microfilariae : Difference between mf. **W. bancrofti** [Fig. 109(a).17] and **Brugia malayi** [Table 109(a)].

Life cycle : When the infected female **culex fatigans** ingests sheathed microfilariae which later cast off sheath and penetrate into intestinal wall, transform in the thoracic muscle into 1st, 2nd and 3rd stage (infective) larva [Fig. 109(a). 9a, b, c, d] and enter mosquito proboscis; the infected larvae [Fig. 109(a) g, d] deposited on punctured skin, migrate settle, grow, sexually mature in lymphatics and fertilised, gravid female discharges, microfilariae into the peripheral blood.

Clinical features : It causes filarial granuloma in soft palate in Kerala, lymphangitis lymphadenitis, elephantiasis, hydrocele, chyluria, in India, the first case of inflammation of retinal epithelium and retinal vasculitis caused by microfilaria of **W. bancrofti** is reported.

Laboratory diagnosis : (a) Microfilariae are demonstrated in Leishman or Acridine orange stained peripheral blood smear. Video microscopy can be used for **B. malayi,** calcified worms can be detected by X-ray.

(b) **Serology :** IFAT, IHA and BF can also be used; but Dot-ELISA is recent sensitive method. New diagnostic skin test gives results within 15 minutes at day or night.

Treatment : Diethylcarbamazine (DEC) mediated salt is strongly indicated as a safe, suitable inexpensive, efficient and practical method of control. Ivermectin (recent anthelminthic agent), single dose of 25-200 mg/kg. body weight is very effective. The excretory secretory

Table 109(a).1. Differences between Mf. bancrofti and Mf. malayi

Mf. bancrofti [Fig. 109(a).3]	**Mf. malayi** [Fig. 109(a).17]
1. Nocturnal periodicity	1. Nocturnal periodicity
2. Anterior end has a stylet	2. Anterior end has 2 stylets
3. Cephalic space is long and broad	3. Cephalic space is broader
4. Length : 24 microns	4. Length : 177 microns
5. Excretory cells : small	5. Excretory cells : large
6. G-cells : small	6. G-cells : larger
7. Tail; tapering to delicate point; no terminal nuclei [Fig. 109(a).10A)	7. Tail : often constricted between 2 terminal nuclei [Fig. 109(a).10c]
8. Appearance : graceful, sweeping curves	8. Appearance : stiff; with secondary kinks
9. Pathology : in all lymphatics	9. Pathology : confined to lymphatics of extremites
10. Intermediate host : **Culex fatigans**	10. Intermediate host : **Mansonia** sp. **Anopheles** sp
ADULT	**ADULT**
11. Posterior end [Fig. 109(a).4; Fig. 109(1).5] of male adult; anterior end [Fig. 109(a).6; Fig. 109(a).7] and posterior end [Fig. 109(a).8] of female adult	11. Anterior end [Fig. 109(a).11; Fig. 109(a).12]; oral papillae [Fig. 109(a).13] and posterior end [Fig. 109(a).14] of female adult; posterior end [Fig. 109(a).15, 16] of male adult
MICROFILARIA	
O. volvulus [Fig. 109(a).18] [Fig. 109(a).20]; **M. ozzardi**	**Loa Loa** [Fig. 109(a).19]; **D. perstans** [Fig. 109(a).21]

antigens of **B. malayi** are effective in inducing resistance against filarial parasites, biological control of mosquito in India is by using **Bacillus sphaerium.**

Onchocerca volvulus

It causes blinding filariasis or river blindness.

Morphology : Adult worm (male—42 mm in length; female—50 cm); is white, opaque and transparent. Microfilariae are unsheathed [Fig. 109(a).10F].

Life cycle : is similar to that of **M. bancrofti;** but its intermediate host, **Simulium** (black fly).

Clinical features : Hard nodule, pruritic dermatitis, conjunctivitis, corneal opacity, damage to optical nerve and blindness.

Laboratory diagnosis : (a) Demonstration of microfilariae in biopsied epidermis, in ocular lesion.

(b) **Serology :** CFT, FAT, Skin test can be used; but Immunoblot is recent test.

Treatment : Ivermectin is very recent effective anthelminthic.

Loa loa

It causes calabar swelling or loasis; it measures 30 mm-50 mm. Its microfilariae are sheathed [Fig. 109(a).10B].

Life cycle is similar to that of other microfilariae, but its intermediate host is **Chrysops dimidiate** (mango fly).

Clinical features : Painful fugitive swelling of hen's egg size.

Laboratory diagnosis : Microfilariae in peripheral blood smear, adult worm in the swelling.

Treatment : DEC is effective against microfilariae.

Dracunculus medinensis (Guinea worm)

Morphology. It is the largest milky white human trematode (male—30 mm in length, 0.4 mm in diameter with coiled posterior end; female-120 cm × 1.7 mm with tapering end). Anterior end (Fig. 109.45), head end (Fig. 109.46) of female adult; posterior end (Fig. 109.47) of male.

Embryos (750 μ × 25 μ) are wiry, coiled with a round head (Fig. 109.48).

Life cycle : Man definite host, ingests, infected cyclops (intermediate host) which is digested in the stomach; the larvae are liberated, migrate through intestine into the retroperitoneal tissue where they grow, sexually mature and are fertilised the gravid female migrates into the skin where blister, then ulcer is formed and discharges embryo, in water is ingested by cyclops (Fig. 109.49)

Clinical features : Allergic reaction and toxaemia due to toxin liberated by migrating worm-erythema, urticaria, pruritus, nausea, diarrhoea and giddiness and blister on the sole of feet, ankles, shoulder etc. which bursts out into ulcer with emerging adult worm from its centre.

Laboratory diagnosis

1. Detection of adult worm in the ulcer and embryo discharged in the water; 2. Skin test; 3. Calcified worm by X-ray. 4. Falcon Assay Screening test (FAST ELISA) is most recent serology for diagnosis of dracunculosis.

Treatment : 1. Removal of adult worm from ulcer by Indian barber technique, 2. The drugs (Niridazole, thiobendazole, mebendazole, metronidazole) reduce duration of emergence and associated pain, lvermectin is under trial.

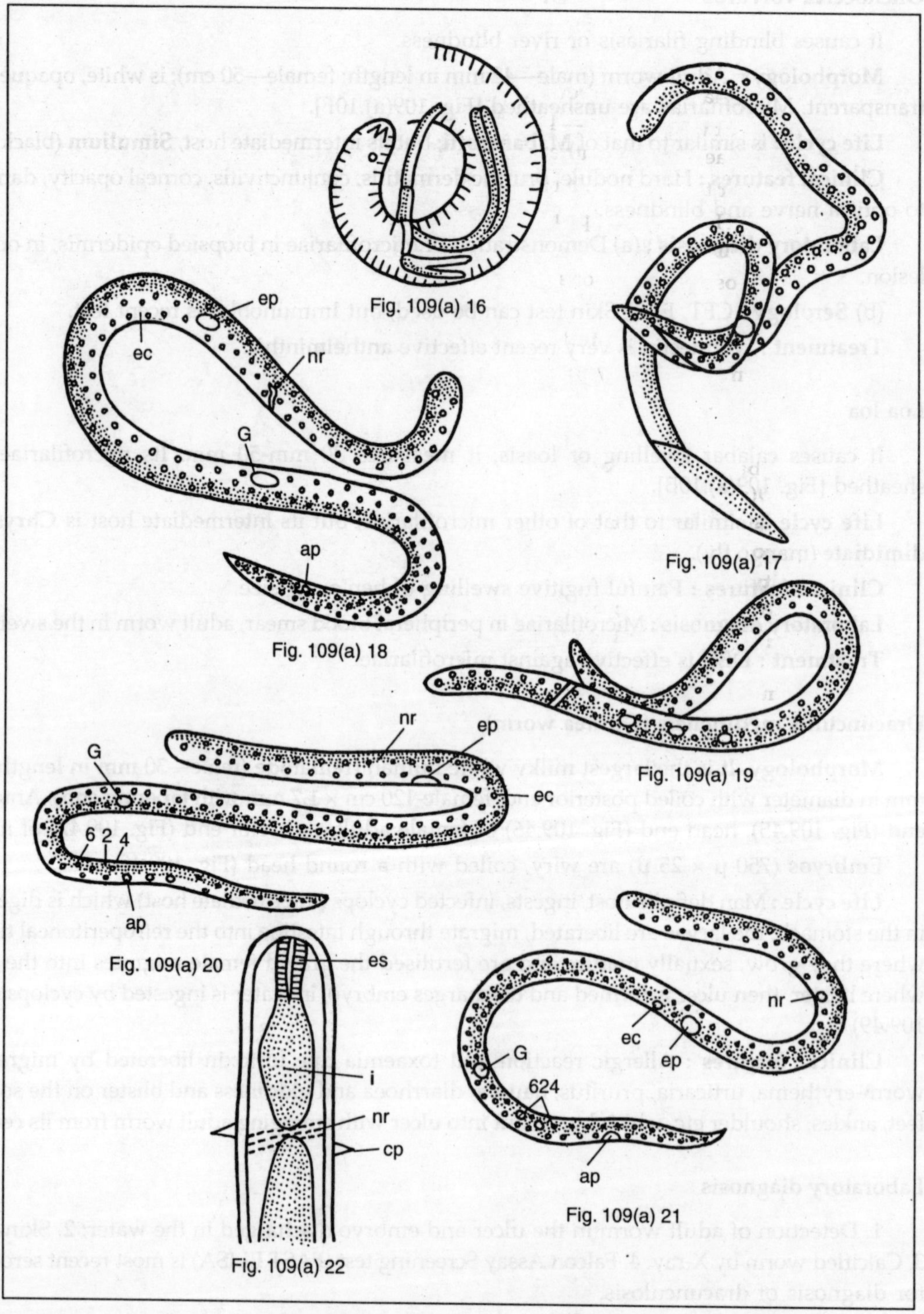

Fig. 109(a) 16-21: Filarial nematodes

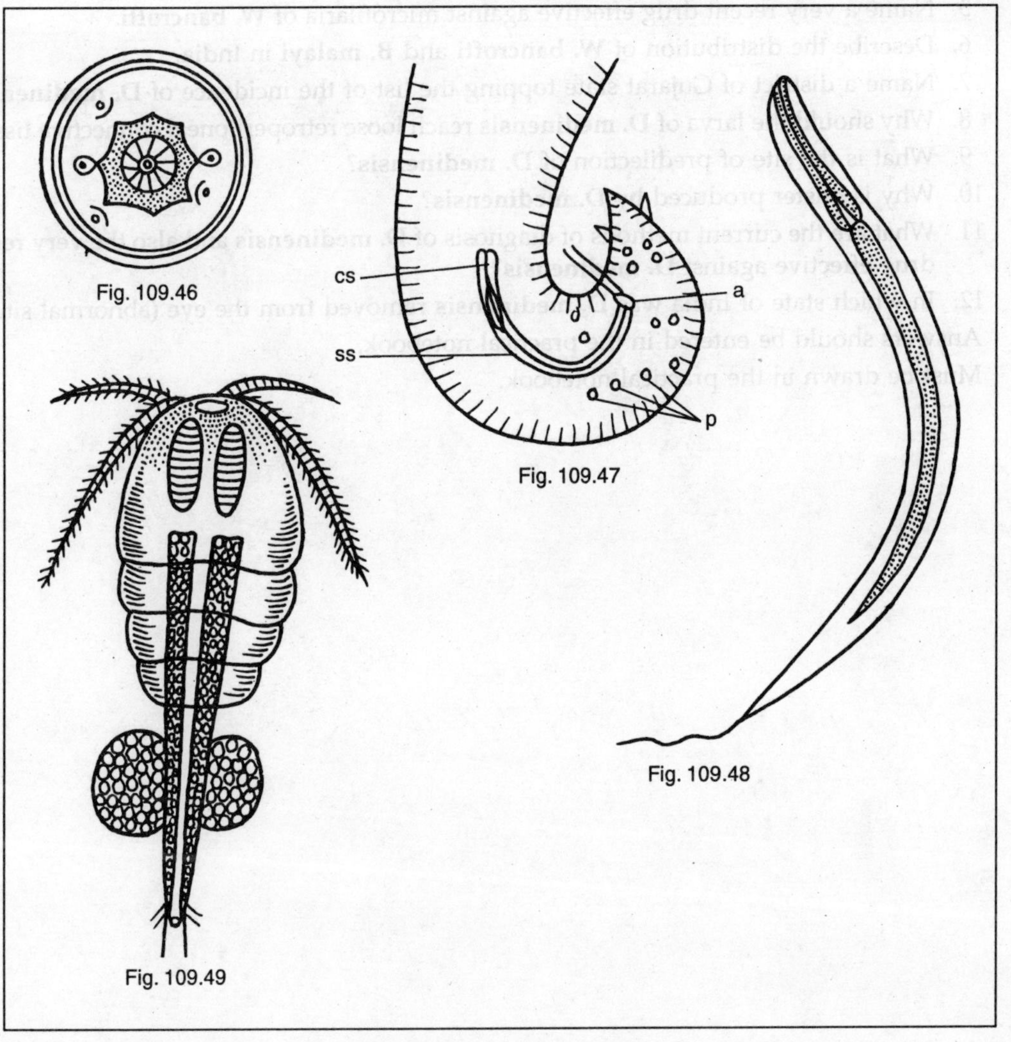

Fig. 109.46-49: Dracunculus medinensis

Demonstration

1. Peripheral blood smear stained with Leishman stain showing microfilaria of **W. bancrofti** (× 1000, [Fig. 109(a).3].
2. Chart representation of posterior end of human microfilariae.
3. Cyclops (representation).

Questions

1. What is nocturnal periodicity?
2. Why is periodicity essential for **W. bancrofti** microfilaria?
3. What are the differences between microfilaria of **W. bancrofti** and **B. malayi**?
4. What are the symptoms of human filariasis?

5. Name a very recent drug effective against microfilaria of **W. bancrofti**.
6. Describe the distribution of **W. bancrofti** and **B. malayi** in India.
7. Name a district of Gujarat state topping the list of the incidence of **D. medinensis.**
8. Why should the larva of **D. medinensis** reach loose retroperitoneal connective tissue?
9. What is the site of predilection of **D. medinensis**?
10. Why is blister produced by **D. medinensis**?
11. What are the current methods of diagnosis of **D. medinensis** and also the very recent drug effective against **D. medinensis**?
12. In which state of India was **D. medinensis** removed from the eye (abnormal site)?

Answers should be entered in the practical notebook.

Must be drawn in the practical notebook.

110
Appendix : Entomology

Adult mosquito : Its body consists of a head, a three segmented thorax and a ten segmented abdomen. The head bears a pair of compound eyes, a pair of fifteen jointed antennae (plumosed in male and pilosed in female), a biting and sucking type of proboscis (Fig. 110. A.1, 2); eggs (110A.3, 4, 5, 6. 7); larva (110 A.8).

Proboscis of the female mosquito is strong like a needle, so that it can pierce through the skin, hence the female is blood sucker; whereas the proboscis of the male is not so strong, so the male is not voracious blood sucker (Fig. 110. A1); Pupa of mosquito (Fig. 110.A9) with trumpet Anopheles, culex (Fig. 110 A.10a, b).

Phlebotomus argentipes (Sandfly) is a delicately built, small insect with lanceolate wings. Both body and wings are covered with hair (Fig. 110 A.11).

Culicoides austeni (biting midges) is a minute insect. Its head is humped over the head. Wings are hairy and dappled (spotted) (Fig. 110 A.12).

Simulium damnosum (black fly) are minute, stout bodied with a humped back and stout and short legs. Eyes are conspicuous. Wings are unspotted (Fig. 110 A.13).

Musca domestica (house fly) is a medium sized, slightly grey fly, with have wings and rectractile rostrum (Fig. 110 A.14).

Glossina palpalis (tse tse fly) is brown and is of the size of a house fly – 8 to 17mm. The wings are folded over one another straight back across the abdomen. Both female and male are voracious blood suckers (Fig. 110 A.15).

Chrysope dimidiata (mango fly) is the size of a house fly or larger. The wings are black, banded. It has secondary eye spots (Fig. 110 A.16).

Triatoma infestans (assassin bug, reduviid bug) is large in size. Its wings are well developed. The head is cone shaped. The abdomen is elongated and is not flattened (Fig. 110 A.17).

Xenopsylla cheopis (rat flea). Its body is laterally flattened and consists of a head, a three segmented thorax and a ten segmented abdomen. The head is roughly triangular and anteriorly rounds, has a pair of pigmented eyes. There is the genal comb at the ventral border of the head, and pronatal combs at the posterior border of the pro-thorax (Fig. 110 A.18). On the ninth abdominal segment, there is saddle shaped structure-pygidium; from the seventh abdominal segment a pair of bristles overhangs the pygidium which is known as antipygidium (Fig. 110 A.18a).

Pediculus humanus (human louse) is dorso-ventrally flattened and has a conical head, three segmented thorax and a ten segmented abdomen. Its three pairs of jointed legs ends in claws. Its abdomen is broad with a festooned border (Fig. 110 A.19).

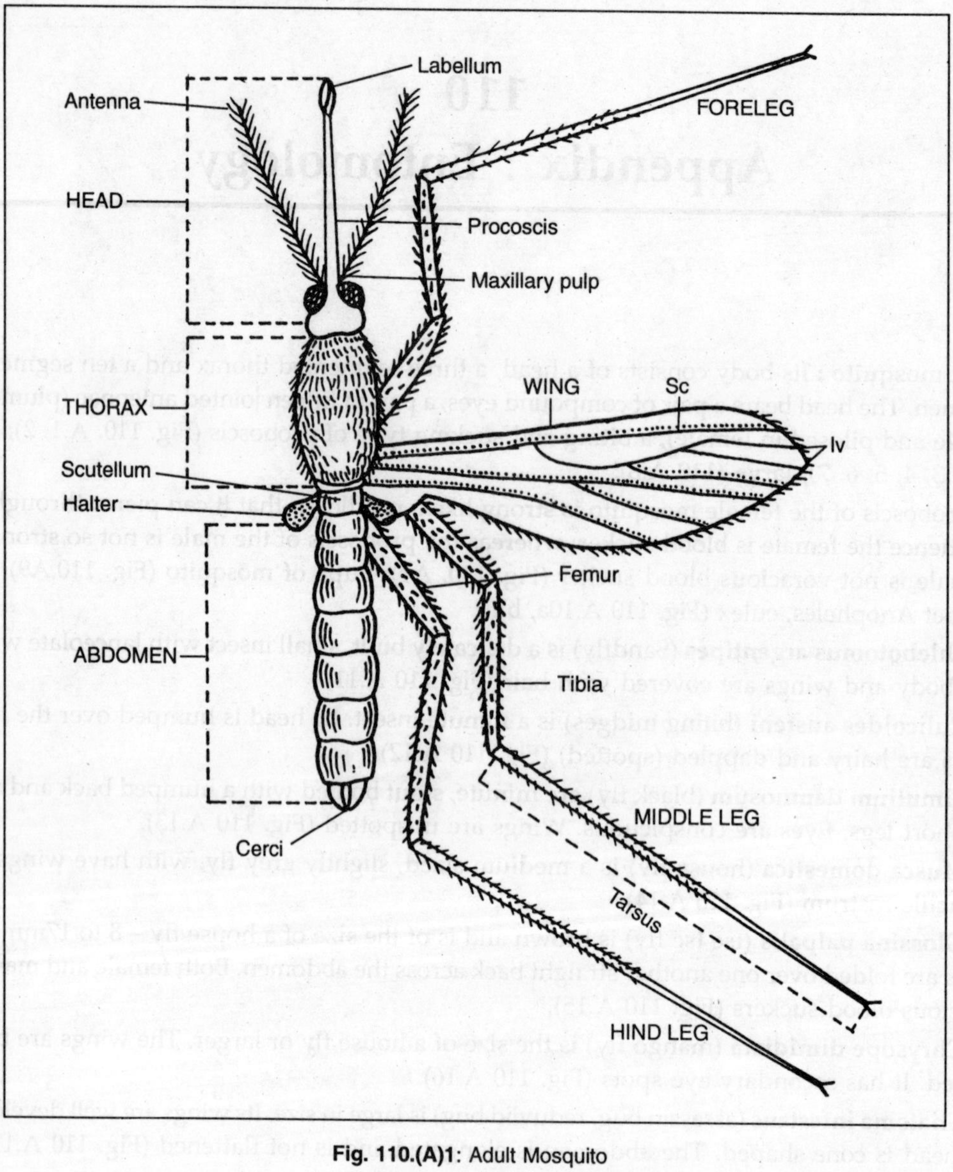

Fig. 110.(A)1: Adult Mosquito

Rhipicephalus sanguineus (tick) is dorsoventrally flattened and has a head, thorax and festooned abdomen, all being contiguous; also has dorsal scutum, short rostrum. Its first coxae is bifid. (Fig. 110 A.20).

Sarcoptes scabei (itch mite). Its body is round, dirty white. Two pairs of anterior legs come out of the margin of the body, the posterior legs remain within the body. The tarsi end in suckers (Fig. 110 A.21).

Demodex fullicularum (mango mite) is anteriority round and posteriorly tapering. Head, thorax and abdomen are clearly differentiated (Fig. 110 A.22).

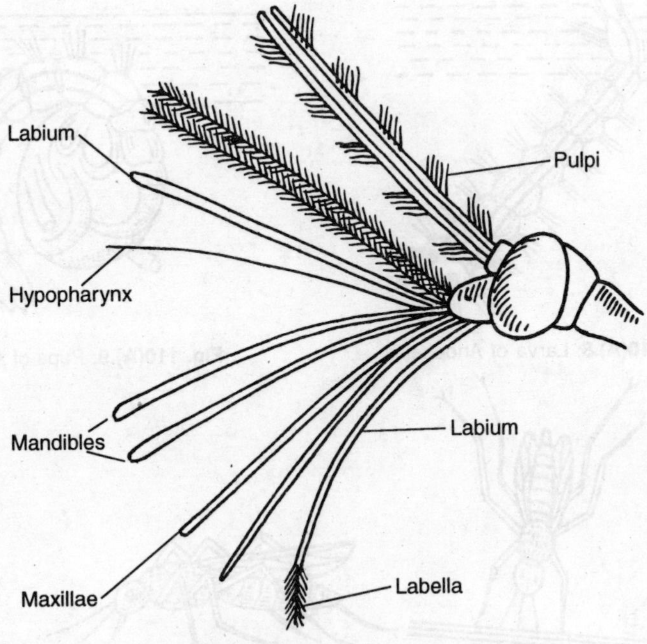

Fig. 110.(A)2: Mouth Part of Mosquito

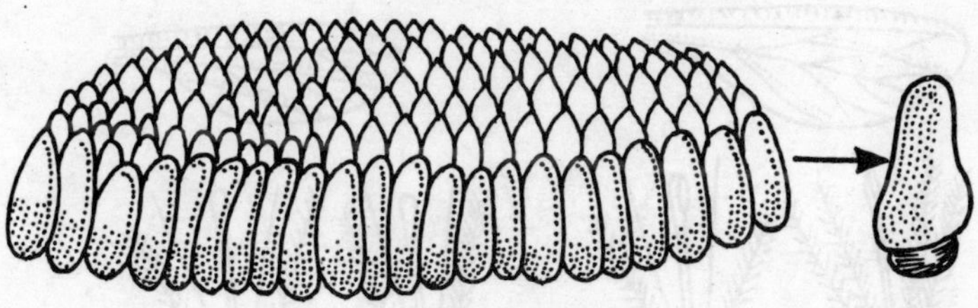

Fig. 110.(A)3: Culex egg

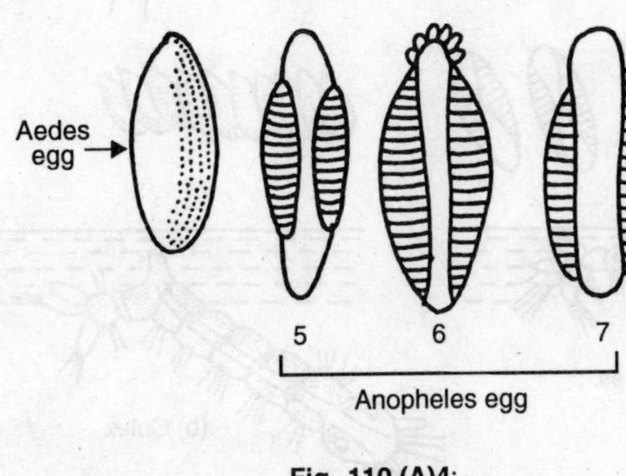

Fig. 110.(A)4:

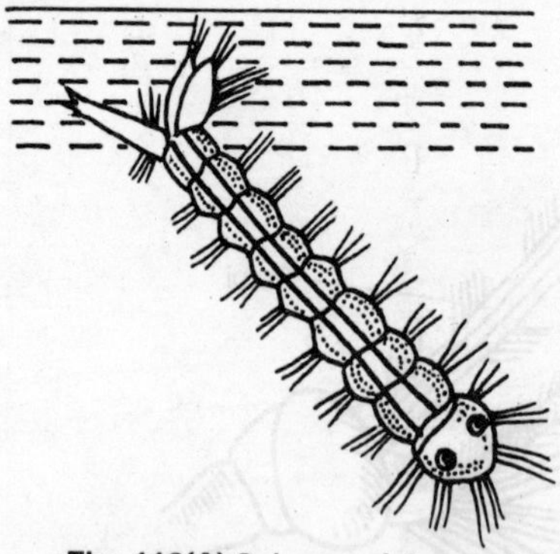

Fig. 110(A).8: Larva of Anopheles

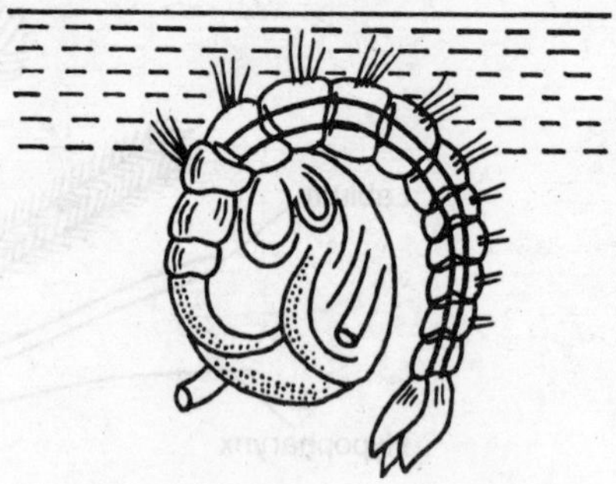

Fig. 110(A).9: Pupa of Anopheles

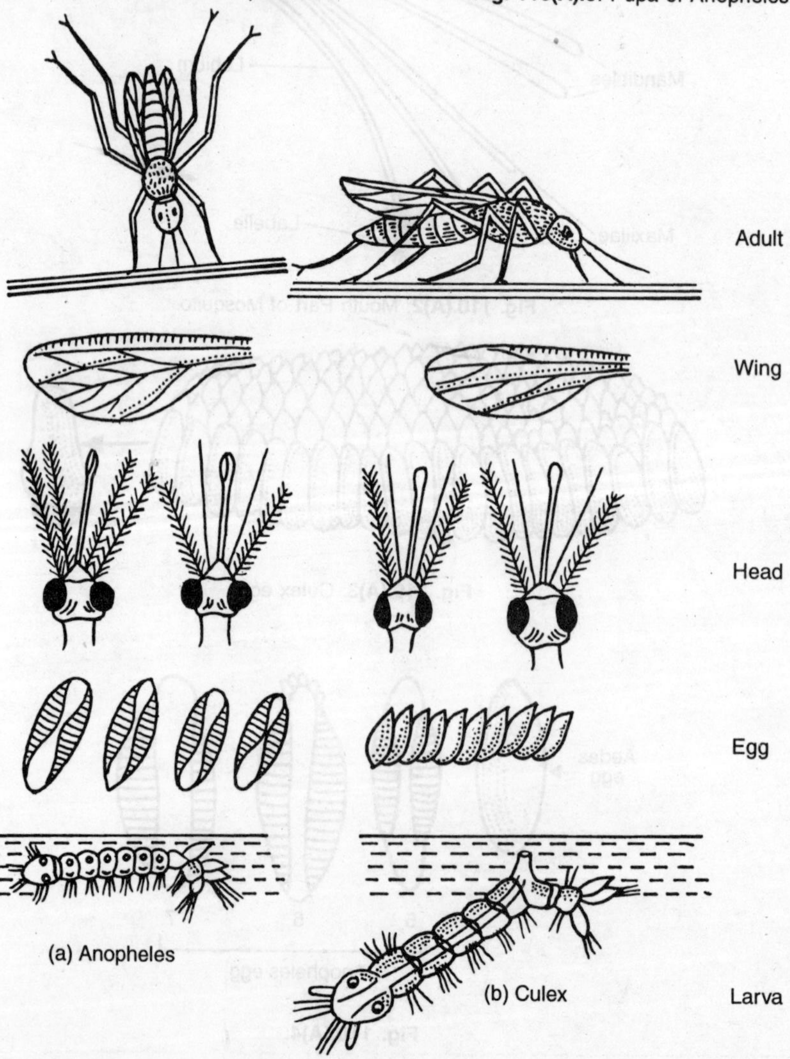

Fig. 110(A).10

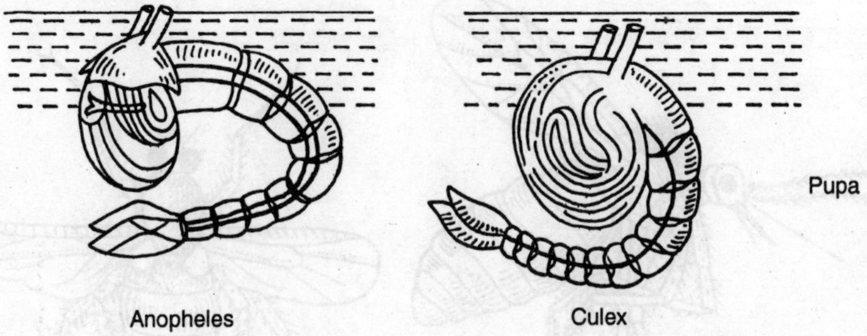

Fig. 110.(A)10: Differential characters of (a) Anopheles and (b) Culex

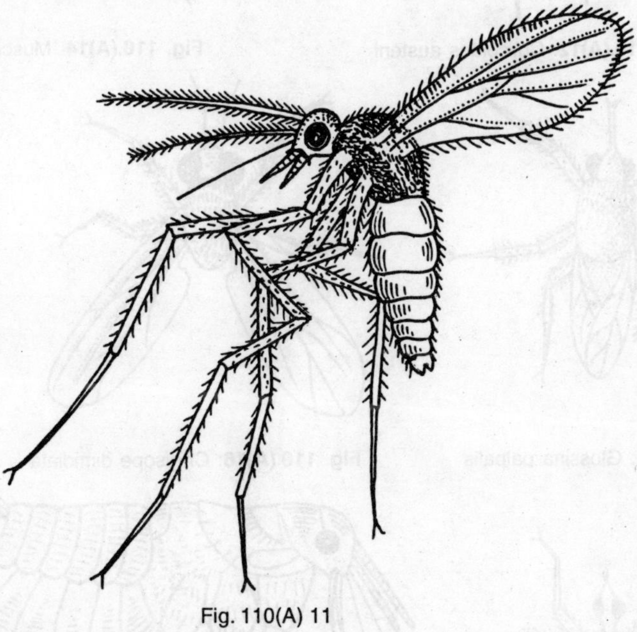

Fig. 110(A) 11

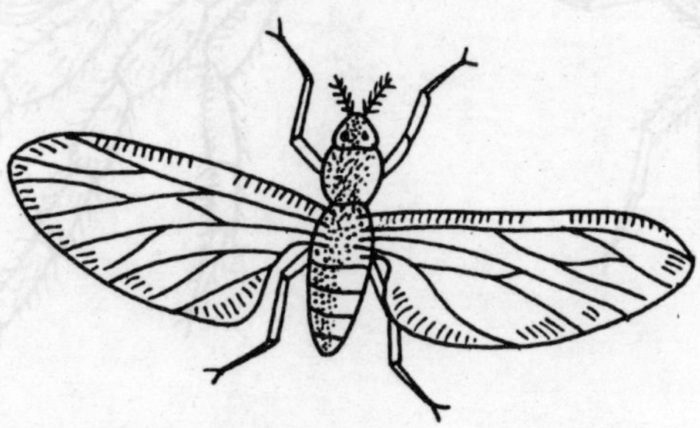

Fig. 110(A) 13

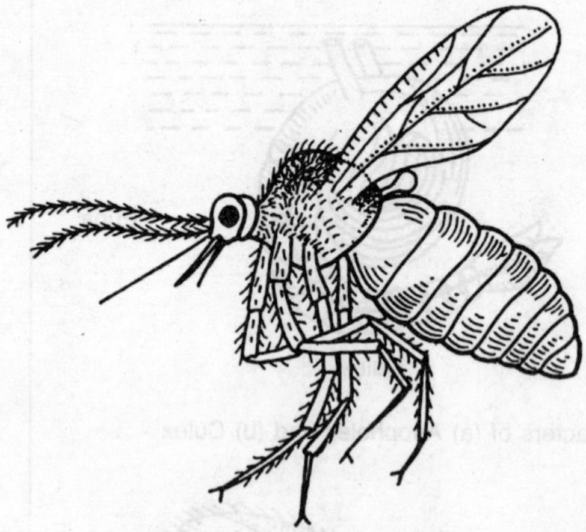

Fig. 110.(A)12: Culicoides austeni

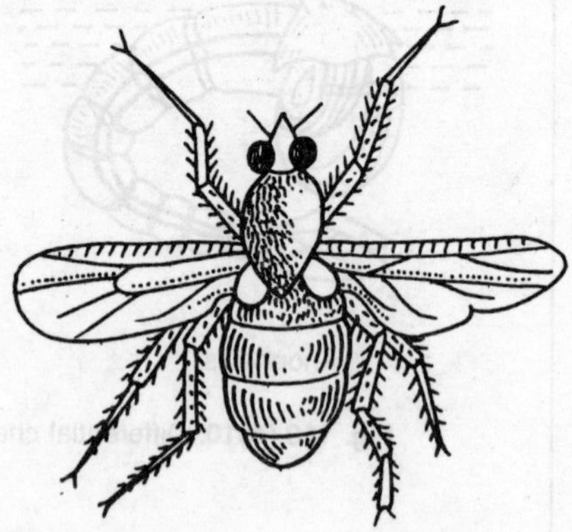

Fig. 110.(A)14: Musca domestica

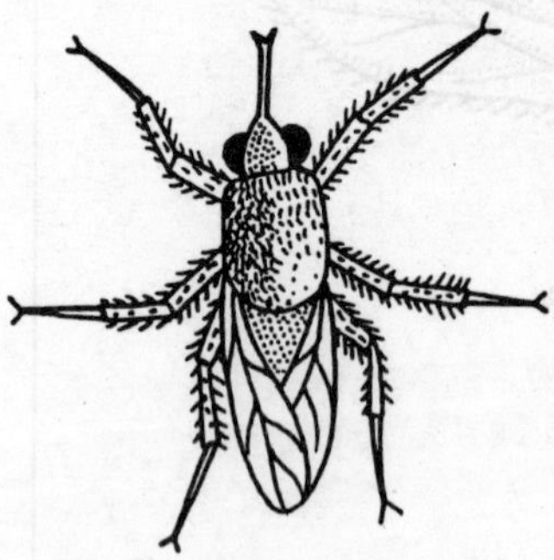

Fig. 110.(A)15: Glossina palpalis

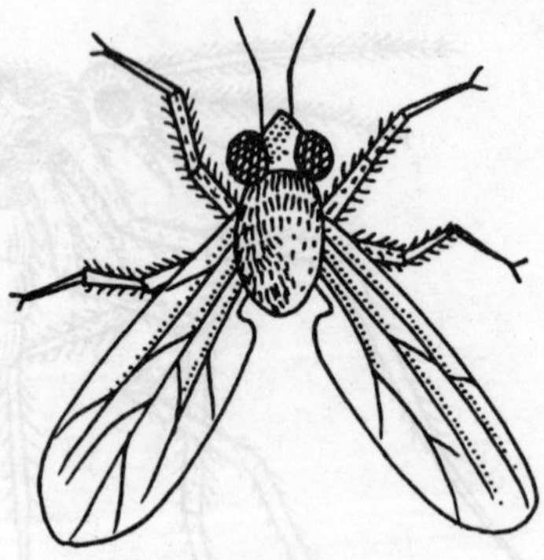

Fig. 110.(A)16: Chrysope dimidiata

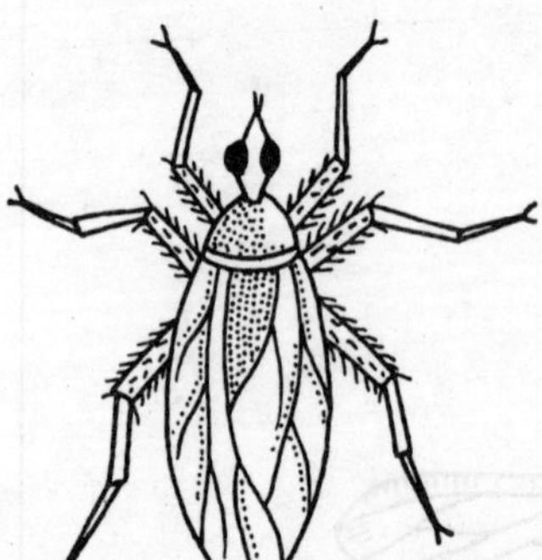

Fig. 110.(A)17: Triatoma infestans

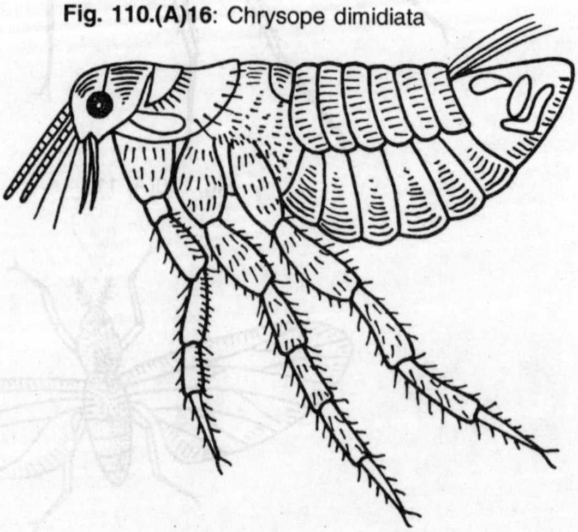

Fig. 110.(A)18: Xenopsylla cheopis

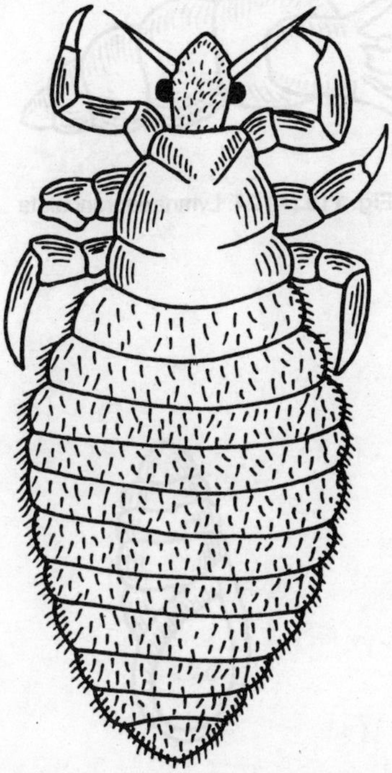

Fig. 110.(A) 19: Pediculus humanus

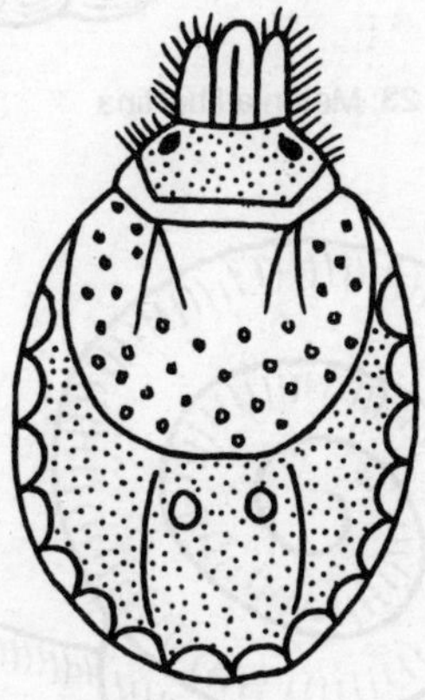

Fig. 110.(A) 20: Rhipicephalus sanguineus

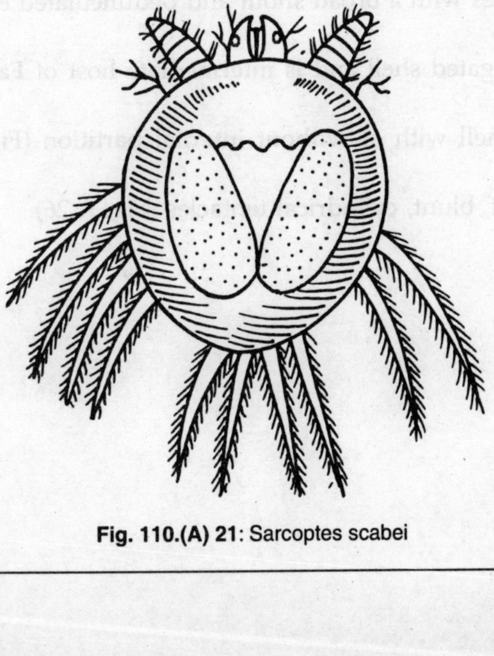

Fig. 110.(A) 21: Sarcoptes scabei

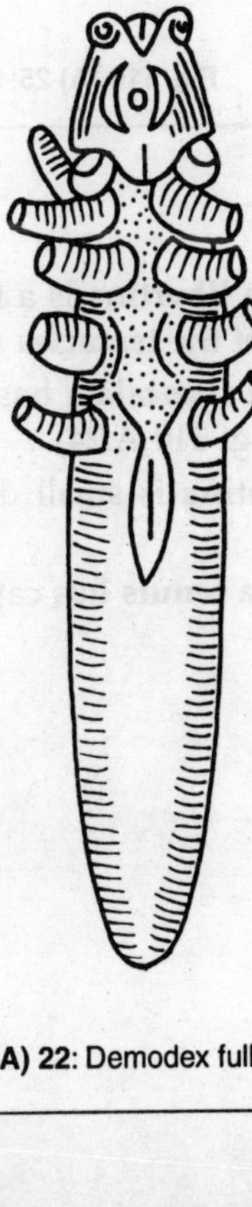

Fig. 110.(A) 22: Demodex fullicularum

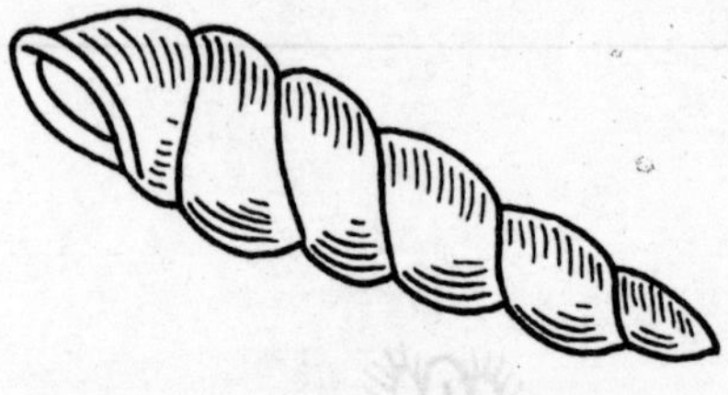

Fig. 110.(A) 23: Melania libertina

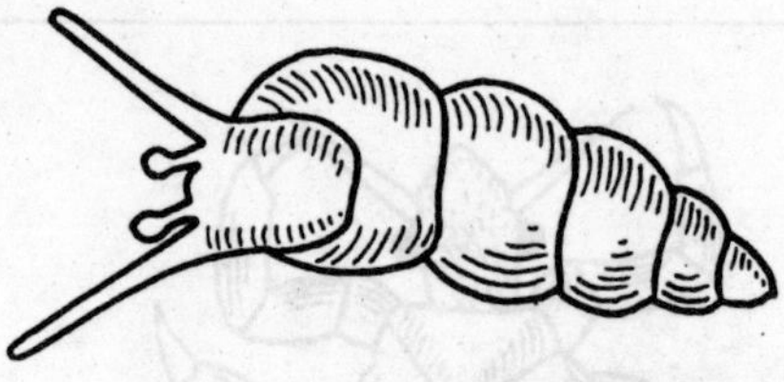

Fig. 110.(A) 24: Lymnaea truncalata

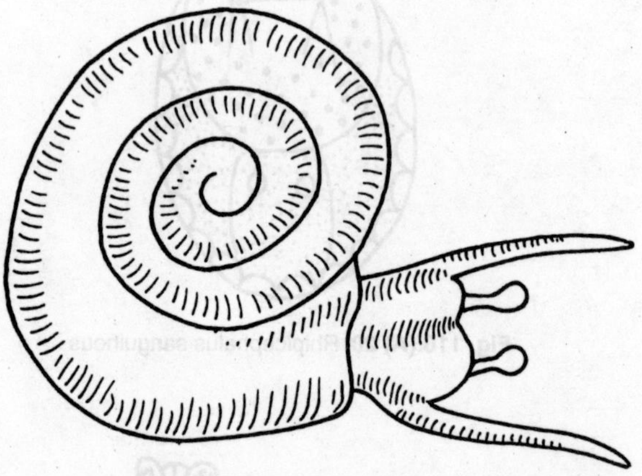

Fig. 110.(A) 25: Segmentina

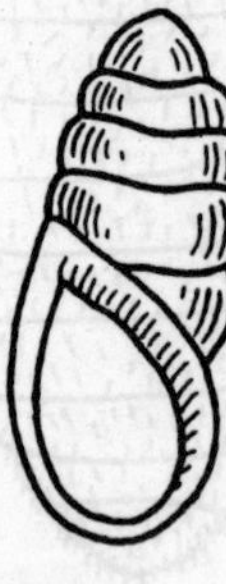

Fig. 110.(A) 26: Ferrissia tenuis

Snails

Melania libertina is a fresh water species with a broad snout and pedunculated eyes at outer base of the tentacles (Fig. 110 A.23).

Lymnea truncalata has an oval or elongated shell and is intermediate host of **Fasciola hepatica** (Fig. 110 A.24).

Segmentina is small discoidal shiny shell with or without internal partition (Fig. 110 A.25).

Ferrissia tenuis has cap like shell, short, blunt, cylindrical tentacles (Fig. A.26).

111
Laboratory Examinations

I. Blood examination for Parasites

Thick or thin blood smear can be stained by Leishman's or Giemsa or Field's or JSB stain to detect blood parasites.

Method of Leishman staining : Leishman's stain should be poured from the dropper bottle and diluted to twice its volume with neutral distilled water. Drying should be prevented by covering the stained slide with a Petri dish for 10-15 minutes. Then the slide should be washed with tap water, dried and examined under oil immersion lens.

II. Stool Examination for Parasites

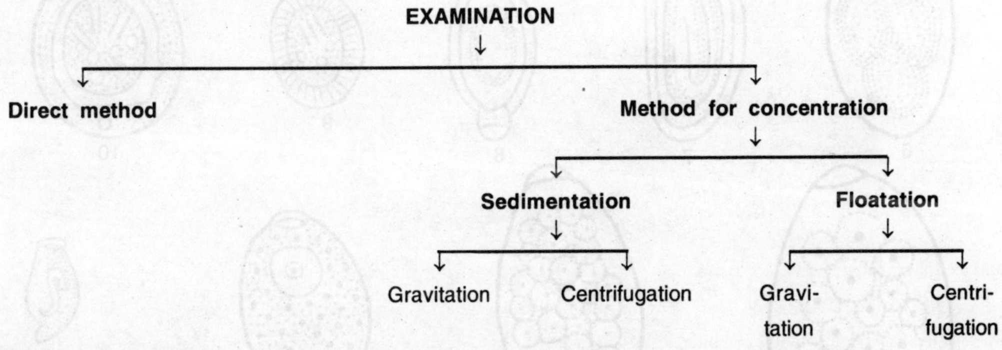

Direct method : Two cover glass preparations are prepared on one microscopic slide far apart from each other : (1) Saline preparation : 1-2 mg of the faecal material should be mixed in a drop or two of physiological salt solution for the left hand preparation; and (2) Iodine preparation : 1-2 drops of iodine solution (Lugol's iodine can be used if it is diluted five times in distilled water). These films should be thin without air bubbles. Cyst can be detected in the saline preparation. While examining the unstained preparation for clearer view, the condenser should be racked down and the iris diaphragm is partially closed to cut down the illumination.

The saline preparation is useful to study living parasites (trophozoites, helminth eggs, chromatoid bar) whereas the iodine preparation to study the characteristic features (nucleus, glycogen mass) of cyst of **E. histolytica** and flagella of parasites.

The direct method is quick, simple and easy; but it cannot detect infections (Fig. B I, II).

Fig. B I-1, 2, 3 cyst of E. histolytica, 2, cyst of E. coli; 3, cyst of G. intestinalis; 4, (fertilised, 5 unfertilised egg of A, lumbricoides; 6, A. duodenale or N. americanus; 7, egg of, E. vermicularis; 8. T. trichiura; 9. T. saginata or solium; 10, H. nana; 11. F. buski; 12. G. hominis,

13, P. westermani; 14, C. sinensis; 15. D. latum; 16. S. japonicum; 17, S. haematobium; 18. S. mansoni, Fig. B-II-1-5, Various yeasts, 6, 7, squamous cell from mucosa; 8. microphage without nuclei; 9, 10, polymorphis; 11, 12, pollen grains; 13, 14, starch granules; 15, plant hair; 16, 17, vegetable materials; 18, vegetable spiral, 19, B. hominis.

1. Aids Assciated parasites (supplement)

Pneumocystis carinii, Toxoplasma gondii, Isospora belli, Leishmania sp. cryptosporidium and Microsporidia.

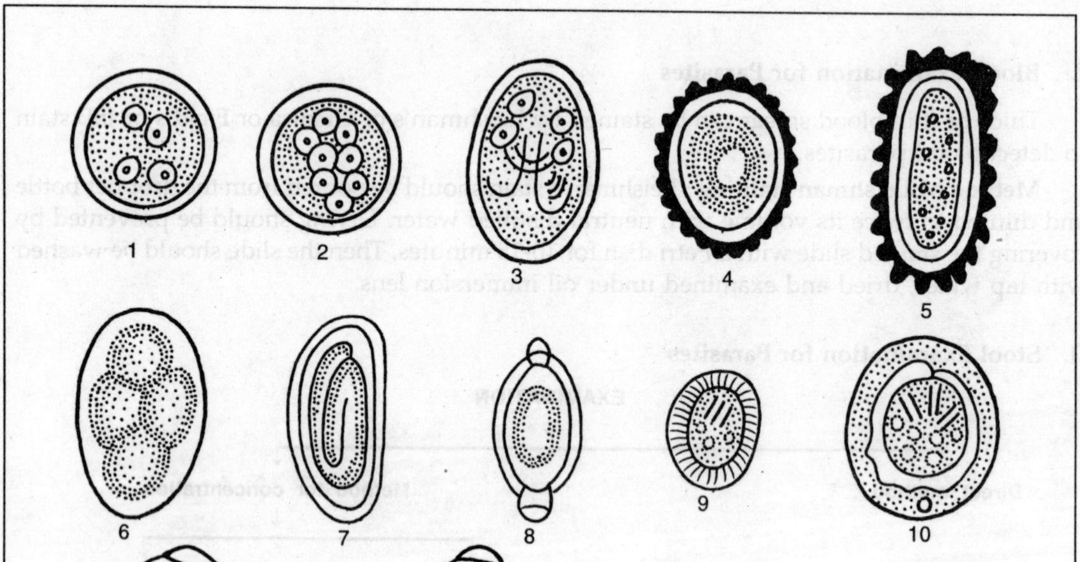

Fig. 111.B. I: Protozoan cysts and helminthic eggs in the stool of man

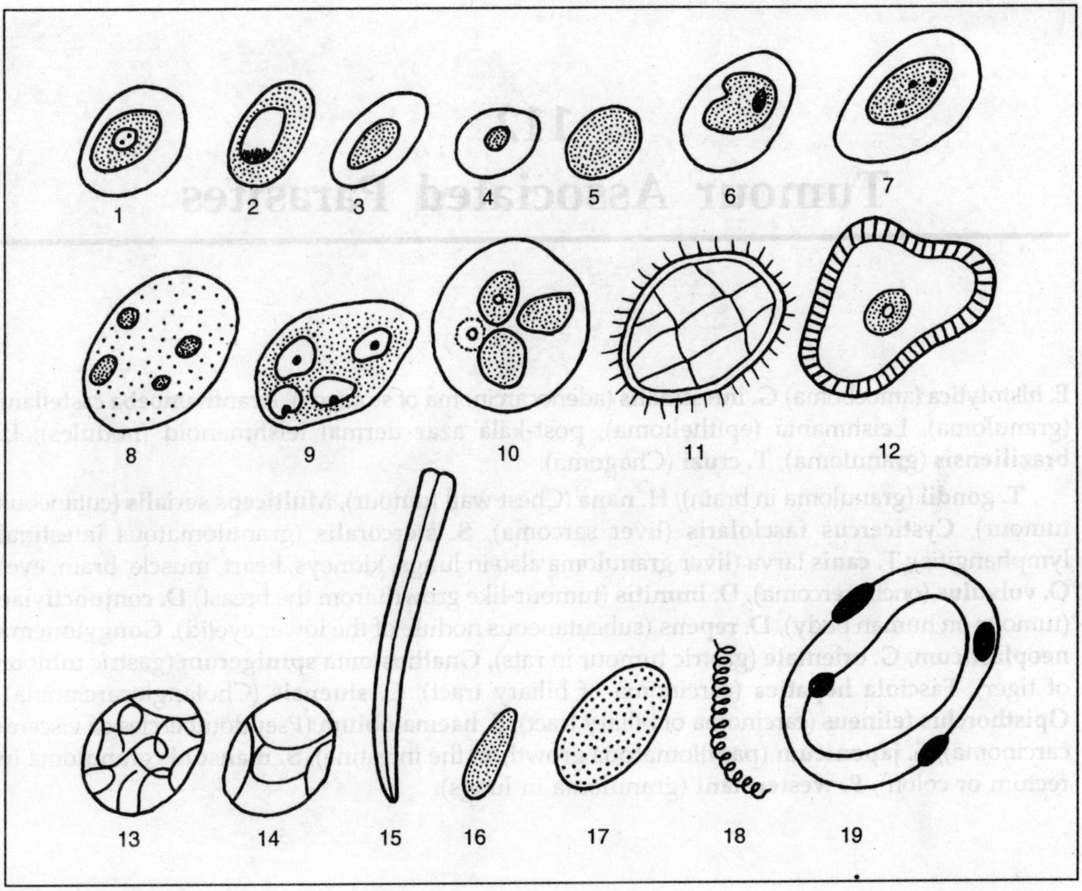

Fig. 111.B. II: Pseudoparasites

112 Tumour Associated Parasites

E. histolytica (amoeboma) **G. intestinalis** (adenocarcinoma of stomach), **Acanthamoeba castellani** (granuloma), Leishmania (epithelioma), post-kala azar dermal leishmanoid (nodules); **L. braziliensis** (granuloma); **T. cruzi** (Chagoma).

T. gondii (granuloma in brain); **H. nana** (Chest wall tumour), **Multiceps serialis** (cutaneous tumour), **Cysticercus fasciolaris** (liver sarcoma), **S. stercoralis** (granulomatous intestinal lymphangitis); **T. canis** larva (liver granuloma also in lungs, kidneys, heart, muscle, brain, eye) **O. volvulus** (onchocercoma), **D. immitis** (tumour-like growth from the breast) **D. conjunctiviae** (tumour on human body), **D. repens** (subcutaneous nodule of the lower eyelid). **Gongylonema neoplasticum, G. orientale** (gastric tumour in rats), **Gnathostoma spinigerum** (gastric tumour of tiger), **Fasciola hepatica** (carcinoma of biliary tract), **C. sinensis** (Cholangiocarcinoma), **Opisthorchis felineus** (carcinoma of biliary tract), **S. haematobium** (Pseudotubercles or visceral carcinoma), **S. japonicum** (papillomatous growth in the intestine), **S. mansoni** (granuloma in rectum or colon), **P. westermani** (granuloma in lungs).

113

Parasites associated with pulmonary diseases

1. **Protozoa. L. donovani.** Pulmonary involvement is usually characterised by signs and symptoms of bronchitis and bronchopneumonia.
2. **Trematodes. S. mansoni.** Pulmonary hypertension and Cor pulmonale induced by pulmonary arteritis as a result of **S. mansoni** egg deposition.

   P. westermani. Pathologically, this lung fluke has a stage of infiltration, encysted stage, non-suppurative chronic granulomatous reaction with numerous ova.
3. **Nematodes. A. lumbricoides, Toxacara canis** and **Capillaria acrophila** cause pulmonary granulomas. Patient may present with a visceral larva migrans syndrome, asthmatic symptoms and eosinophila.

Importance of Parasites in Different Specialities

Parasites of Radiological Importance.

E. histolytica, G. lamblia, P. falciparum, T. gondii, Pneumocystis carinii, E. granulosus; T. solium, S. haematobium, P. westermani, W. bancrofti, D. medinensis.

114
Parasites of Ophthalmic Importance

Naegleria fowleri, Acanthamoeba castellani, Leptomyxid amoeba, T. cruzi, T. gondii, E. ganulosus, Multiceps brauni, T. solium, T. spiralis, Larvae of **T. canis, T. catis, A. lumbricoides,** microfilariae of **O. volvulus,** adult worm of Loa loa, **Thelazia callipaeda, T. californiensis, D. medinensis.**

Parasites of Cardiac Importance

T. cruzi, P. falciparum, T. solium, E. granulosus, C. sinensis, T. sprialis, S. stercoralis, larva of **T. canis and T. catis, A. duodenale, A. lumbricoides.**

Parasites of Gynaecological Importance

T. vaginalis.

115
Parasitology—Protozoology

Chapter 1
SUMMARY

Protozoa are microscopic primitive unicellular animals with

(a) Outer cytoplasm (ectoplasm) responsible for movement, respiration, excretion, protection;

(b) Inner cytoplasm (endoplasm) with nucleus which controls nutrition, reproduction.

(c) Karyosome (minute mass) in the centre of nucleus can be useful to distinguish genera and species.

They are grouped :

(1) **Rhizopoda** move with pseudopodia (false feet) to engulf food (Entamoeba)

(2) **Mastigophora** move with long hair like filaments, flagella (Trypanosoma)

(3) **Sporozoa** do not move (plasmodium)

(4) **Ciliata** move with cilia (short process) — **Balantidium coli**.

Their life cycle stages :

(a) Trophozoite (motile stage) transforms into cyst (encystment)

(b) Precystic stage with blunt pseudopodia

(c) Cystic stage (resistant form) gives rise to trophozoite (excystation).

Solid or liquid food can be engulfed by protozoa, digested by enzymes in food vacuoles. After digestion, it is stored as glycogen, volutin, chromatoid. Waste products are passed out.

Glucose is metabolised into pyruvic acid (end product) by trypanosome and into lactose by plasmodia. Blood protozoa require amino acids, vitamins, salts whereas intestinal protozoa live on bacterial flora.

They reproduce (1) asexually (binary fission of entamoeba; multiple fission or schizogony of plasmodium)

(2) Sexually (temporary union—conjugation-of two protozoa to interchange their nuclear material—ciliata); male and female unite to form a zygote (sporogony or syngamy) which produces sporozoites (infective form).

African trypanosome reproduces asexually by repeated longitudinal fission, whereas American trypanosome occurs in round shape in tissue and elongates into trypanosome and reenters the blood circulation.

QUESTION (Q) – ANSWER (A)

Q. What is protozoa ?

Ans. Protozoa are microscopic single celled primitive animal.

Q. Why protozoa are called primitive animal ?

Ans. Because they are microscopic single cell with animal physiological activities.

Q. What is the function of nucleus ?

Ans. Nucleus controls nutrition, reproduction.

Q. What is the function of ectoplasm ?

Ans. Ectoplasm controls movement, respiration, excretion, protection.

Q. What is Karyosome ? State its use.

Ans. Karyosome is minute mass in the centre of nucleus. It is useful to distinguish genera and species.

Q. What is Rhizopoda ?

Ans. They are motile protozoa moving withe pseudopodia.

Q. What is pseudopodia ? What is its function ?

Ans. It is false feet. It helps the protozoal movement to engulf food material.

Q. What is Mastigophora ?

Ans. They are protozoa moving with flagella.

Q. What is flagella ?

Ans. It is a hair like long filament, arising from the ectoplasm, which helps the movement.

Q. What is sporozoa ?

Ans. They are non-motile protozoa.

Q. What is cilia ?

Ans. Cilia are short processes, they arise from the ectoplasm, they are responsible for the movement of protozoa.

Q. What is trophozoite ? Mention its role.

Ans. Trophozoite is a protozoal developmental stage. It is motile to engulf the food material and to invade the tissue.

Q. What is cystic stage of protozoa ?

Ans. Cystic is a resistant form of protozoa which gives rise to trophozoites (infective forms).

Q. Mention end product of glucose metabolism by African trypanosome and malarial parasite.

Ans. End product of glucose metabolised by African trypanosome is pyruvic acid; whereas in cases of malarial parasite it is lactose.

Q. Which protozoa require amino acids, vitamins, and inorganic salts in the blood for their growth and multiplication ?

Ans. They are blood protozoa.

Q. Which protozoa thrive on bacterial flora ?

Ans. They are intestinal protozoa.

Q. Enumerate different types of multiplication ?

Ans. Different types of asexual reproduction are

(1) Asexual multiplication by protozoa

(a) Binary fission of Entamoeba;

(b) Multiple fission of plasmodium;

(c) Repeated longitudinal fission of African trypanosome

(d) Rounding and elongation of American trypanosome.

(2) **Sexual multiplication**

(a) Conjugation of ciliata; (b) Sporogony of plasmodium in mosquito

Chapter 2

SUMMARY

Rhizopoda, Entamoeba histolytica

Among six species of Entamoeba, **E. histolytica** is pathogenic to man. It causes diarrhoea, dysentery, hepatitis; amoebic abscess in the lungs, brain, spleen, skin.

Infection in man starts within few hours after swallowing of fresh mature four nucleated cysts; these cysts, unaffected by gastric juice, are digested by trypsin in the large intestine where the excystation process is initiated at neutral pH; by binary fission eight uni-nucleated amoeba are liberated to perpetuate their life-cycle. These amoebae (trophozoites) invade the mucosa of the large intestine, multiply and cause **ulceration** (flask-shaped ulcers). Some trophozoites may escape into blood circulation, settle in liver, extra-intestinal amoebiasis.

After multiplication in the mucosa, they reenter in the luman of the gut and transform into cysts (encystation) which are passed out in the stool.

Pathological changes in

(a) Intestine, flask-shaped ulcer

(b) Extra-intestine – Amoebic abscess in lung, brain, spleen, skin.

Amoebic dysentery is characterised by the presence of blood and mucus in the stool as dark red, offensive and copious.

In amoebic liver abscess, the clinical symptom are presence of enlarged liver, pain in the right hypochondrium, epigastrium or lower chest; abdominal mass, fever, sweating.

Cyst in formed stool, trophozoites in diarrhoea (stool can confirm the diagnosis of intestinal amoebiasis, in addition to ultrasonography, X-ray of abdomen and immunodiagnostic tests).

Amoebiasis can be treated by appropriate drugs; it can be controlled by personal, community prophylaxis.

E. coli is non-pathogenic to man and can be identified by the presence of eight nuclei with eccentric karyosome.

QUESTION (Q) – ANSWER (A)

Q. How many species of Entamoeba are in alimentary tract of man ? Enumerate them.

Ans. There are six species : **E. coli, E. gingivalis, Iodamoeba, biitschlii, Dientamoeba, fragilis, E. nana.**

Q. Which species is pathogenic to man ?

Ans. Entamoeba histolytoica is pathogenic to man.

Q. Why other non-pathogenic species are of medical importance ?

Ans. All non-pathogenic species are confused with **E. histolytica,** hence they are medically important for differentiation and identification.

Q. Enumerate the disease caused by E. histolytica.

Ans. It causes diarrhoea, dysentery, hepatitis, amoebic abscess in lung, brain, spleen, skin.

Q. Who discovered first E. histolytica ?

Ans. Lambli discovered first **E. histolytica** in 1859.

Q. Though E. histolytica is distributed worldwide, where is it very common ?

Ans. It is very common in tropics and subtropics.

Q. Where does E. histolytica live ?

Ans. It lives in mucosa and submucosa of large intestine.

Q. What is the importance of karyosome in Entamoeba ?

Ans. Karyosome is important from the diagnostic point of view. Different species can be differentiated by the position of karyosome in the nuclei. In **E. histolytica,** it is in the centre, in **E. coli,** it is eccentric.

Q. What is excystation ?

Ans. It is a process in which the cyst wall retracts, tetra-nucleated amoebae are liberated and by binary fission eight uninucleated amoebae (trophozoites) are produced.

Q. How do trophozoites invade the mucosa of the intestine ?

Ans. They invade the mucosa by production of their cytolysin and symbiosis with gut bacterial flora.

Q. From which structure of E. histolytica the first division starts for their multipliation ?

Ans. First division starts from the nucleus of **E. histolytica.**

Q. How to differentiate E. histolytica from E. coli ?

Ans. The differentiation can be made by the position of Karyosome in nucleus.

Q. Where the lesions are confined in primary light and severe infection of the intestine.

Ans. In primary infection : they are more commonly found at the point of stasis (caecum, hepatic flexure, splenic flexure, rectosigmoid junction).

In light infection : the lesions are restricted to these points only.

In severe infection : more severe lesions are found in the mucosa and submucosa of large intestine.

Q. How are bacteriologically sterile colliquative necrosis and ulcer in the large intestine formed ?

Ans. When the amoebae come in contact with the intestinal mucosa, they secrete a ferment which liquifies cells, ultimately forming sterile colliquative necrosis and flask-shaped ulcer which contains lysed cells and no bacteria.

Chapter 3

SUMMARY

Mastigophora (flagellates) are also single cell animals with several long, delicate, thread-like filaments (organ of locomotion). They are intestinal, oral, genital, blood, tissue flagellates.

Giardia lamblia

Giardia lamblia (intestinal flagellate). Its name is given in honour of Giard and Lambli (1859). It lives in duodenum and jejunum of man. Its life cycle has trophozoite and cystic stages. Trophozoite has two nuclei and a ventral sucking disc and can be cultivated in artificial medium.

Man gets infection within 30 minutes after ingestion of mature cysts in food or drink. These cysts give rise to two trophozoites which multiply enormously and colonise in the duodenum. In large intestine under unfavorable condition they encyst and the cysts are passed out in the stool.

The intestinal function is disturbed because they attach to the mucosal convex surface with their sucking disc causing loose motions with excess fat (steatorrhoea), chronic kerateritis and cholecystopathy.

Diagnosis can be confirmed by the presence of trophozoites or cysts in the stool; or trophozoite in duodenal aspirate; by the hypermotility of the jejunum by fluoroscopy, mucosal defects by X-ray.

Quinacrine, metronidazole can be useful to eliminate the infection; only personal hygiene can control the infection.

Genus Trichomonas

These flagellates have only trophozoite stage in their life cycle. According to their habitat they are grouped into : 1. **Trichomonas vaginalis** (vagina, urinary tract); 2. **Trichomonas hominis** (ileocaecal region); 3. **Trichomonas tenax** (oral cavity).

Trichomonas vaginalis

It was first observed by Donne (1936) in male and female genital tract, prostate gland of man. It is largest protozoa (13 microns) with undulating membrane. It feeds on the vaginal mucosal surface, ingests bacteria and leucocytes with more acidic condition of the vagina. Man gets infected during sexual intercourse with infected woman.

Degeneration and desquamation of vaginal mucosa with leucocytic infiltration are pathological changes. Greenish or yellowish discharge may contain many **trichomonas vaginalis** and leucocytes it is extremely irritating; causes itching and excoriation.

Its infection can be diagnosed by the presence of **Trichomonas vaginalis** in the centrifuged urine and vaginal secretion and by specific indirect haemagglutination test.

Metronidazole is most effective drug; it can be controlled by avoiding sexual intercourse with infected individuals.

Genus Trypanosoma

SUMMARY

It is a spindle-shaped blood flagellate, has a free flagellum at the anterior end and undulating membrane arising from kinetoplast which is at the posterior end and has volutin granules.

Human pathogenic trypanosomes are classified : Trypanosoma brucei –rhodensiense –gambiense group — causes African trypanosomiasis (Sleeping sickness)

2. **T. cruzi** causes South American trypanosomiasis (Chagas disease).

Trypanosoma gambiense

T. gambiense occurs in three forms : long, short, and intermediate. In early stage, it occurs in blood and lymph nodes, in the cerebrospinal fluid (CSF); often cerebral infection.

In their life-cycle, ingested trypanosomes, in the midgut of fly, transform into crithidial forms which migrate to the salivary gland of fly where they develop into metacyclic forms which are infective to man by the bite of **glossina fly.** This type of development in the fly is known as "development at anterior station". In the blood, these metacyclic forms transform into trypanosomes which multiply by longitudinal binary fission.

An elevated, indurated, painful initial "trypanosomal chancre" develops in the skin after glossina fly bite. After invasion in the lymph nodes, spleen, and liver are enlarged and congested.

The chronic or "sleeping sickness" stage of infection is initiated after the invasion of nervous system. The headache is severe, with mental dullness, apathy declination to work, profound sleep – the patient falls asleep while eating, standing, will not be aroused even to take food, ultimately convulsion and death.

Laboratory diagnosis can confirm the infection by demonstration of trypanosomes in blood, lymph node, bone marrow, CSF, by microscopical examination of stained films; by cultivation in media; animal inoculation and by serology.

The infection can be treated by suitable drugs (Trypansamide, suramin, pentamidine) and be controlled by destruction of vectors, isolation of patients.

Trypanosoma cruzi

T. cruzi is a pleomorphic trypanosome occurring in the blood of man, as a typical trypanosome **(trypanomastigote form),** in other tissues as **Leishmania (amastigote form)** whereas in insects, it occurs as **leishmania,** crithidia and metacyclic trypanosomes infective to man. **T. cruzi** an be cultivated in Novy, MacNeal, and Nicolle (N.N.N.) medium.

Life-cycle requires two hosts (man and reduviid bug). The bug **(Triatoma infestans)** ingests trypanosomes, while biting an infected man, which are transformed into amastigote forms which multiply by **binary fission,** and later transformed into epimastigote forms which migrate to the hind gut, multiply by **longitudinal fission** and transform into metacyclic forms which are excreted in the feces of bug. This is the development at the posterior station in the bug.

These metacyclic forms (infective to man) when rubbed into the wound made by the bug, invade the adipose cells of subcutaneous tissue of man, transform into amastigote, promastigote, epimastigote which at last transform into trypomastigote forms which are liberated into the blood of man.

In Chagas disease, primary lesion appears in the skin which is known as "chagoma" which produces oedema by blocking lymphatic capillaries.

Chagas disease occurs in two forms :

(1) **acute form** is common in children with fever lasting for thirty days, swollen face with oedema of eyelids (Romana's sign), keratitis.

(2) **chronic form** is common in adults and is characterised by the disturbance of cardiac rhythm. There is paraplegia, diplegia, spastic paralysis. When motor centres are affected there may be cardiomyopathy complication.

In the laboratory, the infection can be diagnosed by the demonstration of **T. cruzi** and antibodies in the blood. If the blood is negative, guinea pigs can be inoculated for the presence of **T. cruzi** in guinea pig blood. Xenodiagnosis can be done by allowing trypanosome-free laboratory bred triatomids to bite the individuals suspected for the disease. Metacyclic trypanosomes can be detected in the intestinal content of the bug.

Destruction of bugs, avoiding the bug bite, vaccination can control the infection.

Genus Leishmania

SUMMARY

It includes three species :

(a) **Leishmania donovani** which causes Kala azar;

(b) **L. tropica** causes Oriental sore;

(c) **L. braziliensis** causes mucocutaneous leishmaniasis.

Leishmania donovani

Leishman discovered **L. donovani** from spleen smear of a dead soldier at Dum Dum (Kolkata) India; later Donovan reported from Madras (now Chennai).

Though it is common in other countries; in India eastern India–Assam, Bengal, Bihar, Orissa, Madras and eastern Uttar Pradesh, it is often reported.

Leishmania (amastigote form) live in reticulo-endothelial cells of man.

Morphologically, **Leishmania** has two stages :

1. Amastigote (Leishmania) in man; 2. Promastigote (Leptomonas) in sand fly and cultures.

1. **Leishmania** It is an ovoidal body living in mononucleus or polymorphonuclear leucocytes of man. It has a parabasal body (rod-like body) and a delicate filament extending to the anterior tip.
2. **Leptomonas** is long, slender and spindle-shaped with a single flagellum and can be grown on NNN medium.

In their life-cycle, metacyclic; trypanosomes are engulfed by macrophages when they enter into human body after infected sand fly bite. After multiplication by binary fission in the macrophages, they enter into blood circulation, after these host macrophages are destroyed and are drawn up by sand fly during blood meal.

In the intestine of sand fly, they transform into leptomonas forms, which by their longitudinal fission, divide into numerosis leptomonas and migrate into pharynx of the fly. This is known as "development at anterior station". Then they are transmitted by the bite of the infected sand fly to man. Thus the cycle is repeated.

Metacyclic trypanosomes, engulfed by macrophages, metamorphose into Leishmania within the host cells. These parasitised macrophages are carried away from the skin to the viscera by blood stream. In spleen or liver, Leishmania are taken by Kupffer's cells in liver or fixed macrophages and they multiply in these cells and destroy them. These are called as **"kala azar bodies"**. Erythrocytes production is diminished with ensuing anemia when bone marrow is involved.

After an incubation period of 2-4 months, the symptoms (malaise, headache, fever, enlargement of spleen, acute abdominal pain, pigmented, **"darkened"**, rough, dry skin) are observed. Death may be due to complications (tuberculosis, dysentery, pneumonia).

Diagnosis of Kala azar can be done in the laboratory by

(a) Direct method (Demonstration of **L. donovani** in blood or biopsy);

(b) Indirect method (blood count or serology).

Supportive and specific treatment should be undertaken. The infection can be controlled by :

1. Destruction of sand fly by insecticides, 2. Sleeping rooms should be above the ground floor; 3. House should be well lit and ventilated. 4. Mosquito net should be used, 5. All human cases should be treated with effective drug.

Dermal leishmanoid

It is a non-ulcerative cutaneous lesion. It develops in 10 per cent cases of Kala azar after completion of antimony treatment. Skin infection may persist when visceral infection disappears. This lesion may develop also in spontaneously cured Kala azar. It is very common in endemic areas of Kala azar (Assam, West Bengal, Tamil Nadu).

Clinically, the lesions are of three types :

1. Depigmented macules appearing on the face; trunk, extremities.
2. Erythematous patches on the nose, cheek having butterfly distribution.
3. Yellowish pink nodules on the skin, face, eyes, rarely tongue do not ulcerate as in the Oriental sore.

L. donovani can be demonstrated in the smear of the nodular lesion.

This condition can be treated with double dose of antimony.

Leishmania tropica

It was first observed in the tissue of a Delhi boil in Kolkata. It causes cutaneous leishmaniasis or Delhi boil or Oriental sore in man and is distributed in Sri Lanka, Pakistan, Western and West northern India. Oriental sore is limited to the dry parts of India, whereas Kala azar to the moist eastern parts of India. This parasite resides in the capillary endothelial cells of the affected area of the skin, but is not found in the blood. Leishmania identical to **L. tropica** causes Oriental sore in dogs in Mumbai, so it is a parasite of both dog and man and can be grown in NNN medium.

Its life cycle in man and sandflies is similar to that of **L. donovani** except that it does not invade the viscera, but is confined only to reticulo-endothelial cells of skin. It occurs in both Leishmania and Leptomonas forms.

Skin containing numerous parasites breaks down to produce a crateriform lesion with a ulcer at the centre and an indurated periphery. Secondary bacterial infection is common—fever, chills and inflammation are the clinical symptom.

In the laboratory, it can be diagnosed by demonstration of **L. tropica** in the smear prepared from the punctured edge of the ulcer. As **L. tropica** cannot live with bacteria, the scraping from the floor of the ulcer will be negative. They can be cultivated in NNN medium. Skin test (Montenegro reaction) can also be used in the diagnosis.

It can be treated with antimony and can be controlled by following the same prophylactic methods for **L. tropica, L. donovani.**

Leishmania braziliensis

It causes muco-cutaneous Leishmaniasis in man in America, Argentina. Morphologically, it is identical with **L. tropica** and **L. donovani.** These three Leishmania have distinct agglutination and complement fixation reaction, though they are similar in all other characteristics.

QUESTION (Q) – ANSWER (A)

Mastigophora

Q. Define Mastigophora.

Ans. Mastigophora are single celled animals with flagella. They are flagellate protozoa.

Q. What is flagellum (pleural — flagella) ?

Ans. It is a long, delicate thread-like extension of the cytoplasm. It is responsible for motility.

Q. How are these mastigophora (flagellates) classified ?

Ans. They are classified according to their habitat into intestinal, oral, genital, blood and tissue flagellates.

Giardia lamblia

Q. Where do Giardia lamblia live ?

Ans. G. lamblia lives in the duodenum and upper part of jejunum of man.

Q. Enumerate the stages of G. lamblia.

Ans. G. lamblia has 1. Trophozoite, and 2. Cystic stages.

Q. How many flagella do G. lamblia have ?

Ans. Four pairs of flagella arise from ventral side of the body.

Q. Where is sucking disc (concave notch) present in G. lamblia and what is its function ?

Ans. It is ventrally present and attaches to the convex surface of the intestinal epilthelial cells.

Q. How many nuclei are present in trophozoite, immature and mature cyst of G. lamblia ?

Ans. Its trophozoite has 2 nuclei, immature cyst has two nuclei, whereas mature one has four nuclei.

Genus trichomonas

Q. How many additional flagellum are present in Trichomonas ?

Ans. Only one additional flagellum is present.

Q. How is Genus trichomonas classified and on what basis ?

Ans. On the basis of their habitats, they are classified into **Trichomonas vaginalis; 2. T. hominis; 3. T. tenax.**

Q. In what stage it occurs ?

Ans. It occurs only in Trophozoite stage.

Trichomonas vaginalis

Q. What is cylostome and its function ?

Ans. It is a cleft-like structure (depression); cytostome helps to feed on the mucosal surface of the vagina, ingests bacteria and leucocytes.

Q. What are the pathological changes produced by T. vaginal is ?

Ans. Produced by T. vaginalis. They are degeneration, desquamation and leucocytic inflammation of the vaginal epihelium.

Q. What is the colour of vaginal discharge, its content and its effects ?

Ans. Its colour is greenish or yellow, it contains **T. vaginalis** and leucocytes. It is extremely irritating — causing itching, excoriation.

Q. How can T. vaginalis infection be diagnosed in the laboratory ?

Ans. It can be diagnosed by demonstration of **T. vaginalis** in urine and vaginal secretion and by serology.

Q. How can its spread be controlled ?

Ans. It can be controlled by avoiding sexual intercourse with infected individual.

Genus Trpanosoma

Q. What is Trypanosoma ?

Ans. It is a flagellate blood protozoon.

Q. How many flagella do they have ?

Ans. They have only a single free flagellum.

Q. In what stage of infection volutin granules appear in Trypanosoma ?

Ans. The volutin granules appear in chronic stage of infection and relapsed cases.

Q. Enumerate human pathogenic trypanosomes.

Ans. Human pathogenic trypanosomes are classified into :

1. **Trypanosoma brucei — rhodesiensise — gambiense** group causing African trypanosomiasis.
2. **T. cruzi** causing South American trypanosomiasis.

Trypanosoma gambiense

Q. In what stage is T. gambiense found in cerebrospinal fluid ?

Ans. It is found after cerebral symptoms.

Q. Name the definite host and intermediate host involved in the life cycle of T. gambiense.

Ans. Man is definite host, Glossina fly or tse tse fly is the invertebrate intermediate host.

Q. Which forms of T. gambiense are infective to man ?

Ans. Metacyclic forms are infective to man.

Q. Where does T. gambiense live in man and how does it multiply ?

Ans. It lives in blood of man and it multiplies by longitudinal binary fission in the blood.

Q. Describe the multiplication of T. gambiense in intermediate host.

Ans. After ingestion of **T. gambiense** trypanosomes by fly bite, these flagellates reach the intestine of fly, multiply in the lumen, **not intracellularly,** and transform into crithidial forms which migrate to salivary gland of fly for further development into metacyclic forms which are infective to man. This type of development in the fly is known as development at anterior station as in case of sand fly (intermediate host of **L. donovani**).

Q. What is trypanosomal chancre ?

Ans. At the site of glossina fly bite, an initial (indurated, elevated painful to touch) trypanosomal chancre develops.

Q. When does sleeping sickness stage of infection develop ?

Ans. This stage develops when the nervous system is affected.

Q. Describe the symptoms of sleeping sickness.

Ans. Severe headache, mental dullness, apathy, disclination to work, sleepiness, becomes so pronounced that patient cannot be aroused even to take food — convulsion and ultimate death are the last symptoms.

Q. How to diagnose the disease in the laboratory ?

Ans. The infection can be diagnosed by microscopic examination of stained blood, lymph node bone marrow, cerebrospinal fluid; by cultivation in NNN medium, animal inoculation and by serological tests.

Q. How is this disease treated and controlled ?

Ans. The disease is treated by effective drug and can be controlled by destruction of vector (glossina fly), isolation of infected individuals.

Trypanosoma cruzi

Q. How can T. cruzi be differentiated from T. gambiense morphologically in stained smear under microscope ?

Ans. T. cruzi has a characteristic C-shape, whereas **T. gambiense** is elongated, spindle shaped.

Q. Name the intermediate host of T. cruzi.

Ans. Reduviid bug **(Triatoma infestans)** is the intermediate host of **T. cruzi** in which amastigote, epimastigote, metacyclic trypanosome forms are found.

Q. In which life cycle of Trypanosome, epimastigote form is found in both the hosts ?

Ans. In life cycle of **T. cruzi.**

Q. In which host of the life cycle of T. cruzi, a mastigote, promastigote, epimastigote forms are found ?

Ans. All these three forms are found in vertebrate definite host (man).

Q. What is Chagoma ?

Ans. It is a characteristic primary lesion in the skin of Chagas' disease caused by **T. cruzi.**

Q. What is Romana's sign ?

Ans. Romana's sign is usually found in acute form of Chagas' disease in children and is characterised by high fever, swollen face, marked oedema of eyelids and keratitis.

Q. When paraplegia, diplegia and spastic paralysis occur in chronic form of Chagas disease ?

Ans. When motor centres are destroyed.

Q. What is xenodiagnosis ?

Ans. It is employed by allowing trypanosoma-free laboratory bred triatoma (bug) to bite suspected individuals for Chagas' disease. If trypanosomes are recovered from the intestinal content of bug, then it is positive for Chagas' disease.

Genus leishmania

Q. What is Leishmania ?

Ans. It is a tissue flagellate.

Q. How many species of Leishmania cause disease in man ?

Ans. 1. **Leishmania** donovani causes Kala azar.

2. **L. tropica** causes Oriental sore.

3. **L. braziliensis** causes mucocutaneous Leishmaniasis.

Leishmania donovani

Q. Where was L. donovani first discovered in India ?

Ans. L. donovani was first discovered in the spleen smears of a dead soldier at Dum Dum, Kolkata, later it was reported from Chennai as it is limited to the most eastern parts of India.

Q. How was L. donovani named ?

Ans. It was named in honour of Leishman and Donovan (discoverers).

Q. In how many stages L. donovani occurs in its life-cycle ?

Ans. L. donovani occurs in two stages : (1) Aflagellar Leishman (amastigote) stage in man and reservoir.

(2) Leptomonas (promastigote) in the sand fly.

Q. Where Leishmania lives in man ?

Ans. It lives intracellularly in polymorphs of man and is an ovoidal body.

Q. Where are Leptomonas found in its life cycle ?

Ans. They are found in the intestine of sand fly, later migrate to the salivary gland and buccal cavity.

Q. Why should leptomonas migrate to salivary gland ?

Ans. Because they migrate to salivary gland for further development to infect man.

Q. Why is this type of development called "anterior station development" ?

Ans. Because it develops at salivary gland of sand fly.

Q. What is rosette form ?

Ans. Rosette form occurs when several leptomonas are arranged with their innermost flagella entangled. This form is seen in insect or culture.

Q. Why are leptomonas carried away from the victim's skin after their inoculation into the skin by the bite of infected fly ?

Ans. Leptomonas are set free into the blood stream, after parasitised macrophage are ruptured they are carried from the skin to spleen, liver via blood for their multiplication in fixed macrophages which will be destroyed to produce **"Kala azar bodies"** — later anemia when bone marrow is affected.

Q. Describe in brief the clinical features of Kala azar.

Ans. Symptoms are fever, malaise, headache, abdominal pain, oedema of skin, emaciated chest, dysentery, skin is dry, rough, **"darkened"** death is due to complication (tuberculosis, dysentery).

Q. How will you diagnose Kala azar in the laboratory ?

Ans. Kala azar can be diagnosed directly and indirectly : In direct method, by demonstration of **L. donovani** in blood smear, culture, biopsy; in indirect method by blood count, serology.

Q. How can Kala azar be treated ?

Ans. Treatment can be specific and supportive. Control by destroying sand fly, using mosquito net, sleeping quarter should be above ground floor.

Leishmania tropica

Q. Who first observed L. tropica and where ?

Ans. Cunningham (1885) first observed **L. tropica** in the tissue of Delhi boil in Kolkata.

Q. Where is it confined in India ?

Ans. It is confined in dry parts of India (western and north western India) causing Oriental sore or cutaneous.

Q. How does Leishmaniasis L. tropica differ from L. donovani ?

Ans. Though **L. tropica** is identical to **L. donovani,** it differs mainly by its limiting multiplication in the reticulo-endothelial cells of the skin, not invading into the viscera.

Q. What is Crateriform lesion in Oriental sore and how is it produced ?

Ans. Crateriform lesion is the depressed ulcerated centre covered with granulating tissue and indurated periphery. It is produced when skin cells containing a large number of **L. tropica** breakdown to produce this lesion.

Q. Describe the clinical features.

Ans. Symptoms are fever, chills and inflammation. A reddish papule develops first, later transforms into shallow ulcer.

Q. How can Oriental sore be diagnosed in the laboratory ?

Ans. L. tropica can be demonstrated microscopically in the stained smear prepared from the punctured indurated edge of the sore, **NOT** in the **blood** smear.

Q. Why is scraping of the floor of the ulcer negative ?

Ans. Because **L. tropica** cannot exist along with the bacteria in the ulcer.

Q. When smear from the floor of smear is negative where L. tropica can be demonstrated ?

Ans. It can be demonstrated in the biopsy material of Lymphoid under ulcer.

Dermal Leishmanoid

Q. Define Dermal leishmanoid and how is it developed ?

Ans. It is non-ulcerative cutaneous lesion which develop in 10% Kala azar patients after completion of antimony treatment.

Q. Where is it distributed in India ?

Ans. It is common in endemic areas of Kala azar (Assam, Tamil Nadu, West Bengal).

Q. How can it be diagnosed and treated ?

Ans. It can be diagnosed by demonstration of Leishmania in the nodule and treated with pentavalent antimony.

Leishmania braziliensis

Q. How is the name L. braziliensis derived ?

Ans. It is so named because Lindenberg (1909) first found Leishmania in patient's ulcer in Brazil.

Q. What disease is caused by L. braziliensis in man ?

Ans. It causes muco-cutaneous leishmaniasis in man.

Q. How can all these three species (L. donovani, L. tropica, L. braziliensis) be distinguished as they are morphologically identified ?

Ans. They can be differentiated by agglutination and complement fixation reactions.

Q. Among all these three species of Leishmania, which one can be cultivated in chorio-allantoic membrane (CAM) of the chick embryo ?

Ans. L. braziliensis can be grown in CAM of chick embryo, though all species can be grown in NNN medium.

Q. Among all these species of Leishmania, which species can also be transmitted by direct contact ?

Ans. Only **L. braziliensis** can be transmitted by direct contact, though it is transmitted by sand fly as in other cases.

Q. Name a common skin test for all these three species.

Ans. Montenegro intradermal test is common to all.

Q. Where is the primary lesion commonly found in mucocutaneous leishmaniasis and how does it heal up ?

Ans. The primary lesion is mostly found on the ear lobe and it tends to be self-healing in six months.

Chapter 4
SUMMARY

Sporozoa are protozoa showing no locomotion. They produce spores and have a life cycle characterised by alternation of generation, one sexual and one asexual occurring completely in one host **(Eimeria, Isopora)** or an alternation of host **(Plasmodium).**

Genus Isopora

Isorpora belli and **Isopora hominis.** They produce oocysts and sporocysts. Oocysts are elongated, or ovoidal, have two layers; inner layer is thin and outer layer is hard. At one end, they have a small micropyle and have two sporocysis with four sporozoites which sporocysis are long, crescent shaped with a single nucleus. It causes self-limited disease in man.

Genus Eimeria

This genus produces oocysts containing four sporocysts. Each sporocyst contains two sporozoites (schizogony). It is an animal parasite causing coccidiosis (common disease) in calf, human infection is accidental after ingestion of contaminated food with oocysts of Eimeria and self-limited.

Genus Plasmodium

This genus consists of the following species :

1. **Plasmodium vivax** causing vivax or tertian malaria,
2. **P. ovale** causing ovale malaria,
3. **P. falciparum** causes malignant tertian or falciparum malaria.

Laveran (1880) first observed **P. vivax,** Romanowsky (1891) developed staining method for malarial parasites. Big mani et al (1898) described mosquito life cyle of human plasmodium.

Endemic areas of these plasmodia is tropical zone **P. falciparum** is common in tropics and subtropic plasmodia develop in liver cells, reside in red blood cells and they are carried to various organs via blood stream.

Two hosts are required for their life cycle :

1. Man (intermediate host)
2. Mosquito (definite host).

In man, plasmodia reside in hepatic cells and red blood cells and multiply **asexually** (schizogony). Man is also intermediate host for hydatid disease (caused by tapeworm). In mosquito (female anopheles definite host) plasmodia multiply **sexually;** male and female gametocytes are ingested by the mosquito from the human blood, of infected man and form zyote in the mosquito intestine after fertilisation, later become ookinete (motile zygote). **After** reaching the salivary gland of mosquito, they liberate sporozoites **infective** to man.

Human cycle

Sporozoites injected by the infected mosquito bite into man enter directly into liver cells (Not RBCs)–pre-erythrocytic schizogony. Macromerozoite re-enter liver cells (in P. vivax, P. malariae, P. ovale – **there is Relapse**); No relapse in P. falciparum. Micro-merozoites enter RBCs, develop into trophozoites, schizonts, merozoites (erythrocytic schizogony) then at last into gametocytes (gametogony) which are ingested by mosquito.

The individuals who harbour these gametocytes are called 'carriers'.

Phanerozoites are merozoites liberated from the liver cycle.

Sporozoites are infective forms of malarial parasites. Their shapes vary from narrow curved (vivax), thick (malariae), sickle-shaped (falciparum). They have apical cup, mitochondria, paired organelles.

Ookinete is enveloped by two layers : the inner one is smooth, the outer one is corrugated, has cytoplasmic inclusions (mitochondria, black pigment granule).

Malarial parasite feeds on its host cytoplasm by pyknocytosis; it gets energy by phosphorylation of glucose; oxidative process is maintained by the oxyhaemoglobin of erythrocytes. The globin of hemoglobin is split by enzymes into amino acids and peptides to form the parasite's protein. Its metabolites are derived from the hemoglobin and blood plasma.

The malarial parasite is malnourished when the host is starved. Restriction of thiamine, riboflavin, biotin may inhibit the growth of their parasite. **P. falciparum** heavily infect West African children restricted to a milk diet.

Glucose 6 phosphate dehydrogenase deficient (G6 PD) trait may confer some protection to against **P. falciparum** infection.

Sickle cell anemia trait may also cause resistance to **P. falciparum** infection as this parasite cannot utilise the abnormal hemoglobin (rod-shaped masses) which distorted blood cells into sickle-like shape.

Thalassemia hemoglobin and hemoglobin E can provide protection against **P. vivax** and human fetal hemoglobin against all plasmodia.

P. vivax

Vivax (Latin *vivere*—to live) **P. vivax** has worldwide distribution and is common in India.

Gametes. Its microgamete penetrates into the small projection of the macrogamete and forms ookinete. This process takes ten minutes to one hour in the mosquito's gut.

Schizogony forms of **P. vivax** in peripheral blood after 48 hours after staining :

Trophozoites (ring forms), 2-5 µm, cytoplasm opposite to nucleus is thicker,

Growing form irregular with a vacuole, actively amoeboid.

Schizont (mature) 9-10 µm, regular, completely fills enlarged RBCs.

Merozoites 12-24 arranged in an irregular grape like cluster.

Pigment. Yellowish brown fine granules. Infected RBCs are enlarged, pale, Schuffner's dots present.

Gametocyte is spherical much larger than a RBC. Cytoplasm of female ganetocyte is blue, nucleus is small and compact. Cytoplasm of male is pale blue, its nucleus is large and diffuse.

Plasmodium falciparum

The name falciparum (Latin, falx, a sickle) is derived from sickle shaped gametocyte of **P. falciparum.** Its distribution is worldwide. It is very common in India.

Gametes Microgamete is spherical, with its nucleus approaching the edge of the parasite forming a protruberance into which a microgamete will penetrate. Sporozoites are sickle shaped.

Schizogony forms of **P. falciparum** in the peripheral blood after 48 hours (after staining) : Trophozoite (ring form) 1.25 µ m-1.5 µm. Cytoplasm fine, regular **accole form** nucleus growing form assumes compact form, pigments collect into a single mass early.

Schizont (mature) 4.5 µm-5 µm, fills two third of RBCs which are not enlarged.

Merozoites 18-24 or more, arranged in a grape like cluster.

Pigments are dark brown or blackish, (one or two solid blocks).

Infected RBCs are unaltered, crenated, reddish violet colour Maurer's dots.

Gametocytes are spherical, much larger than RBCs. Host cells are hardly recognisable cytoplasm of female gametocyte is blue, nucleus is small and compact.

Cytoplasm of male gametocyte is pale blue, nucleus large and diffuse.

Plasmodium malariae

Schizogony forms of **P. malariae** of the peripheral blood.

Trophozoites same as P. vivax.

Growing forms are band-like, slightly amoeboid, their vacuoles disappear early.

Schizont (mature) measures 5-7 µm, regular, almost fills a normal sized RBC.

Merozoites are 6-12, arranged around a central mass of pigment like a "daisy" or rosette. Pigments are dark brown, coarse granules. Infected RBCs are not enlarged, not pale and have no dots.

Gametocyte is round, oval, size of RBC. The cytoplasm of male is pale blue; its nucleus is large and diffuse; whereas that of female is blue and its nucleus is large and diffuse.

Plasmodium ovale

Its name is derived from its shape—ovale. Its schizogony forms :

Trophozoite (ring form) is same as **P. malariae.** Growing form has no ribbon shape, slightly amoeboid.

Schizont (mature) is 6.2 µm, fills three quarters o RBC which is slightly enlarged.

Merozoite 6-12, is irregularly arranged.

Pigment is dark yellowish brown, coarser than **P. vivax.** Infected RBCs are enlarged, oval with James's dots. Gametocyte is oval, size of RBC. Host cell is slightly enlarged with James's dots. Male gametocyte cytoplasm is stained pale blue by Leishman stain, its nucleus is large and diffuse; whereas that of female one is stained blue, its nucleus is small and compact.

Pathogenicity of Plasmodium

Intermittent fevers caused by plasmodium infection are called "malaria" (Lal. ***mala*** and ***aria*** means "bad air".)

Each species causes characteristic fever

1. Quotidian fever (daily fever) is caused by vivax and malariae malaria.
2. Tertian fever (every third day) occurs in **P. falciparum** malaria.
3. Quartan fever (recurring every fourth day) is caused by malariae malaria.

Sporozoites injected into blood by mosquito bite leave the blood stream and enter the liver cells without any host reaction. **Micromerozoites** liberated from the liver cells after schizogony enter into red cells and pathogenic effects will become noticeable.

The infection may cause disturbance of oxygen usage which may occur in two ways : (1) Oxygen supply may be reduced below physiological level resulting into a state of **anoxic anemia**; (2) because of pathological changes in the metabolising cells, the host may not utilise adequate oxygen supply which is responsible for a state of **cytotoxic anoxia.**

Acute severe malaria (algid malaria) may cause a state of shock in which there will be local anoxic anemia with liver or kidney damage. The incubation period is 10-14 days in **P. vivax, P. ovale** and **P. falciparum;** whereas in **P. malariae,** it is 18 days to 6 weeks (longest period).

Fever is main clinical features and has three stages : cold, hot, and sweating stage. Total duration of fever is 6-10 hours.

During schizogomy of **Plasmodium** in red cells, these RBCs break-down and cause microcytic hypochromic type anemia with iron deficiency which occurs after paroxysomes.

Splenomegaly is a main sign showing a steady enlargement of spleen; after 2 weeks, it is much enlarged and palpable.

Shivering with high fever (104°F), headache, muscular pain, are main symptoms. **Pernicious symptoms** (coma, convulsion, cardiac failure) are frequently observed in falciparum malaria. Because of its protean manifestations, malaria may simulate other diseases.

Blackwater fever develops in falciparum malaria due to repeated falciparum infection which is inadequately treated with quinine.

Congenital malaria is due to intra-uterine transmission of malaria and is common in infected mother, whose placentae are heavily loaded with **P. falciparum.**

Congenital malaria is acquired during parturition. Laboratory diagnosis can be done by :

Direct detection of Plasmodium in stained blood smears is an easy accurate method; when parasites are scanty, thick smears are prepared, while thin smears can be used to identify plasmodium species.

(2) Various serological methods :

Treatment may be **curative** or **prophylactic** :

(a) **Curative ;** Padbhanaban (2005) obtained one of the ingredients of Turmeric (Haldi;-hindi word) found to be effective against human malaria it is a very cheap anti-malarial drug still under trial.

(b) **Prophylactic. Anti-malarial vaccine** prepared by DNA recombinant technique is proved successful in animal experimentation and is under human trial (Padbhanaban, 2005).

Babesia

It is a protozoan parasite affecting mostly cattle however few human cases were reported. This protozoa is similar to **P. falciparum** and found in the blood smear. Babesia is pear shaped, divides within red cells and no pigment. Complement fixation and latex agglutination tests can detect Babesia antibodies. Chloroquine has some value in human babesiosis.

Toxoplasma gondi

Its name is derived from gondi (gondi means a small rodent). It has a worldwide distribution.

It is an obligatory, intracellular, **coccidial** parasite occurring in two forms :

1. Extracellular form is sickle, crescent shaped
2. Intrcellular form has mitochondria, conoid.

Its life cycle may be (a) enteric, and (b) exo-enteric.

(a) Enteric cyclic occurs in the epithelial cells of ileum of the cat (i.e. schizogony, gametogony). Oocysts similar to those of Isopora may be detected in the infected cat's faeces.

(b) Exo-enteric cycle. Isopora (oocysts containing two sporozoites) are excrted in the cat's faeces. Sporozoites liberated from the oocysts infect mucous membrane of the ileum and carried by blood to various organs (brain, eyes, lymph node, liver, heart, placenta of pregnant uterus where they produce **pseudocysts.** The parasites inside these pseudocysts are known as **endozoites** which escape to continue their multiplication in the cells and cause damage to the tissues and transform into **tissue cysts.** Both pseudo-cysts and tissue cysts are infective to man and animals.

T. gondi has predilection for reticuloendothelial cells causing **lymphadenopathy;** for central nervous system causing encephalitis, chorioretinitis; for heart (cardiomegaly, myocarditis); for uterus (abortion). Clinically, toxoplasmosis may be congenital or acquired :

(1) **Congenital toxoplasmosis** is common in children characterised by encephalitis, chorioretinitis, hydrocephalus, mental retardation and convulsion; enlarged liver and spleen. This infection passes from the infected mother in late pregnancy through the placenta to the foetus.

(2) **Acquired toxoplasmosis** is often fatal and very rare in adults (prolonged remittent fever with erythematous rash).

Laboratory diagnosis : Complement fixation test, dye test of Sabin and Feldman are useful in addition to radiological diagnosis.

Treatment is not satisfactory and the prevention can be done by the proper disposal of cat's faeces.

Sarcoystis lindermanni

Linderman first discovered **Sarcocystis lindermanni** (which was so named in honour of its discoverer). This parasite is worldwide in distribution. In India (Mumbai) only one case (40 year old labourer) was reported.

It is a cylindrical, elongated body lying in the affected muscle, contains crescent shaped spores known as "Miscsher's tubes". Each tube contains "Rainey's corpuscle" or spores. Known as trophozoites (banana shaped).

Man gets infection by ingestion of infected meat or drink containing the trophozoites which pass through the intestinal wall and blood to striated muscle where they produce round bodies enclosed in acyst.

Sercocystin (toxic by product) affects CNS, heart, adrenals and intestinal wall. The infection in animals is fatal. Mischer's tubes do not produce serious injury. Best method of diagnosis is the demonstration of Micscher's tube in the affected muscles. Serology can also be useful. Treatment is non-specific and the infection can be controlled by avoiding the ingestion of food contaminated with the trophozoites.

Pneumocystis carinii

It causes interstitial plasma cell pneumonia in suckling infants. It is a single cell parasite with foamy appearance found in the alveoli of lung enclosing the spores.

The sporozoites after escaping from the spores enter into gut wall. After repeated schizogony, the merozoites spread to kidney, lungs where sporogony occurs. Oocyst contains eight sporozoites. Clinically the disease is acute. Death may be due to asphyxia.

Detection of this parasite is the best method of laboratory diagnosis, in addition to radiology and serology can be used. **Pentamidine isothionate** is very effective and there is no specific preventive measure.

QUESTION (Q) – ANSWER (A)

Q. What is sporozoa ?

Ans. Sporozoa is a non-motile protozoa which produces spores.

Q. Why sporozoa requires an alternation of generation ?

Ans. Because they multiply both sexually and asexually in their life-cycle.

Q. Name a species of sporozoa which requires an alternation of hosts for its life cycle.

Ans. Plasmodium requires an alternation of host (man—intermediate host; mosquito—definite host).

Q. For what multiplication Plasmodium requires mosquito ?

Ans. Plasmodium requires mosquito for sexual multiplication.

Q. What is sporogony ?

Ans. Sporogony is sexual multiplication which occurs after fertilisation of female gametes by male gametes in the gut of mosquito where oocysts are formed.

Q. What is schizogony ?

Ans. Schizogony is asexual cycle of development, multiplies by segmentation in RBCs in man (intermediate host).

Q. Differentiate Isospora and Eimeria.

Ans. Eimeria is identified by its oocyst containing four sporocysts, each one has two sporozoites.

Isospora is identified by its oocyst containing two sporocysts with four sporozoites (in each sporocysts which undergoes schizogony — Trophozoite, schizont, merozoites) and, eventually, sporogony with the development of oocysts.

Q. Describe in brief the clinical features of Isospora and Eimeria.

Ans. Isopora causes anorexia, nausea, abdominal pain, and diarrhoea. Human infection is self-limited. Eimeria causes coccidiosis (common) in calf and is found in the human stool during its transit after accidental ingestion.

Plasmodia

Q. Who recommended that the term malarial parasites should be restricted to the family plasmodiae.

Ans. World Health Organisation (WHO).

Q. How many species of Plasmodium cause malaria ?

Ans. There are 4 species : **Plasmodium vivax; Plasmodium falciparum, P. ovale** and **P. malariae.**

Q. Who discovered first the following : (1) P. vivax;

(2) Staining method for plasmodium

(3) Mosquito cycle of human plasmodia; avian plasmodia.

Ans. (1) **P. vivax** by Laveran (1880)

(2) Staining method by Romanowsky (1891)

(3) Mosquito cycle of human plasmodia by Bigmani et al (1898)

(4) Mosquito cycle of avian plasmodia by Ross in Kolkata (India).

Q. Where do plasmodia undergo a development and reside ?

Ans. Plasmodia undergo a development stage in the parenchyma cells of the liver, reside in RBCs of man, and are carried via blood-stream to the various organs.

Chapter 5

SUMMARY

QUESTION (Q) – ANSWER (A)

Q. Name two diseases in which man acts as intermediate host.

Ans. 1. Malaria; (2) Hydatid disease.

Q. Why the mosquito represents the definite host of malarial parasites ?

Ans. Because of the sexual method reproduction of malarial parasites.

Q. What forms of plasmodia are required to initiate the mosquito cycle ?

Ans. To initiate the mosquito cycle, sexual forms (male and female gametocytes) are first developed in the human host and they are transferred to definite host **(female anopheles mosquito)** where they develop further and transform into sporozoites **infective** to man.

Q. Why only female Anopheles mosquito can transmit malaria ?

Ans. Because they have stout proboscis which can pierce the skin of man like a needle.

Q. Why proboscis of female mosquito is stout ?

Ans. Because of the presence of well developed serrated maxillae and mandibles in the proboscis.

Q. Why male anopheles mosquito cannot bite man ?

Ans. Because the proboscis of male is not stout, but it is flexible, hence it cannot pierce through the skin.

Q. How is host specificity observed in plasmodium ?

Ans. Host specificity is determined by the presence or absence of certain amino acids in the mosquito required by plasmodium for its sexual development.

Q. How many stages of human cycle are involved and cite them ?

Ans. There are four stages.

They are : 1. Pre-erythrocytic schizogony;

2. Erythrocytic schizogony; 3. Gametogony;

4. Exo-erythrocytic schizogony.

Q. Why do not the sporozoites (infective forms) enter directly into RBCs to initiate the infection ?

Ans. Because they have to undergo the development stage in the parenchyma cells of liver (tissues of man). This is known as **pre-erythrocytic schizogony.** After this schizogony the merozoites are liberated.

Q. What are cryptozoites ?

Ans. Merozoites liberated from liver are called Cryptozoites or phanerozoites (both micro-merozoite and macro-merozoite).

Q. What is the main function of cryptozoites or merozoites ?

Ans. Merozoites give rise to micromerozoites and macromerozoites.

Q. What is the role of macromerozoite and macromerozoite ?

Ans. Micromerozoites enter RBCs to initiate the infection, whereas macromerozoites re-enter the liver cells for exo-erythrocytic schizogony which is responsible for **relapse** of vivax, ovale and malariae malaria.

Q. What is Relapse ? Why there is no relapse in P. falciparum ?

Ans. P. vivax, P. ovale and P. malariae pre-erythrocytic schizogony persists in its form of a focal liver cycle (tissue phase) which is necessary for Relapse of malaria.

In case of **P. falciparum,** there is no relapse because it has no exo-erythrocytic schizogony or liver cycle.

Q. When the blood is sterile in malaria ?

Ans. The blood is sterile when the parasites (plasmodia) are not found in the peripheral blood during pre-erythrocytic schizogony.

Q. When is there no clinical manifestations and pathological damage in malaria ?

Ans. When plasmodia develop inside the liver.

Q. Why is liver cycle in malaria necessary ?

Ans. Liver cycle is necessary for the development of micromerozoites which can only enter into RBCs to initiate the infection. No micromerozoites if no liver cycle.

Q. How many stages of plasmodium are seen in the RBCs during erythrocytic schizogony?

Ans. Three stages (trophozoites, schizont and merozoites) are seen in erythrocytic schizogony.

Q. When does clinical attack of malaria (overt malaria) occur ?

Ans. Clinical attack of malaria occurs during the parasite multiplication in erythrocytic phase.

Q. When plasmodia have the urge for sexual multiplication ?

Ans. They have the urge for sexual multiplication when they are exhausted with asexual multiplication and when there is spontaneous destruction of the parasites (plasmodia).

Q. After erythrocytic schizogony, why some of the merozoites do not develop directly into trophozoites ?

Ans. Because some of the merozoites transform into sexual forms which are capable of sexual reproduction outside the human host. These forms are known as gametocytes. These gametocytes are required to propagate and continue their life cycle in the mosquito. This stage is called as **Gametogony.**

Q. What is carrier ?

Ans. Individual who harbour these gametocytes is called as "carrier".

Q. Why pre-erythrocytic schizogony disappears ?

Ans. Once the merozoites enter the erythrocyte they never reinvade the liver.

Q. What is exflagellation in mosquito cycle ?

Ans. Exflagellation is a process of development in which the male microgametocyte gives rise to form to eight thread-like filamentous structures known as microgametes which move toward female by the process of chemotaxis.

Q. Where male gamete will get attached to the female one ?

Ans. Male gamete will get attached to the site of projection which is at the periphery of the female.

Q. What is zygote ?

Ans. Zygote is formed when male gamete penetrates into the projection of female and fertilises thus forming zygote.

Q. What is ookinete ?

Ans. It is a small zygote with pseudopodium; it enters into the mucosa of mosquito intestine, it forms oocysts which burst to give rise to sporozoites.

Q. What is sporozoite ?

Ans. Sporozoite is a sickle shaped single-nucleated structure liberated from the oocyst and is spread throughout the body of mosquito except ovaries. It is infective to man and is injected to man by mosquito bite.

Q. When is plasmodium malnourished ?

Ans. When the host is starved.

Q. When is the growth of malarial parasites inhibited ?

Ans. The growth of plasmodia is inhibited when the food elements (thiamine, riboflavine, biotin) are restricted.

Q. In which country the children are heavily parasitised by P. falciparum when they are restricted to a milk diet?

Ans. Africa.

Q. What are the traits responsible for the resistance to malaria ?

Ans. They are G6PD deficient trait, sickle cell anemia trait.

Q. How will you differentiate between male and female gametocytes of P. falciparum ?

Ans. The male microgametocyte is more banana shaped than crescentic, is thicker and blunder the female macrogametocytes which stain darker blue with small and compact nucleus.

Q. What is average number of merozoites of P. falciparum and their size inside RBCs ?

Ans. Average number of merozoites is 18-24 inside RBCs. It measures 0.5-0.7 micron in diameter (less than size of bacteria (cocci)).

Q. How is the word "malaria" derived ?

Ans. It is derived from Italian words, ***mala*** and ***aria***, meaning "bad air".

Q. Can you notice host reaction when the destruction of liver cells occurs ?

Ans. Host reaction is most noticeable when the liver cells are destroyed during liver cycle of **Plasmodium.**

Q. When pathogenic effect is significant ?

Ans. The pathogenic effect is significant when the exo-erythrocytic merozoites (micromerozoites) invade RBCs and multiply.

Q. What is a major factor in the pathogenesis of malaria ?

Ans. A major factor is the disturbance in oxygen usage caused by the infection : 1. Oxygen supplies may be reduced; 2. Adequate oxygen supply may not be utilised by the host due to pathological changes in the metabolising cells.

Q. What is algid malaria ?

Ans. Algid malaria is acute severe malaria with low blood pressure, low cardiac output, and vasoconstriction leading to liver or kidney damage with a state of shock.

Q. How many types of fever are common in malaria ?

Ans. There are three types : 1. quotidian, 2. tertian, 3. quartan fever.

Q. What type of anemia develops in malaria ?

Ans. Anemia of the microcytic hypochromic type with iron deficiency develops.

Q. In malaria which organ is much enlarged and palpable after second week of infection ?

Ans. The spleen is much enlarged and palpable after second week (splenomegaly).

Q. Describe in brief the symptoms of malaria.

Ans. Symptoms are : sudden onset; shivering succeeded by fever (104°F), headache, muscular pain, malaise, increased pulse and respiration. In **P. falciparum** malaria, pernicious symptoms (coma, convulsion, cardiac, failure) are observed.

Q. What is Black water fever ?

Ans. It is a manifestation of repeated infections with falciparum malaria inadequately treated with quinine.

Q. What is congenital malaria ?

Ans. It is an intra-uterine transmission of malaria and is common in non-immune mothers whose placentae are heavily parasitised with **P. falciparum schizonts.**

Q. What is connatal malaria ?

Ans. Connatal malaria is malaria acquired by babies during parturition.

Q. What is certain method of laboratory diagnosis of malaria ?

Ans. Certain method is the demonstration of plasmodium in the blood smear under microscope.

Q. When is thick blood smear required ?

Ans. It is required for quick detection of **Plasmodium.**

Q. When is thin blood smear required ?

Ans. It is required for the identification of the species.

Q. When does the detection of plasmodium become difficult ?

Ans. It becomes difficult if the blood films are taken 1. after anti-malarial drug use; 2. during an apyrexial period of **P. falciparum;** 3. during the first 2-3 days of primary infection.

Q. Enumerate the serodiagnostic methods for malaria.

Ans. The serological methods (serology) are complement fixation, slide flocculation, Latex agglutination, indirect haemagglutination and fluorescent antibody tests.

Q. Cite other methods which are under study.

Ans. They are sedimentation, centrifugation, flurochrome, stain, new side angle microscope objectives, new genetic engineering method.

Q. Describe in brief new genetic engineering method of Padmanabhan for detection of P. falciparum.

Ans. Padmanabhan (1989); Indian scientist, Bangalore, can detect very specifically falciparum malaria by using the radioactive chemicals in his genetic engineering method. This method is very accurate and can detect as low as 50 parasites in the blood sample.

Q. How can malaria be treated ?

Ans. Malaria can be treated by

(1) Curative treatment, Chloroquine, Amodiaquine (drug of choice), Mefloquine and Quinine (for drug resistant **P. falciparum** Primaquine can be used to prevent **relapse** in malaria).

(2) **Prophylactic treatment :** Chloroquine, amodiaquine in weekly doses will prevent the acute attack of malaria.

Q. How primaquine can prevent relapse in malaria ?

Ans. Primaquine can prevent relapse in malaria by acting on the exo-erythrocytic phases of the parasites inside the liver. It also acts on the gametocyte but has little action on the erythrocytic stages of the parasites.

Q. What are the recent (2005) findings of malaria treatment by Padmanabhan at Bangalore (India) ?

Ans. (a) Curative treatment of malaria by turmeric (Hindi—***Haldi***) is under experimentation with great hope.

(b) Prophylactic treatment : Anti-malarial vaccine prepared by the use of DNA recombinant technique is very effective in animal experimentation and is under human trial.

Q. How can prophylaxis of malaria be carried out ?

Ans. It can be done by personal prophylaxis and community.

(a) Personal prophylaxis by protection against mosquito by using mosquito net and by systemic anti-malarial drugs.

(b) Community prophylaxis by destruction of mosquito by spraying insecticides; DDT or by the use of larvicides (DDT dissolved in oil) by treating carriers by anti-malarial drugs.

Q. Is there any hope for malarial vaccine in near future ?

Ans. There is a great hope for successful malarial vaccination in near future.

Babesia

Q. What is Babesia ?

Ans. It is a protozoa affecting mostly cattle, very rarely human being; it resembles **P. falciparum** and is found in RBCs. Chloroquine has some value in the treatment of human babesiosis.

Toxoplasma gondii

Q. What is gondii ?

Ans. It is a protozoa affecting small rodent, **gondi.** It is an obligatory, intracellular, **coccidial** parasite.

Q. How many hosts it requires ?

Ans. It requires two hosts : cat and man.

Q. How does man get the infection ?

Ans. Man gets the infection by ingestion of food contaminated with oocysts in cat's faeces, trophozoites liberated from oocyst infect/penetrate into the ileum of man and carried by blood stream to various organs (brain, liver, placenta of woman) which are damaged. It causes abortion in pregnant woman.

Q. How many clinical toxoplasmosis are seen ?

Ans. (a) Congenital; and (b) Acquired toxoplasmosis.

Sarcocystis lindemanni

Q. Where was the parasite reported in India ?

Ans. It was reported in Mumbai (India) in a 40-year old labourer.

Q. How does man get infected ?

Ans. Man gets infection by ingestion of infected meat or drink containing the trophozoites which pass the mucosa of the intestine, enter blood stream and are carried to the striated muscles where they form round bodies enclosed in a cyst which enlarges. Their toxic product, **sarcocystin,** affects CNS, heart and intestine.

Q. How can it be diagnosed and treated ?

Ans. It can be diagnosed by demonstration of Miescher's tube in the affected muscles and there is no specific treatment.

Pneumocystis carinii

Q. Describe in brief P. carinii.

Ans. It resembles a protozoon. It causes interstitial plasma cell pneumonia in suckling infants and is common in AIDS patients as secondary invader. It is enclosed in a sphere which is foamy in appearance in the alveoli of lung. This foamy mass causes asphyxia leading to death. It is diagnosed by detection of **P. carinii** in lung tissue by radiological examination of lung and by complement fixation test. Pentamidine isothionate is effective drug for **P. carinii.**

Chapter 5

SUMMARY

Class Ciliatea

Ciliata are motile protozoa which move with the help of cilia (short hair-like extensions of its cytoplasmic membrane). They are covered with cilia, have two distinct nuclei (large macronucleus and small micronucleus). Their shape is by a cell membrane.

Balantidium coli

Malmstein (1857) first observed this protozoa in two human patients; Panjarathinan (1972) first reported from pig in Pondicherry (India), though this protozoon (**B. coli**) has worldwide distribution. It is the largest protozoon of the large intestine of man, pig. Its trophozoites feed on the intestinal mucosal cells, bacteria and mucus. Pig is the reservoir of **B. coli** and does not suffer from infection. It has two stages : Trophozoites and cysts.

1. Trophozoite is found in acute dysentery patient's stool.
2. Cyst is detected in chronic cases and carriers.

The cyst (infective) ingested by man liberates only one trophozoite which gives rise to two trophozoites. These free trophozoites burrow into the intestinal mucosa with the help of hyaluronidase enzyme and form an **ulcer** with short neck and broad base containing pus and necrotic material. These trophozoites are harmless to pigs as they feed on abundant starchy food in the pig's intestine.

Clinically, dysentery is accompanied by abdominal pain, **tenesmus,** nausea and vomiting. Besides, loss of appetite, headache, insomnia, loss of weight are observed.

Diagnosis can be done by the microscopic demonstration of trophozoites and cysts in the stool.

Carbarsome can be used for human treatment.

Tetracycline, Diiodohydroxyquin can eliminate the parasite.

Prophylaxis. It can be prevented by the methods used for **E. histolytica.**

QUESTION (Q) – ANSWER (A)

Q. What is ciliata ?

Ans. Ciliata are protozoa which move with cilia.

Q. What are cilia ?

Ans. Cilia are short hair-like extensions of cytoplasmic membrane.

Q. How many nuclei do they have ?

Ans. They have two nuclei (large macronucleus and small micronucleus).

Q. Which species of ciliata is pathogenic to man ?

Ans. Balantidium coli is pathogenic to man.

Balantidium coli

Q. Who observed B. coli in man first ?

Ans. Malmstein first observed **B. coli** in man in 1857.

Q. Who first reported B. coli in pig in Pondicherry (India) ?

Ans. Panjarathinam (1972) first reported **B. coli** in pig in Pondicherry (India).

Q. What is the largest protozoon infecting the large intestine of man, pig ?

Ans. B. coli is the largest protozoon of intestine of man, pig.

Q. On what cells trophozoites of B. coli feed ?

Ans. They feed on intestinal cells, bacteria, mucus.

Q. Why pig does not suffer from this infection, though it is reservoir of B. coli ?

Ans. Because **B. coli** feeds on intestinal starchy food, as a result it does not enter the intestine.

Q. How many stages has B. coli ?

Ans. It has two stages : Trophozoite, cyst stage.

Q. Describe Trophozoite of B. coli.

Ans. Trophozoite is oval, covered with cilia. It has two nuclei — cytostome, cytopyge.

Q. Where is the smaller nucleus (micronucleus) of B. coli situated ?

Ans. It is situated in the centre of inner curvature of the large nucleus (macronucleus) of **B. coli.**

Q. What is the function of micronucleus ?

Ans. It is believed to function as kinetic organel and divided first.

Q. What is cytostome ?

Ans. Cytostome is a deep, slightly curved, inverted conical depression situated on one side of the longitudinal axis of the pointed anterior end of **B. coli.**

Q. What are adoral cilia ?

Ans. Adoral cilia are longer cilia which line the mouth part of **B. coli.**

Q. What is Cytopyge ?

Ans. Cytopyge is a small opening in the membrane at the posterior end of **B. coli.**

Q. What are the positions of contractile vacuoles in B. coli ?

Ans. One contractile vacuole is near the middle of the body and the other at the posterior end.

Q. What contains food vacuole ?

Ans. Food vacuole contains debris of RBCs and WBCs. It can be grown in various nutrient media with or without associated bacteria.

Q. Cite a protozoon which has only one host in its life cycle.

Ans. B. coli has only one host (man or pig) in its cycle.

First Report of Protozoa

E. histolytica – Lamb (1859)

G. lamblia – Leeuwenhock (1681)

T. vaginalis – Dorne (1836)

Trypanosoma gambiense – Forde (1901)

T. cruzi – Chagas (1909)

L. donovani – Leishman (1900)

L. tropica – Cunningham (1885)

L. braziliensis – Lindenberg (1909)

I. hominis (belli) – Kjellberg (1860)

P. vivax – Laveran (1880)

P. ovale – Ingram (1917)

P. falciparum – Short et al (1949)

Babesia – Garnham (1969)

T. gondii – Nicolle and Manceaux (1908)

Sarcocystis lindemanni – Lindemann (1868)

B. coli – Malmsten (1857)

Section II

HELMINTHOLOGY

All species of Helminths (Greek, ***helminth*** means "worm") belong to subkingdom of the Metazoa, which are provided with tissues, organs derived from the embryonic endoderm, ectoderm and mesoderm. Helminths of medical importance are : They may be phylum–

I. Plathelminthes (class Cestodea and Trematoda)

II. Nemathelminthes (Class Nematoda).

Phylum plathelminthes

They are leaf or tape-like, segmented, hermaphrodite, and have no alimentary canal and no body cavity.

Phylum nemathelminthes

They are elongated, cylindrical, unsegmented, and they have separate sexes, body cavity, alimentary canal.

Chapter 6

SUMMARY

Cestodes

They are long, dorso-ventrally flattened, segmented, tape like. So they are also called "Tapeworm", they measure from a few millimetres to several metres, are found in the intestine of man and animal. They have 3 regions : (a) head (**scolex**); (b) body (**strobila**); (c) segments (**proglottid**); suckers (slit like or cup like) have no separate sexes; no body cavity and alimentary canal; they have reproductive excretory and nervous systems.

They are pseudo-phyllidean and cyclo-phyllidean cestodes.

A. Pseudophyllidean cestodes

Species Diphyllobothrium latum.

It is a parasite of man, has worldwide distribution, but not yet reported from India. It lives in the intestine of man, dog, cat.

It is yellowish, measures 3-10 metres. Its head is small, spoon-shaped and long; has two bothria (slit-like grooves) on both ventral, dorsal surfaces; has no rostellum (or beak like projection on the head) and no hooklets. Its neck is longer than head; has 3,000 proglottids. Each proglottid is broader and is filled with male and female genitalia. Operculated eggs are discharged through uterine pore of mature proglottid.

One definite host (man, dog, cat) and two intermediate hosts (first in the cyclops, second in fish) are required by **D. latum** to complete its life cycle. When the egg of **D. latum** comes in contact with water, **Coracidium** (first stage larva, ciliated embryo) escapes through the **opercular opening** of the egg, swims in the water and is ingested by cyclops in the midgut of cyclops, the ciliated embryo casts its ciliated coat, transforms into **procercoid** larva (second stage larva). If the fresh water fish ingests the infected cyclop, the procercoid larva grows into **plerocercoid** or in the muscle fibres of fish. On ingestion of infected raw or insufficiently cooked fish the man (definite host) becomes infected, because **plerocercoid** is infective to man which develops into an adult worm, in the intestine of man, which lays eggs. It takes five or six weeks for the development from plerocercoid to egg appearance in the feces.

When **D. latum** gets attached to the ileum, brings out the pernicious type of anemia. It contains large amount of vitamin B_{12} and deprives the host of essential nutritional components which also cause pernicious anemia.

Clinically, non-specific symptoms and vitamin B_{12} deficiency develop.

Demonstration of operculated egg of **D. latum** is accurate laboratory diagnosis.

Treatment with broad spectrum anthelmintic drugs is effective. Pernicious anemia can respond well with Folic acid therapy.

D. latum infection can be prevented by : thorough cooking of infected fish; proper disposal of sewage to avoid pollution of water; not feeding dogs with infected fish.

Taenia saginata (Beef tapeworm)

It is called common unarmed tapeworm. It was known to infect man since ancient times. It has cosmopolitan distribution. In India, it is prevalent in Muslim community due to their beef eating habit.

It lives with its head embeded in the intestinal mucosa of man. It is white and semi-transparent measuring 5-10 metres. It may live up to 10 years.

Its head is quadrate with suckers situated at four angles of the head and is not provided with rostellum. Its neck is narrow followed by 2,000 proglottids. The mature gravid segments are narrow and longer with uterus filled with eggs and atrophied reproductive organs. The central longitudinal stem has 15-30 lateral branches.

Because of absence of uterine pore the eggs are liberated after the rupture of the gravid segment. Its eggs are spherical (31-43 microns in diameter). The egg has a thin outer transparent shell and the inner brown, thick walled, radially striated embryophore; it contains a **oncosphere** (14-20 microns in diameter) with three pairs of hooklets. Oncosphere is **infective** to man.

When cattle (intermediate host) graze the polluted ground with eggs in human feces, ingest the eggs which hatch out after rupture of the embryophore caused by gastric juice. The oncosphere liberated from the embryophore penetrates the intestinal wall of cattle, reaches the mesenteric venules or lymphatics and carried to various organs (liver, right side of the heart; lungs, left side of heart, systemic circulation in that order). This marked oncosphere is filtered in the striped muscle where it transforms into **cysticercus bovis.**

On ingestion of beef containing cysticercus (called as **"measly beef"**), man (definite host) gets infected. The larva (cysticercus) develops into adult worm liberating eggs to repeat its life cycle.

Taenia solium (Pork tapeworm)

This "armed tapeworm" was known since Hippocrates time, has worldwide distribution, is not common in Muslims who do not eat pork. Its larval infection is common in population infected with **T. solium,** causing cysticercosis in the brain. It is much similar to **T. saginata.** Its length is 2-7 metres. Its head is small, globular, with rostellum, and hooklets. Its proglottid number is under 1,000 and expelled in chains of 5-6. Its uterus has 5-10 thick lateral branches on each side. The gravid proglottid is longer than broad.

Its vaginal sphincter is absent. Its ovaries are two in number with an accessory lobe. Its testes have 150-200 follicles. It lives attached to the intestinal wall of man about 25 years.

Its life cycle is similar to that of **T. saginata.** The definite host is man. The intermediate host is pig. The pork "measle" or "measly pork" or "bladder worm" (**Cysticercus cellulosae**) is an opalescent ovoidal body measuring 10 mm is length and 5 mm is width. It can live for 8 months in the flesh of pig and sometimes in man.

Clinically, the adult worm produces no serious damage, but it can cause vague abdominal pain, hunger, diarrhoea. It causes less frequently intestinal obstruction as in **T. saginata.**

The larva of (**Cysticercus bovis**) of **T. saginata** is not found in man, but the larva (**Cysticercus cellulosae**) of T. solium is found in man.

Cysticerus cellulosae produces cysticercosis cellulosae in man. It is found in every organ and tissue of the body. Finally in brain it develops into visible nodules without any disturbance during its life time. As soon as the larva dies, a variety of symptoms develop : Epileptiform seizures and fatal outcome. Sometimes man may get infected, as in the pig, by ingestion of food or drink contaminated with eggs.

Treatment is by specific recent anthelminthic drugs. Prophylaxis is by (1) personal hygiene; (2) community sanitation; (3) avoiding the ingestion of pork or beef (4) rigid inspection in slaughter houses.

Ecchinococcus granulosus (dog tapeworm)

This cestode is also called dog tapeworm. It was known since ancient time causing hydatid disease in man. It is widely distributed. In Punjab (India), dogs (28.8 per cent) and cattle (90 percent) has born hydatid cysts.

The adult worm lives attached to the small intestinal villi of dog. Its larval form develops only in man (the intermediate host).

It is minute (dwarf) worm. It comprises three regions (scolex, neck, strobila) measures 3-6 cm in length, has a pyriform scolex with four suckers and a protrusible rostellum armed with two circular rows of hooklets. Its neck is short. The strobila consists of one immature, one mature and one gravid proglottid. The gravid proglottid is the broadest and longest. Its uterus resembles a loosely twisted coil. Its egg is similar to other Taenia egg and infective to man, cattle, sheep. It contains a hexacanth embryo (oncosphere).

Its larval form is within hydatid cyst developing in the intermediate host. It represents the scolex of the future worm and is invaginated. When ingested by the definite host (dog), the scolex with its four suckers and rostellar hooklets evaginates and develops into an adult worm.

For perpetuation of life cycle, sheep, cattle while grazing on the ground contaminated with the eggs in dog's feces; man while playing with the dog, ingests the eggs which later hatch out oncospheres in the duodenum oncospheres enter into the intestinal wall and venules, are first filtered in liver, next in lungs and then various organs, hydatid cysts develop in viscera. These hydatid cysts in cattle, sheep viscera are ingested by dog, the scolex is evaginated and develops into adult worm which lays eggs. These eggs are passed out in dog's faeces to repeat the life cycle.

The adult worm of **E. granulosus** may not cause much disturbance in the intestine of dog. The damage caused by its hydatid is both toxic and mechanical. The cysts in the vital organs may interfere with the function of the organ, damage the organ and even cause the death. The osseous cyst may erode the bony structure. If the cyst is increased to a tremendous size it may cause physical burden to the patient and bursts, precipitating an anaphylactic reaction cyst in the brain, heart valve may cause death.

Hydatid fluid is clear, colourless, slightly acidic with low specific gravity, is antigenic and is highly toxic causing anaphylaxis.

Hydatid sand contains brood capsules, scolices and hooklets and settle in the fluid as granular deposits.

Diagnosis can be done by Intradermal test, Casoni's test (routine test).

Serological and other diagnostic test (roentgenogram, exploratory cyst puncture).

Treatment : Although all non-surgical procedures are unsuccessful, Ivermectin injection was found effective on adult worm **E. granulosus** in dog (Panjarathinam 2005) is published.

Prophylaxis can be by 1. avoiding infected dog. 2. ingestion of polluted vegetables, drink, 3. personal hygiene; 4. preventing dogs from eating infected carcasses, 5. strict inspection in slaughter house.

Hymenolepis nana

Its common name is Dwarf tapeworm. The name Hymenolepis is derived from Greek ***hymen*** — membrane — and ***lepis, nanus*** — nana. Though it is cosmopolitan in its distribution, it is common in India. It remains attached to the villi of small intestine of man, and rodents (rats, mice), lives for about two weeks. It is small (25-30 nm in length). Its scolex is minute, globular with four hemispherical suckers with a short retractile rostellum armed with 20 hooklets in one single row which can invaginate into the apex. These hooklets are shaped like tuning forks. Its neck is long. Proglottids are about 200 in number. The general contour of the distal end of strobila is rounded. The genital pores are marginal on the same side. Its uterus is transverse and there are three testes.

Eggs liberated after disintegration of distal proglottid are spherical, contains an oncosphere enclosed in an inner envelope (embryophore) with two polar thickenings from which four or more polar filaments arise. The oncosphere contains 3 pairs of tuning fork shaped hooklets. The space between outer and inner envelopes is filled with yolk granules and **polar filaments.**

Its life cycle requires **only one host,** no intermediate host. It is an exception to general rule that the helminth does not multiply inside the definite host.

Man ingests eggs in human's faeces. These eggs are hatched out in the intestine; the free oncospheres penetrate villi, transform into cerocysts or **cysticercoids,** migrate further down in other villi and transform into adult worm which lays eggs; some eggs are passed out in faeces, some restart life cycle in the same host.

H. nana irritates the intestinal mucosa. The absorption of parasitic metabolic wastes by the patient's system may cause generalised toxemia, headache, anorexia, pruritus of nose and anus, diarrhoea and abdominal pain.

Demonstration of eggs with typical polar filaments in the stool is an accurate diagnosis. Prophylaxis is similar to that of other cestodes.

Hymenolepis diminuta (rat tapeworm)

It is mainly the tapeworm of rat. Some human cases have been reported in India. It lives in the intestine of rat for about 13 years is morphologically similar to **H. nana.** Its eggs are similar to those of H. nana, except that they have **no polar filaments.** Then six lanceolate hooklets are arranged in a **fan shape** on the oncosphere.

It requires two hosts : man (definite host) and xenopsylla cheopis — **rat flea** (intermediate host). In the intestine of rat flea, the eggs are hatched out. The free oncospheres penetrate into the hemal cavity and develop into **cysticercoid.** Accidental ingestion of infected rat flea causes the infection in man. The cysticercoids liberated from rat flea develop into adult worm. Cachexia is common symptom. Demonstration of typical eggs and adult worm in the stool is a definite diagnosis.

Accidental swallowing of ectoparasites should be avoided.

Dipylidium caninum

Its common name is double pored dog tapeworm. It is the common tapeworm of dog (Panjarathinam 1989)) is small. Its scolex is small with four cup shaped oral suckers. Gravid proglottid is pumpkin seed shaped, is filled with uterine blocks. Each block contains 8-15 eggs.

Eggs are spherical, thin-shelled and hyaline have delicate hooklets.

Dog flea (**Ctenocephalides canis**) ingests eggs deposited on the ground. Dog flea is similar to rat flea. These eggs are hatched out in the intestine of dog flea, migrate into the hemal cavity, develop into cysticercoid larvas when these infected fleas are ingested by the definite host, they produce the infection.

Clinical manifestations (intestinal disturbance, indigestion, loss of appetite, toxic nervous system) are noticed when the metabolic wastes of the worm are absorbed into the human system. Diagnosis is by the demonstration of characteristic eggs in the mother's capsules.

Treatment by effective drugs

The disease can be prevented by distinction of dog flea by insecticides and by avoiding the dogs.

QUESTION (Q) – ANSWER (A)

Q. What is helminth ?

Ans. Helminth means worm.

Q. What is metazoa ?

Ans. It is a subkingdom to which all species of helminths belong.

Q. Classify helminths.

Ans. Helminths are I. Platyhelminthes (cestodes, trematoda).

2. Nemathelminthes (Nematoda).

Q. Define Cestodes.

Ans. Cestodes are long, dorso-ventrally flattened, segmented and tape-like. They are also known as 'Tapeworm'.

Q. What is the meaning of the following :

scolex, strobila, proglottid, sucker, hook, hermaphrodite ?

Ans. Scolex means head; strobila means body or trunk; proglottid – segment; sucker – slit-like, cup-like depression or groove; hook - organ of attachment; hermaphrodite – sexes are not separate, bothria – groove.

Q. How many types of cestodes are there ?

Ans. There are two types of cestodes : 1. Pseudophyllidean, 2. Cyclophyllidean cestodes.

Q. What is coracidium, procercoid, plerocercoid ?

Ans. Coracidium – first stage larva of **Diphyllobothrium latum** or ciliated embryo liberated from operculated egg in the water; procercoid – its second stage larva, in cyclops : plerocercoid third stage larva in fish flash. This third stage larva is also called as sparganum which is infective to man.

Diphyllobothrium latum

Q. What is the common name of D. latum ?

Ans. Its common name is broad fish tapeworm.

Q. Why is it called Diphyllobothrium ?

Ans. Because it has bothria on both surfaces.

Q. What is the shape of its scolex ?

Ans. It is spoon-shaped.

Q. How are its eggs discharged ?

Ans. Its eggs are discharged through the uterine pore.

Q. How many eggs can one single worm discharge ?

Ans. It may discharge about one million eggs per day.

Q. How is pathogenic effect produced ?

Ans. The pathogenic effect is due to the absorption of parasite waste products.

Q. How is pernicious anemia caused ?

Ans. Pernicious anemia is due to deprivation of host with the essential nutritional compounds, thus **D. latum** contains a large amount of vitamin B_{12}.

Q. What are the clinical symptoms ?

Ans. Clinical vitamin B_{12} deficient symptoms develops if the adult worms are attached to the jejunum. Adult worm in the intestine may cause no symptom.

Q. How will you treat pernicious anemia associated with D. latum ?

Ans. It can be treated by folic acid administration.

Taenia saginata

Q. What is the common name of T. saginata ?

Ans. It is called 1. Beef tapeworm, or 2. Unarmed tapeworm.

Q. Why is it called 1. Beef tapeworm or 2. Unarmed tapeworm ?

Ans. 1. Since its larva is lodged in the beef.

2. Since its scolex is not provided with the rostellum.

Q. Why is T. saginata very common in Muslims in India ?

Ans. Since Indian Muslims consume beef.

Q. How many years the adult worm may live ?

Ans. It may live for 10 years.

Q. How many gravid proglottids are present in a adult worm ? How is it expelled ?

Ans. It may range to 2,000 and is expelled singly at a time.

Q. Since it has no rostellum how does it get attached to the intestine ?

Ans. It gets attached to the intestine with the suckers.

Q. Why are its eggs liberated after rupture of gravid segment ?

Ans. Because of the absence of uterine pore.

Q. For how many weeks their eggs remain viable ?

Ans. They remain viable for eight weeks.

Q. Why is hatching of their eggs necessary ?

Ans. Hatching is necessary to liberate oncosphere.

Q. What is the function of oncosphere ?

Ans. It is infective to cattle and is carried through the circulation to various organs and transforms into **cysticercus bovis** in the beef.

Q. For how many months can this cysticercus live ?

Ans. Cysticercus can live for 8 months in the muscle of cattle.

Q. What is "measly Beef" ?

Ans. Beef containing the cysticercus is called "measly beef" and can become infective to man.

Taenia solium

Q. What is common name of T. solium ?

Ans. Its common name is "pork tapeworm" or "armed tapeworm".

Q. Why is it called "pork tapeworm" or "armed tapeworm" ?

Ans. 1. Since its larva is found in pork it is called pork tapeworm.

2. Since its scolex is armed with a double row of large and small hooklets.

Q. What is the shape of hooklet ?

Ans. Hooklet is dagger shaped.

Q. Why is T. solium rare in Muslim community ?

Ans. It is rare in Muslims as they do not eat pork.

Q. How many number of proglottids are produced ?

Ans. It produces 1,000 and it is produced in chain of 5-6 at a time.

Q. How many lateral branches are present on each side of a median longitudinal stem of the gravid ?

Ans. (1) There are 5-10 thick lateral branches in **T. solium.**

(2) There are 15-30 thin lateral branches of T. saginata.

Q. What is measle ?

Ans. It is a bladder worm found in muscle. If it is found in beef, it is called "measly beef" **(cysticercus bovis)**, if it is found in pork it is called "measly pork" or bladder worm **(cysticercus cellulosae).**

Q. Is intestinal obstruction by T. solium is frequent ?

Ans. Intestinal obstruction is less frequent, but it may cause a lot of irritation, when compared to **T. saginata** which cause a considerable disturbance because of its large size.

Q. What are the symptoms of T. solium ?

Ans. T. solium produces no serious damage, but it causes vague abdominal discomfort hunger pain, diarrhoea, sometimes appendicitis.

Q. Which is cysticercus found in man ?

Ans. Cysticercus cellulosae is found in man, but **Cysticercus bovis** of **T. saginata** is not found in man.

Q. When do brain symptoms in man develop in cysticercosis, caused by Cysticercus cellulosae ?

Ans. As soon as larva (**Cysticercus cellulosae**) dies, the tissue reaction begins around the dead larva and symptoms develop.

Q. What are the brain symptoms ?

Ans. Symptoms : Epileptiform seizures are common and may produce fatal outcome.

Q. How auto-infection takes place in man ?

Ans. Auto-infection may occur in man harbouring an adult worm and is due to the gravid segments being thrown back into the stomach by the reversal peristaltic movement of the intestine.

Echinococcus granulosus

Q. What is its common name ?

Ans. Its common name is dog tapeworm.

Q. Where was it reported in animals in India ?

Ans. It was reported in Punjab.

Q. What is the name of the disease caused by E. granulosus ?

Ans. It is hydatid disease.

Q. Name a minute tapeworm.

Ans. E. granulosus is minute like a grain.

Q. What type of rostellum has this tapeworm ?

Ans. It has a protrusible rostellum.

Q. Name a tapeworm with a strobila consisting of only three segments.

Ans. It is **E. granulosus.**

Q. Why is E. granulosus the smallest tapeworm ?

Ans. It is the smallest because of its minimum number of **three** segments.

Q. What is the function of larval form of E. granulosus found within the hydatid cyst ?

Ans. It represents the scolex of the future worm and is invaginated into its own body to protect its rostellar hooklets.

Q. What is hydatid cyst ?

Ans. It is a cystic cavity formed by the developing oncosphere in the viscera, it may transform into a bladder worm (Greek ***hydatis*** meaning a "drop of water").

Q. What is hydatid sand ?

Ans. Free brood capsules and free scolices set free in the fluid of cystic cavity are called hydatid sand.

Q. What is acephalocyst ?

Ans. The cyst which produces brood capsules only never produces scolices.

Q. What are the pathological effects produced by hydatid cyst ?

Ans. The young cyst lodged in the vital center may interfere with the function of the organs and even cause death. The cyst may grow to tremendous size, may become a physiological burden and burst — causing an anaphylactic reaction. Osseous cyst may erode the bone with multiple fractures. Thus hydatid cyst may cause both mechanical and toxic damage; it may damage even the brain and heart valve.

Hymenolepis nana

Q. What is its common name ?

Ans. It is also called dwarf worm.

Q. Is it common in India ?

Ans. It is common in India.

Q. How are its eggs set free ?

Ans. Its eggs are set free due to distintegration of the proglottid.

Q. What are the characteristics of its egg ?

Ans. It is spherical. Its oncosphere is enclosed by embryophore with **two polar thickenings** from each arising **4-8** polar filaments. Within oncosphere there are three parts of **tuning fork shaped hooklets.**

Q. Name the tapeworm bearing egg containing oncosphere with tuning fork shaped hooklets.

Ans. H. nana can only liberate such an egg with tuning fork-shaped hooklets.

Q. Which oncosphere metamorphoses into young cerecocysts or cysticercoids ?

Ans. Oncosphere of **H. nana** transforms into cysticercoids after penetrating the villi of the small intestine.

Q. Cite a tapeworm which does not utilise an intermediate host.

Ans. H. nana has no intermediate host.

Hymenolepis diminuta (rat tapeworm)

Q. Cite another species of Hymenolepis having an intermediate host.

Ans. H. diminuta has an intermediate host **(Xenopsylla cheopis).**

Q. What is its common symptom ?

Ans. Cachexia is a common symptom.

Dipylidium caninum

Q. What is the common name of this tapeworm ?

Ans. It is called double pored dog tapeworm.

Q. Who reported this tapeworm in dog in India ?

Ans. Panjarathinam reported this tapeworm in dog in India.

Q. How are the eggs of this tapeworm passed out in faeces ?

Ans. Groups of eggs within the mother embryonic membrane are passed in faeces.

Q. How pathogenic effect is produced ?

Ans. Due to absorption of the metabolic wastes of the worm.

Q. What are its clinical manifestations ?

Ans. They are intestinal disturbance, indigestion, loss of appetite, toxic nervous symptoms.

First Report of Cestoda

D. latum – Linnaeus (1758)

T. saginata – ? (1782)

T. solium – ? (1782)

E. granulosus – Hippocrates and Galen

H. nana – Bilharz (1851)

D. caninum – Linnaeus (1758)

H. diminuta – Rudolphi (1819)

Chapter 7
SUMMARY

Trematoda

It is a flatworm with suckers. Its name is derived from Greek *trematos* — means pierced with holes.

The trematodes are unsegmented, dorso-ventrally flattened or leaf-shaped and are called "flukes". Their size is variable, the largest human trematode is **Fasciolopsis buski.** They have two cup shaped (ventral and oral) suckers which are organs of attachment. They are hermaphrodite, except **schistosoma.** They lay operculated eggs except Schistosoma. Their life cycle requires one or more intermediate hosts.

According to their habitats, they are classified into : 1. blood trematode; 2. hepatic trematode; 3. intestinal trematode; 4. lung trematode.

Schistosoma haematobium

It is commonly called vesical blood fluke causing schistosomiasis heamatobia. In India, Gadgil and Shah identified an autochthonus focus at Ratnagiri district of Maharashtra. Panjarathinam (1972) reported **Schistosoma nasalis** in the nasal washing of the nasal granuloma of cattle for the first time in Pondicherry (India).

Schistosoma haematobium lives in the vesical plexuses of venous circulation. The **male** adult is shorter and has ventral and oral suckers and has at the end a **gynaecophoric canal** in which the female is held during copulation and oviposition. The **female** is long and slender. Its suckers are small and its tuberculations are confined.

Its definite host is man; its intermediate host is fresh water snail **(Ferrisia tenuis** in India) involved in its life cycle.

Its **eggs** have a distinct terminal spine. When its eggs are discharged into the water, the ciliated larva (**miracidium,** the first stage larva) is hatched out. This **miracidium** swims in water, comes in contact with the snail, penetrates into the snail, reaches the liver and other organs where it looses its cilia, transforms into the first and second generation of **sporocysts** (second larval stage), finally a generation of **fork-tailed cercariae** breaks out of the snail, swims in water, penetrates into human skin, casts off its tails.

This tailless cercaria is called metacercaria or **schistosomula.** It is **infective** to man. It enters into peripheral venules then right heart, pulmonary capillaries, left heart, systemic circulation, abdominal aorta, mesenteric arteries, mesenteric capillaries, portal circulation. This larva feeds, grows in intra-hepatic vessel becomes sexually differentiated, migrates against the blood stream, enters in inferior mesenteric veins, rectal, pelvic venous plexuses, at last vesical plexuses of veins, it becomes sexually mature. The male worm holds the female within the gynaecophoric canal. After fertilisation the eggs are passed in urine to restart its life cycle. Its pathogenic effects are due to : 1. generalised and localised reaction to metabolites of growing and mature worm, 2. trauma with haemorrhage as their eggs escape from the venules, 3. pseudo-abscess and pseudo-tubercle formation around lodged eggs in the tissues.

Clinically, there is irritation, minute haemorrhage at the site of entry on the skin, followed by toxic symptoms (anorexia, headache, malaise, pain, rigor, night sweating, urticaria), liver and spleen are hypertrophied, **hematuria** at the end of micturition.

In the laboratory, the diagnosis is by microscopic demonstration of terminal spined eggs in urine deposits by serological tests.

Treatment is by the use of specific drug (antimony compound).

Prophylaxis is by eradication of snails; sanitary improvement; prevention of pollution of water by infected persons; by avoiding wading in polluted water; proper disposal of human excreta.

Schistosomal Cercarial Dermatitis

There are 3 types :

1. **Schistosome dermatitis Type I** is caused by **Tricho-bilharzia ocellata.** Its intermediate host is **Lymnea** snail. It is also reported in India. Clinically, there is pricking sensation, followed by urticaria, at the initial stage. After several hours, intense itching of the area develops with oedema, and the papule transforms into pustule.
2. **Schistosome dermatitis Type II** is caused by an avian species of **Trichobilharzia** cercaria.
3. **Schistosome dermatitis Type III** is caused by the penetration of into human skin by cercaria of mammalian species of blood fluke **(Schistosoma spindalis)**. Oral trimperazine is effective.

Schistosoma mansoni

It is commonly called Manson's blood fluke. It causes Manson's intestinal schistosomiasis (bilharziasis). It is found in the mesenteric veins of the sigmoid-rectal area and lives for 26 years.

It resembles **S. haematobium** but it is smaller, its egg has a characteristic lateral spine. Its **miracidium** is larger than that of **S. japonicum** and **S. haematobium.**

Its life cycle in the snails is similar to that of **S. japonicum** and **S. haematobium.** The definite host is man; the intermediate host is the fresh water snail **Biomphalaria glabrata.**

The lesion produces by **S. mansoni** are smaller to those of **S. haematobium** and **S. japonicum.** The colon and rectum are mostly involved.

Initially, there is papular rash, with pruritus over the skin of feet, fever, dysentery, abdominal pain.

Diagnosis can be by demonstration of characteristic lateral spined eggs in the stool, by various serological tests and by blood examination.

Antimony compounds are effective and the prophylaxis is similar to that of **S. haematobium.**

Schistosoma japonicum

Its common name is Oriental blood fluke. It lives in the radicles of the superior mesenteric veins draining the ileo-cecal region, cause Oriental schistosomiasis. It is similar morphologically to other two schistosoma, but it lacks tuberculations. Its egg has an abbreviated spine on the upper right border of the shell.

Its life cycle is also similar to that of other two schistosoma; but its intermediate host is fresh water snail of the genus **Oncomelania.** Its **miracidium** is smaller in size.

Its pathogenic lesions are also similar to those of other two schistosoma. Intestine and liver are mostly affected. The intestinal and hepatic schistosomiasis in Orient is also called Katayama disease.

Its clinical features are dysentery, hepatic cirrhosis, splenomegaly, appendicitis, intestinal obstruction, pneumonitis, cerebral syndrome, intoxication, urticaria, fever — diagnosis, treatment and prophylaxis are same as in other schistosome.

Gastrodiscoides hominis

Human infections have been reported from India (Assam, Bengal, Bihar, Orissa) and other countries. Rhesus monkeys have also been found to be infected in India. Pig is the common reservoir host. It lives in large intestine of the definite host (man). It is pyriform, has a conical anterior portion and a discoidal posterior portion. Its eggs are ovoidal, operculated. This worm causes a mucous diarrhoea. Typical egg can be demonstrated in faeces. Treatment by effective drug.

Fasciola hepatica

It is commonly known as sheep liver fluke causing fascioliasis hepatica. It was first trematode to be described alongwith its complete life cycle. It lives in the biliary passage for 13 years in man.

It has a cosmopolitan distribution including India. It is a fleshy fluke, with oral and ventral suckers. The oral sucker is the conical projection.

Its eggs are large, ovoidal and operculated. They contain a large unsegmented ovum.

Definite host (sheep, goat, cattle or man) and intermediate host (snail – **lymnaeidae**) are involved in its life cycle.

Life cycle : Eggs, passed in faeces, mature in water. The miracidium escapes from the egg, swims, enters into the snails, forms sporocyst after loosing its cilia. This sporocyst produces first and second generation rediae finally cercariae (**redia** is formed only in all trematodes in snail, but not in Schistosoma). These cercariae liberated from snail, swim in water, encyst into metacercaria (infective form) on the grass. Cattle get infected by grazing, man by accidental swallowing of metacercariae which excyst in duodenum, enter into the intestine, peritoneal cavity, liver capsule, liver parenchyma, at last settle in the biliary passage and mature into adult worm — liberating eggs in faeces.

During migration its larvae produce traumatic, necrotic changes; inflammation, oedema of biliary epithelium, fibrosis of biliary ducts.

Clinically, obstructive jaundice, coughing, vomiting, abdominal pain, urticaria, fever, diarrhoea, anemia. Cholelithiasis is a complication.

Diagnosis is by recovery of eggs from stool or biliary drainage. Its egg is similar to that of **Fasciolopsis buski.** It can be treated by suitable drug (Albendazole is recent effective drug). Prophylaxis is by eradication of worm; by killing of snails by chemicals; education of public.

Fasciolopsis buski

It is called as giant intestinal fluke causing fasciolopsiasis in man and pig. It is a fleshy, elongated, ovoidal, has no cephalic cone. It lives for six months attached to the duodenum. It has a worldwide distribution including India (Assam, Bengal).

Its life cycle is similar to that of **F. hepatica** except its intermediate host **Segmentina trichoideus.** Its cercariae encyst on the seed pod of the water caltrop – **Trapa bispinosa,** commonly found in India (Bengal). Man gets infected by swallowing the metacercariae, on the seed pod, which get attached to duodenum and transform into adult worm laying eggs similar to those of **F. hepatica.**

All other characteristics are similar to those of **F. hepatica.**

Clonorchis sinensis

It is commonly known as Chinese Liver fluke, producing clonorchiasis. It was first identified by McConnell (1875) in the bile passage of a Chinese carpenter who died in Kolkata (India). It lives in biliary passage of man, pig, cat. It is distributed worldwide.

It is flat, transparent and spatulate.

Its eggs are ovoidal, resemble an electric bulb with terminal hook-like spine; has an operculum. They are finally embryonated (miracidium) and are infective to man.

Three intermediate hosts are required : one definite host (man, cat, dog); first intermediate host snail (**Bulinidae**); second intermediate host Cray fish (**Cyprinidae**).

Life cyle : When fully embryonated eggs are ingested by snail (**Bulimus, Arlocinma**), the miracidium hatches out from the egg. Within snail the rediae are developed, produce cercariae which come out of snail, swim in water, get attached to the fish, looses its tail, enter into the flesh. Man gets infected by ingestion of infected fish. The metacercariae excyst in the duodenum and enter into the common duct through ampulla of Vater, mature into adult worm whose eggs are discharged with the faeces. Proliferation, inflammation, fibrosis of bile duct may ensue.

Clinically, there are three stages : mild, progressive and severe. Cholangitis may occur. It can be diagnosed by recovery of its characterstic egg from the stool. It can be treated by effective drugs.

The infection can be prevented by properly cooking infected fresh water fish; sterilising nights soil, avoiding pollution of water with faeces.

Opisthorchis felineus

Its common name is cat liver fluke. Though it is prevalent in many countries, it was reported from India (Bengal). It is morphologically similar to **C. sinesis,** except that its testes are lobed. Its egg is also similar to **C. sinesis,** but there is a minute tubercular thickening.

In all other aspects, it is similar to **C. sinensis** but there is no specific treatment.

Heterophyes heterophyes

It is a minute fluke causing electro-phylaxis. It is distributed in many countries including India where a worm was recovered from a dog. It is elongated and pyriform.

Its eggs are minute, operculated and ovoidal. Well developed egg has miracidium.

Definite host (man, dog, fox) and intermediate host (marine water, snail, fresh water fish) are required for its life cycle. Snail ingests the eggs which are hatched out. A sporocyst or two rediae are developed from which the cercariae emerge out and encyst in the mullet fish. On ingestion of this infected fish, man gets infected. Adult worm deposits eggs.

Mild inflammation at the sites of intestinal attachment by worm. Colic pain, mucous diarrhoea, some eggs may enter into the circulation, filter into the cardiac valves and myocardium causing tissue reaction and cardiac failure, if carried to the brain, cause fatal cerebral hemorrhage.

Recovery of typical egg from feces is correct laboratory diagnosis. It can be treated by effective drug.

Prevention by eating cooked fresh water fish and destroying the snail.

Metagonimus yokogawai

It causes metagonimiasis. It is attached to the intestine. It resembles **H. heterophyes.** Its egg cannot be distinguished from **H. heterophyes.**

Three hosts (1) Definite host (man, pelican); (2) First intermediate host (snail); (3) Second intermediate host (fresh water fish). Snails ingest fully embryonated eggs. These eggs develop into first sporocyst, them into two rediae generation. At last cercariae escape from the snail swim in the water, encyst in the fish skin or flesh of fresh water fish. Man gets infected by consuming infected fish. Adult worms lay eggs. Later found in feces.

Pathogenicity and clinical features are similar to those of **H. heterophyes.**

Diagnosis, treatment and prophylaxis or same as in case of **H. heterophyes.**

Paragonimus westermani

Its common name is Oriental lung fluke. It causes paragonimiasis.

Many countries are heavily infected with this fluke including India (Assam, Bengal, Chennai).

It is a reddish brown, plump, ovoidal fluke. Its eggs are ovoidal and have a flattened operculum.

Three hosts are involved in its life cycle :

1. Definite host (man, tiger, leopard, Indian monkeys); 2. First intermediate host (snail); 3. Second intermediate host (fresh water fish-cray fish, crab).

Miracidium hatched out from eggs swims in the water, enters into the snail. Within the snail, a sporocyst, two generations of rediae and cercariae are produced, liberated, swim in the water, enter the muscle of cray fish and encyst. After ingestion of infected cray fish, man gets infected. The metacercariae excyst in the duodenum; migrate through the abdominal cavity, diaphragm, pleural cavity and to lungs, finally settle in the bronchioles, mature into adult worm which deposits eggs. The eggs are coughed up, voided in the feces to repeat. Its life cycle granulomatous reactions may take place around the worm, abscess may take place around the worm, abscess in the abdominal cavity, with pseudotubercles around the eggs. The cysts may be found in the liver, intestine, muscle, brain, pleura.

QUESTION (Q) – ANSWER (A)

Q. Define Trematode.

Ans. Trematode is flat worm with suckers.

Q. Why are they called flukes ?

Ans. Because they are unsegmented, dorso-ventrally flattened or leaf-shaped.

Q. What is the largest human trematode ?

Ans. Fasciolopsis buski is the largest human trematode.

Q. Why are all trematodes hermaphrodite ?

Ans. Because they do not have separate sexes.

Q. Why are Schistosome (blood fluke) not hermaphrodite ?

Ans. Because they have separate sexes.

Q. Which trematode does not produce operculated eggs ?

Ans. Schistosoma do not produce operculated egg.

Schistosoma haematobium

Q. What is the common name of S. haematobium ?

Ans. The common name is vesical blood fluke.

Q. Where was S. haematobium reported in India ?

Ans. S. haematobium was reported from Ratnagiri district of Maharashtra state (India).

Q. What is gynaecophoric canal ?

Ans. Behind the ventral sucker, the body of the **male** schistosoma is folded all the way to the caudal extremity to form the gynaecophoric canal in which the female is held during copulation.

Q. What is miracidium ?

Ans. Miracidium is ciliated larva of Schistosoma and is first larval stage.

Q. What is the function of miracidium ?

Ans. Its function is to infect the snail (intermediate host).

Q. What is sporocyst ?

Ans. It is second larval stage of schistosoma.

Q. What is schistosomula ?

Ans. It is cercaria without tail.

Q. Where do Schistosoma feed, grow and become sexually differentiated ?

Ans. In the intra-hepatic portal vessels.

Q. Where is the site of predilection of S. haematobium ?

Ans. The site of prediction of **S. haematobium** is the vesical venule.

Q. What is the use of the terminal spine of egg of S. haematobium ?

Ans. It helps the eggs to work their way through the vessels and mucosa of urinary bladder.

Q. How is an allergic reaction provoked in the patient ?

Ans. It is due to discharge of metabolites of schistosoma.

Q. How are fibrosis and miliary pseudo-tubercle formed in schistosomiasis haematobium infection ?

Ans. They are formed due to infiltration of eggs into the tissues.

Q. What is the main clinical features of schistosomiasis haematobium ?

Ans. There is painless passage of small volumes of blood at the end of micturition-haematuria, burning sensation and increased frequency of micturition.

Q. What is the synonym of cercarial dermatitis ?

Ans. It is also called swimmer's itch or cercarial itch.

Q. How many types of cercarial dermatitis are reported ?

Ans. There are three types : Schistosome Types I, II, III.

Q. What type is reported in India ?

Ans. Type I is reported in India.

Schistosoma mansoni

Q. What is its common name ?

Ans. It is also called Manson's blood fluke.

Q. What is Bilharziasis ?

Ans. Manson's intestinal schistosomiasis is also called bilharziasis.

Q. What is the site of predilection of S. mansoni ?

Ans. It is found in the mesenteric veins of the sigmoidorectal area.

Q. What is its life span of S. mansoni ?

Ans. It lives for 26 years.

Q. Which schistosoma can be kept in the laboratory for research purpose ?

Ans. S. mansoni is used for research purpose.

Q. Why is the production of the granuloma around the eggs delayed in case of S. mansoni ?

Ans. Production of granuloma is delayed because of the smaller number of eggs produced by **S. mansoni.**

Q. Which schistosoma was recovered from the anterior chamber of the eye of a patient ?

Ans. S. mansoni.

Schistosoma japonicum

Q. What is its common name ?

Ans. Its common name is Oriental blood fluke.

Q. What is the site of predilection of S. japonicum ?

Ans. It inhabits in the radicles of superior mesenteric veins draining the ileo-cecal region.

Q. How adult worm of japonicum differs morphologically from other schistosoma ?

Ans. Adult worm of **S. japonicum** lacks integumentary tuberculations.

Q. What is katoyama disease ?

Ans. It is intestinal and hepatic schistosomiasis of the Orient.

Gastrodiscoides hominis

Q. In which states of India is G. hominis prevalent ?

Ans. It is prevalent in Bengal, Bihar and Orissa.

Q. In which country is Rhesus monkey infected with G. hominis ?

Ans. In India, Rhesus monkey is infected with **G. hominis.**

Q. In which country is life cycle of G. hominis known ?

Ans. In India, its life cycle is known.

Q. What disease is produced by G. hominis ?

Ans. G. hominis produces mucous diarrhoea.

Fasciola hepatica

Q. What is its common name ?

Ans. It is known as sheep liver fluke.

Q. For how many years it lives in man ?

Ans. It lives for 9-13 years in man.

Q. In which trematode is redia formation observed ?

Ans. Redia formation is observed in **Fasciola hepatica.**

Q. What is redia ?

Ans. Redia is the third larval stage of cell trematodes in the snail except in Schistosoma.

Q. What is Cerceria ?

Ans. It is the final larval stage after redia.

Q. What is metacercaria ?

Ans. Metacercaria is encysted cercaria and is infective to cattle or man.

Q. How metacercaria of F. hepatica migrates from the intestine to its site of predilection (biliary passage) ?

Ans. It migrates from the intestine, peritoneal cavity, liver capsule and parenchyma to biliary passage.

Q. Why should metacercaria of F. hepatica settle down in the biliary passage ?

Ans. It settles to grow to maturity.

Q. How much time it takes to reach the site of predilection (biliary passage) ?

Ans. It takes one month.

Q. What are the lesions produced during migration of the larva of F. hepatica ?

Ans. Traumatic and necrotic lesions are produced in the liver parenchyma.

Q. What are the pathological changes produced by adult worm of F. hepatica in the bile duct and gall bladder ?

Ans. Inflammatory and oedematous changes of the biliary epithelium with fibrosis of the bile ducts and gall bladder are produced.

Q. What are the clinical features of F. hepatica ?

Ans. Hepatic, obstructive jaundice, coughing, vomiting, abdominal pain, diarrhoea, fever, anemia, hemoglobinuria.

Q. What is the frequent complication of F. hepatica infection ?

Ans. Cholelithiasis is frequent complication.

Fasciolopsis buski

Q. What is its common name ?

Ans. It is also known as giant intestinal fluke.

Q. In which states of India F. buski is prevalent ?

Ans. it is prevalent in Assam, Bengal, Orissa (India).

Q. What is the largest intestinal trematode ?

Ans. F. buski is the largest intestinal fluke.

Q. What is the life span of F. buski ?

Ans. Its life-span is six months.

Q. On which plant do cercariae of F. buski encyst ?

Ans. They encyst on seed pods of the water caltrop (plant).

Q. Where is this water caltrop (water plant) common in India ?

Ans. It is common in Bengal (India).

Q. Why adult worms of F. buski obstruct the passage of food ?

Ans. Because of their giant size, many adult worms may obstruct the food passage.

Q. Why is there oedema of face, abdominal wall and lower limbs and eosinophilia in F. buski infection ?

Ans. Because of the generalised toxic and allergic reactions provoked by adult worm of **F. buski.**

Clonorchis sinensis

Q. What is its common name ?

Ans. Its common name is Chinese liver fluke.

Q. What is the appearance of egg of C. sinensis ?

Ans. Its egg looks like an electric bulb.

Q. In which country were twenty one thousand worms recovered from one patient ?

Ans. In China.

Q. How many stages are there in clinical manifestions in C. sinensis infection ?

Ans. There are three stages : (1) mild symptomless stage (2) progressive stage; (3) the severe stage.

Q. In which stage portal cirrhosis syndrome occurs in C. sinensis infection ?

Ans. In severe stage.

Q. How catarrhal cholangitis occurs in C. sinensis infection ?

Ans. Catarrhal cholangitis occurs due to occlusion of the bile passage by sticky masses of eggs and by tissue proliferation.

Q. Why do the following symptoms (palpitation of heart, tachycardia, vertigo, tremor, cramps, mental depression) occurs in C. sinensis infection ?

Ans. These symptoms occur due to systemic toxemia.

Q. How are the detoxifying properties of the liver impaired in C. sinensis infection ?

Ans. These properties are impaired by the by-products of adult worms of **C. sinensis.**

Opisthorchis felineus

Q. How is it called commonly ?

Ans. It is commonly called cat liver fluke.

Q. In which place of India was the adult worm of O. felineus recovered ?

Ans. In Kolkata.

Q. Cite two passages in which O. felineus lives.

Ans. It lives in the biliary and pancreatic passages of man.

Heterophyes heterophyes

Q. Why are clinical manifestations (colicky pain, mucous diarrhoea with excess mucous production) produced ?

Ans. These clinical manifestations are due to mild inflammation at the sites of attachment of adult worms to the intestine.

Q. How is cardiac failure caused in H. heterophyes ?

Ans. Sometimes its èggs may enter the mesenteric lymphatics, filter into the cardiac valve and myocardium where they produce tissue reactions, ultimately causing cardiac failure.

Q. What will happen if these eggs are carried to the brain ?

Ans. They cause fatal cerebral haemorrhage.

Metagonimus yokogawai

Q. What changes will take place if the eggs of M. Yokogawai are carried to myocardium, brain, spinal cord etc. ?

Ans. Granulomatous changes will take place.

Paragonimus westermani

Q. What is its common name ?

Ans. Its common name is Oriental lung fluke.

Q. Cite the places in India where P. westermani is reported.

Ans. It is reported in Assam, Bengal, Malabar, Chennai (Tamil Nadu).

Q. For how many years is P. westermani alive in the lungs ?

Ans. It lives for six to seven years.

Q. How do metacercaria of P. westermani migrate from the intestine to bronchioles (site of predilection) ?

Ans. It travels through the abdominal cavity, diaphragm, pleural cavity, lungs, bronchioles.

Q. What will happen if the adult worm of P. westermani is present in the lungs ?

Ans. In the lungs, if it is present, there will be a thick, cystic encapsulation of the parasite. Similar change may also be observed in other organs.

Q. What will happen if the adult worm of P. westermani is in the brain of adult or children ?

Ans. It causes epilepsy of the Jacksonian type as in cerebral cysticercosis in adult; in children, infantile paralysis, cerebral hemorrhage, encephalitis and meningitis are observed.

First Report of Trematodes

Q. Who reported for the first time the following trematodes :

S. haematobium, S. mansoni; S. japonicum, S. nasalis, Gastrodiscoides hominis, F. hepatica; F. buski; C. sinensis; O. felineus; H. heterophyes; M. yokogawai, P. westermani.

Ans. S. hematobium – Bilharz (1851)

S. mansoni – Figinami (1904)

S. japonicum – S. nasalis (animal trematode) Panjarathinam (1972) in Pondicherry

G. hominis – Lewis and Mc Connell (1876)

F. hepatica – de Brie (1379)

F. buski – Busk (1843)

C. sinensis – McConnell (1875)

O. felineus – in 1892

H. heterophyes – Bilharz (1851)

M. yokogawai – Katsurada (1912)

P. westermani – Ringer (1879).

Class Nematoda

The nematodes are elongated, cylindrical, tapering at both the ends; non-segmented. Their sizes range from smallest (**Trichinella spiralis, Strongyloides stercoralis**) to the largest (**Dracunculus medinensis).** They have cuticula (protective covering). They have nervous system, complete genitalia, digestive tract with both oral and anal openings. The oral cavity has teeth or cutting plates. If the oesophagus is uniform, it is called filariform oesophagus; if it is expanded into a bulb, it is referred to rhabditiform oesophagus.

The free-living stages of the worm have rhabditiform oesophagus; the parasite forms have filariform oesophagus.

In contrast to parasitic trematodes and cestodes, the nematodes may be (1) viviparous, (2) oviparous; (3) ovo-viviparous.

1. Viviparous (**Dracunculus medinensis** giving birth to larva); (2) oviparous (**Ascaris lumbricoides** laying eggs); (3) ovo-viviparous (**Strongyloides stercoralis** laying eggs containing larva).

The sexes are separate. So nematodes are **"diecious helminths".** The male worm is smaller than femlae, seminal vesicle, an ejaculatory duct opening into cloaca. In some males, accessory organs (spicule, gubernaculum) are also present. In some other males their posterior end is expanded into a copulatory bursa supported by rays. Female has two cylindrical ovaries, uteri which may open to the exterior through a single vulva or a common vagina. The vulva is near the middle of the body, but its position varies in different species.

Trichinella spiralis

It is commonly known as "trichina" worm. It causes trichinosis. It was first discovered by Peacock (1828). It has worldwide distribution. Adult worm of **T. spiralis** remains buried in the duodenal or jejunal mucosa. Its larva encysts in the striated muscle of man, pig harbouring the adult worm. It is one of the "smallest" nematode infecting man. Its anterior end is delicate. The caudal extremity, the cloaca, is evertible and guarded by two conspicuous conical papillae. The female is twice longer than male. It is viviparous and discharges embryo (larva).

Mode of human infection is by ingestion of raw meat infected with the cysts of **T. spiralis.** In stomach, these cysts are digested out of the meat; in the duodenum they excyst, these larvae invade into the mucosa of duodenum and jejunum and develop into minute adult female and males. The female burrows into the villi and males die after fertilising the females. These fertilised females discharge 1,500 progenies. Some escape into lumen and the majority enter the circulation via mesenteric lymphatics, are lodged in various tissues (myocardium, brain, cerebrospinal fluid and body cavities). From these tissues they re-enter the blood stream and are distributed in striated muscle where they encyst. The cyst wall formation is due to tissue reaction, but it is not due to larval secretion. Diaphragm, muscles of the pharynx; tongue, biceps, deltoid are mostly infected. Pathogenicity has three stages : (1) invasion (incubation); (2) migration of larvae; (3) encysation and tissue repair.

In first stage, clinical symptoms are : nausea, vomiting, toxic diarrhoea; colic pain and profuse sweating.

In second stage, muscular pain, oedema, enlarged lymph nodes, fever, encephalitis, meningitis, ocular disturbance, deafness may occur.

In third stage, cachexia, oedema, dehydration, low blood pressure, collapse of patient are observed.

In the laboratory, demonstration of :

larvae in the muscle, adult worm and larvae in the faeces, larvae in the blood, spinal fluid and mother's milk can be useful.

Following serological tests can also be done : intradermal test, precipitin test, flocculation test, fluorescent antibody test, xenodiagnosis can be useful during surveys.

Curative and supportative treatment can be undertaken, the infection can be prevented by destruction of carcasses, viscera of dead pigs, by consumption of thoroughly cooked pork, destruction of rat, mice.

Trichuris trichiura

This "whipworm" causing trichuriasis was first discovered by Linnaeus (1771). It has a cosmopolitan distribution, remains attached to the wall of cecum of man. Its anterior end is thin hair-like. Its posterior portion is fleshy, thick and stout. It contains intestine, sex organs. So, it looks like a whip with a handle.

The caudal extremity of male worm is coiled ventrally. Its genitalia ends into the cloaca. A single spicule protrudes through a refractile penial sheath.

Posterior end of adult female is rounded. Its genitalia end into the external pore. Female is oviparous.

Its egg is barrel shaped with mucoid plugs at both the ends. About 5,000-7,000 eggs are liberated per day.

Eggs passed in the stool are embryonated in moist soil. Embryonated eggs containing rhabditiform larva are infective to man. After ingestion by man, these eggs are digested in the small intestine, the larva emerges out of the egg. This larva gets attached to small intestine for nourishment and migrates to the cecum (site of predilection) where it grows into adult worm which lays eggs in the stool of man.

The process of infection may be traumatic or allergic. Though many worms block the lumen of intestine, they cause irritation and inflammation of the cecum and produce colitis and secondary anemia and allergic reaction.

Clinical symptoms are abdominal pain, vomiting, constipation and systemic intoxication. The patient is emaciated with dry skin. Clinically, this infection resembles hookworm diseases, acute appendicitis, or amoebic dysentery.

Typical egg of **T. trichiura** can be detected in the stool.

The infection can be treated by effective drugs and can be prevented by personal hygiene and community prophylaxis.

Capillaria philippinensis

This parasite was first reported in 1963 and is common in Philippines. It remains burrowed in jejunal mucosa with both ends free. The male has caudal alae. The anterior part of female has oesophagus with glands whereas its posterior part has intestine, reproductive organs.

Only man gets infected by consuming raw fish though its life cycle is not yet established. Epithelium of jejunum shows degenerative changes. The clinical symptoms are diarrhoea, emaciation, weakness, abdominal pain. Death may be due to cachexia.

Adult worm and eggs can be detected in the stool. Skin test is sensitive and specific.

Treatment is by effective drugs. Prevention is by thoroughly cooking the fish.

Strongyloides stercoralis

This nematode is also named "threadworm". It produces strongyloidiasis in man and was first discovered by Normand (1876). Like **T. spiralis,** it remains buried in the mucosa of duodenum and jejunum.

Anterior third of the body of female contains cylindrical oesophagus, the posterior two-thirds is filled with intestine and anus opens mid-ventrally. Two sets of genitalia extend from vulva. It is ovo-viviparous.

The parasitic male adult worm is shorter than the female, it does not penetrate the intestinal mucosa and remains in the lumen of man.

Its egg is transparent, thin and oval. As soon as the eggs are laid, the rhabditiform larvae are hatched and come out of the human intestinal mucosa, then enter into the lumen and passed out into the stool.

There are two types of larvae : 1. rhabditiform larvae, 2. filariform larvae. The **male** rhabditiform larva has two spicules, a gubernaculum and no caudal alae; its posterior end is curved ventrally, the **female** has a two horned uterus and vulva opening in the middle of the ventral side of the body.

The rhabditiform larva is developed directly from the gravid female and is found in the lumen of the intestine. It transforms into filariform larva, which penetrates into the mucosa of the intestine to cause internal re-infection. Sometimes they penetrate perianal, perineal skin of the host causing auto-infection (hyper-infection).

Some other rhabditiform larvae passed out into the soil may develop in filariform larva, which may penetrate the skin when man walks bare footed, enter venous circulation, right heart, lungs, bronchi, trachea, larynx, epiglottis, are swallowed back and enter the intestine.

The free living rhabditiform larvae have two types of cycles : 1. Direct cycle – in the soil they develop into filariform larvae;

2. Indirect cycle – the male and female free-living rhabditiform larvae copulate and produce a batch of rhabditiform larvae similar to those produced by parasite females.

Skin lesions (petechial hemorrhage, pruritus, congestion, oedema, urticarial rash) are produced by the filariform larvae at the site of entry.

Pulmonary lesions (hemorrhage and cellular infiltration in air sacs and bronchioles) are produced when the larvae break out of pulmonary capillaries into the alveoli.

Recovery of adult worms and larvae of **S. stercoralis** is correct direct diagnosis from stool and sputum samples; serological tests are not satisfactory.

Treatment is effective.

1. Human body should be protected from contaminated soil and feces, and by personal hygiene.

Super Family Strongylodea

General Character

This super family has

(a) buccal capsule (well developed mouth cavity) which may contain teeth or cutting plates.

(b) bursa (copulatory bursa) of male

(c) egg with unsegmented ovum develops in soil

(d) two subfamilies : (A) subfamily Ancylostomadinae (tooth like processes) I. Two pairs of teeth – **Ancylostoma duodenale**

II. One pair of teeth – **A. braziliense**

III. Three pairs of teeth – **A. caninum**

B. Super family Uncinarinae (cutting plates) – **Necator americanus.**

Ancylostoma duodenale

It is commonly named old world hookworm causing ancylostomiasis. It was first reported by Dubini (1843). It has worldwide distribution including India (Punjab and Uttar Pradesh). Ancylostomiasis in dogs was first reported in Pondicherry (India) in 1972 by Panjarathinam. It lives in the jejunum.

Adult worm is larger and thicker. Its anterior end bends dorsally like a hook, hence the name "hookworm", even its oral aperture is also bent dorsally. Its buccal capsule has six teeth : four hook-like on the ventral surface and two knob-like on the dorsal surface. Its digestive system is connected with the oesophageal gland secreting an enzyme which prevents the clotting of blood. The posterior end of **male** has a copulatory bursa expanded in an umbrella-like fashion. Its genital opening is connected with the cloaca.

Dorsal ray of copulatory bursa is single. Total number of rays – 13.

The **female** has tapering end and no expanded bursa. Its genital opening is at the middle third of the body. Insemination occurs when the male applies its copulatory bursa around the vulva. Its posterior end has a spine. During copulation worm assumes a Y-shaped figure because of the position of genital opening. In human intestine, it lives for four years.

The rhabditiform larva has a midgut, a short rectum, a small genital opening. The filariform larva is long, delicate with short oesophagus and is infective to man. Its egg contains segmented ovum with four blastomeres, and is not infective to man.

Life cycle. Eggs with four blastomeres are passed in feces. In soil, eggs are hatched out rhabditiform larvae. These larvae develop into filariform larvae which cast off their sheaths come in contact with skin of bare foot. They invade the blood stream, are carried to right hert, lung then break out from pulmonary trachea, larynx, epiglottis, oesophagus and are swallowed back, enter into the intestine, develop into adult worms which lay eggs. The eggs are passed out in the feces.

Ancylostome adult worm or larvae may cause pathogenic effects : cutaneous lesions ancylostome dermatitis and creeping eruption, pulmonary lesion (minute hemorrhage, bronchitis; broncho-pneumonia).

Filariform larvae of **A. duodenale** and **Necator americanus** penetrate the skin, produce "ground itch" characterised by itching and burning, oedema, erythema, papular eruption, then a vesicle; they also produce cutaneous larva migrans (creeping eruption); anemia, iron deficiency.

Clinical symptoms are of three types : mild, moderate, and severe types.

In mild type, anemia is negligible; in moderate type, heart burn, flatulence, epigastric pain, they are relieved by eating clay/mud (which is known as pica or geophagy) mild fever, dyspnea, palpitation of heart.

In severe type, constipation, diarrhoea, food is undigested, dry skin, the patient is cold even in hot climate, oedema of face and around the eyes. Pot belly is typical sign in children. Finally, cardiac failure and anasarca.

1. Direct demonstration of adult worm and its egg microscopically.
2. Blood examination can be done to find out indirectly the nature of anemia and the presence of eosinophilia. **A. duodenale** and **N. americanus** can be differentiated by the morphological examination of adult worm and mature filariform larva.

Supportive treatment should be followed by curative treatment.

Prevention is by personal hygiene using gloves, boot and by community prophylaxis.

Necator americanus

Its name is "New World hookworm" or American hookworm. It causes necatoriasis, was first described by Stiles (1902). It is prevalent in many countries including southern India. Its life cycle, morphology, pathogenicity, diagnosis, treatment are same.

Ancylostoma braziliense

It is similar to **A. ceylanicum.** Male is smaller than female. Its eggs are similar to those of other ancylostoma.

The filariform larvae of **A. braziliense** cause creeping eruption in man and they also produce a serpiginous tunnel as they cannot penetrate below the stratum germinativum of the human skin.

A. Ceylanicum

It does not produce creeping eruption.

A. Malayanum

It is the largest hookworm found in India and Malaysia—in bears—and was reported once in man.

A. Caninum

It was reported once in man in Philippines and in dogs in India (Pondicherry) by Panjarathinam (1972).

Enterobius vermicularis

Human pin worm or seat worm is the common name. It causes enterobiasis or human oxyuriasis; known since ancient times, it has a cosmopolitan distribution. A gravid female was recovered from the perianal skin of a child (Panjarathinam 1978) in Ahmedabad (India).

Its adult worm remains attached to the mucosa of cecum, appendix, colon and ileum. It is small, white, spindle-shaped, has no buccal capsule but is provided with three lips; has a cervical alae, has a characteristic double bulb oesophagus.

The male has ventrally curved posterior end, with spicule. Without it lacks a gubernaculum, it dies after fertilisation, hence it is rarely seen.

The female has sharply pointed posterior end. Its vulva opens mid-ventrally. Its vagina is long and extends from vulva. Its cloaca is near the copulatory spicule. It has a paired genitalia (uteri, oviducts, ovaries). The gravid female gets detached from the intestinal mucosa migrates freely in the lumen and crawls out the anus onto the perianal or perineal skin, and dies after oviposition.

Its eggs are colourless, plano-convex in shape, contain motile embryo.

When fully embryonated eggs (infective) are ingested by man, they reach the duodenum and are digested by digestive juice. The larvae hatch out and pass down the intestine. Without migrating through lungs, they moult, lodge into villi of jejunum and ileum, become sexually mature and are fertilised in the intestine.

The male dies after fertilisation. The gravid female then migrate down the cecum, colon and appendix and remains there till the eggs are developed, then crawls on the perianal region for oviposition. Its eggs are transmitted from anus to mouth (auto-infection).

Minute intestinal ulcers with hemorrhage caused by : adult worm may get infected with pathogenic bacteria. Submucosal abscess and appendicitis may be produced. When metabolites of adult worms are absorbed, a generalised helmintic toxemia may ensue. Gravid female may deposit eggs on the perianal region and causes severe pruritus with scratchings. It may enter the genital tract causing salpingitis, encysts in the peritoneal cavities. It may cause urethritis, nocturnal enuresis. Clinical symptoms are insomnia, nervousness, nail biting, nose picking; grinding of teeth at night may be observed in children. Laboratory diagnosis can be done by demonstration of adult worm and its eggs under microscope. Treatment is by specific drugs and prevention can be done by personal hygiene.

Superfamily Ascaridoidea

The worms of this super family are large and stout. They have no buccal capsule, but they have three lips in their mouth. Males have no copulatory bursa.

Ascaris lumbricoides

It is also called giant intestinal roundworm. It causes ascariasis. It is common in children of rural area in China and India. It was also recovered from the infected calves in Pondicherry (India) by Panjarathinam (1972).

The adult worm is the **largest** nematode of the intestine. It is elongate, cylindrical. Its anterior end has **three** small-toothed lips. **Each lip** has minute papillae; has a small triangular buccal cavity.

The male has ventrally curved posterior end, its genitalia has testes, vas deferens, ejaculatory duct opening into cloaca, has copulatory spicule, no gubernaculum.

The vulva of the **female** is mid-ventrally situated near the junction of anterior and middle third of the body. It is narrow and is called as **"vulvar waist"**. Its vagina is connected with two genitalia consisting of uterus, oviduct, ovary. Its body fluid is irritant due to ascaon or ascarase which is responsible for allergy. It deposits about 2,00,000 eggs per day. Its life-span is two years. Its **fertilised** egg is ovoidal, transparent; the ovum is unsegmented.

The **unfertilised** egg contains a small, atrophied ovum with various sized refractile granules. It is heaviest.

Fertilised eggs in the soil embryonate in soil. These embryonated (containing rhabditiform larva) eggs are ingested alongwith food by man. The egg shell is digested by digestive juice in the duodenum. The rhabditiform larvae are liberated, penetrate into the intestine. Instead of becoming adult worm, they enter the circulation, reach the lungs, break through the pulmonary capillaries into the alveoli. They crawl up the bronchioles, bronchi, trachea and epiglottis and are swallowed. They develop into adult worm in the intestine. The female is fertilised and discharges eggs in the stool.

Some trauma and petechial hemorrhage may occur when the larvae escape into alveoli. As a result, consolidation of the lobules, spasms and coughing, bronchial rales, urticaria, fever and difiiculty in breathing.

This condition is known as **Ascaris pneumonitis** (Loeffler's syndrome). While in circulation, the larvae filter out in the brain, spinal cord, eyelid, kidneys where they cause physiological disturbance. Microorganisms are carried by these migrating larvae from the larvae to other organs and set up the infection. They deprive the host of its nutrition. They cause vitamin A deficiency (night blindness). Generalised toxemia and mechanical effects are also observed.

Common symptoms are vague, abdominal discomfort, acute colicky pain in the upper gastric region, diarrhoea, fever, meningitis, epilepsy. Adult worm and eggs can be detected in the stool.

Blood examination and allergic tests can also be undertaken for diagnosis.

Effective anthelminthic drugs can be used. Prevention by personal hygiene, community prophylaxis.

Anisakis marina

This nematode is a parasite of sea mammal and fish. Man acquires the infection (anisakiasis) by consuming the raw fish.

The fish is digested; the liberated larvae enter mucosa of the stomach and intestine producing a growth simulating malignancy. Its life cycle is not yet known. Colicky pain and obstruction of the intestine are the symptoms.

Demonstration of larvae from the incised tissue growth and HA test are useful for diagnosis.

Superfamily Filarioidea

Filariform larvae have a circular simple mouth surrounded by papillae, buccal cavity without lips and caudal alae. They are : **Wuchereria bancrofti, Brugia malayi, Onchocerca volvulus, Dipetalonema perstans, D. streptocercum, Mansonella ozzardi and Loa loa.**

Wuchereria bancrofti

Though symptoms of filariasis were known since antiquity, Microfilariae were demonstrated by Demarquay only in 1963. The name **Wuchereria bancrofti** was given in honour of discoverers Wucherer and Bancrofti.

This parasite is distributed in many countries including India (Rajasthan, Punjab, Uttar Pradesh, Delhi, Gujarat) along the Indian sea coast and banks of rivers (except Indus).

Adult worm is long, minute thread-like nematode. The tail end of **male** is curved ventrally with two spicules and gubernaculum. It has no caudal alae. The male worm is very rare.

The vulva of the **female** is cervical in position. Its female genitalia consists of short vagina, uterus.

Its tail end is pointed. It is ovo-viviparous, it liberates active embryo with the sheath (i.e. **microfilariae.** These microfilariae enter into lymph and blood circulation. Their anterior end is round with a stylet and posterior end is tapering. The anatomical "landmarks" in the central column of their nuclei extending from head to tail can differentiate different species **Wuchereria bancrofti, Brugia malayi** and **Loa loa** are sheathed; whereas **O. volvulus, Dipetalonema, Mansonella ozzardi** are unsheathed.

Microfilariae **Wuchereria bancrofti** appears in the peripheral circulation between 10 pm and 2 am (**nocturnal periodicity**) and adapt themselves to the feeding habits of the mosquito,

Culex pipiens, a night feeder; its length is 244 microns; tail end has no terminal nuclei. They require two hosts in their life cycle : (1) the definite host—man, and (2) the intermediate host—mosquito (culex).

When mosquito bites infect man, it ingests the sheathed microfilariae. These microfilariae cast off their sheath in the proventriculus (stomach) of mosquito, penetrate into mosquito's intestinal wall, reach into the mosquito's thoracic muscle, transform into first, second, third stage (infective) larva when infected mosquito bites the man, the infective larvae are deposited on punctured skin, they migrate into the punctured wound and settle into the lymphatics (inguinal, scrotal, abdominal), grow and sexually mature in lymphatics, fertilise; gravid female discharges microfilarvae which enter into peripheral circulation.

The filarial granulation tissue is pathognomonic of the disease. As the worm dies, lymphangitis ensues and results into elephantiasis. Following symptoms are common :

1. Lymphangitis : In this condition, the lymphatics of the testicle, epididymis are involved, they are red, congested, palpable and painful.
2. Lymphadenitis : It is the inflammation of the regional lymph nodes which precedes an attack of lymphangitis. It is mostly found in groin or axilla, is soft not painful and tender.
3. Elephantiasis is due to obstruction of the lymphatic tracts caused by recurrent attacks of lymphangitis.
4. Hydrocele is due to repeated attacks of wuchererial orchitis and epididymitis.
5. Chyluria is the escape of chyle through the urine. The urine is milky.

Filariasis can be diagnosed :

1. Directly by the demonstration of microfilariae in the peripheral blood.
2. Indirectly by various serological tests.

Effective drug is available for treatment; Prophylaxis is by destruction of mosquito and protection from mosquito bite.

Brugia malayi

It is prevalent in many countries including India (Assam, Andhra Pradesh, Orissa, Madhya Pradesh, Kerala).

It resembles **W. bancrofti,** has non-labiate mouth. Anterior end of the **female** has the reproductive organ; its posterior end has cuticular bossing; but that of **male** has peri-anal papillae, has copulatory spicules and gubernaculum.

Microfilariae of **B. malayi** have the nocturnal periodicity; their anterior end has two stylets, cephalic space is broader; length is 177 microns, tail is often constructed between two terminal nuclei; their appearance is stiff with secondary kinks. They are confined to lymphatics of extremities and their intermediate host is Mansonia, Anopheles. Its life cycle is same as that of **W. bancrofti.**

B. malayi; lymphangitis and elephantiasis of the lower extremities. Scrotal swellings are present in **B. malayi;** but chyluria is absent. Microfilariae can be demonstrated in the peripheral blood.

Treatment and prophylaxis are similar to those of **W. bancrofti.**

In addition, certain water plants should be destroyed as **Mansonia** grows on these plants. These plants are grown in Kerala, India.

Onchocerca volvulus

Convulated filaria, blinding filaria (common name) causing onchocerciasis. It was reported by Brumpt (1919) remains coiled in nodules (tumours) eleven years. It is wire-like filiform, and bent at both ends.

The **male** of **O. vulvulus** is smaller than the female. Its posterior end is re-curved ventrally and has perianal and caudal papillae, it has vulva, uterus. The microfilariae are unsheathed, both ends are nuclei-free.

Man is definite host and Simulium is intermediate host in its life cycle. The development of the microfilariae (Mf) of **O. vulvulus** is same as that of **Mf. bancrofti** in the mosquito.

It produces primary lesion which is a non-abscessing fibrous tumours. Pruritus is due to toxic metabolites of the embryo. The microfilariae circulate in the eyeball and cause corneal opacity. Clinical manifestations are simple conjunctivitis, corneal opacity, keratitis, secondary glaucoma.

Microfilariae can be demonstrated in the biopsy of a small piece of the epidermis. They can be detected in ocular lesion.

Serological tests can also be useful.

Treatment is by effective drugs.

Spraying of DDT in the breeding places of **Simulium.**

Dipetalonema perstans

D. perstans (persistent filaria) causes dipetalonemiasis. It was found by Daniels (1898), distributed in Africa and America, lives in peritoneal and pleural cavities.

Male adult worm is smaller than female. Its posterior end has caudal papillae, and copulatory spicules. The female has vulva situated in the cervical region. Its tail end presents cuticular thickening.

Microfilariae of **D. perstans** are sub-periodic (i.e. they are found in the circulation in the day time and at night). Then tail end is blunt and the nuclei extend upto tail tip. Like **O. volvulus,** it requires two hosts; like other microfilariae, **Mf. perstens** larval development is the same in Culicoides (intermediate host).

Symptoms are fatal pericarditis, local irritation, toxic oedema of the eyelid, dyspnea, pericardial pain.

Detection of **Mf. perstens** in the peripheral blood at night and day. Serological tests can be employed.

Treatment by suitable drugs.

Prophylaxis is not possible by the eradication of **culicoides** as they breed in the jungle.

Mansonella ozzardi

M. ozzardi (Ozzard's filariae) produces mansonelliasis. Its microfilariae were recovered for the first time by Ozzard.

It lives embedded in the visceral adipose tissue **Male** adult worm is smaller than the female. Its posterior end is strongly curved ventral. **Female** has smooth cuticula. Its head is unarmed. Its posterior end has a pair of fleshy lappets. **M.f ozzardi** are unsheathed, non-periodic and resemble **Mf perstens** during larval development in **culicoides** (intermediate host).

No clinical manifestations are observed. There are some reports of associated hydrocele, enlarged lymph nodes with tissue reaction.

Laboratory diagnosis is by the detection of **Mf. ozzardi** in peripheral blood. Hetrazan has no effect on microfilariae. Prophylaxis is not yet established.

Loa Loa

Loa loa (eye worm) produces loasiasis. It was identified by Mongin from the eye of an African national. It has an extensive distribution.

It lives in subcutaneous tissue.

Adult worm is thread-like and whitish with tapering cephalic end. Its anterior end is unarmed but it has small papillae. The **male** is smaller than female. Its caudal end is curved ventrally and with "cuticular bosses", has perianal papillae and unequal copulatory spicules. The vulva of **female** is in the cervical region. Adult worm may live for 15 years.

Its microfilaria is sheathed, has diurnal periodicity. Its tail is tapering. Its caudal nuclei are continuous with those of the trunk. For its life cycle, it requires the definite host (man) and intermediate host (**chrysops dimidiata**-mango fly or deer fly). Its larval development is same as that of other microfilariae in the intermediate host.

After migration through the subcutaneous tissue of the body, the adult worms reach the eye (site of predilection) where they creep in and around the eyes. Temporary swelling (fugitive or calabar swelling) are caused by wandering worms. They reach the size of hen's eggs, are painful. The worm metabolites cause the local reaction. The worms are troublesome when they cross the bridge of the nose. Reddened giant urticaria of the skin, fever and high eosinophila are the common symptoms.

The microfilariae can be demonstrated in the peripheral blood in day and the adult worm in the swellings. Immunological tests are same as those adopted for **W. bancrofti. Treatment** is by surgical removal of adult worm and by effective chemotherapy.

Prophylaxis : Detection and treatment of human case; spray antilarval insecticides in breeding places of **chrysops;** protection from **chrysops** bites; use of fly repellant.

Loa inquirenda

It was recovered from a European woman's neck in India by Mapestone (1938).

Human Dirofilariasis

Dirofilaria of animals (**D. immitis, D. conjunctivae) D. tenuis, D. repens** may become adult without producing microfilariae.

Superfamily Dracunculoidea

These worms are long, cord like; have

(a) simple pore like mouth; surrounded by double circles of papillae.
(b) oesophagus and intestine are rudimentary.
(c) females are larger than males.
(d) with vulva at the middle of body, and uteri are divergent.
(e) they are viviparous, rhabditoid larvae are discharged.

Dracunculus medinensis

D. medinensis (serpent worm; dragon worm) cause dracunculiasis. It is known since antiquily. It is widely distributed including India (Rajasthan—Jodhpur, Mumbai; Karnataka,

Andhra Pradesh, Gujarat). Gujarat has highest incidence. Adult worms are mostly lodged in the legs, arms and back. Its anterior end is round and blunt. So far only one **male D. medinensis** was recovered in India. Its posterior end is coiled with spicule and gubernaculum. **Female** is largest nematode, has paired ovarian tubules, ulcers and a **single vagina.** Gravid female has no vulva. Its poserior end is hook like, discharges embryos. Its body is toxic and causes blisters when it invades the tissue. Its life-span is one year, but that of male is six months.

Their rhabiditoid larvae are coiled, wiry with tapering tail.

In their life cycle, they require two hosts : man (definite host); cyclops (intermediate host). If man drinks water contaminated with infected cyclops. In stomach the cyclops are digested and their larvae are set free. These larvae migrate through the intestinal wall and reach retroperitoneal connective tissue where they grow, sexually mature male die after fertilisation. The gravid females migrate and select those parts of body which come in contact with water and form "blister" due to secretion of toxin and the blister ruptures producing ulcer. The female discharges embryos in the water. Allergic reaction occurs when **D. medinensis** migrates under skin; secretes a toxin which causes blister and may also produce systemic reaction (erythema, urticaria will pruritus, nausea, vomiting; diarrhoea and giddiness) due to toxemia.

Detection of adult worm in the ulcer, embryos in water when gravid females ejaculate them into water.

Skin test, X-ray of dead calcified worms and blood examination.

Treatment by effective drugs; removed of the whole parasite by Indian barber technique.

Prevention of infected persons from stepping into water sources; drinking of filtered water or boiled water; converting step wells into draw wells.

Gnathostoma spinigerum

It causes gnathostomiasis. It was first reported by Owen from the gastric tumour of tiger, later Chandter (1927) from India. It lives in the gastric tumours of dog, cat). The **male** of adult worm is smaller than female. The male has pseudobursa and copulatory spicules. The female has vulva which is posto-equatorial, paired genital tubes.

Its eggs are ovoidal, transparent pitted and have mucoid plug at one pole and are embryonated.

Eggs of **G. spinigerum** are extruded out from the lesions , evacuated into faeces, into the water where they embryonate and hatch. These larvae are ingested by cyclops, transform into the second stage larva. Where these infected cyclops are eaten by fish, frog, they transform into third stage in the flesh of these animals. When suitable host eats the third larval host, the larva develops to maturity in the stomach of wall of the host.

Third stage larva is responsible for human **gnathostomiasis.** Immature worms cause superficial lesions in the skin, subcutaneous tissue. Advanced larval stage causes breast abscess. The formation of tunnels in which the worms are migrating is "larva migrans" causing creeping eruption (**Gnathostomiasis externa**). Toxic and allergic reactions are responsible for these lesions. The erratic migration of the larva in eye or brain is also encountered.

In dogs and cats, adult worms are coiled inside the tumours of the digestive tract. This is referred as **gnathostomiasis interna.**

Removal and identification of adult worm is specific diagnosis; skin test is also useful.

Treatment is not effective.

Gnathostoma hispidum

It is stouter than **G. spinigerum.** It is a common parasite of the stomach wall of pigs.

Angiostrongylus cantonensis

A. cantonensis (rat lung worm) causing eosinophilic meningo-encephalitis or human angio- strongylosis was first reported by Nemura and Lin (1945). It is distributed in some countries. It is found in the lung of rat.

It is a delicate, filiform worm. Its cuticular is smooth. Its cephalic end is simple has three lips, no buccal capsule, mouth opens into the oesophagus. The **male** is smaller than female. The copulatory capsule is curved ventrally. The posterior end of the **female** is like a blunt horn with anal pore and a vulva.

Its eggs are elongated, ovoidal. A single female may lay 15,000 per day. Its eggs are hatched out in the lung of the rat and the larvae into trachea. After swallowing, the first stage larvae are expelled in the feces. Then they infect a molluscum (intermediate host) in which they develop into third stage larva. This infective larva migrates to the brain and matures migrates to the pulmonary arteries and begins to lay eggs.

In human infection, eosinophilic meningo-encephalitis is the main pathological change; symptoms are chronic brain syndrome, low grade fever, headache, difficulty in urination, later semi-unconscious and death. Detection of mature and immature worms and skin test are useful diagnosis.

QUESTION (Q) – ANSWER (A)

Q. Define nematode.

Ans. Nematode parasite is elongated, cylindrical, tapering at both the ends; are unsegmented. Their size is variable, smallest to largest, have protective cuticula.

Q. What is filariform oesophagus of nematode ?

Ans. Certain nematode has oesophagus of uniform calibre—it is called as filariform oesophagus. Parasitic nematode has filariform oesophagus.

Q. What is rhabditiform oesophagus of nematode ?

Ans. If the oesophagus is expanded posteriorly into a bulb with valve mechanism, it is called as rhabditiform oesophagus. Free living types of nematode have rhabditiform oesophagus.

Q. What is diecious helminth ?

Ans. Diecious helminth is helminth with separate sexes.

Trichinella spiralis

Q. What is its common name ?

Ans. Its common name is "trichina" worm.

Q. Where does its adult worm remain buried ?

Ans. It remains buried in the mucosa of duodenum and jejunum.

Q. Where does its larva encysts ?

Ans. Its larva encysts in the striated muscles of man, pig harbouring the adult worm.

Q. Which nematode is smallest ?

Ans. T. spiralis is the smallest nematode.

Q. How long is T. spiralis viviparous ?

Ans. It is viviparous as long as it is alive.

Q. What is viviparous, oviparous, ovo-viparous ?

Ans. Viviparous – giving birth to larva

Oviparous – laying eggs

Ovo-viviparous – laying eggs containing larvae which are hatched out immediately.

Q. How many hosts are required for the life cycle of T. spiralis ?

Ans. T. spiralis requires only **one** host for its life cycle. (man or pig or rat).

Q. What happens to males of T. spiralis after fertilisation of females ?

Ans. Males will die after fertilisation.

Q. How many progenies are discharged by females of T. spiralis ?

Ans. They discharge 1,500 progenies during sixteen weeks.

Q. Where are the progenies of T. spiralis are temporarily lodged in body cavities before they re-enter into circulation for their final distribution in the striated muscle ?

Ans. They are lodged in various tissues and body cavities.

Q. For how many years these encysted larvae remain alive ?

Ans. For many years.

Q. How is cyst wall formed ?

Ans. Cyst wall is formed due to host tissue reaction.

Q. How many principal maintenance cycles are there ?

Ans. There are three principal maintenance cycles. (1) pig to pig; (2) rat to rat; (3) sylvatic.

Q. How many stages are there in their pathogenicity ?

Ans. There are three successive stages : (1) invasive; (2) migration of the larvae; (3) encystation and tissue repair.

Q. What are the symptoms during invasion stage ?

Ans. The symptoms are nausea, vomiting, toxic, dysentery or diarrhoea, colic, sweating.

Q. What is the correct diagnosis of T. spiralis ?

Ans. Demonstration of adult worm in feces, larvae in blood or mother's milk.

Q. Can xenodiagnosis be useful in the diagnosis ?

Ans. It can be useful.

Q. Cite main pathological changes produced by T. spiralis.

Ans. Skin lesion, pulmonary lesion and intestinal lesion are the main pathological changes.

Q. Why T. spiralis filariform larvae should enter lungs before entering the intestine ?

Ans. For further development, these filariform larvae should pass through the lungs.

Trichuris trichiura

Q. What is its common name ?

Ans. It is called whip worm.

Q. Why is it called whip worm ?

Ans. It resembles a whip with a handle.

Q. Where was the egg of T. trichiura first observed ?

Ans. It was first observed in the feces of preserved dead girl who had died 450 years ago.

Q. Which nematode has a retractile penial sheath ?

Ans. T. trichiura has a retractile penial sheath.

Q. What is the shape of the egg of T. trichiura ?

Ans. It is barrel shaped with mucoid plugs at both ends.

Q. What is egg laying capacity of T. trichiura ?

Ans. Its egg laying capacity is 5,000-7,000 per day.

Q. What is its site of predilection ?

Ans. Its site of predilection is the cecum.

Q. What are the symptoms of T. trichiura ?

Ans. Symptoms are abdominal pain, vomiting, constipation and systemic intoxication.

Capillaria philippinensis

Q. How C. philippinensis remain burrowed in the mucosa of the jejunum ?

Ans. They remain burrowed in the mucosa with both ends free.

Q. Wht is the mode of infection ?

Ans. Its mode of infection is fecal-oral route.

Q. What are its symptoms ?

Ans. Its symptoms are diarrhoea, emaciation, weakness and abdominal pain. Death may be due to cachexia.

Strongyloides stercoralis

Q. What is its common name ?

Ans. Its common name is threadworm.

Q. What is its site of predilection ?

Ans. Its predilection site is duodenum or jejunum.

Q. What type of larvae is hatched out from the egg of S. stercoralis ?

Ans. Rhabditiform larvae are hatched out.

Q. Enumerate different types of larvae of S. stercoralis.

Ans. (1) Rhabditiform larvae; (2) Filariform larvae.

Q. What is rhabditiform larvae ?

Ans. If the oesophagus is expanded posteriorly into a bulb, which contains a valve mechanism, it is referred as rhabditiform larvae.

Q. What is filariform larva ?

Ans. If the muscular oesophagus is of uniform calibre throughout, it is called filariform larva. It is infective.

Superfamily Strongyloidea

Q. What does the mouth cavity of this super family contains ?

Ans. The mouth cavity contains teeth or cutting plates.

Q. How many families are under this superfamily ?

Ans. There are two families : (1) Family Ancylosto-matidiae; (2) Family Strongyloidae.

Q. How many subfamilies are in the family Ancylostomatidae ?

Ans. There are two subfamilies : (1) Subfamily Ancylostomatinae; (2) Subfamily Uncinarinae.

Q. Give example of subfamily.

Ans. Subfamily Ancylostomatinae contains :

Ancylostoma duodenale (with two pairs of teeth);

A. braziliense (with one pair of teeth);

A. caninum (with two pairs of teeth);

Subfamiliae uncinarinae – Necator americanus (with cutting plates).

Ancylostoma duodenale

Q. What is its common name ?

Ans. Its common name is old world hookworm.

Q. Where does adult worm live ?

Ans. Adult worm lives in the jejunum.

Q. Why is living worm pinkish in colour ?

Ans. It is pinkish due to ingested blood.

Q. Why A. duodenale is called hookworm ?

Ans. It is called hookworm as its anterior end is bent dorsally like a hook.

Q. How is blood clotting prevented in ancylostomiasis ?

Ans. Blood clotting is prevented by an enzyme secreted by its esophageal gland.

Q. During copulation why does the worm assumes a Y-shaped figure ?

Ans. Because of genital opening.

Q. How are rhabditiform larvae of a duodenale distinguished from the strongyloides larvae and other free living nematodes ?

Ans. Because it has a long, narrow buccal chamber, a flask shaped muscular oesophagus, a midgut, short rectum.

Q. When does the segmentation of ovum to form blastomeres takes place ?

Ans. The segmentation takes place when the fertilised egg passes through the bowel.

Q. How many stages are there in their life cycle ?

Ans. There are four stages.

Q. During its life cycle, why its larvae should migrate through lungs ?

Ans. They further develop during their migration through lung.

Q. What are the common sites of entry of filariform larvae of A. duodenale ?

Ans. The common sites of entry are : 1. the thin skin between the toes; (2) dorsum of the feet; (3) the inner sides of the soles.

Q. What are the pathogenic effects of A. duodenale ?

Ans. They are (1) cutaneous lesions; (2) pulmonary lesions.

Q. What is ground itch ?

Ans. At the site where the filariform larvae of **A. duodenale** penetrate the skin they produce ground itch.

Q. What are the characteristics of ground itch ?

Ans. The ground itch is characterised by itching and burning, oedema, erythema which develops into papule, then a vesicle.

Q. What is cutaneous larva migrans ?

Ans. Cutaneous larva migrans (creeping eruption) is a skin lesion produced by the entry of feline or canine ancylostoma.

Q. Why larvae of A. braziliense produces itchy papule at the site of invasion ?

Ans. Because they cannot enter below stratum germinativum of the human skin.

Q. What is serpiginous tunnel in stratum germinativum ?

Ans. It is a tunnel formed with a coriam as floor and stratum germinativum as the roof.

Q. Why are they called larva migrans ?

Ans. Since these larvae move at the rate of several millimeters to a few centimeters per day within the tunnel is called as larva migrans.

Q. Why cannot these larvae penetrate below the stratum germinativum ?

Ans. It may be due to its partial physiological inadaptability of the particular strain of Ancylostoma of man.

Q. What type of anemia is observed in A. duodenale ?

Ans. Microcytic hypochromic type of anemia is observed, which may be due to chronic loss of blood or nutritional defects.

Q. What are the different types of anemia and how are they caused ?

Ans. In microcytic hypochromic anemia, there is iron deficiency, in macrocytic type there is deficiency of folic acid and vitamin B_{12}; in diamorphic type there is both iron, vitamin B_{12} or folic acid deficiency.

Q. Why blood loss is more in A. duodenale ?

Ans. Because **A. duodenale** is larger worm which is armed with teeth and is highly migratory therefore leaving more bleeding points.

Q. How many types of symptoms are there ?

Ans. There are three types of symptoms : mild, moderate or, severe types.

Q. Describe severe type of symptoms.

Ans. Severe type is classical picture of hookworm disease. There is constipation or diarrhoea and the food is undigested. The skin is dry. Even in hot climate, the patient is cold. The patient eats clay to relieve the abdominal pain.

Q. What is Pica or Geophagy ?

Ans. Pica or Geophagy is eating clay or mud to relieve abdominal pain.

Necator americanus

Q. What is its common name ?

Ans. Its common name is New World Hookworm.

Enterobius vermicularis

Q. What is its common name ?

Ans. It is called pin worm or seat worm.

Q. What is its site of predilection ?

Ans. The site of predilection is mucosa of cecum, appendix, colon and ileum.

Q. Do E. vermicularis larvae migrate through lungs for their moulding ?

Ans. Larvae of **E. vermicularis** do not migrate through the lungs for their moulding; but they mould twice en route in the intestine.

Q. How many eggs does a single female adult worm deposit ?

Ans. It deposits 11,105 eggs.

Superfamily Ascaridoidea

Q. Describe the mouth of this super family.

Ans. Its mouth has three lips without the buccal capsule.

Q. Describe the posterior end of male adult worm of this superfamily.

Ans. Males do not have bursa copulatrix and caudal alae.

Ascaris lumbricodes

Q. What is the common name of A. lumbricoides ?

Ans. Its common name is giant intestinal roundworm.

Q. What is ascarase ?

Ans. Ascrase is proteose and is responsible for the allergy in the infected person. It is present in the body fluid of **A. lumbricoides.**

Q. What is the life-span of the adult worm ?

Ans. Its life-span is less than two years.

Q. What is the indication of the presence of unfertilised eggs in the feces ?

Ans. It shows the host is harbouring the female.

Q. How long will Ascaris egg remain infective ?

Ans. It may remain active for many months.

Q. Why should larvae of A. lumbricoides migrate through the lungs ?

Ans. They migrate through the lungs for further development.

Q. What is the migration period through the lungs ?

Ans. Its migration period is about 15 days.

Q. How many eggs are deposited by each female ?

Ans. Each female deposits 2,00,000 egg per day.

Q. What are the pathological effects produced by migrating larvae, adult worm ?

Ans. During migration through lungs, larvae cause trauma, hemorrhage, coughing, urticaria, fever.

Adult worm obtains its food by sucking liquid nutrient — thus it deprives the host of its nutrition.

Q. What is Ascaris pneumonitis (Loeffler's syndrome), night blindness; spoliative action ?

Ans. Ascaris pneumonitis is a condition where will be consolidation of the lobule, spasms of coughing, urticaria, fever, difficulty in breathing. Night blindness is caused by vitamin A deficiency caused by adult worm. Spoliative action occurs when the adult worms obtain their food by sucking liquid nutrient from the intestine by depriving the host of its nutrition.

Q. How are the adult worms protected from enzymatic digestion ?

Ans. Because of the anti-enzymes liberated by them in the intestine.

Q. What is ectopic ascariasis ?

Ans. Ectopic ascariasis occurs when the adult worms enter the Eustachian tube and cause otitis media due to fever which may cause the worms to be passed out.

Q. What are the symptoms due to generalised toxemia ?

Ans. Symptoms are insomnia, twisting, restlessness, meningitis, paraplegia, urticaria, cerebral symptoms in children.

Q. In whom can visceral larval migrans be seen ?

Ans. Visceral larval migrans can be seen in children.

Superfamily Filarioidea

Q. What are the characteristics of this superfamily ?

Ans. Its mouth is circular, simple and dorso-ventrally elongated and surrounded by papillae.

Wuchereria bancrofti

Q. What is nocturnal periodicity ?

Ans. In the night (between 10 pm and 2 am) the microfilariae of **W. bancrofti** appear in the circulation. This period is called nocturnal periodicity.

Q. Why microfilaria of W. bancrofti appear in the circulation at night ?

Ans. Because the microfilariae may migrate to the periphery at night when human body is relaxed at night; they respond to CO_2 and O_2 supply; they may adapt to the feeding habits of the mosquito; **Culex** is night feeder and Aedes is daytime feeder; they retire in the capillaries of the lung during the daytime.

Q. How the third stage larvae migrate into the wound ?

Ans. Because they are attracted by the warmth of the skin.

Q. Why W. bancrofti requires mosquito in its life cycle ?

Ans. For the complete development of their microfilariae.

Q. What are the pathological changes produced by the microfilariae lodged in the lymphatic vessels ?

Ans. There will be reticulo-endothelial cell infiltration to attack these microfilariae, thickening, folding of endothelial layer of lymph vessel with fibrin deposition.

Q. What is pathogonomic of this disease ?

Ans. Filarial granulation tissue is pathognomic.

Q. Enumerate the symptoms of W. bancrofti filariasis.

Ans. They are (1) Lymphangitis, (2) Lymhadenitis, (3) Elephantiasis, (4) Chyluria, (5) Hydrocele.

Q. Why is urine of chyluria milky in colour ?

Ans. Because it contains fat, albumin, fibrinogen.

Q. In complement fixation test, what antigen is used ?

Ans. In CFT, alcoholic extract antigen of **Dirofilaria immitis (D. immitis** — dog heartworm) is used.

Q. Why is D. immitis used as antigen ?

Ans. Because **D. immitis** and **W. bancrofti** are antigenically related.

Brugia malayi

Q. What is its common name ?

Ans. It is called Malayian filarial worm.

Q. Describe the main characteristics of Mf. malayi.

Ans. Its anterior end has two stylets; cephalic space is broader; its tail is constricted between two terminal nuclei, its appearance is stiff with secondary kinks. It is enveloped in a sheath.

Q. What are the main clinical features of B. malayi ?

Ans. It causes lymphangitis and elephantiasis of lower extremities.

Q. How is Malayian filariasis characterised ?

Ans. It is characterised by the absence of chyluria and by the presence of scrotal swellings.

Q. Where does Mansonia sp. grow ?

Ans. Mansonia sp. grows on water plant (**Pistia stratioides**).

Q. In which state of India does Mansonia grow ?

Ans. Since water plant (**Pistia stratioides**) grows well in Kerala state, **Mansonia** sp. breeds well and multiplies.

Q. How is Mansonia sp. controlled ?

Ans. It can be controlled by destroying the water plant.

Onchocerca volvulus

Q. What is the common name of filaria of O. volvulus ?

Ans. Its common name is blinding filaria.

Q. What is the name of the disease caused by O. volvulus ?

Ans. Its name is blinding filariasis, river blindness.

Q. Where does its adult worm remain coiled ?

Ans. It remains coiled in the subcutaneous tissue connective tissue tumours (nodules).

Q. For how many years does the adult female of O. volvulus live ?

Ans. It lives for more than eleven years.

Q. What is its intermediate host ?

Ans. Its intermediate host is Simulium (Black fly).

Q. What are the ocular symptoms in O. volvulus infection ?

Ans. They are conjunctivitis, corneal opacity, keratitis, iridocyclitis, glaucoma.

Dipetaonema perstans

Q. How is it called commonly ?

Ans. It is called as persistent filaria.

Q. Where does it live ?

Ans. It lives in the body cavities (periitoneal, pleura, pericardium).

Q. What is its intermediate host ?

Ans. It is **Culicoides austeni.**

Q. What are the symptoms of D. perstans ?

Ans. They are–fatal pericarditis, local irritation, toxic oedema of eyelid.

Mansonella Ozzardi

Q. How is it known ?

Ans. It is known as New World filaria or Ozzard's filaria.

Q. What is its intermediate host ?

Ans. Its intermediate host is **Culicoides furens.**

Loa loa

Q. What is its common name ?

Ans. Its name is Loa loa worm or eye worm.

Q. What does it produce ?

Ans. It produces fugitive swelling or calabar swelling.

Q. What is its life-span ?

Ans. Its life-span is fifteen years.

Q. What is its intermediate host ?

Ans. Its intermediate host is **Chrysops dimidiata** (deer fly or mango fly).

Q. What are the symptoms of Loa loa infection ?

Ans. Creeping in and around eye, calabar swelling of a hen's egg size, reddened giant urticarial swellings in the skin and mucous membrane, fever with eosinophilia.

Q. Enumerate human dirofilaria.

Ans. They are **Dirofilaria immutis, D. conjunctiveae, D. tenuis, D. repens.**

Superfamily Dracunculoidea

Q. Describe in short this superfamily.

Ans. It is long, cord-like worm, has pore like mouth surrounded by papillae. The females are larger than males. Its vulva is in the middle of the body.

Dracunculus medinensis

Q. What is its common name ?

Ans. It is also called medina worm, guinea worm, serpent worm.

Q. Why Arabian physicians named this nematode vena medina ?

Ans. Because it was common in Medina.

Q. Which state of India has highest incidence of D. medinesis, and why ?

Ans. Gujarat has the highest incidence of **D. medinensis.** Stepwells are very common in Gujarat.

Q. In which state of India adult worm of one metre long was removed from the eye of a patient ?

Ans. It is Orissa state.

Q. Where does the adult worms live ?

Ans. They live in the subcutaneous tissue of the legs, arms and back.

Q. In which country a single specimen of male D. medinensis was recovered from a natural infection of man ?

Ans. From India.

Q. How are blisters caused in the subcutaneous tissue ?

Ans. Toxic body fluid of **D. medinensis** causes blisters.

Q. Where are blisters formed ?

Ans. Blisters are formed only in those parts of the body which come in contact with water.

Q. When larvae of D. medinensis are discharged into water, why do they swim ?

Ans. They swim in search of minute fresh water cyclops for their further development.

Q. What will happen if they are not taken up by cyclops ?

Ans. They will die.

Q. Where do their larvae grow and become sexually mature ?

Ans. They grow and become sexually mature in the retro-peritoneal connective tissue.

Q. What is the duration period of migration of larvae from the intestine to retroperitoneal connective tissue ?

Ans. Migration period of larvae is one year.

Q. Where does copulation of D. medinensis takes place ?

Ans. Their copulation takes place in deeper connective tissue, not in the intestine.

Q. What is the fate of male D. medinensis after copulation ?

Ans. Male **D. medinensis** dies after copulation.

Q. What is the duration period for the complete development of the embryo ?

Ans. It is two weeks.

Q. How many larvae can kill the cyclops ?

Ans. More than 5-6 larvae can kill the cyclops.

Q. What is the life-span of the cyclops ?

Ans. Its life-span is about three months.

Q. Within how many days heavy infection of larvae can kill the cyclops ?

Ans. Heavy infection may kill within fifteen days.

Q. When will there be allergic reaction in D. medinensis infection ?

Ans. When the gravid female worms begin to migrate to the skin, there will be allergic reaction.

Q. When will there be systemic reaction ?

Ans. Before the formation of the blister, there will be systemic reaction.

Q. What are the symptoms of systemic reaction ?

Ans. They are erythma, urticaria, intensive pruritus, nausea, vomiting, diarrhoea and giddiness.

Gnathostoma spinigerum

Q. Where does its adult worm live ?

Ans. They live in the tumour of the stomach wall of cat and dog.

First Report of Nematodes

Trichinella spiralis – Peacock (1828)
Trichuris trichiura – Linnaeus (1771)
Strongyloides stercoralis – Normand (1876)

Ancylostoma duodenale – Dubini (1843)

Ancylostoma caninum – Panjarathinam (1972), Pondicherry, India

Nector americanus – Stiles (1902)

Enterobius vermicularis – Panjarathinam (1978) in Gujarat, India

Ascaris lumbricoides – Known since ancient times

A. lumbricoides in calf – Panjarathinam (1972), Pondicherry

Wuchereria bancrofti – Demorquay (1863)

Brugia malayi – Brug (1927)

Onchocerca volvulus – Brumpt (1919)

Dipetaonema perstans – Daniels (1898)

Mansonella ozzardi – Ozzard ?

Loa loa – Mongin ?

Dracunculus medinensis – In Bible (since antiquity)

Gnasthostoma spinigerum – Owen; Chandla

Angiostrongyloides cantonensis Chen (1935)

Q. What happens to the eggs of G. spinigerum when they are evacuated with feces ?

Ans. In the water the embryo is formed and hatched out. These larvae are ingested by cyclops where second stage larva is formed when the infected cyclops is ingested by fish, where third stage larva is formed in the flesh of fish. When the definite host (cat) eats fish flesh with infective larvae, cat gets infected and tumour is formed in the stomach of cat.

Q. What is (1) Gnathostomiasis externa, and (2) interna ?

Ans. (1) **Gnathostomiasis externa** is characterised by development of abscesses pockets; formation of subcutaneous tunnels in which larva migrates (larva migrans causing creeping eruption).

(2) **Gnathostomiasis interna** occurs when the adult worms are coiled in the tumour of digestive tract.

Gnathostoma hispidium

Q. In India, how many times it was found in human infection ?

Ans. It was found twice in human infection.

Angiostrongyloides cantonensis

Q. What its common name and what causes it in man ?

Ans. It is called rat lung worm. It causes eosinophilic meningo-encephalitis.

Q. How many eggs may a simple female lay ?

Ans. A single female may lay up to 15,000 eggs per day.

Q. Where are these eggs hatched out after ingestion by rats ?

Ans. They hatch out in the lung of rat.

Q. What is its intermediate ?

Ans. Its intermediate host is cyclops.

Q. What happens in the rat when the rat ingests the cyclops containing infective larvae ?

Ans. The third (infective) stage larvae migrate to the rat brain, mature, migrate to the pulmonary alveoli, and begin to lay eggs. After swallowing, the larvae are passed out in the feces.

Glossary

At the end of chapter 1

Protists are unicellular organisms that are typically neither plant and animals.

Prokaryote is one group of organisms with nucleus NOT bounded by nuclear membrane (e.g. bacteria).

Eukaryote is another group with nucleus bounded by nuclear membrane (algae, protozoa).

At the end of Chapter 2

Capsule is protective gelatinous layer on the bacterial cell wall.

Flagella are filamentous appendages protruding from the cell wall and are organs of locomotion.

Fimbriae are hair-like appendages and are organs of adhesion (syn. **pili**).

At the end of chapter 4

Sterilisation is the process of freeing of an article from all living microorganisms alongwith their **spores. Sterility** is an absolute state.

Disinfection is a relative term indicating a mere removal of the pathogenic microorganisms.

At the end of chapter 5

Culture media are mixtures of suitable food materials for growth of bacteria.

At the end of chapter 6

Isolation is the process by which a single bacterium is obtained from a mixture of bacteria.

Pure culture is the one which contains only one kind of microorganism.

At the end of chapter 8

Serology is the study of reaction between antigen-antibody.

Agglutination is a serological reaction in which the antigen used is particulate in nature.

Precipitation is also a serological reaction in which water-soluble antigen is used.

Roundworm (Ascaris lumbricoides) is the largest common intestinal nematode causing vague abdominal discomfort acute colicky pain, diarrhoea and fever.

At the end of chapter 10

Elephantiasis, hydrocele, chyluria are caused by microfilaria of Wuchereria bancrofti.

Blinding filariasis, river blindness caused by Onchocerca volvulus.

Calabar swelling caused by **Loa loa.**

Guineaworm (Dracunculus medinensis) causes erythma, urticaria, pruritus, blister on the sole.

At the end of chapter 12

Innate (native) **immunity** is a resistance with which a person is born. It is non-specific.

Antigen usually protein in nature; when introduced into a living animal evokes specific immune response.

Hapten is incomplete antigen unable to induce an immune response, but can become immunogenic only when linked to protein (called **carrier protein**).

Heterophilic antigen, certain antigen of similar nature present in different tissues of more than one species are called **heterophilic antigens.**

Chapter 13

Complement is non-specific protein present in normal serum of man which has got the ability to lyse or damage cells (bacteria, virus, tumour cells) and to stimulate antigen antibody reaction.

Chapter 18

T-lymphocytes are called Thymus dependent lymphocytes.

B-lymphocytes mature in cloacal bursa of chickens and birds.

Monokines are soluble proteins produced by monocytes and macrophages.

At the end of chapter 21

Transplantation is a useful procedure in surgical repair or replacement of diseased tissues or organs.

At the end of chapter 22

Tumour antigens are present on the membrane of cancer cells. When syngenic animal is injected with such tumour specific antigen it rejects tumour transplantation in immunised hosts.

At the end of chapter 23

Coagulase is an enzyme produced by pathogenic **Staph. aureus.**

At the end of chapter 26

Morning drop of **secretion** is suppurative inflammation of male urethra with purulent discharge.

At the of chapter 30

Swarming (concentric circles) **growth** produced by proteus.

At the end of chapter 31

Pyocyanin, fluorescein are pigments produced by pseudomonas.

At the end of chapter 32

Rose spots appear on the skin during second or third week of typhoid fever.

At the end of chapter 34

Cholera — acute profuse diarrhoea — "rice water" diarrhoea of sudden onset due to vibrio cholerae, string test, cholera red reaction for identification of **vibrio cholerae.**

Choleraphage — bacteria infecting **vibrio cholerae.**

At the end of chapter 35

Acute infantile diarrhoea is caused by Campylobacter enteritis, recent pathogen.

At the end of chapter 36

Bubonic plague is characterised by **bubo** (greatly enlarged tender lymph node).

At the end of chapter 38

Diphtheria, localised inflammation in the throat.

At the end of chapter 42

Spore, resistant of bacilli.

Inverted fir-tree appearance growth in gelatin stab by **Bacillus anthracis.**

At the end of chapter 43

Trismus — when the muscles of jaw are affected the **trismus** occurs as an early sign of tetanus.

Drum stick appearance of **Clostridium tetani** is due to spherical, terminal spore.

At the end of chapter 44

Stormy clot appearance in litmus milk medium is due to fermentation of sugars with gas and acid by **Cl. welchii.**

At the end of chapter 49

Hydrophobia (Rabies) is caused by neurotropic virus.

At the end of chapter 55

Blood donation associated infections, are serum hepatitis (HBV)-hepatitis B virus, Human Immunodeficiency virus (HIV).

At the end of chapter 69

Typhus, arthropod borne rickettsial infection, is characterised by fever and rash.

At the end of chapter 70

Frei test — a delayed hypersensitivity skin test once useful in the diagnosis of chlamydial infection.

After end of chapter 71

Fried egg colony in solid medium is produced by Mycoplasma.

At the end of chapter 72

Chancres are primary sores on genitalia in syphilis caused by **Treponema pallidum.**

At the end of chapter 75

Gastroenteritis is manifested by frequent loose motions with mucus, with or without vomiting and with inflammation of mucous membrane of the intestine.

Dysentery is characterised by the presence of blood mucus in stool.

Food poisoning is due to consumption of preformed bacterial toxin in the food contaminated with bacteria (**staph. aureus; Cl. botulinum**).

At the end of chapter 76

Sore throat is an acute pharyngitis or tonsillitis characterised by painful swelling, congested tonsils, pyrexia.

Diphtheria is caused by toxigenic strains of **C. diphtheriae** and is manifested by pseudomembranous exudate in the faeces.

Nosocomial pneumonia is hospital acquired infection by patients admitted in the hospital for more than 48 hours.

At the end of chapter 77

Bacteriuria is the multiplication of bacteria in the urinary tract infection by more than hundred thousand (10^5) per ml of mid stream urine. Pyuria is the presence of pus cells in the urine.

At the end of chapter 78

Meningitis is the inflammation of the membrane surrounding the brain; spinal cord.

At the end of chapter 79

Nosocomial infection is also known as Hospital acquired infection.

Susceptible patients are Hospitalised patients with diabetes, immunosuppression with preexisting diseases.

Exogenous sources are people or immediate objects in the environment.

Iatrogenic infection occurs when the natural barrier is damaged by contaminated urethral or intravenous cathethers.

Aerosols are produced by air conditioner and can transmit certain pathogen (Legionella) to the respiratory tract if air conditioner water is contaminated.

At the end of chapter 80

Pasteurisation is the process in which the milk is heated at a particular temperature for fixed period required to destroy any pathogens.

Holder method Pasteurisation temperature employed is 63°-66°C for 30 minutes followed by rapid cooling to 5°C.

Flash method Pasteurisation Temperature employed is 72°C for 15 seconds and then rapidly cooled to 4°C.

Dacroadenitis is the infection of lacrimal gland due to endogenous source.

At the end of chapter 81

Bacteremia is a condition in which the bacteria are simply present in the blood without multiplication.

Septicaemia is a condition in which the bacteria circulate without multiplication in the blood.

Endotoxaemia is the presence of bacterial endotoxin in the blood of infective endocarditis is caused by bacteria.

At the end of chapter 84

Transmissibility is the spread of disease from one host to a fresh host.

Infectivity or ability to breach the new hosts defences.

Pathogens Pathogenic microorganisms causing disease in man.

At the end of chapter 94

Pyrexia of unknown origin. In spite of investigations, the cause of a febrile illness remains uncertain, hence it is called as Pyrexia of unknown origin (PUO).

At the end of chapter 96

Genetics is the study of inheritance except for RNA viruses, because hereditary characteristics are encoded in DNA.

Plasmids are extra-chromosomal DNA molecules.

Genetic engineering is the recombinant DNA technology by which any genetic system can be analysed.

At the end of chapter 97

Putrefaction is the decomposition of proteins (animal matter) under anaerobic conditions.

Fermentation — under anaerobic conditions, the microorganisms decompose, by their saccharolytic activities, the sugars into gas and acid.

At the end of chapter 100

Vaginal thrush is vaginitis caused by candida albicans.

Oral thrush occurs in bottle fed infants.

At the end of chapter 104

Amoebic dysentery, or amoebiasis, is caused by Entamoeba histoytica.

At the end of chapter 105

Malignant tertian malaria caused by **Plasmodium falciparum.**

At the end of chapter 106

Trypanosomal chancre, elevated and painful swelling caused by the bite of infected tse tse fly with **Trypanosoma gambiense.**

Chagoma — primary skin lesion, due to **Trypanosoma cruzi** transmitted by reduviid bug (**Triotoma infestans**).

Kala azar (Dum Dum fever) — caused by **Leishmania donovani; Delhi boil** or **Oriental sore** caused by Leishmania **tropicalis.**

Vaginal discharge which is greenish and yellow is seen in Trichomonas vaginalis.

At the end of chapter 107

Coracidium is ciliated embryo from the egg of **Diphyllobothrium latum.**

Plerocercoid or **sparganum** larva of D. latum is infective to man.

Beef tapeworm (**Taenia saginata**); Pork tapeworm (**Taenia solium**) are Cestoda.

Cysticercus bovis — (measly beef) not found in man; **C. cellulosae** (measly pork) found in man — are bladder worm.

Hydatid cyst of **Echinococcus granulosus** (dog tape worm) can cause damage by their mechanical and toxic effect.

Cercocysts or **Cysticercosis** larvae of **Hymenolepsis nana** migrate and get attached to the lumen of small intestine and develop into adult worm.

At the end of chapter 108

Giant intestinal fluke, common name of **Fasciolopsis buski.**

Sheep liver fluke, common name of **Fasciola hepatica.**

Oriental lung fluke, common name of **Paragonimus westermani.**

Blood fluke, common name of genus schistosoma.

Miracidium ciliated first stage larva of schistosoma.

Terminal spine is present at the terminal end of egg of **S. haematobium.**

Gynaecophoric canal in which the female is held during copulation by schistosoma.

At the end of chapter 109

Trichina worm, common name of **Trichinella spiralis** (smallest nematode).

Whip worm, common name of **Trichuris trichiura.**

At the end of chapter 109

Threadworm, common name of **Strongyloides stercoralis,** causes enteritis.

Ancylostoma duodenale (old world hookworm); **Necator americanus** (New world hookworm) cause, a severe type constipation or diarrhoea, cardiac failure and anasarca. In moderate type, there is epigastric pain which is relieved by eating clay or mud which is known as **pica** or **geophagy.**

Pinworm or **seat worm** (Enterobius vermicularis) may cause salpingitis in female, severe pruritus, salpingitis around anus.

Roundworm (Ascaris lumbricoides) is the largest common intestinal nematode causing vague abdominal discomfort, acute colicky pain, diarrhoea and fever.

At the end of chapter 110

Elephantiasis hydrocele, chyluria are caused by microfilaria of Wuchereria bancrofti.

Blinding filariasis, river blindness caused by Onchocerca volvulus.

Calabar swelling caused by **Loa loa.**

Guinea worm (Dracunculus medinensis) causes erythma, urticaria, pruritus, blister on the sole.

TECHNICAL TERMS

(a) Microbiology

Acid fast. Retaining the initial stain and difficult to decolourise with acid alcohol. A property of certain bacteria.

Actinomycetes (ak-tin-o-mye-seets) Gram-positive bacteria that are characterised by the formation of branching filaments.

Active immunity. Specific resistance to disease acquired by individuals as a result of their own reactions to pathogenic microorganisms or to the products of such organisms.

Adaptive enzyme. An enzyme produced by an organism in response to the presence of the enzyme's substrate or related substance. Also called induced enzyme.

Adenovirus. A group of icosahedral double stranded DNA viruses.

Adijuvant. A substance that when infected together with antigen increases antibody production and can grow under an air atmosphere. Compare **anaerobe.**

Aerosol. Atomised particles suspended in air.

Agar. (ah gar). A dried polysaccharide extract of red algae used as a solidifying agent in microbiological media.

Agglutination (uh-gloo-tin-ay-shunt). The clumping of cells.

Alga. pl. **algae** (an-guh-**al**-jee) Any member of a heterogeneous group of eukaryotic, photosynthetic and unicellular or multicellular organisms.

Allergy. A type of antigen-antibody reaction marked by an exaggerated physiological response to a substance is sensitive.

Aminoglycoside antibiotics. A class of antibiotics which disrupt the normal synthetic sequence of protein synthesis.

Amphitrichous (am **fit**-rik-us). Having a single flagellum at each end of a cell.

Anaerobe (an uh-robe) An organism that does not require O_2 to obtain energy, cannot grow under an air atmosphere and for which O_2 is toxic compare aerobe.

Anamestic response (an-am-**ness** tik). The heightened immunologic reaction to a second exposure to an antigen.

Anaphylatoxin. A complement derived peptide that causes the release of histamine mast cells.

Anaphylaxis (an-Up-Fi-**Lak**-sis). Hypersensitivity in an animal following the parenteral injection of an antigen.

Angstrom (A^0) 1/10 of nanometre. Conventionally used for measuring wavelengths. Also used to express dimensions of some intracellular structure of microbes.

Antibiosis (an-tee-bye-o-sis). An antagonistic association between two organisms in which one is adversely affected.

Antibiotic (an-tee-bye-ot-ik) A substance of microbial origin that has antimicrobial activity in very small amount.

Antibody (an-ti-bod-ee). Any of a class of substances (Proteins) produced by an animal in response to the introduction of an antigen.

Antigen (an-ti-jen). A substance that, when introduced into an animal body, stimulates the production of specific substances (antibodies) that react or unite with the substance introduced (antigen).

Antimicrobial agent. Any chemical or biological agent of that microorganisms.

Antiserum. Blood serum that contains antibodies.

Antitoxin. An antibody capable of uniting with and neutralising a specific toxin.

Arthropod. An invertebrate with jointed legs (insect).

Arthrospore. An asexual spore formed by the fragmentation of the mycelium.

Ascitic fluid. Serous fluid that accumulates abnormally in the peritoneal cavity.

Asepsis. A condition in which harmful microorganisms are absent.

Aseptic technique. Precautionary measures taken to prevent contamination.

Assay. The quantitative or qualitative estimation of the components of a drug.

Asymptomatic. Exhibiting no symptoms.

Autoclave. An apparatus using pressurised steam for sterilisation.

Autoimmune disease. A condition in which the body develops an immunological reaction against its own tissues.

Autoysis. The disintegration of cells by the action of their own enzymes.

Bacillus. Any rod-shaped bacterium.

Bacteriaemia. A condition in which bacteria are present in the blood-stream.

Bactericidal. An agent that destroys bacteria.

Bacteriolysin. An agent or substance that causes the disintegration of bacteria.

Bacteriostasis. The inhibition of the growth and reproduction of bacteria without killing them.

Bacteriostatic. Inhibiting the growth of bacteria without killing them.

Bacterium. Any of a group of diverse and ubiquitous prokaryotic single-celled microorganism.

BCG vaccine. Bacillus Calmette-Guerin Vaccine, an attenuated strain of Mycobacterium tuberculosis bovis strain against tuberculosis.

Bergey's manual. An international reference work which classifies and describes bacteria.

Binomial nomenclature. The scientific method of naming plants, animals and microorganisms, because species names consist of two terms.

Blood plasma. The fluid portion of fresh blood.

Blood serum. The fluid expressed from clotted blood.

BOD – biochemical oxygen demand.

Botulism. Food poisoning due to the toxin of **Cl. botulinum.**

Bronchi – Branches of trachea.

Brownian motion. A peculiar dancing movement shown by fine particles or bacteria.

Bubo. Swollen infected lymph nodes.

Capsid. The protein of a virus.

Capsomere. A morphological subunit of a capsid seen under electron microscope.

Capsule. An envelope or slime layer surrounding the cell.

Calalase. An enzyme that converts hydrogen peroxide into water and oxygen.

Cell. The microscopic functionally and structurally basic unit of all living organisms.

Cell wall. A rigid external covering of the cytoplasmic membrane.

Chemotherapy. Treatment of the disease with the use of chemicals.

Chromatid body. Bacterial nuclear material.

Coagulase. An enzyme of staphylococci that causes the coagulation of blood plasma.

Colony. A microscopically visible growth of microorganisms on a solid culture medium.

Commensalism. A relationship between members of different species living in the same cultural environment in which one organism benefits from the association but the other is not affected.

Competitive inhibition. The inhibition of the action of an enzyme by a non-substrate molecule occupying the site on the enzyme that would otherwise be occupied by the substrate.

Complement. A normal thermolabile protein constituent of blood serum, that participates in antigen-antibody reaction.

Complement fixation. The binding of the complement to an antigen-antibody complex so that the complement is unavailable for a subsequent reaction.

Conjugation. A mating process of temporary fusion of the mating partners and the transfer of gene and it occurs in unicellular organisms medium.

Cytoplasm. The living matter of a cell between the cell membrane and the nucleus.

Cytoplasmic membrane. A thin layer under the cell wall consisting of phospholipids and proteins, and responsible for the selective permeability properties of the cell. Also called **plasma membrane**.

Diplococci. Cocci occurring in pairs.

Disinfection. An agent that frees from infection by killing the vegetative cells of microorganism.

Ecology. The study of the interrelationships that exist between organisms and the environment.

Edema or oedema. The excessive accumulation of fluid in body tissue.

Electrophoresis. An electrochemical process in which suspended particles with an electric charge migrates in a solution under the influence of an electric current.

Endemic. With reference to a disease, one that has a low incidence but which is constantly present in a particular geographic region.

Endospore. A thick walled spore formed in the bacterial cell. Highly resistant to physiological and chemical agents.

Endotoxin. A heat stable toxin which consists of lipo-polysaccharide — located in the outer membrane of Gram-negative bacteria and liberated only when the bacteria disintegrate.

Enteric. Pertaining to the intestine.

Enterotoxin. A toxin specific for cells of the intestine.

Epidemiology. The study of the occurrence and distribution of disease.

Etiology or Aetiology. The study of the cause of a disease.

Exotoxin. A toxic protein excreted by a microorganism into the surrounding medium.

Facultative anaerobe. An organism which does not require O_2 for growth (but may use it if available) which grows well under both aerobic and anaerobic conditions and for which oxygen is not toxic.

Fastidious organisms. An organism that is difficult to isolate or cultivate on ordinary culture media because of its need for special nutritional factors.

Fermentation. The anaerobic oxidation of compounds by an enzyme action of microorganisms, neither gaseous oxygen nor a respiratory chain is involved in this energy-yielding process. An organic compound is the electron acceptor.

Fibrinolysin. A substance produced by haemolytic streptococci that can liquefy clotted blood plasma or fibrin clots. Also called streptokinase.

Fimbriae. Surface appendages of certain Gram-negative bacteria composed of protein subunits. They are shorter and thinner than flagella. Also called **pili.**

Flagellum. (pl. flagella). A thin filamentous appendage on cells responsible for swimming motility.

Fluorescence microscopy. Microscopy in which cells or their compounds are stained with a fluorescent dye and thus appear as glowing objects against a dark background.

Fomites. Inanimate objects that carry viable pathogenic microorganisms.

Frei test. A skin test to determine sensitivity to the agent that causes lymphogranuloma venereum.

Fungicide. An agent that kills or destroys fungi.

Fungus. A microorganism that lacks chlorophyll and is usually filamentous, a mold or yeast.

Gamma globulin. A fraction of serum globulin that is rich in antibodies.

Gastroenteritis. Inflammation of the mucosa of the stomach or intestine.

Genome. A complete set of genetic material, i.e., a complete set of genes.

Genus. A group of very closely related species.

Germ. A microbe, usually a pathogenic one.

Germicide. An agent that kills pathogenic microorganism.

Giardiasis. Disease of human small intestine caused by **Giardia lamblia.**

Globulin. A protein soluble in dilute solution of neutral salts but insoluble in water. Antibodies are globulins.

Glucan. A polymer of glucose.

Gram-negative bacteria. Bacteria that do not retain crystal violet iodine complex when subjected to the Gram-technique and thus acquire the colour of the dye (usually red dye) that is used to counterstain the cells.

Gram-positive bacteria. Bacteria that retain the crystal violet-iodine complex when subjected to Gram technique and appears violet.

Gram-stain. A differential stain by which bacteria are classed as Gram-negative or Gram-positive.

Growth curve. A graphic representation of the growth of bacteria in a culture medium.

Hanging drop technique. A technique in which microorganisms are observed suspended in a drop of fluid.

Hapten. A simple substance that reacts like an antigen, in vitro, by combining with antibody but cannot induce the formation of antibodies by itself.

H antigen. A type of heat-labile protein antigen found in the flagella of certain bacteria.

HeLa cells. A pure line of human cancer cells used for the cultivation of viruses.

Helix. A coiled spiral form.

Hemagglutination or **Haemagglutination.** The agglutination (clumping) of red blood cells.

Hemoglobin or **Haemoglobin.** The constituent of red blood cells that gives them their colour and carries oxygen.

Hemolysin or Haemolysin. A substance produced by microorganisms that lyses red blood cells liberating hemoglobin. Also can refer to a type of antibody that acts in conjunction with complement to cause the lysis of red blood cells.

Hemolysis or Haemolysis. The process of dissolving of red blood cells.

Hemorrhagic or **Haemorrhagic.** Showing evidence of hemorrhage (bleeding). The tissue becomes reddened by the accumulation of blood that has escaped from capillaries into the tissue.

Heterophilic antibody. An antibody that reacts with microorganisms or cells that are unrelated to the antigens that stimulate production of the antibody. The agglutination is stimulated by unrelated species.

Heterotroph. A microorganism that is unable to use the carbon dioxide as its sole source of carbon and requires one or more organic compounds.

Humoral immunity. Immunity arising from the formation of specific antibodies that circulate in the blood-stream in response to the introduction of an antigen.

Hyalurinadase. An enzyme that catalyses the breakdown of hyaluronic acid. Also called spreading factor.

Hypersensitivity. Extreme sensitivity to foreign antigens, e.g., allergens.

Hypha. One filament or thread of mycelium.

Icosahedron. A solid formed of 20 triangular faces and 12 corners, the geometrical shape of many virions.

IDU. An antiviral agent, 5-iodo-2-deoxyuridine.

Immune serum. Blood serum that contains one or more specific antibodies.

Immunity. A natural or acquired resistance to a specific disease.

Immunisation. Any process that develops resistance (immunity) to a specific disease.

Immunoelectrophoresis. A technique which employs a combination of immunodiffusion and electrophoresis to identify various antigens.

Immunogenicity. The capacity to stimulate the formation of specific antibodies.

Immunoglobulin. Any of the serum proteins such as gamma globuin that possess the antibody activity.

Inactivate. To destroy the activity of a substance, e.g., to heat blood serum to 60°C for 30 min. to destroy complement.

Inclusion bodies. Discrete assemblies of virions and/or viral components that develop within virus-infected cells.

Incubation. In microbiology, the subjecting of cultures of microorganisms to conditions (especially temperatures) favourable to their growth.

Incubation period. The time between the exposure to an infection and the appearance of symptoms, or the time period during which microorganisms inoculated into a medium are allowed to grow.

Indicator. A substance that changes colour as conditions change, e.g., pH indicates reflecting changes in acidity or alkalinity.

Infection. A pathological condition due to the growth of microorganisms in a host.

Infections. Capable of producing disease in a susceptible host.

Inflammation. A tissue reaction resulting from irritation by a foreign material and causing a migration of leucocytes and an increased flow of blood to the area producing swelling, reddening, heat pain, and tenderness.

Inhibition. In Microbiology, the prevention of the growth or multiplication of microorganisms.

Inoculation. The artificial introduction of microorganisms or other substances into the body or into a culture medium.

Inoculum. The substance containing microorganisms or others such.

in situ. In the original or natural location.

Interferon. An antiviral substance produced by animal tissue.

in vitro. Literally, 'in glass'. Pertaining to experiments carried out in test tubes.

in vivo. Within the living organisms. Pertaining to the laboratory testing of agents within living organisms.

Isoantibody. An antibody found only in some members of a species that acts upon cells or cell components of other members of the same species.

Isoantigen. A tissue specific antigen present in one individual of a species but not in another. Also called allo-antigen.

Kahn test. A flocculation test for the diagnosis of syphilis.

Lag phase. A period of slow orderly growth when a medium is first inoculated with a culture.

Laminar airflow. The flow of air currents in which streams do not intermingle, the air moves along parallel flow lines.

Liquefaction. The transformation of a gel into a liquid.

Litmus. An indicator for pH and oxidation or reduction.

Lophotrichous. Having a polar tuft of flagella.

Lyopholisation. The preservation of biological specimens by rapid freezing and rapid dehydration in high vacuum.

Lysin. An enzyme, antibody or other substance capable of disrupting or disintegrating cells (lysis).

Lysogenic bacteria. Bacteria that carry prophages.

Lysogeny. The state of a bacterium that is carrying a bacteriophage (often as a prophage) to which it is not itself susceptible.

Medium. pl. Media. A substance used to provide nutrients for growth of microorganisms.

Mesosomes. Membrane invaginations in the form of convulated tubules and vesicles.

Metachromatic granules. See **Granules, metachromatic**.

Microaerophile. An organism that requires low levels of oxygen for growth but cannot tolerate the level of 21 per cent oxygen present in an air atmosphere.

Microbe. Any microscopic organism, a microorganism.

Microbiology. The study of organism of microscopic size (microorganisms) including their culture economic importance, pathogenicity etc.

Microorganism. Any organism of microscopic dimensions.

Mold. A fungus characterised by a filamentous structure.

Monoclonal antibody. A specific antibody produced by hybridoma cells.

Mordant. A substance that fixes dyes.

Morphology. The branch of biological science that deals with the study of the structure and form of living microorganism.

Mycology. The study of fungi.

Mycoplasma. A member of a group of bacteria lacking cell wall.

Mycosis. A disease caused by fungi.

Mycotoxin. Any toxic substance produced by fungi.

Naked virion. A non-enveloped virus.

Nanometer. A unit of length equal to one billionth of a meter, or 10^{-9} m; 1 millimicrometer. Abbreviation: nm.

Negri bodies. Minute pathological structures (inclusion bodies) found in certain brain cells (hippocampus) of a human or animal infected with rabies virus.

Nomenclature. Any system of scientific names such as those employed in biological classification.

Nosocomial disease. Disease acquired in hospital.

O antigen. Polysaccharide antigen found in the body of bacterial cell. Also called **somatic antigen**.

Ocular micrometer. Eyepiece of a microscope with a scale in divisions.

Oxidase. An enzyme that brings about oxidation.

Pandemic. A worldwide epidemic.

Passive immunity. Immunity produced by injecting serum containing antibodies.

Pasteurisation. The process of heating a liquid food or milk to a controlled temperature to destroy harmful or pathogenic microorganisms.

per os. Through the mouth.

pH. A symbol for the degree of acidity or alkalinity of a solution.

Phagocyte. A cell capable of digesting microorganisms or foreign particles.

Pilus pl. **Pili.** Any filamentous appendage other than flagella on certain Gram-negative bacteria. Also called **fimbria**.

Pinocytosis. The uptake of fluid and soluble nutrients through small invaginations in the cell membrane that form intracellular vesicles.

Precipitin. An antibody causing precipitation of soluble antigen.

Psychrophile. A cold loving microorganism growing at 0°C.

Pus. The fluid product of inflammation containing serum, protein, bacteria, dead cells, and leucocytes.

Putrefaction. The decomposition of proteins by microorganisms producing disagreable odour.

Reagin. Antibodies against cardiolipin.

Reticuloendothelial system. A system of cells in various organs and tissues (spleen, liver, bone marrow) that are important in resistance and immunity.

Rickettsiae. Obligate parasitic bacteria of arthropods — many are pathogenic to human and other animal.

PPR test. Rapid plasma regin test, a macroscopic precipitation screening test for detection of Wassermann antibodies in the serum of syphilitic patients.

Salmonellosis. An infection by salmonella species that affects the gastrointestinal tract.

Schick test. A skin test used to determine the susceptibility of a person to diphtheria.

Schultz-Charlton reaction. A skin test used to diagnose scarlet fever.

Sepsis. Poisoning by the products of putrefaction, a severe toxic state resulting from an infection with pyogenic microorganisms.

Septicaemia. A systemic disease caused by the invasion and multiplication of pathogenic microorganisms in the blood-stream.

Serology. Study of reaction between antigen and antibody in the laboratory.

Serotype. A subdivision of species based on its antigenic culture spread on a glass slide for microscopic examination. Also called **film.**

Species. The basic taxonomic group.

Spirillum. A rigid helical bacterium.

Spirochaete. A helical bacterium which is flexible and has periplasmic flagellum.

Staphylococci. Spherical cocci occurring in grape-like clusters.

Sterile. Free of living organisms.

Sterilisation. The process of making sterile, the killing of all forms of life.

Stock culture. Known species of microorganism maintained in the laboratory.

Strain. All descendents of a pure culture.

Streak-plate method. A procedure for separating cells on a sterile agar surface so that individual cells will grow into distinct separate colonies.

Streptobacilli. Rod shaped bacteria in chain.

Streptococci. Spherical bacteria in chain.

Streptokinase. See **fibrinolysin.**

Subclinical. Pertaining to infection so minor that there are no detectable clinical signs or symptom of the infection.

Subcutaneous. Beneath the skin.

Substrate. The substance acted upon by an enzyme.

Suppuration. Formation of pus.

Susceptibility. A state of being exposed to infection.

Symbiosis. The living together of two or more organisms.

Syphilis. A venereal disease caused by Treponema pallidum.

Terminal disinfection. The disinfection of a room or building after it has been vacated by a patient who had a contagious disease.

Terminal infection. An infection with pathogenic microorganisms that terminate into the death of the host.

Tetanus. A disease caused by Clostridium tetani.

Thermolabile. Destroyed by heat at temperatures below 100°C. Opposite : thermostable.

Tinea. Ringworm which is caused by fungi.

Tissue. A collection of cells causing a structure.

Toxaemia. The ability to produce a toxin.

Toxin. A poisonous substance such as bacterial toxin elaborated by a bacterium.

Toxin-Antitoxin. A mixture of toxin and antitoxin containing slightly more toxin than antitoxin. This was formerly used to produce active immunity.

Toxoid. A toxin that has been treated to destroy the toxic properties without affecting its antigenic properties.

Tyndallisation. A process of fractional sterilisation with flowing steam.

Urease. An enzyme that catalyses the hydrolysis of urea.

Vaccination. Inoculation with a biological preparation (in vaccine) to produce immunity.

Vaccine. A preparation of killed or attenuated microorganisms.

VDRL test. Venereal Disease Research Laboratory test used to screen reagin antibodies in serum of syphilitic patients.

Vector. An agent (insect) which transforms a pathogen from one organism to another.

Venereal. Sexually transmitted.

Viable. Capable of living, growing and developing alive.

Vibrio. A curved or comma shaped bacterium.

Vincent angina. Ulcerative condition of gums caused by a spirochaete with a fusiform bacillus.

Viraemia. The presence of virus in the blood.

Virion. Complete mature virus particle.

Viropexis. Phagocytosis of whole virion by phagocytic cells.

Virucide. An agent that kills the viruses.

Virulence. The degree of pathogenicity exhibited by a microorganism.

Virus. An obligate intracellular parasitic entity that is similar to bacteria — can be seen only under electron microscope.

Voges-Proskauer test. A test for the presence of acetylmethyl carbinol to assist in distinguishing between species of coliform groups.

Volutin. See **Granule, metachromatic.**

Wasserman antibodies. Antibodies against cardiolipin. Also called reagins.

Wasserman test. A complement fixation test for syphilis.

Widal test. An agglutination test for typhoid.

Yeast. A kind of fungus that is unicellular and lacks typical mycelium.

Yolk sac. The membrane covering the yolk of an egg.

Zoonosis. An animal disease transmitted to human being.

(B) PARASITOLOGY

Abscess. Latin : *abscedere* — to go away, to separate circumscribed collection of pus in tissue.

Acole. French : *accoler* — to embrace. Referring to the form of **plasmodium falciparum** which adhere to the surface of red cells as a thin strip of cytoplasm.

Acetabulum. Latin : *acetabulum* — a little cup to hold vinegar. The sucking cup of flukes.

Aedes. Greek : *cedes* — odious, annoying. A genus of mosquitoes.

Alae. Latin : *ala* — wing. Referring to the hyaline wings at the anterior end of Enterobius.

Amoeba (Ameba) Greek : *amoibe* — change. A genus of protozoa which changes shape by extending pseudopodia.

Ancylostoma Greek : *agkylos* — curved, bent, *stoma* — mouth. Referring to the head which is bent backward. A genus of hookworms.

Anopheles. Greek : *an* — without, *opheles* — help. The harmful one. A genus of mosquitoes.

Antenna. Latin : *antenna*. The feeler of insects.

Arthropoda. Green : *arthron* — joint, *poda* — plural of *pous* — foot. The phylum of animals having jointed limbs.

Ascaris lumbricoides. Greek : *askaris* — intestinal worm. Latin : *lumbricus* — earthworm, Greek. *eidos* — form. The large intestinal roundworm.

Axonema. Greek : *axon* — axis, *nema* — thread. The intracellular portion of the flagellum in flagellates.

Axostyle. Greek : *axon* — axis. *stylos* — pillar. The axial supporting structure in flagellates.

Babesia. In honour of Victor Babes, Rumanian bacteriologist — 1854-1926. A genus of Haemosporidia, which contains the species causing Texas cattle fever.

Balantidium. Greek : *balantidion* — little bag. A genus of ciliata.

Bilharziasis. After Theodor Bilharz, helminthologist — 1825-62. Infection with **Schistosoma haematobium.**

Binary. Latin : *Bini* — two at a time. Referring to the equal parts into which protozoa divide.

Bursa Latin : *bursa* — purse, sac A posterior expansion of the cuticle of some nematodes which serves as a clasper.

Calabar. A district, river, and town in Southern Nigeria.

Casoni's test. After Tommaso Casoni, Italian physician, Skin test for hydatid disease.

Cercaria. Greek : *Kerkos* — tail. The tailed larval stage of flukes.

Cestoda. Greek : *Kestos* — girdle, *eidos* — form resembling Tapeworm.

Chagas disease. After Carlos Chagas, Institute Oswaldo Cruz, Rio de Janeiro, 1879-1934. Infection with **Trypanosoma cruzi.**

Charcot-Leyden crystals After Jean Martin Charcot, French neurologist, 1825-93, and Ernst Victor Von Leyden, German physician, 1832-1910. Colourless, pointed crystals found in sputum in bronchial asthma and in faeces in amoebic dysentery and other ulcerative disease of the colon.

Chromatin. Greek : *Chroma* — colour. The deeply staining protoplasmic material within the nucleus of the cell.

Chromatoidal. Greek : *Chroma* — colour eidos form, Resembling chromatin in affinity for stains.

Chrysops. Greek : *Chrysos* — gold, *ops* — face. A genus of biting flies.

Ciliata. Latin : *Cilium* — eyelash. A class of protozoa.

Cirrus. Latin : *Cirrus* — curl. Slender, flexible appendage, the male copulatory organ of flatworms.

Clonorchis sinensis. Greek : *Klon* — branch, **orchis** testicle; pertaining to *sinae,* i.e. Latin name for oriental people or Chinese. The Chinese liver fluke.

Coccidiosis. Greek : diminutive of *kokkos* — berry infection with Coccidia. e.g. **Isospora hominis.**

Commensal. Latin : *Cum* — together, *mensa* — table. Companion at the table. An organism living in or on another, partaking of its food but not harming it.

Copepoda. Greek : *Kope* — oar, *pous* — foot, *poda* — feet. Small Crustacea.

Coracidium. Greek : diminutive of *Korax* — hooklet (originally crow) — Larval stage of **Diphyllobothrium latum.**

Cosmopolitan Greek : *Kosmos* — word. *polites* — citizen. At home in any country.

Crithidia. Greek : diminutive of *Krithal* — barley. A stage in the life cycle of **Trypanosoma.**

Crustacea. Latin : *Crusta* — crust, the hard surface or shell of a body. Class of Arthropoda including lobster, crab, shrimp.

Cryptozoite. Greek : *Kryptos* — hidden, *zoion* — animal. A stage in the life cycle of plasmodium.

Culex. Latin. *Culex* — gnat. A genus of mosquitoes.

C. fatigans. Latin : *fatigare* — to hunt down.

C. pipiens. Latin : pipire to chirp.

C. quinquefasciatus. Latin. *quinque* — five, *fasciatus* — past participle of **fasciare** to envelop with hands (**fascia band**).

Culicoides. Latin : *Culex* — gnat, Greek : *eidos* — form.

Resembing Culex. The punkies or biting midges.

Cyclops. Greek : *Kylops* — round-eyed. A genus of small crustacea, the intermediate host of **Diphyllobothrium latum** and **Dracunculus medinensis.**

Cyst. Greek : *Kystis* — bladder. The immotile, resistant stage of protozoa. In pathology a sac with a distinct wall containing fluid or other material.

Cysticercoid. Greek : *Kystis* — bladder, *kerkos* — tai, eidos form. Resembling a cysticercus, but with a small bladder without fluid. A stage in the life cycle of **Hymenolepis nana.**

Cysticercosis. Infection with cysticercus, the larval stage of **Taenia.**

Cysticercus. Greek : *bos* — cattle. The larval stage of **Taenia saginata.**

C. cellulosae : Latin diminutive of *cella* — cell. The cysticercus of "Cell tissue." The larval stage of **Taenia solium.**

Cytoplasm. Greek : *Kytos* — hollow vessel, hence cell, *plasma* — a thing molded, hence the viscous matter of a cell. The cytoplasm of a cell other than that of the nucleus and inclusions.

Cytopyge. Greek. *Kytos* — hollow vessel, cell, *pyge* — bullock. The excretory orifice of certain protozon.

Diaptomus. Greek : *diaptoma* — from *diapiptein* — to slip away. A genus of small Crustacea, the intermediate host of **Diphyllobothrium latum.**

Diphyllobothrium latum. Greek : *dis* — double, *phylon* — leaf, *bothrion* — groove; Latin : **latus** broad. The broad fish tapeworm.

Diptera. Greek : *dis* — double *pteron* — wing. The order of the Arthropoda which includes the mosquitoes and flies.

Dirofilaria imitis. Latin : *dirus* — terrible, *fium* — thread; imitis merciless. The filaria of the dog, the dog heart worm.

Diurenal. Latin : *dies* — day. Relating to the day time.

Donovania. In honour of C. Donovan, born 1863, pathologist in the-then Madras (Chennai), India. Bacteria causing granuloma inginale.

Dracunculus medinensis : Greek : diminutive of *drakon* — dragon; probably from Medine, French Sudan, or Medina, Saudi Arabia. A tissue roundworm, the Guineaworm.

Echinococcus granulosus. Greek : *echinos* — hedgehog, *Kokkos* — berry; Latin *granulum* — a little grain, a small particle. The hydatid worm.

Ectoplasm. Greek : *ektos* — outside, external, *plasma* — a thing molded, hence the viscous matter of a cell. The outer, more compact layer of the cytoplasm.

Endemic. Greek : *en* — in, *denos* — the people. Constantly present in the people of a certain area.

Endoplasm. Greek : *endon* — within *plasma* — a thing molded, hence the viscous matter of a cell. The inner portion of the cytoplasm of a cell.

Entamoeba hisolytica. Greek : *entos* — within *amoibe* — change, histos web, hence the tissue, **lyein** to dissolve. The causative organism of amoebiasis.

Enterobius vermicularis. Greek : *enteron* — intestine, *bios* — life; Latin : *vermicularis* — diminutive of *vermis* — worm. The seat worm or pinworm.

Entomology. Greek : *entomon* — insect, past participle of *entemmein* — to cut in, because insects appear cut in, or almost divided, *logos* — word, science. The study of insects or of arthropods in general.

Espundia. Spanish : Tumour, ulcer. Mucocutaneous leishmaniasis.

Estivoautumnal malaria. Latin : *aestivus* — belonging to the summer **autumnus** fall. Falciparum malaria.

Fasciola. Latin diminutive of *fascis* — bundle, referring to the appearance of the reproductive organs. A genus of hermaphroditic flukes.

Fasciolopsis buski. Latin : diminutive of *fascis* — bundle, Greek : *Opsis* — appearance, after George Busk, surgeon in London, 1807-86. The giant intestinal fluke.

Faeces. Latin. plural of *faex* — yeast, i.e. residue after fermentation. Faeces are the excrement.

Filaria. Latin : *filum* — thread. The tissue roundworms.

Fuadin. Antimony compound named in honour of Ahemd Fuad, Pasha, King of Egypt from 1922-36. Used in the treatment of a number of parasitic infections.

Gamete. Greek. *gamei* — to marry. The mature sexual cell in the life cycle of **plasmodium.**

Gametocyte. Greek : *gamein* — to marry. *Kytos* — hollow vessel, hence cell. The sexually differentiated but immature cell in the life cycle of **Plasmodium.**

Genal Latin : *gena* — cheek. Pertaining to the cheek, the anterior part of the side of the head of an insect.

Giardia lamblia. In honour of Professor Alfred Ciard, biologist in Paris, France, 1846-1908, and Dr. Wilhelm Dusan Lambi, Bohemian physician, 1824-95. An intestine flagellate.

Glossina. Greek : *glossa* — tongue. A genus of biting flies. **G. palpalis.** Latin : *palpare* — to touch.

Guinea worm. Guinea, a coast region of West Africa, Dracunculus **medinensis.**

Helminths. Greek : Plural of helminth worms. The parasitic worms.

Haematuria. Greek : *haina* — blood. *ouron* — urine. Discharge of bloody urine.

Hermaphrodite. Greek : *Hermaphroditos* — the son of Hermes and Aphrodite, Organism with male and female reproductive organs.

Hexacanth; Greek : **hex** six, **pous** foot, poda feet.

Hyalie. Greek. **hydatis** a watery vesicle. The larva of **Echinococcus granulosus.**

Hydrocephalus. Greek : *hydor* — water, *kephale* — head. A condition in which the amount of cerebrospinal fluid is increased.

Hymenolepis nana. Greek : *hymen* — membrane, *lepsis* — shell; Latin : *nanus* — dwarf. The dwarf tapeworm, the eggs of which have a thin membrane.

Infect. Latin : *in* — and *facere* — to put into. The establishment of a pathogenic organism (except arthropods) upon or within a host.

Infest. Latin : *Infestare* — to attack, to molest. The establishment of arthropods upon or within the host.

Kala-azar. Hindi : *Kala* — black, *azar* — febrile disease infection with **Leishmania donovani.**

Karyosome. Greek : *Karyon* — Kernel, hence nucleus, *soma* — body. The nucleolus like body within the nucleus of Protozoa.

Kinetoplast. Greek : *Kinetos* — movable, *plastos* — formed. Kinetonucleus closely associated with the blepharoplast of haemoflagellates.

Leishmania donovani. After Sir William Boog Leishman, British Army Surgeon, 1865-1926, and C. Donovan — 1863, pathologist in the-then Madras (Chennai), India. Species of haemoflagellates causing kala-azar.

Leptomonas. Greek : *leptos* — delicate, *monas* — unit. The flagellate stage of Leishmania.

Loa : Congo dialect : worm. A genus of filarial worm.

Macrogametocyte. Greek : *makros* — large, *gamein* — to marry, *kytos* — hollow vessel, hence cell. The female sexual stage in the life cycle of Sporozoa.

Malaria. Italian : *mala* — bad, *aria* — air. Infection with Plasmodium sp.

Mastigophora. Greek : *mastix* — whip, flagellum, *pherein* — to bear. A class of Protozoa.

Maurer's dots. After Georg Maurer, 1860-1919, German physician in Sumatra (1888-1905). Irregular, red-staining dots or lines in erythrocytes infected with **Plasmodium falciparum.** Maurer's dots were discovered and described by Schuffner in 1889. Maurer devised an important staining technique for them in 1902.

Merozoite. Greek : *meros* — part, *zoion* — animal A stage in the life cycle of plasmodium.

Metacercaria. Greek : *meta* — after, *kerkos* — tail. The larval stage of flukes which follows the cercaria stage.

Metazoa (singular metazoon). Greek : *meta* — after, beyond, *zoion* — animal. Animals that came after the Protozoa, characterised by segmentation of the ovum.

Microgametocyte. Greek : *mikros* — small, *gamein* — to marry, *kytos* — hollow vessel, cell. The male sexual stage in the life cycle of sporozoa.

Miracidium. Greek : *meirakidion* — little boy. The ciliated larva which hatches from the egg of flukes.

Mosquito. Spanish : diminutive of musca fly.

A member of the family culicidae, order Diptera.

Necator. Latin : *necator* — killer, slayer. A genus of hookworm.

Nemathelminthes. Greek : *nema* — thread, *helmins* — worm. The roundworms.

Nematoda. Greek : *nema* — thread, *eldos* — form. Roundworms.

NNN Medium. Devised for the culture of haemoflagellates by Novy and Mcneal in 1904 and modified by Nicolle in 1908.

Onchocerca volvulus. Greek : *Onkos* — hook, tumour, Kerkos tail. Latin *volvere* — to twist. A filaria worm.

Onchosphere. Greek : *Onkos* — hook, tumour, *sphaira* — sphere. A stage in the life cycle of tapeworm.

Oocyst. Greek : *Oion* — egg, *kystis* — bladder. A stage in the life cycle of sporozoa.

Ookinete. Greek : *Oion* — egg, *Kinesis* — motion. A stage in the life cycle of Plasmodium.

Operculum. Latin : *Operculum* — cover, lid. Referring to the lid of eggs of certain flatworms.

Paragonimus. Greek : *para* — bed side, *gonimos* — generative. A genus of flukes.

Parasite. Greek : *parasitos* — he who eats at some one else's table. An animal or plant which lives upon or within another organism.

Parasitology. Greek : *para* — beside, *sitos* — food, *logos* — word, science. The study of parasites.

Paroxyam. Greek : *Paroxynein* — to sharpen. A sudden severe attack in a disease.

Pathogenesis. Greek : *pathos* — disease, *genesis* — origination. The origination and development of a disease.

Pathogenic of or pertaining to pathogenesis. Causing disease.

Pathognomonic. Greek : *pathos* — disease, *gnone* — a sign. Characteristic of a disease, distinguishing it from other diseases.

Plebotomus argentipes. Greek : *phlebs* — vein, *tommein* — to cut. Latin : **argentum** silver, **pedes** feet. A genus of blood sucking flies, the sandflies.

Phlanorbis. Latin : *planus* — flat, *orbis* — circle. A genus of snails, the intermediate host of **schistosoma mansoni.**

Plasmodium. Greek : *plasma* — a thing molded, hence the visco matter of a cell, *eldos* — form, resemblance. A game of sporozoa which contains the parasites causing malaria.

Plasmodium falciparum. Latin : *falx* — sickle, *parfo* — to bring forth.

Plasmodium vivax. Latin : *vivax* — vigorous.

Platyhelminthes. Greek : *platys* — wide, flat, *helmins* — worm. Flatworms.

Proboscis. Greek : *proboskis* — trunk (of an elephant). The tubular process of the head, especially of insects and arachnids, made up of various mouth parts.

Procercoid. Greek : *pro* — (occurring) before *kerkos* — tail, *eldos* — form. A stage in the life cycle of some tapeworm.

Proglottid. Greek : *proglottis* — the tip of the tongue. A segment of Taenia.

Protozoa : (Singular protozoon). Greek : *protos* — first, *zoion* — animal. The phylum of uninuclear animals.

Pseudopodia. Greek : *pseudes* — false, *poda* — plural of *pous* — foot. Footlike. A temporary protrusion of the cytoplasm of amoeboid cells serving locomotion and feeding.

Pyrogenic. Greek : *pyr* — fire, hence fever, *gannan* — to produce. Producing fever.

Redia. After Francasco Redi, Italian naturalist, 1626-97. Larval stage of flukes, found in snails.

Rhabtifirorm. Greek : rhabdos rod, *eidos* — form. A stage in the life cycle of some roundworms.

Rhizopoda. Greek : *rhiza* — root *poda* — plural of *pous* — foot.
The class of Protozoa which move by means of pseudopodia the amoeba.

Rostellum. Latin : *rostellum* — the little beak. A prolongation of the scolex.

Schistosoma. Greek : *Schistos* — split, *soma* — body.

A genus of flukes, the blood flukes.

Schistosoma haematobium. Greek : *haima* — blood. *bios* — life.

Schistosoma mansoni. After Sir Patrick Manson, 'the father of Tropical Medicine,' 1844-1922.

Schizogony. Greek *Schizein* — to split, *gonos* — generation. Asexual multiplication by multiple fission. The nucleus divides into several, after which the cell divides into as many as they are nuclei.

Schizont. Greek : present participle of *schizein* — to split. The stage in the life cycle of plasmodium, which precedes the merozoite stage.

Schuffner's dots or **granules.** After Wilheim Schuffner, German pathologist, 1867-1949, who discovered and described. Acidophilic stripping of erythrocytes parasitised by **Plasmodium vivax or ovale.**

Scolex. Greek : *Sltolex* — worm (Plural succlices). The anterior end of a tapeworm, by which it attaches to the wall of the intestine, commonly referred to as head.

Simulium. Latin : *simulare* — to stimulate. This genus includes the black flies and buffalo gnats.

Sparganum. Greek : *spargana* — diaper referring to early childhood. The larval stage of the fish tapeworm, which is infective to man.

Sporocyst. Greek : *Sporos* — seed, *kytos* — cell. The oocyst of plasmodia after sporozoites have developed within it the larval stage of flukes in snails from which eventually cercariae develop.

Sporogony. Greek : *sporos* — seed, *gonos* — generation. Sexual reproduction by the formation of spores. The life cycle of plasmodium in the mosquito.

Sporozoa. Greek : *Sporos* — seed, zoion animal. The class of Plasmodium that form spores in their life cycle.

Sporozoite. Greek : *sporos* — seed, *moin* — animal. The end product of sporogony. The stage of Plasmodium transmitted to man by the mosquito.

Stoma. Greek : *stoma* — mouth. A minute opening.

Strobila. Greek : *Strobile* — twisted. The complete tapeworm including scolex, neck and proglottides.

Stroma. stroma bed. The supporting framework of an organ.

Strongyloides stercoralis. Greek : *Strongylos* — round, *eidos* — form. Latin; *stercus* — drug. An intestinal roundworm, the cause of strongyloidiasis.

Symbiosis. Greek : *Symbiosis* — living together. The mutually advantageous association between organisms of different species.

Taenia. Greek : *taina* — ribbon. A genus of tapeworm.

Taenia saginata. Latin : *seginare* — to fatten. The beef tapeworm.

Taenia solium. Arabic *sosi* — chain. The pork tapeworm.

Tenesmus. Greek : *tainein* — to strain. The painful straining to empty the bowels or bladder, without the evacuation of faeces or urine.

Toxoplasma gondii. Greek : *toxon* — bow, *plasma* — a thing molded, hence the viscous matter of a cell; the gondii is a small North African rodent : A protozoon.

Trematoda. Greek : *trema* — hole, *eidos* — form, i.e., having holes. Referring to acetabula. The flukes.

Triatoma. Latin : *tria* — three; Greek : *tomos* — sectioned. A genus of Hemiptera (true bugs).

Trichinella. Greek : diminutive of *thrix* — hair. The Trichina worm.

Trichocephalus trichiurus. Greek : *thrix* — hair, *kephale* — head, *thrix* — hair, *oura* — tail. Synonyms of **Trichiuris trichiura**. The whipworm.

Trophozoite. Greek : *trypanon auger* — borer, *soma* — body. A genus of haemoflagellates.

Tsetse. South African Dutch from Bantu. **Onomatopoeic** (imitative in origin) 'fly'. species of genus Glossina.

Vacuole. Latin : *Vacuns* — empty. Cavity in the cytoplasm.

Wuchereria bancrofti. After Otto Wucherer 1820-73, who described the microfilaria, in 1866, in Bihar, Brazil; after J. Bancroft, English physician, 1836-94, who discovered the adult worm of this species in 1876, in Australia. A species of the filarial worm.

Xenodiagnosis. Greek : *Xenos* — foreign, *diagnoskein* — to learn thoroughly. Diagnosis by finding the causative organism in an arthropod infected from the patient.

Xenopsylla cheopis. Greek : *xenos* — foreign, guest, *sylla* — flea; *cheopi* — king of Egypt, 2900-2877 B.C. The tropical rat flea.

Zoonosis. Greek : *zoon* — animal, *nosos* — disease. Disease of animals transmitted to man.

Zygote. Greek : *Zygon* — yoke. A stage in the sexual life cycle of sporozoa. The cell resulting from the union of microgamete and macrogamete.

Bibliography

1. Benenson As (ed) 1980 Control of communicable diseases in man. 13th Edn. American Public Health Association.
2. Block S.S. (1983) Disinfection, sterilisation, preservation, 3rd Edn. Philadelphia, Lea and Febiger.
3. Cassel, GH Gole, B.C (1981) : Mycoplasma agents of human disease. New Engl. J. Med. 304 : 80
4. Chalmers, C.H. (1962) Bacteria in relation to Milk supply. 4th Edn. London, Edward Arnold.
5. Chakravorty, P (1995) A text book of Microbiology 1st Edn. New Central Book Agency, Kolkata.
6. Cooper MD (1987) B-Lymphocytes. Normal Development and function, New Engl. J. Med. 17 : 1452.
7. Cruick Shank, R. et al (1975) Medical Microbiology. The Practice of Medical Microbiology Vol. II 12th Edn. London, Churchill Livingstone.
8. Ducttt; H.A. (1967) Airborne Microbes, Cambridge University Press.
9. Finegold, SM (1985) Anaerobic bacteria in human disease, New York Academic Press.
10. Goodfellow, M. Board, R.G. (1980) Microbiological Classification and, Identification London Academic Press.
11. Grange, JM (1988) Mycobacteria and Human Disease. London, Edward Arnold.
12. Greenwood, D. Stack R.C.B. (1980) Peutherer, J.F. (eds) 1992 Medical Microbiology, 14th Edn. Edinbrugh, Churchill Livingstone
13. Hardy K. (1986) Bacterial Plasmid, 2nd Edn. American Society for Microbiology Washington.
14. Isenberg, MD (1988) Pathogenesis and virulence. Another view, Clin Microbiology Rev. 1 : 40
15. Johnson RB Jr. (1988) Monocytes and Macrophages, New Engl. J. Med. 316 : 747
16. Lancefield R.C. (1933) A serological differentiation of human and other groups of haemolytic streptococci. J. Exp. Medicine 57 : 571.
17. Linton AH. Dick HM (eds) 1990 Topley and Wilson's Principles of Bacteriology, Virology and Immunology, 8th Edn. London, Edward Arnold p. 154-210.
18. Mims, CA (1987) The pathogenesis of infectious disease, 3rd Edn. London, Academic Press.
19. Morgan D. (ed.)\Infection Control, British Medical Association Guide, London. Edward Arnold.
20. Parker, MT Coller, LH (eds) 1990). Topley and Wilson's Principles of Bacteriology, Virology and Immunity 8th Edn. London, Edward Arnold.
21. Pollitzer R. (1954) Paque WHO monograph series N° 5 22 Geneva 1954.
22. Read SC and Zabriskie, J.B. (1980) Streptococcal Diseases and Immune response, New York Academic Press.
23. Roitt, I.M. (1988) Essential Immunology, 6th Edn. (ELBS) Oxford, Blackwell Scientific Publication.
24. Smith, S.R. and Scotland SM (1958) Verocytotoxic producing strain of **Esch. coli**, J. Medical Microbiology 26 : 77.
25. Shrinivash (1991) Hospital acquired infection guidelines for control, Ministry of Health and Family Welfare, Government of India, New Delhi.

Index